Pregnancy, Childbirth & the Newborn

Revised by Dr Jonathon Morris

Specialist in Maternal Fetal Medicine

MB ChB MM FRACOG DDU CHFM PhD

HINKLER BOOKS

Published and edited for the Australian market by Hinkler Books Pty Ltd.

ISBN 1 8651 5700 7

The illustrations in this book were developed by Shanna Dela Cruz, © 1994, 1999 Ruth Ancheta, from the *Labor Progress Handbook,* Blackwell Science (2000); Childbirth Graphics, a division of WRS Group, Ltd.; Susan Aldridge © 1999, from *The Nursing Mother's Companion,* 4th ed., reprinted with permission from the Harvard Common Press (Boston, MA); Medela Inc.; and Terri Moll. Illustrations by Karen Martin Tomaselli and Bill Farley © 1991 by Childbirth Graphics, Ltd.

Previously published by Meadowbrook Press, 5451 Smetana Drive, Minnetonka, MN 55343.

www.meadowbrookpress.com

First published in the UK 1991.

Reprinted 2003

The contents of this book have been reviewed and checked for accuracy and appropriateness by medical doctors, midwives, nurses and physical therapists. However, the authors, editors, reviewers and publisher disclaim all responsibility arising from any adverse effects or results that occur or might occur as a result of the inappropriate application of any of the information contained in this book. If you have a question or concern about the appropriateness or application of the treatments described in this book, consult your health care professional.

Printed in Australia.

Dedication

To our husbands Peter Simkin, Doug Whalley and Jerry Keppler.

To our children and their families: Andy, Bess, Freddy, Charlie and Eva Rose Simkin;
Linny Simkin and Jeff, Peter and Callie Jobson;
Mary Simkin-Maass and Greg, Sara Jane and Amelia Maass; Lizzie Simkin;
Scott and Heidi Whalley; Mike Whalley; Kristin Platt; Brian Platt;
Eric Keppler and Heidi Keppler.

To the thousands of expectant and new parents whom we have taught
and who have taught us so much.

And to the Childbirth Education Association of Seattle, which since 1950 has educated, supported and encouraged families in their transitions to parenthood.

Acknowledgments

This book, originally conceived as a class manual called *Becoming Parents,* was first published by the Childbirth Education Association of Seattle (CEAS) in 1976. Gillian Mitchell and the three authors of this book wrote and edited it. In 1984, Meadowbrook Press published the first edition of *Pregnancy, Childbirth and the Newborn* (an extensive revision of the original book) with the help of editor Tom Grady. The second edition was published in 1991 with the help of editor Kerstin Gorham. After several years and hundreds of thousand of copies sold, it became time to update and revise our book again.

We wish to thank our editors for this edition, Joseph Gredler, Nancy Campbell and Christine Zuchora-Walske, for their thoughtfulness and expertise. Each has uniquely contributed to the development of this expanded version.

Many other people have helped with the 2001 edition by reading the text for clarity, content and medical accuracy. We are grateful to the following readers:

Thoughtful parents Lisa Anderson, Jennifer Ernst, Susanne Fahey, Emily Fisher, Wendy Gross, Margarita Halverson, Sondra Kornblatt, Robin Lang, Vicky Latz, Robin Marshall, Kymmberly Myrick, Cathy Rankin, Kathy Sheldon, Lorre Thorpe, Wendy Van Koevering and Stacy White.

Fellow childbirth educators Trish Booth, M.A., L.C.C.E., F.A.C.C.E.; Wendy Dean, D.V.M.; Carmel Elliott, R.N.; Kris Haldeman, R.N., M.N.; Judy Higgins, R.N.; Connie Leibow, P.T.; Mimi Malgarini, P.T.; Susan McDonald; Janet McGuigan, R.N.; Heidi Mellen, R.N.; Barbara Orcutt, R.N., M.N.; JoAnne Rendall, R.N.; Heather Sargent, I.C.C.E.; Susan Paul Sasnett, O.T.R.; Candice Schuchardt, R.N.; Sandra Szalay, A.R.N.P.; and Marla Timm, P.T.

Professional consultants Roger Anderson, M.D.; Sally Avenson, C.R.N., C.N.M.; Judith Babcock, M.D.; Thomas Benedetti, M.D.; Steven Bird, Pharm.D.; Susan Blackburn, R.N., Ph.D.; Dana Blue, M.S.W.; Margie Bone, M.D.; Katie Brock, R.N., M.N., I.B.C.L.C.; Collette Crawford, R.N., certified yoga instructor; Steven Dassel, M.D.; Michelle Grandy, R.N., C.N.M.; Mary Beth Hasselquist, M.D.; Karen Ilika, M.D.; Tim Jernberg, M.D.; Donna Johnson, Ph.D.; Sandra Jolley, A.R.N.P., M.S., I.B.C.L.C.; Amy Irene Keyser, P.T.; Debbie Kinton, M.S., R.D.; Judy Lazarus, C.N.M.; Ourania Mallaris, M.D.; Suzy Meyers, L.M., M.P.H.; Ralph Neighbor, M.D.; Peggy Odegard, Pharm.D.; Nancy O'Neil, M.D.; Janine Plifka, Ph.D.; Kathryn Ponto, M.D.; Robert Resta, M.S.; Susan Rutherford, M.D.; Barbara Schinzinger, M.D.; Jeanne Schneider, R.N., I.B.C.L.C.; Debora Sciscoe, M.D.; Donna Smith, M.D.; Tanya Sorensen, M.D.; Lin Thoennes, M.N., A.R.N.P.; Ginna Wall, R.N., M.N.; Kathe Wallace, P.T.; Rebecca Zacharias, M.S., C.G.C.; and Kristine Zelenkov, M.D.

We also wish to thank the following people for their contributions to the artwork of this edition:

Photographers Paul Joseph Brown, Jan Dowers, Susan Ewbank, Katie McCullough, Bruce Miyake, Marilyn Nolt, Patti Ramos, Penny Simkin, Michael Spafford (Spike Mafford), David Stein and David Swain.

Models Ellen Cecil and Glenn Atwood; Ann and Gregg Bury; Sheila, Fred and Elijah Capestany; Katherine and Sam Coleman; Karen and Peter Contreras; Rosemary Garner and Lucinda Brown; Jennifer and Ry Middlestadt; Brenda, Bruce, Max, and Jem Miyake; Angela and James Oliver; Terry Payson and Dave Marquis; Linny Simkin and Callie Jobson; Mary Simkin-Maass and Greg, Sara Jane and Amelia Maass; Pamela, David and Jordan Swain; Sandra Szalay; and Shifra and Peter Weiss-Penzias.

Illustrators Shanna Dela Cruz/Ruth Ancheta; Childbirth Graphics, a division of WRS Group, Ltd.; Susan Aldridge for Harvard Common Press; Medela Inc.; and Terri Moll. We also want to remember the illustrators whose contributions to the last edition appear in this edition: Jamie Bolane of Childbirth Graphics for coordinating the creation of certain illustrations and Karen Martin Tomaselli for the shaded pencil drawings.

We also wish to thank the CEAS Board of Directors, the CEAS office staff (Judy Higgins, Cheri McMeins, Barbara Orcutt, Megan Sasnett, Susan Sasnett, Lois Stettner and Bronwen Vetromile) and the Penny Simkin, Inc. staff (Jan Dowers, Brenda Sutherland Field, and Cinda Weber) for their help and support during this revision.

Lastly, we wish to acknowledge our mentor, the late Virginia Larson, M.D., the founder of the Childbirth Education Association of Seattle, whose years of work with new families continue to inspire us.

Contents

Preface

Although society and culture change, maternity care practices change, families change and our book changes, the birth process itself does not change. This third edition of *Pregnancy, Childbirth & the Newborn* reflects the changes in our society and in maternity care that have taken place since the 1991 edition. The most significant changes involve how we communicate with each other and how the Internet and television inform us about pregnancy and birth. Numerous web sites offer opportunities to learn about childbearing from experts, highly opinionated would-be experts and other expectant parents. In addition, besides the sensationalised births portrayed on television in soap operas, sitcoms and dramas, you can watch edited versions of real births of all kinds almost every day.

In this era of abundant information, you might wonder if there is a need for a book like *Pregnancy, Childbirth & the Newborn*. Our resounding response is, 'Yes, more than ever!' As expectant parents, you should have a portable, comprehensive and unbiased source of factual information and sound advice. We hope *Pregnancy, Childbirth & the Newborn* will give you the insight and wisdom you need to sift through the information and make the choices that are best for you.

The continuing trend towards busier lifestyles—both in work and leisure—may leave you with little time to focus on your pregnancy. You may suddenly realise one day that your baby is coming whether you are ready or not! This book can be used both as a quick reference for answers to specific questions when you are rushed, and also as a single, complete resource for the entire childbearing year from conception through the first months of your baby's life.

What's new with this edition? We have updated and expanded every section of the book. We have added a new chapter, 'Planning for Birth and Post Partum', new charts on infections in pregnancy and childhood immunisations and information on over-the-counter medications. The chapters on nutrition, pain medications and obstetrical interventions and procedures have been updated. New photos and illustrations throughout the book add visual appeal, interest and clarification.

We present a new approach to self-help comfort measures in labour, based on our observations of the real experts—women in labour. We have noted both the similarities and differences in how women cope with the discomfort and stress of labour. Our observations have helped us simplify and individual- ise labour coping techniques. We name our approach 'The Three Rs' (relaxation, rhythm and ritual), which describe the behaviours we always see in women who deal well with the demands of labour and birth. You will learn how to adapt the Three Rs to suit your individual needs and desires.

Emotional support during labour receives even more attention in this edition and we have also covered in detail *new* comfort aids, such as the birth ball and use of the bath.

We have added important new material on post-partum adjustment, including advice on getting enough sleep, information on post-partum mood disorders, and advice for grandparents and other loved ones. The chapter on feeding your baby has been completely updated and expanded.

In addition to the updates, we have preserved the features that were so highly praised in previous editions: the clear and readable writing style, the concise at-a-glance tables and charts and the emphasis on what you as a consumer of maternity services need to know in order to make informed and personally meaningful choices.

We have used inclusive language to reflect various family configurations including traditional mother-father-children families, single-parent families, blended families formed by second marriages, families with gay and lesbian parents, and families formed by open adoption or surrogate mothers. We have tried to avoid assumptions about the gender of the woman's partner. At the same time, we did not want to neglect the unique contributions and needs of the biological father. In addition, we have avoided gender assumptions regarding the baby and caregivers; references to the baby's gender alternate by section or by chapter.

You will never forget the day you give birth and hold your baby in your arms for the first time. We want your childbirth to be safe, satisfying and a marvellous memory you will want to share with your child and each other for years to come.

This is the third time the three of us have joined to create or recreate *Pregnancy, Childbirth & the Newborn*. It has been a pleasure working with the Childbirth Education Association of Seattle and our editors and publisher to realise our goal of helping make your birth experience and transition to parenthood the smoothest, safest and most satisfying possible.

Penny Simkin, Janet Whalley, Ann Keppler

Introduction

Birth is more than the birth of a baby. It is the birth of a mother, a father, siblings, grandparents and others. In one day (more or less), many lives are transformed, but none more than the parents' and, of course, the baby's.

For the baby, birth ends nine months of rapid growth and preparation for life outside the wonderful, warm, watery womb. For the parents, birth ends nine months of wondering, waiting and worrying. When the parents and baby meet face-to-face for the first time, they may react as if they have always known each other, or—just the opposite—they may be totally surprised by each other.

And then the process of discovery begins. They stare, stroke, sniff, suckle and snuggle together, falling in love as only parents and their baby can. Amazement, awe and total engrossment mark the first few hours and days as the parents come to fully appreciate that this little person is the same little mystery child they knew in the womb.

And then reality sets in. Babies are dependent; their needs are almost constant and sometimes hard to understand. Is she hungry, wet, cold, sleepy, lonely, in pain? How do I soothe him, hold him, change him, bathe him, feed him? How do I know I am doing a good job? How can I get enough sleep? Will we ever have time for each other again?

Life will never be the same. It used to be simple, and now it is full of uncertainty. Able, intelligent, skilled adults feel puzzled, clumsy and ignorant around their baby. They may wonder how the human species has survived when birth, baby care and breastfeeding are so challenging. Somehow, with all the questions and doubts and demands, some powerful, non-rational drive gives them the willingness to keep giving, keep responding and keep trying.

And then the rewards start to come. The baby settles when cuddled. His nappy stays on. She gains weight. He smiles. She coos. He cannot take his eyes off his parents, and they cannot take their eyes off him. She stops crying when they sing to her. He sleeps for five hours straight. She knows they are the best parents ever, and they know their baby is the most special baby ever.

And then they realise that, even if they could, they would probably never want to go back to life as it was before their baby arrived.

The time spanning pregnancy, childbirth and the newborn's first weeks presents some of the greatest challenges and the greatest rewards you will ever experience. It is our privilege to offer you some guidance during this mysterious and wonderful time in your lives. We hope this book will help set the stage for you to become wonderful parents by helping you discover that you already know how to grow a baby, how to give birth to a baby and how to nourish and nurture a baby.

Chapter 1

Becoming Parents

Pregnancy is a state of becoming: an unborn baby is becoming capable of living outside the safe, protective and totally sufficient environment of the mother's body, and you and your partner are becoming parents. This state lasts about nine months and allows you the opportunity to learn, adjust, plan and prepare for parenthood. For most people, becoming parents is a greater life change than any other they will experience. Parenthood is permanent. The physical, emotional and spiritual nurturing of a child is both a delightful opportunity and a heavy responsibility.

Like most parents-to-be, you and your partner are probably looking forward to the rewards and joys of parenthood. You want to produce the healthiest baby possible and bring up a happy, secure person. In fact, you may find yourselves spending much time individually and together thinking and dream-ing about your child. What kind of person will your child become? What kind of guidance, role models, examples and discipline will be best for your child? As you both begin examining yourselves and evaluating your strengths and weaknesses as parents, you may wonder whether you have the qualities of the ideal parent. You may use the time during pregnancy to develop the characteristics you believe are essential in fulfilling your new roles.

Pregnancy is a positive growth experience for most expectant parents. This is a time to draw on or develop your support system—to talk to other pregnant women, expectant fathers or partners, or new parents; to find prenatal care and get referrals for any special needs; to strengthen bonds or mend fences with your own parents; to take childbirth preparation and parenting classes; and to read relevant books. This is a time to assess your lifestyle and make necessary changes to improve the chances of optimal health for mother and baby—changes in diet, exercise and any use of harmful substances.

Birth as Transition

Childbirth represents the transition from pregnancy to parenthood. Within a day or less, the nine-month-long state of pregnancy is over and the permanent state of parenthood begins. Cultures worldwide perceive birth as a life event equal to death in its significance. Birth is celebrated almost everywhere as a joyous event and is surrounded by rituals associated with hope, promise and new life.

For you, however, the anticipation of birth and motherhood brings up questions and deep feelings—positive and negative—about such things as your sexuality, your childhood, your own mother, your parents' relationship, and your expectations of yourself and of your partner—both during labour and then as a parent. Partners also look at these factors in themselves and in their own backgrounds as they anticipate parenthood.

Your need to complete this major life transition with safety and satisfaction leads you and your partner to seek advice, guidance and help. You may turn to your own parents, other experienced parents, doctors, midwives, nurses, counsellors, childbirth

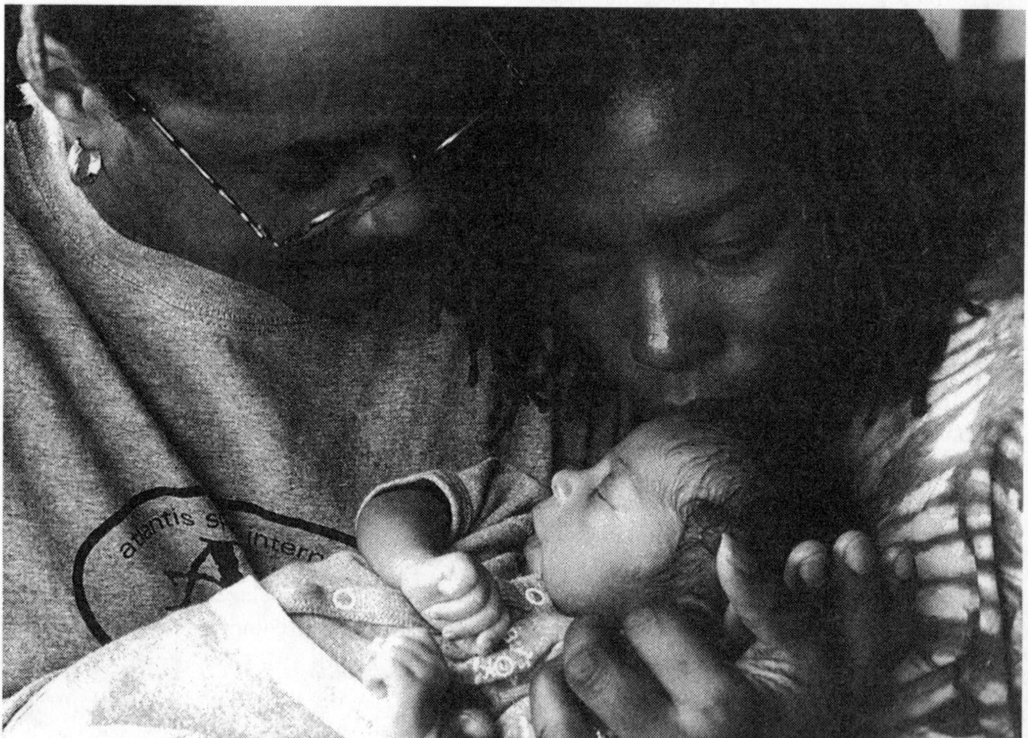

Photograph by Marilyn Nolt

It is hard to believe that soon you will be kissing your baby.

educators, authors of books, and organisations and individuals on the Internet. After considering their suggestions in light of your own experience, knowledge, common sense and priorities, you will begin to discover and follow your own path in preparing for childbirth.

You may be surprised by the vast amount of information available, the number of experts ready and willing to advise you, and the number of decisions to make. Perhaps this reflects the fact that pregnancy, unlike other medical conditions, is normal and healthy. It is also a highly personal and emotionally significant event. Your active participation in your care and the presence of competent, kind, respectful caregivers help ensure maximum safety for you and your baby and a sense of satisfaction and fulfilment after the birth.

Pregnancy is not a disease, although its extra demands on your body make you more vulnerable to medical complications than you are at other times in your life. For this reason, you and your baby benefit from prenatal (before birth) care and regular checkups throughout pregnancy. Neither is the birth process an acute illness that ends when the baby is born. Birth is a time of stress, however, and sometimes exceeds normal boundaries and requires medical intervention (assistance by health care professionals to solve problems for mother and baby to ensure optimal outcomes). Whether medical interventions are needed must be carefully considered. If used without evidence of problems or complications, medical interventions can interrupt the normal process of labour and birth.

Birth as a Long-term Memory

The day you give birth will, most likely, be vividly etched in your memory for the rest of your life. Ask your mother and your partner's mother for details about your birth and that of your partner. What did your fathers do? What did the nurses and doctors or midwives do and say? How do your mothers feel as they recall your births? What did your mothers feel when they first saw and held you and your partner as newborns? Research on women's long-term memories of their birth experiences shows that these memories are vivid and deeply felt.[1]

Unless your mothers were heavily drugged during labour, chances are they will have clear and detailed memories of their birth experiences. The amount of emotion they express when telling their stories may surprise you. Some women have very positive, fulfilling, even empowering memories of giving birth and love to talk about it, while others remember with shame, anger, remorse or resignation. Positive, satisfying memories are likely if the mother was cared for kindly, respectfully and with consideration of her personal priorities and concerns, even if her labour was long and complicated.

You, too, will probably recall your upcoming childbirth vividly and with profound emotion. And your memories are likely to be greatly influenced by the way you are cared for by your doctors, midwives and nurses. Knowing all this may motivate you to do whatever you can ahead of time to ensure that your memories of this childbirth will be good ones. The choices you make—about where to have your baby, who will be your caregiver, who else to have with you during labour and birth, and your preferred general approach to birth management—will largely determine whether you will have the kind of care that leads to long-term satisfaction or dissatisfaction. The remainder of this chapter and Chapter 7 will help you with these choices.

Childbirth Choices

There is no universal agreement among medical professionals or the general public on the single best, safest and most satisfying way to give birth, especially for the healthy woman experiencing a normal pregnancy. Many types of care are offered. You and your partner should investigate the choices available and decide what kind of care seems appropriate for you depending on your needs, desires and priorities.

Health Care Coverage

If you have health insurance, be sure to find out the extent of your maternity care coverage. Caregiver fees and hospitalisation for normal birth may or may not be fully covered, while care of the mother or baby with complications may be more fully covered. Procedures like epidural anaesthesia (a regional nerve block used for pain relief) and circumcision may or may not be covered or covered in part. With these procedures there may be two charges, one for the equipment used and another for the services of the physician who performs the procedure. Check on the length of hospital stay that is covered after both a vaginal birth and a caesarean birth. Your doctors are obliged to provide you with a schedule of fees for antenatal care and confinement. Ask the providers of those services how to submit a request for reimbursement of your costs for such services. If, as you read your health insurance policy, you do not understand the extent of your coverage, contact your agent or a company representative for clarification.

Choosing the Place of Birth

In a Hospital

While most women in Australia give birth in hospitals, these institutions vary widely in the services they offer, their staffs' attitudes towards patients and their philosophies of care. Depending on your health care coverage and where you live, you may or may not have a choice of hospitals. If you have a choice, you should try to learn about several hospitals, take their tours and carefully choose the one that best meets your needs.

Hospitals committed to family-centred maternity care strive to be flexible and responsive to the mother's needs and the family's wishes. Some hospitals provide a birthing room where the woman labours, gives birth and may remain with her baby and partner until they go home. Birthing rooms may have comfortable furniture, televisions and other amenities. Many newer or remodelled birthing units have baths or showers. Some hospitals have gardens or outdoor areas where patients can walk or sit during labour. The staff members of some hospitals take pride in providing individualised service to their patients, while staff members of other hospitals tend to operate on a more rigid and routine protocol in which they treat all patients alike and allow parents little or no say in their care and that of their baby.

While all hospitals know the value of a low ratio of patients per nurse, not all guarantee that you will have one-to-one nursing care in active labour. You may want to inquire about each hospital's staffing policies for low- and high-risk women in labour. How often do they rely on 'floating' nurses—that is, nurses who work in several departments and who may not be experienced in maternity nursing? How often do they use practical nurses or nursing assistants, either of whom may be limited in the tasks they are legally allowed to perform?

If you want or need an epidural, knowing something about who will give you anaesthesia—may be important to you. In public hospitals a registrar, who is a doctor training to be a specialist, may administer the epidural. Anaesthesiologists are medical doctors who specialise in administration and maintenance of anaesthesia and recovery from it. You cannot choose the individual who gives the anaesthesia (whoever is on call at the time you need anaesthesia is the one you get), but you can find out the credentials of the anaesthesia staff members who work at the hospital that you have chosen.

Hospitals vary in the overall level of maternity care they provide—from primary care for healthy, low-risk women having normal pregnancies to tertiary care that ensures the availability of intensive care for women with highly complicated pregnancies or for very ill babies. If you are having a difficult pregnancy or if complications are anticipated in labour or birth, you may need a hospital that provides tertiary care with complete obstetrical, anaesthetic, blood bank and laboratory services available twenty-four hours a day.

An efficient way to find out about each hospital's procedures and policies (called 'routines') is to inquire about them while on a hospital tour. You can also discuss them with your caregiver, as your doctor's or midwife's orders determine your care while you are in the hospital. (See Chapter 7 on birth planning for ideas about specific features to check when comparing hospitals.) Knowing the philosophy, policies and services of each of the hospitals you are considering will help you choose wisely. You will know whether changes can be made to meet your individual needs, or at least you will know what to expect.

The Hospital Tour

Most hospitals' maternity departments schedule tours regularly. To find out specifics, call the hospital's prenatal education department or the labour-and-delivery unit. Scheduled tours are often led by a volunteer. Some hospitals will conduct a personal tour whenever they have a nurse available to show a prospective patient around. If this is the case, call when you wish to take the tour to see if a nurse is available. Tours typically involve visiting an empty birthing room, a post-partum room if it is separate, the nursery and the family waiting area. You usually do not see the room where caesarean births are performed. The tour guide discusses some usual routines and policies and gives you a chance to ask questions.

Possible Questions to Ask

- How many doctors and midwives attend births here?
- On average, how many births per month take place here?
- Which entrance should I use to enter the hospital during the day or at night?
- What is the ratio of patients to midwives during early labour, active labour, birth and post partum?
- Do you encourage the use of birth plans (a written list of the parents' preferences for care during birth and post partum)?
- What equipment is used to monitor the foetal heart rate during labour?
- Do most labouring women have intravenous (IV) fluids?
- Is anaesthesia available at all times?
- If there are bathtubs, how often are they used for comforting a woman in labour? How many tubs do you have? Do women ever give birth in the tubs?
- If I have a caesarean, where will it take place? How many people are allowed to attend? Who decides who can attend?
- What are your visitor policies during labour and post partum?
- Do you have lactation consultants on staff twenty-four hours daily, including weekends? May I call them after I go home if I have breastfeeding questions?
- How long is the usual post-partum stay after a vaginal birth or a caesarean birth? May I stay longer? Is there a set time for checkout?
- What security measures do you employ to protect my baby's safety?
- Does this hospital offer any post-partum and newborn follow-up after I go home? What is available?

If your tour guide cannot answer some of these questions, ask him or her to find out who can. The answers will give you a better idea of what to expect at the hospital and how flexible and skilled the staff can be in individualising your care. In some cities childbirth education organisations, other consumer groups or the hospitals themselves have published information answering some of these questions.

Outside a Hospital

A small percentage of low-risk Australian women give birth outside the hospital in birth centres, or at home with midwives or doctors in attendance. In these settings, there are fewer routines and less medical equipment because they are usually not needed for normal, uncomplicated births. The cost of such care is usually lower than the cost of hospital care.

With a planned out-of-hospital birth, you are unlikely to need medical interventions such as IV fluids, medications and electronic foetal monitoring. (See Chapter 10 for more on medical interventions.) Because it is more difficult to get some of these same interventions if they become desirable or necessary, throughout your pregnancy your caregiver should screen carefully for signs of problems. You will be transferred to in-hospital care if there are warning signs such as a rise in blood pressure, bleeding, high blood sugar, protein in the urine, anaemia, foetal problems or premature labour contractions. Even with careful pregnancy screening, 15–27 percent of women who intend to give birth outside the hospital are transferred to the hospital during labour or post partum for problems judged to require obstetrical intervention.[2] Most transfers during labour are for non-emergencies such as prolonged labour, meconium in the amniotic fluid or prolonged ruptured membranes—situations in which procedures or medication will be helpful or needed but are not immediately necessary for the welfare of the baby or mother.

For most low-risk women with good prenatal care, the outcomes of planned out-of-hospital births are as good as those of planned hospital births. Emergency transfers are extremely rare for women who have been screened and who have had uncomplicated, normal pregnancies. The principal unpredictable, potentially dangerous conditions that can arise during labour and that require immediate medical action include cord prolapse (when the cord slips out of the uterus before the birth), haemorrhage and deprivation of the foetus's oxygen supply during labour (due to bleeding, cord compression and other factors). After delivery, the main reasons for emergency transfer are haemorrhage, retained placenta and serious newborn problems. These problems, which can occur in both hospital and out-of-hospital births, are discussed in Chapters 3 and 10.

The best place for you is the place where you will feel safe and comfortable and where you can get the help and expertise you want and need as you make the transition to parenthood.

Choosing a Caregiver

Many types of caregivers—obstetricians, general practitioners, midwives and others—provide maternity care to the childbearing woman. (For more on choosing a health care provider for your baby, see Chapter 7, pages 155–157.)

Obstetricians/gynaecologists have graduated from medical school. They have had six or more years of additional training in obstetrics (medical care before, during and after birth) and gynaecology (medical care of women). Much of their education focuses on detection and treatment of obstetrical and gynaecological problems. To qualify for board certification, they must pass an exam administered by the Royal Australian New Zealand College of Obstetricians and Gynaecologists (RANZCOG).

Maternal-foetal medicine specialists are obstetricians/gynaecologists who have received further training and certification in managing high-risk pregnancy and birth. They often consult with or accept referrals from other physicians and midwives. These specialists practice only in major medical centres in urban areas.

General practitioners have graduated from medical school and have completed additional training in family medicine, including, in some cases, maternity care. Their education focuses on the health care needs of the entire family. They refer to specialists if their patients develop serious complications. To qualify to offer maternity care general practitioners may have undertaken a Diploma in Obstetrics and Gynaecology. Some hospitals require continuing accreditation for general practitioners to participate in shared care programmes. Not all general practitioners include maternity care in their practice.

Certified midwives (CM) have usually graduated from a school of nursing, passed an examination to become registered nurses and completed additional training in midwifery. Direct entry midwifery courses are being evaluted in Australia. Midwives' education and the care they provide focus on normal health care during the childbearing year, psycho-social and emotional aspects of childbearing, parent education, prevention of and screening for possible problems, and newborn care. They specialise in the care of women with uncomplicated, normal pregnancies and births. Referrals are made to an obstetrician when needed. To become certified, they must complete recommended assessments and examinations as determined by their training university and approved by the respective State and territory Nursing Board.

Independent midwife practitioners practice autonomously and may deliver at home or in hospitals. Most hospitals do not have independent midwives on the staff.

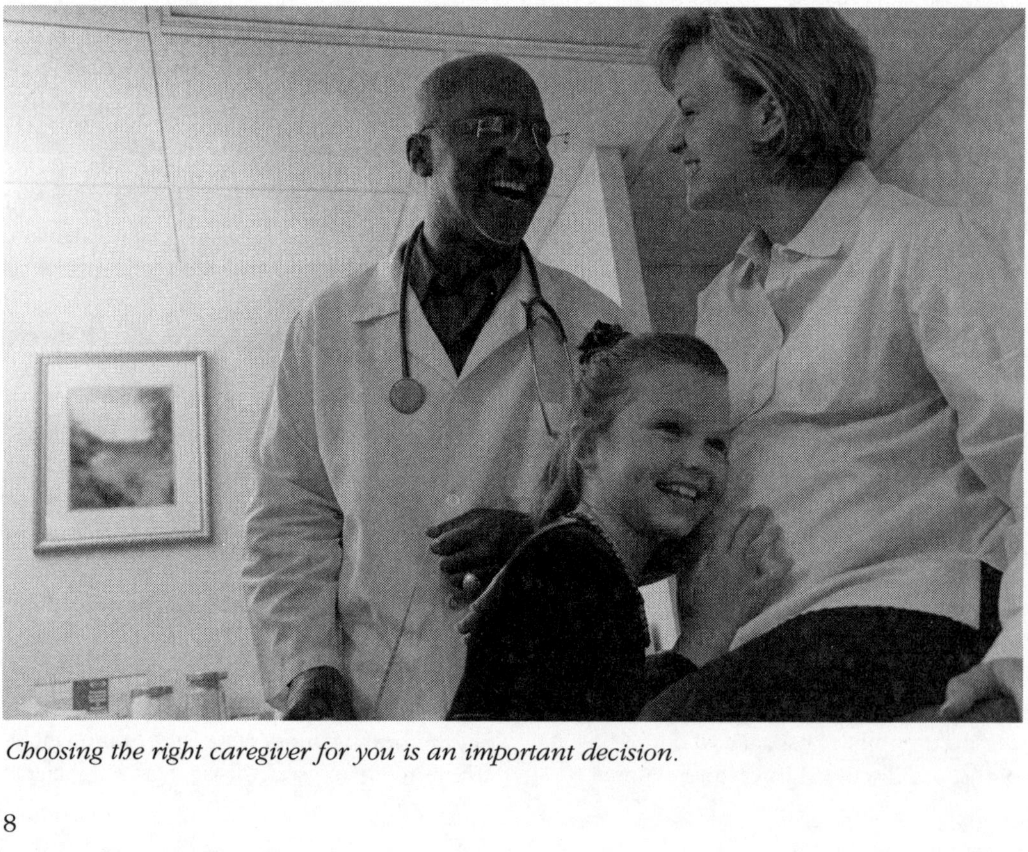

Choosing the right caregiver for you is an important decision.

You will want to know the educational background, credentials, training and experience of any possible caregiver, especially if you are considering one whose practice is unregulated. Learn about the caregiver's backup and referral arrangements should you need to transfer to a specialist.

One important consideration in choosing your caregiver is the state of your health. A healthy pregnant woman experiencing a normal pregnancy will have different needs than a woman with health problems or one who is experiencing complications during pregnancy. A healthy pregnant woman can choose from any of the specialties offering maternity care. If your pregnancy is complicated or if problems are anticipated during labour or birth, your options are more limited. In such cases, an obstetrician or maternal-foetal medicine specialist should be involved in your care either as your sole caregiver or as a consultant co-managing your care along with your family physician or midwife. Co-management is most likely if you live far away from a specialist or if you are being cared for in a group practice that provides both midwifery or family practice and obstetrics.

In Australia, obstetricians provide most of the care to childbearing women. However, many general practitioners provide maternity care, which appeals to some expectant parents because general practitioners provide medical care for the entire family, including the new baby. Midwives are the usual caregivers in most other countries of the world and are becoming increasingly popular in the United States. Midwives are available in some parts of Canada as well.

Gender of Your Caregiver

You may have a preference regarding the gender of your caregiver. Today many women prefer a female maternity caregiver. Many women feel more comfortable allowing examination of their sexual parts by and discussing intimate issues with a female than a male. Some may believe that such issues are better understood by other women. However, you may have a problem finding a physicians' group practice that contains only women. While some groups of physicians are all men or all women, most include both. Most midwives are women. If you feel strongly about the gender of your caregiver, you need to recognise that the person whom you choose from a group is not necessarily the person who will be present during labour and birth. In fact, in some large groups the chances that you will have your own caregiver are very small.

When making your selection, we suggest that you look beyond gender to the personal qualities, philosophy of care and professional qualifications of caregivers. While it is true that many female caregivers are sensitive, caring, understanding and competent, so are many males. By the same token, females and males alike could be impersonal, rushed and uninterested in you as an individual. Do not assume that having a female caregiver is a guarantee of more sensitive care.

General Considerations in Choosing a Caregiver

In narrowing your possibilities for maternity care providers, your first questions should be:

1. What options are available to me?
If you live in a rural area there may be only one hospital and very few caregivers available to you. If you belong to a health maintenance organisation or have health care coverage by an insurance company or a government assistance program, your choices are restricted to those covered by your third-party payer, unless you are willing to pay more for a caregiver practicing outside their system. Once you have a list of available caregivers and know which hospitals and birth centres (and whether home births) are covered, your next step is to consult a knowledgeable person (a trusted nurse, doctor, midwife, childbirth educator or friend who is a new parent) to narrow your list further.

2. Where do I want to give birth? In a hospital, birth centre or at home?
If you have the option, you may choose the birth setting before selecting your caregiver. If you choose a hospital or birth centre, tour the facility, learn about its routines and policies, meet one or more midwives, and talk to families who have recently given birth there. You may find a big difference among various birth settings. Select a caregiver who attends births at the setting you prefer.

3. Am I selecting a single caregiver or a group?
The fact is that when you choose a caregiver, you are most often choosing a group. Your appointments may rotate among members of the group, or you may see one or two caregivers throughout your pregnancy but not at your birth. In most cases, the caregiver at your labour is the person who happens to be on call at the time—and she or he could very well be a stranger to you.

With your preliminary questions answered, your next step is to evaluate available caregivers. Be aware that the general philosophical approach of different caregivers to pregnancy and childbirth may vary and is influenced by their education, training and personal experiences. Some caregivers think of pregnancy and birth as a normal family-centred event that seldom requires medical intervention. Others rely heavily on technology and interventions when caring for a healthy childbearing woman. Such interventions may include inducing or speeding labour, continuous electronic foetal monitoring, intravenous fluids, medications, episiotomy, vacuum extraction or the use of forceps.

Look for a caregiver whose philosophical approach appeals to you and who is qualified to provide care appropriate to your health needs. Some caregivers are more holistic in their approach than others. In other words, they focus not only on the medical aspects of your pregnancy but also on your emotional, spiritual and physical wellbeing. If your caregiver does not provide holistic care, you may find other people with whom to discuss the non-medical issues. Talk with your friends and relatives, other pregnant women or your childbirth educator. They are likely to be interested in you and have the time to help with these non-clinical matters.

Initial Interview

As you consider your options, feel free to shop around. Interview more than one caregiver, if necessary, before choosing. Because you will probably be charged for an office visit, you may want to do some initial screening over the telephone. Inquire about the qualifications and experience of the doctor or midwife. Ask about fees, who takes calls when the caregiver is off duty, and whether he or she attends births at more than one hospital. Some attend births in homes or birthing centres. Ask your local childbirth education group for suggestions and referrals.

Think of your first appointment as a consultation (a chance to interview the caregiver) and make that clear when setting up the appointment. One appointment need not commit you to remaining in his or her care. Try to have a general idea of what you are seeking in a caregiver. Once you decide to make an appointment with a doctor or midwife, be prepared to ask questions that will help you discover the philosophy and type of care offered.

Since an initial interview will probably last only ten to thirty minutes, you will need to select only a few key questions. Choose from the following list or develop your own.

Possible Questions to Ask

Become as knowledgeable as possible about your questions before interviewing a caregiver. Doing so will help you more quickly understand terminology and options that may be a part of the answers. This book will provide background for your questions. Your interview will help you decide if the caregiver is suitable for you.

- What do you see as my role and responsibilities during pregnancy and childbirth?
- Are there any restrictions on my partner being with me throughout labour, vaginal or caesarean birth and during my hospital stay?
- How do you feel about other family members (children, grandparents and so on) or friends attending prenatal appointments or being present at the birth?
- What recommendations do you make on nutrition during pregnancy (foods to eat/avoid, weight gain and so on)? Do you provide nutritional counselling? Do you have specific recommendations on exercise, sex and the use of medicines and drugs (including over-the-counter drugs; caffeine; tobacco; alcohol; and marijuana, cocaine and other street drugs)?
- What are your feelings about childbirth preparation classes and natural, non-medicated childbirth? Approximately what percentage of your clients or patients are interested in natural childbirth? How many of those actually have it?
- Do you have routine standing orders for your patients in labour about IV fluids, pain medications and so on? What are they? Can these routines be altered to conform to my needs and desires? Would you encourage and help me prepare a birth plan? (See Chapter 7.) Will you check my birth plan for safety and compatibility with your practices and hospital policies?
- What are the chances you will be present when I deliver? If you are not there, who covers for you? Will I have a chance to meet that person? Will that person and the hospital staff respect the arrangements I have made with you?
- How often and under what circumstances do you find it desirable or necessary to use labour induction or augmentation, IV fluids, artificial rupture of the

membranes, continuous electronic foetal monitoring, episiotomy, forceps and vacuum extraction?

- What is your caesarean rate or how often do you find it necessary to do a caesarean birth? What are the most common reasons for caesareans among the women in your practice? What, if anything, can I do before and during labour to help reduce the likelihood of a caesarean? Will you perform a caesarean should I request one?
- If I should develop complications during pregnancy or labour, would you manage my care? If not, to whom would you refer me?
- What usually happens to the baby immediately after birth? Does the baby go to the nursery or may she stay with us? May I/we hold her for her initial assessments? Who will examine the baby after birth? When is this usually done?
- What is the usual hospital stay after a vaginal birth or a caesarean birth?
- Is follow-up care routinely available for me and the baby? If so, how soon after discharge may I expect the follow-up? Who initiates the follow-up? Would it include home or clinic visits with a nurse, midwife or doctor, or just phone follow-up?

As you discuss these questions, listen as much to *how* the caregiver answers as to *what* he or she actually says. Is the caregiver impatient and defensive with you or open and comfortable with your questions? Do the answers satisfy you? Does this person inspire your confidence and trust? Often your overall feeling about the interview will provide as much information as the direct answers to your questions. An interview like this will help you discover how the caregiver feels about prospective parents who take their responsibilities seriously.

Dissatisfaction with Your Present Caregiver

What if you have been seeing a caregiver for some time and then, after getting a better idea of his or her practice, you feel uncomfortable with your choice? You should heed those feelings and act on them in one of the following ways:

1. Express your discomfort and explain what would make you feel more at ease. Using 'I-messages', calmly describe your discomfort. In other words, tell your caregiver how you feel and what you need without blaming your caregiver or using accusatory language about his or her shortcomings. Consider the following two approaches:

- Dr Jones, you're always in a rush and you don't let me ask any questions. You don't even care about your patients.
- Dr Jones, this is hard for me to say, but I get the impression that my questions are an inconvenience to you. I need to know more about (a test, my problem and so on), but I feel brushed off and that I should not ask you anything.

The first approach will likely make Dr Jones feel angry or defensive and will not result in better communication, whereas the second is more likely to evoke an apology or an effort to improve communication and to work together as equals. After you have stated your needs, you should try to negotiate in areas where you and your caregiver have differences. Effective negotiation means respectfully communicating your wishes and needs and the reasons for them, considering your caregiver's response, and then coming to an agreement. You might practice this conversation ahead of time with your partner or a friend, if it seems challenging. Sometimes clearer communication leads one of you to change your mind, or it may lead to compromise. Your birth plan should contain these joint decisions. (See Chapter 7 for a discussion of birth plans.)

2. If the first approach does not succeed and if you have a choice, consider changing caregivers. It's best not to switch to another caregiver in the same group, since your caregiver might be on call when you are in labour. Try to get recommendations from knowledgeable people who know what you are looking for, and try to interview the new caregiver before making your decision. Although it is always uncomfortable to change caregivers, it is better to act than to stay with someone who makes you feel uneasy.

3. If you cannot or do not want to change caregivers and you are unable to discuss your feelings, you will have to find a way to minimise a negative experience. If possible, talk with a midwife, a childbirth educator or others. They may be able to help. Your midwife in labour may also be able to help you, so you might tactfully share some of your concerns with him or her.

Choosing Your Childbirth Classes

Many institutions, nonprofit community organisations, groups of doctors or midwives and independent childbirth educators offer childbirth preparation classes. Their programs vary in size, philosophy, cost, topics covered and number of classes in the series. The background and training of the teachers also vary, as does the quality of the classes. Some classes are consumer oriented with the goal of preparing parents to take responsibility in decision-making and self-care. Others are more provider oriented; they inform parents about the type of care provided by a hospital or caregiver group but avoid discussion of alternatives

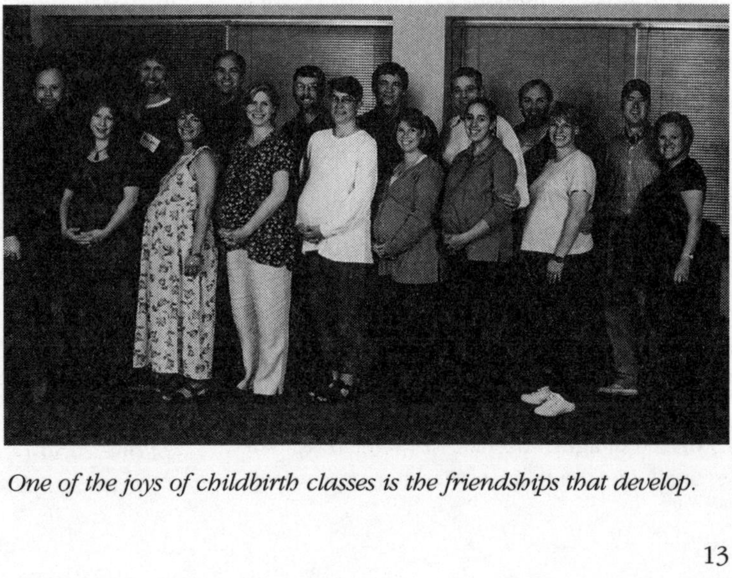

Photograph by David Swain

One of the joys of childbirth classes is the friendships that develop.

or controversial aspects of maternity care. If you have a choice, compare the classes to determine which one best suits your needs.

Possible Questions to Ask

- Who sponsors the classes? (Sponsors may include a hospital, your physician or midwife, an independent childbirth education association, the Red Cross, a public health department, a non-affiliated individual and so on.) Are the classes consumer or provider oriented?
- What is the instructor's background? The instructor may be a midwife or physiotherapist. What is the instructor's training? The instructor may have completed a credentialled Australian antenatal eduction program. This is not a requirment of all antenatal progams.
- What is the instructor's experience with birth and childbirth education? If the instructor is a woman, has she given birth? If a man, has he participated in a birth? Has the individual cared for or supported women in labour? How long has she or he been teaching? Does the teacher participate in continuing education in the field?
- What is the philosophy and approach of the instructor? Does she or he cover normal childbirth and variations from normal? Does she or he describe all choices available and their pros and cons? Are comfort measures and techniques for natural childbirth (also called prepared childbirth) taught? Does the instructor describe disadvantages and risks as well as advantages and benefits of various procedures and medications? Does she or he emphasise the parents' right and responsibility to be informed and to make decisions?
- Does the instructor cover topics other than childbirth, such as nutrition, foetal development, emotional aspects of pregnancy and parenthood, baby care and feeding? Are other classes available on early pregnancy, pregnancy fitness, breastfeeding, parenting, baby care, sibling preparation, caesarean preparation and preparation for vaginal birth after a caesarean? Are refresher courses available for those who already have children?
- How many weeks does the class meet? How long is each session? How much time is spent in lecture and discussion? How much time is spent in practising exercises, relaxation and comfort measures?
- What is the cost of the series? (Some private health insurers and government assistance programs cover the cost of childbirth preparation classes.)
- Does the educator teach a particular method (such as Lamaze or Bradley), or has she or he developed a method from many sources (like the Three Rs described on pages 174–176)?
- What is the ratio of students to teachers? If classes are large, are there assistants or other teachers available to ensure individual attention?
- Is there a reunion class after all class members' babies are born?
- Is the instructor available to students by phone or in person for questions outside of class and after the course?

After investigating the options, you will likely find the class that is most suitable for you. If there is little or no choice in your community, it is still a good idea to take whatever class is available and to supplement your preparation with reading materials and videotapes. The resource list at the end of this book will help.

Conclusion

Once you have made these important choices of caregiver, birth setting and childbirth classes, you can settle in to your pregnancy, take care of yourself, and learn about the profound changes taking place in your body and happening for your baby. The rest of this book can be your guide in preparing for the giant steps ahead.

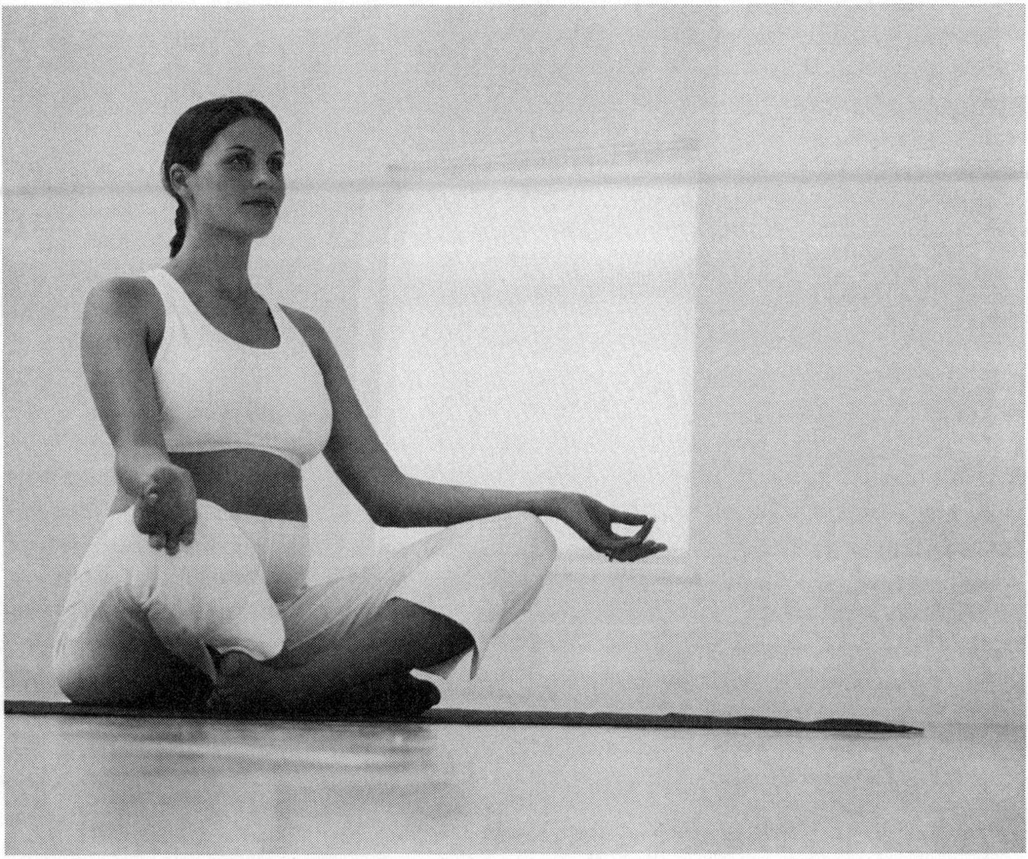

There are many different types of childbirth classes available.

Chapter 2

Pregnancy

The normal and healthy process of pregnancy brings profound physical and emotional growth for the expectant mother and psychological changes for the expectant father or partner. This chapter explores the many changes you are likely to experience during pregnancy and the dramatic foetal growth and development that will take place from conception to birth. The discussion begins with an explanation of reproductive anatomy and the process of conception.

Anatomy of Reproduction

The Male

The external *genitalia* of the male include the *scrotum* and the *penis*. The scrotum contains two *testicles* (testes or male sex glands), which produce *sperm* or *spermatozoa*. Each testicle contains over 800 small, tightly coiled tubes known as *seminiferous tubules*, which produce hundreds of millions of sperm in response to a hormone produced by the *pituitary gland*, which is located in the brain. Another hormone from the pituitary gland stimulates the testicles to produce the male sex hormone *testosterone*, which is responsible for the male's sexual characteristics (deep voice, facial and body hair, and others). Testosterone also ensures adequate development of sperm.

The seminiferous tubules join to form the *epididymis*, a wider coiled tube that stores the sperm for a few weeks until they are mature and ready to make their way out of the scrotum. As the epididymis leaves the scrotum and enters the pelvic cavity, it becomes the *vas deferens*, a duct that carries and stores the sperm. Into this duct the *seminal vesicles*, *prostate gland* and *Cowper's glands* secrete fluids that enhance fertility by nourishing the sperm and aiding their motility (movement). Together with the sperm, these secretions make up the *semen*

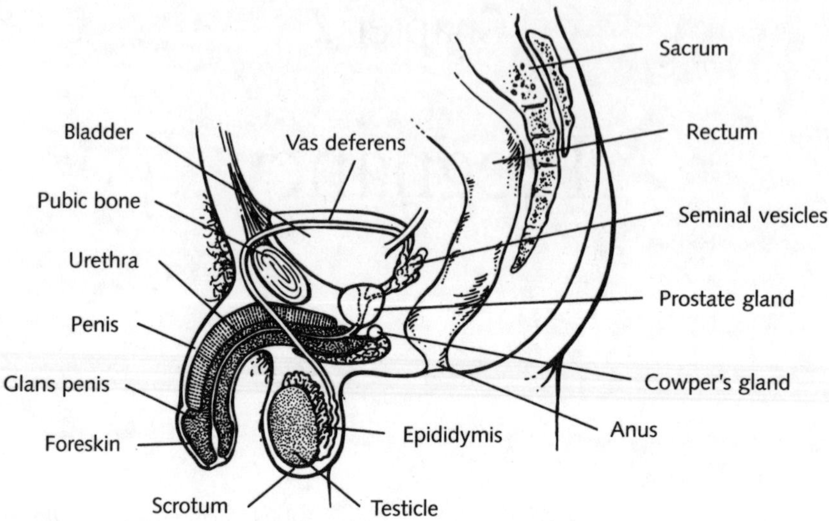

Male anatomy

that is ejaculated into the vagina during sexual intercourse.

The vas deferens empties into the male *urethra*, which leads from the bladder to the end of the penis. The urethra transports both urine and semen from within to outside the man's body. During urination and most other times, the penis is soft or flaccid. With sexual excitement, blood rapidly fills the tissues of the penis, causing it to expand and become firm and erect, facilitating insertion into the vagina during intercourse. With sexual excitement, muscles contract to close the duct to the bladder, keeping urine out of the semen. During orgasm, ejaculation triggers involuntary muscle contractions, which propel 2–6 millilitres (1 teaspoon is 5 millilitres) of semen through the urethra. The ejaculate contains approximately 150 million to 400 million sperm.

The Female

The following description and the accompanying illustrations of the female's reproductive anatomy and physiology provide the background for later discussion of conception, pregnancy and birth.

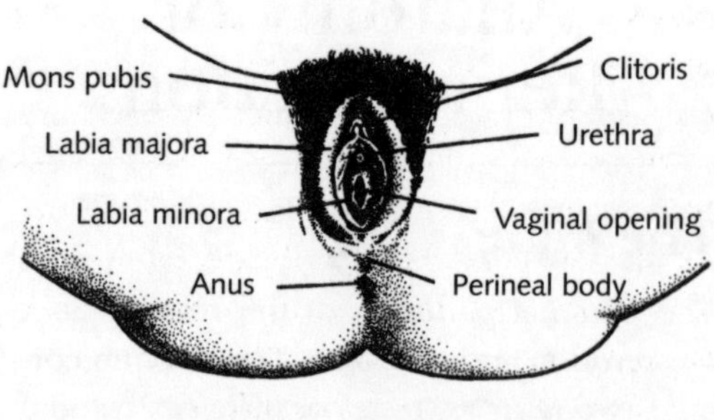

External female anatomy

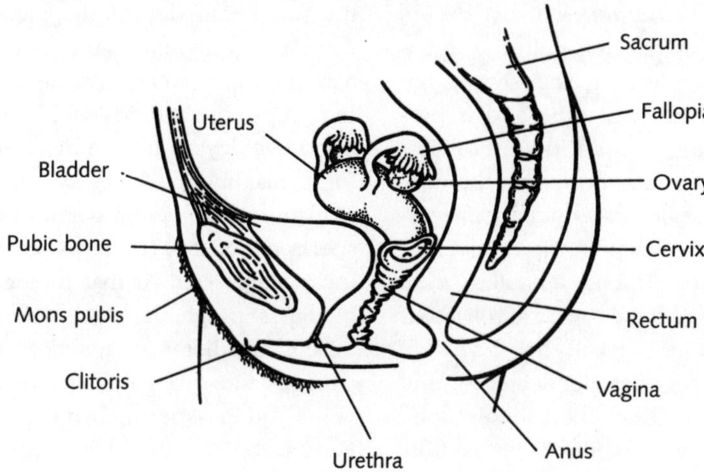

Internal female anatomy

A woman's *perineum* includes the pelvic floor muscles, external *genitals*, urethra, anus and *perineal body* (the area between the vagina and anus). The external genitals (called the *vulva*) include the vaginal opening, *clitoris, labia majora, labia minora* and *mons pubis* (the fatty tissue over the pubic bone). The internal reproductive organs are the *uterus* (or womb), *vagina, fallopian tubes* and *ovaries*. The uterus is a hollow, muscular, pear-shaped organ situated in the pelvis—behind the bladder and in front of the rectum. Divided into two parts, the uterus has an upper part called the *body* and a lower part called the *cervix*, which protrudes into the vagina, the stretchy canal connecting the internal and external genitals. Two fallopian tubes extend from the upper sides of the uterus towards the ovaries.

The two ovaries, located on each side of the uterus, are a woman's sex glands. One of their functions is to produce the female sex hormones *oestrogen* and *progesterone*. During adolescence, oestrogen, along with other hormones from the pituitary and adrenal glands, stimulates the development of secondary sexual characteristics in the female, such as enlarged breasts and body hair. The ovaries also expel ripe *ova* (eggs). Of the hundreds of thousands of ova present in the ovaries, only about 400–450 ripen and are expelled (ovulated) in a woman's lifetime.

During a woman's reproductive years, except during pregnancy, the ovaries undergo cyclic changes, which usually occur monthly. The *menstrual cycle* is influenced by pituitary hormones, which cause an ovum to mature and its *follicle* (the sac surrounding the ovum) to enlarge and secrete oestrogen. This process then stimulates the growth of the *endometrium* (the lining of the uterus).

Usually only one ovum ripens and is released from its follicle each month in a process called *ovulation*, which occurs approximately halfway through the menstrual cycle. After leaving the ovary, the ovum enters the fallopian tube and is propelled slowly to the uterus. Under the influence of another pituitary hormone, the now empty follicle begins producing progesterone, which stimulates further development of the uterine lining, enabling it to receive and nourish the ovum, if fertilised. If fertilisation does not occur, the levels of oestrogen and progesterone decrease, and the uterus sheds its unneeded lining along with the unfertilised ovum. This monthly shedding process is called *menstruation*.

Becoming Pregnant: Conception

Conception occurs as a result of sexual intercourse or, if that is not possible, by *artificial insemination (AI)* or by other alternative procedures.

Artificial insemination is a procedure by which previously collected semen is placed at the cervix or in the uterus with a special catheter. Artificial insemination is used when sperm are needed from another source, as in cases of infertility or impotence in the male partner, or if a woman without a male partner wants to become pregnant.

After sexual intercourse or artificial insemination, sperm travel from the vagina through the opening of the cervix, into the cavity of the uterus, and along the fallopian tubes. When cervical mucus thins around the fourteenth day of the menstrual cycle, even more sperm are able make the journey towards the awaiting ovum. Sperm can live in fertile cervical fluid inside the woman for up to five days, while an ovum remains alive for a maximum of twenty-four hours after ovulation. Conception occurs when a single sperm penetrates (fertilises) an ovum, forming a single cell. At that moment a woman becomes pregnant. Once an ovum is fertilised, a chemical reaction occurs that changes the surface of the ovum and prevents other sperm from penetrating it. Fertilisation usually takes place in the outer part of the fallopian tube near the ovary. Then the fertilised ovum continues down the fallopian tube to the uterus and, several days later, embeds in the uterine lining.

Alternative methods of conception include *in vitro fertilisation (IVF), gamete intra-fallopian transfer (GIFT), zygote intra-fallopian transfer (ZIFT)* and *intracytoplasmic sperm injection (ICSI)*. With most of these procedures, the physician prescribes drugs to stimulate ovulation, surgically gathers many mature eggs from the ovaries, and collects the sperm, possibly mixing it with a culture medium to enhance sperm motility. Depending on the chosen procedures, fertilisation occurs in a laboratory container (IVF, ZIFT), in the woman's fallopian tube (GIFT) or by injecting a single sperm directly into an ovum (ICSI). If fertilisation occurs outside the woman's body, the physician places the fertilised ovum in her fallopian tube (ZIFT) or her uterus (IVF or ICSI).

Achieving a successful pregnancy may require several attempts at fertilisation or implantation. The extremely high cost of

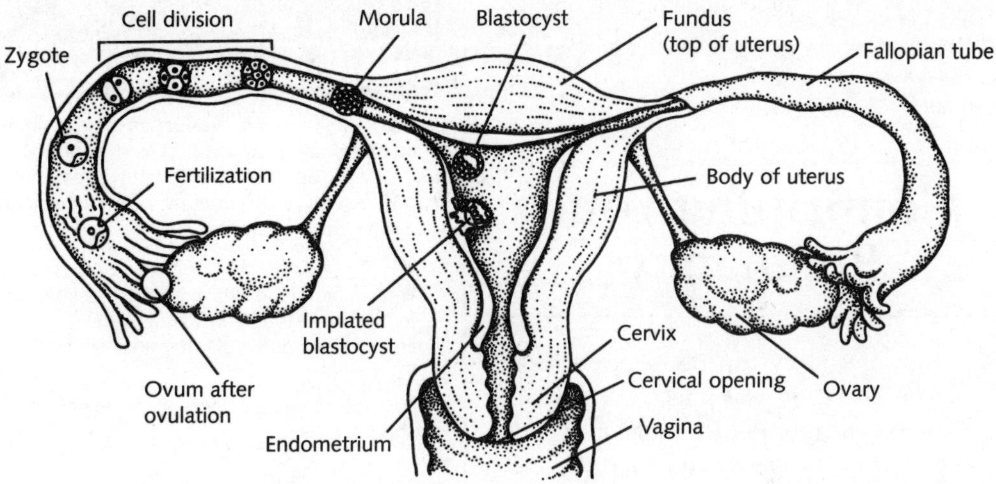

Fertilisation

alternative methods of conception limits their availability. These procedures have the potential of producing a multiple pregnancy. (See page 38.)

At conception, all the inherited characteristics of your child are established. Each ovum and sperm contains twenty-three *chromosomes* (which contain the genetic material), half the number contained in all other human cells. The union of egg and sperm gives the fertilised ovum the full complement of forty-six chromosomes (twenty-three from the mother and twenty-three from the father). These twenty-three pairs of chromosomes combine to form a unique blueprint for your child's development. Your child's body build, physical appearance, sex, blood type, some personality traits, some mental characteristics and much more are decided immediately. The remainder of growth and development during pregnancy, infancy, childhood—in fact, your child's entire lifetime—is guided to a great extent by this original genetic blueprint.

Only one pair of chromosomes determines the sex (or gender) of the baby. Women have a matching pair of X chromosomes (XX); all your ova carry X chromosomes, meaning that your baby will always get one X chromosome from you. Men have one X and one Y chromosome in their set of sex chromosomes, so some sperm carry X chromosomes and others carry Y chromosomes. Consequently, the sex of your unborn child is determined by the chromosome that the father contributes. For example, if a sperm carrying an X chromosome fertilises the egg, the baby is a girl (XX); if the sperm carrying a Y chromosome fertilises the egg, the baby is a boy (XY).

Occasionally, a woman releases more than one egg at ovulation, and each is fertilised by a separate sperm, resulting in *fraternal* or nonidentical twins (or triplets, quadruplets and so on). Sometimes, a single fertilised egg divides into two or more, resulting in *identical* multiples.

Confirming Your Pregnancy

Although pregnancy can be detected soon after you conceive, you might not suspect you are pregnant or test for pregnancy until you have missed a menstrual period. A pregnancy test checks your urine or blood for *human chorionic gonadotropin (hCG)*, a hormone produced only during pregnancy.

Do-it-yourself pregnancy test kits are available in drug stores. Many kits provide supplies for two tests; you can test a week or so after missing a menstrual period and again a few days to a week later. Using two tests gives a higher rate of accuracy than using only one. Laboratory blood tests can be performed as early as two to four weeks after ovulation (or at about the time you miss a menstrual period) and are more accurate than do-it-yourself kits.

If you suspect you are pregnant, whether or not you have used a home pregnancy test, have your pregnancy confirmed by a medical professional. Also, begin prenatal care, avoid environmental hazards and pay special attention to your nutritional needs.

Early Signs and Symptoms of Pregnancy

Changes in hormone production begin almost immediately after conception and help ensure optimal development of your baby. Most of the following signs and symptoms of pregnancy are caused by these hormonal changes:

- Missed menstrual period
- Breast changes: a heavy and full feeling, tenderness, tingling in the nipple area and a darkened areola (the area around each nipple)
- Fullness, bloating or ache in the lower abdomen
- Fatigue and drowsiness
- Faintness
- Nausea, vomiting or both ('morning sickness')
- Frequent urination
- Increased vaginal secretions
- Positive pregnancy test

Calculating Your Due Date

Your doctor or midwife must know your due date in order to judge whether the growth rate of the foetus is appropriate. Knowledge of your due date is also essential in deciding whether the baby is preterm (before thirty-seven weeks of pregnancy) or post-term (after forty-two weeks of pregnancy). Also, it can provide an early clue that you may be carrying twins.

At your first prenatal appointment, your caregiver will determine your due date by asking the date of your last menstrual period. (Conception takes place about two weeks after your last period.) To calculate the due date, he or she subtracts three months from the first day of your last menstrual period and adds seven days. (Although it is more accurate to count ahead 266 days from the exact date of conception, this date is rarely known.) Pregnancy, sometimes called gestation, lasts an average of 280 days or 40 weeks after the last menstrual period. When the doctor or midwife says you are twelve weeks pregnant, it means that the foetus is ten weeks old. However, the gestational age of the foetus is said to be twelve weeks.

If you cannot remember the date of your last menstrual period or if your last period was scant or unusual, your doctor or midwife will use other methods to determine your due date. An ultrasound scan between nine and eleven weeks is the most accurate and common of these methods. (See the discussion of ultrasound on page 53.)

Remember, normal pregnancies vary in length. Think of your due date as approximate, and expect the baby from two weeks before to two weeks after that date. Two-thirds of all babies are born within ten days of their due dates, but only about 4 percent are actually born on their due dates.

Hormonal Changes during Pregnancy

Pregnancy brings profound changes in your body, emotional adjustments for you and your partner, and dynamic growth and development of the foetus. Many of the physical changes that occur are caused by changes in hormone production. The major source of these hormones is the *placenta*, an organ formed (along with the unborn baby) in the uterus from the fertilised ovum.

Human chorionic gonadotropin (hCG), produced by the developing placenta, ensures that your ovaries produce oestrogen and progesterone until your placenta matures and takes over production of these hormones in approximately three to four months. (See page 26 for more on the placenta.)

Oestrogen promotes the growth of reproductive tissues by increasing the size of the uterine musculature, by promoting growth of your uterine lining and its blood supply, by increasing the production of vaginal mucus, and by stimulating the development of the duct system and blood supply in your breasts. The high levels of oestrogen in pregnancy probably influence water retention, subcutaneous fat build-up and skin pigmentation.

Progesterone inhibits smooth muscle contractions. It relaxes the uterus, keeping it from contracting excessively. It also has a relaxing effect on the walls of blood vessels, helping to maintain a healthy low blood pressure, and on the walls of the stomach and bowels, allowing for greater absorption of nutrients. Progesterone stimulates secretion of the ovarian hormone *relaxin*, which relaxes and softens ligaments, cartilage and the cervix, allowing these tissues to spread during the birth.

Besides oestrogen and progesterone, other hormones are produced in greater quantities and cause many physical changes during pregnancy. These hormones influence growth, mineral balance, metabolism, levels of other hormones and onset of labour.

First Trimester Changes for Mother and Baby

Pregnancy is divided into three trimesters, each one lasting approximately three months. We call the first trimester the 'formation' period, since by the end of this period all the foetal organ systems are formed and functioning. For you, the first trimester is a time of physical and emotional adjustment to being pregnant. (For a summary of the changes during this period, see the Calendar of Pregnancy on pages 45–48.) During your pregnancy, the terms used to describe the unborn baby change to reflect its age and development, as follows: *ovum, zygote, morula, blastocyst, embryo* and *foetus*. In the first trimester, the unborn baby's age after conception (sometimes called foetal life or foetal age) will be used when scientific milestones occur in the early weeks of pregnancy. In the second and third trimesters and in the Calendar of Pregnancy chart, gestational age is used, which is the same as weeks of pregnancy and includes the two weeks from the last menstrual period (LMP) to conception.

The First Four Weeks of Pregnancy

(conception through two weeks of foetal life or four weeks gestational age)

Unborn Baby

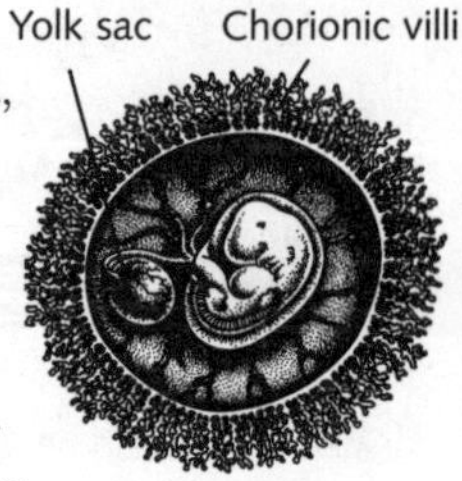

Five weeks

After it has been fertilised, the ovum, now called a *zygote*, quickly changes from one cell to many by dividing into two cells, then four, eight, sixteen and so on. By the end of two days the cluster of cells is known as a *morula*. Within five days the morula has made its way along the fallopian tube to the uterus and is now called a *blastocyst*. By the end of the first week, it implants in the uterine lining, usually in the upper part of the uterus. By two weeks it is called an *embryo*, and another part of the fertilised ovum has developed tiny, root-like projections that penetrate the uterine lining and draw nourishment from it.

Expectant Mother

While these changes are taking place for your baby, you may have noticed only some breast swelling or tenderness or a slight ache in your lower abdomen. And you are about to miss your menstrual period! The remarkable changes that you will experience have just begun.

The Fifth through Fourteenth Weeks of Pregnancy

(third through twelfth weeks of foetal life)

Unborn Baby

During the fifth through fourteenth weeks of pregnancy, the baby develops rapidly. In this time period the baby's scientific name changes from *embryo* to *foetus.* A primitive nervous system with a brain and a spinal column begins to form. The circulatory system also develops, and the heart is beating by the twenty-fifth day after conception. By this time the embryo is only half the size of a pea, with eyes, ears and a mouth beginning to form. The embryo has simple kidneys, a liver, a digestive tract and a primitive umbilical cord. On the twenty-sixth day, arm buds appear. Two days later, leg buds appear.

Although your baby's sex is determined at conception, the anatomy of the male and female baby appears the same until the embryo is about seven weeks old. Between the developing leg buds, there is a slit with a knob of tissue called the *genital tubercle.* Within the embryo's abdomen are two embryonic sex glands. During the seventh week, if the embryo is male, the Y chromosome stimulates these sex glands to begin producing androgens, male hormones that cause the two sides of the slit to join, forming the scrotum. Androgens also cause the genital tubercle to develop into a penis. Before birth, the sex glands descend from the abdomen into the scrotum as testicles. In a female embryo, the absence of male hormones causes the slit to become the vulva (external genitals) and the genital tubercle to develop into a clitoris. The sex glands remain within a girl's abdomen as ovaries.

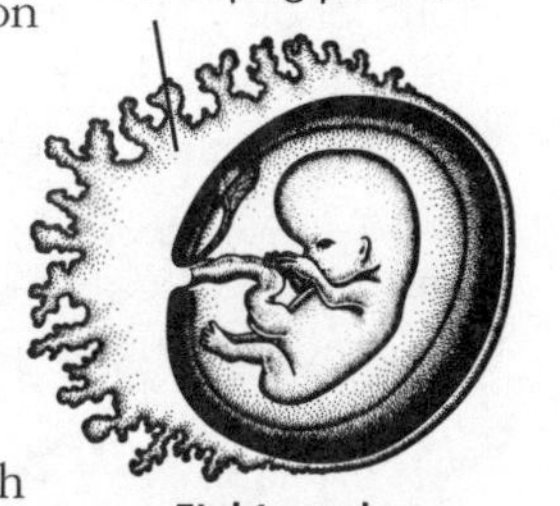

Eight weeks

By the eighth week after conception (tenth week of pregnancy), the embryo is structurally complete. The face has eyes, nose, ears, and a mouth with lips, a tongue, and teeth buds in the gums. The arms have hands with fingers and fingerprints. The legs have knees, ankles and toes. The arms and legs move at eight weeks, but coordinated movements do not begin until about fourteen weeks of development. The brain, although still quite immature, sends out impulses that begin to influence the functions of other organs; the heart beats strongly; and the liver manufactures red blood cells. The embryo grows about 1 millimetre a day, with different parts developing on different days. At nine weeks foetal age (or eleven weeks gestational age), the embryonic period is complete and the developing baby is now called a *foetus.*

During the first three months of foetal life, the foetus has become quite active, although you probably do not yet detect any movements. Legs kick and arms move. The foetus can frown or smile, suck his thumb, swallow amniotic fluid and urinate drops of sterile urine into the amniotic fluid. The fluid is completely exchanged about every three hours. Vocal cords are complete and the foetus makes breathing movements (the chest rises and falls), but of course no air exchange takes place because the foetus is in amniotic fluid. Breathing amniotic fluid into the lungs, however, may actually aid lung development. By ten to twelve weeks, the heartbeat is strong enough to be detected with a foetal ultrasound stethoscope (often called a Doppler). Eyelids cover the foetus's eyes and remain closed until the sixth month. By fourteen weeks of pregnancy, the foetus is about 8 centimetres long and weighs 28 grams.

Placenta and Uterus

During the early weeks of pregnancy, the uterine lining *(endometrium)* becomes thicker and the blood supply increases, providing a rich source of nourishment. At the end of the first month of development, the projections (now called *chorionic villi*) that had formed two weeks earlier extend into the uterine lining, becoming a primitive placenta. Foetal blood (blood for the unborn baby) circulates through this root-like formation while your blood circulates into the spaces (intervillous spaces) surrounding the villi. A thin layer of tissues separates the two bloodstreams, which normally do not mix.

Through a complex process of cell division and differentiation, the baby, placenta, *membranes* (amnion and chorion) and *amniotic fluid* are formed from the single-celled fertilised ovum. The membranes, also called the amniotic sac, surround the embryo and eventually the foetus. The amniotic fluid within the sac will benefit the foetus by absorbing bumps from the outside, by maintaining an even temperature inside and by providing the foetus with a medium for easy movement.

By twelve weeks of pregnancy, the *placenta* is completely formed and serves as an organ for producing hormones and exchanging nutrients and waste products. The *umbilical cord* links the placenta to your unborn baby. The cord extends from the foetus's navel to the approximate centre of the placenta. It is through the placenta and umbilical cord that oxygen and nutrients—such as simple sugars, protein, fat, water, vitamins and minerals—are passed from your blood supply to the foetus's. The placenta also provides protection against most bacteria in your bloodstream, although most viruses and drugs will cross to the foetus. Waste products from the foetus are exchanged through the placenta and are carried by your blood to your kidneys and lungs for excretion.

With a multiple pregnancy, there may be one or more placentas. Most identical twins share the same placenta, although occasionally they have separate ones. Fraternal twins have separate placentas, although the placentas sometimes fuse into one large organ.

By fourteen weeks of pregnancy, your uterus is about the size of a grapefruit. Amniotic fluid fills the uterine cavity and is cleaned continually by the small blood vessels in the membranes that surround the fluid. The cervix of the uterus is about 2–4 centimetres long and, though softer than before pregnancy, is fairly firm. The mucous plug that fills the cervical opening provides a barrier to help protect the unborn baby.

Expectant Mother

During this period, you may feel unusually tired and require more sleep because of the new demands on your energy supply and because of the accompanying shift in your metabolic rate. You may also experience nausea and vomiting during the early months of your pregnancy. Although this is usually called 'morning sickness', it may occur at any time of the day. Though the exact cause is unknown, it is thought that human chorionic gonadotropin (hCG), produced by the developing placenta, plays a role. (Ways to cope with the nausea and vomiting are discussed in Chapter 4.)

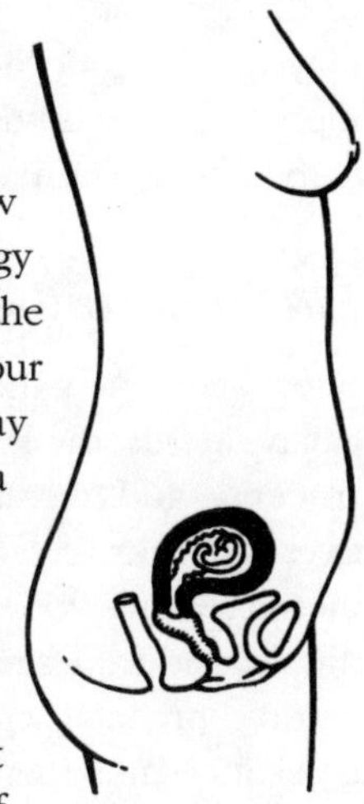

First trimester

Some women notice a metallic taste in their mouths during this time, but its cause is unknown. Although your breasts develop in puberty, the glandular tissue that produces milk does not fully develop until you become pregnant. As the levels of oestrogen, progesterone and other hormones increase during pregnancy, your breasts change in preparation for providing milk for your baby. They will enlarge, and you may notice tenderness, more prominent veins and a tingling sensation in your nipples. The nipples and *areola* (area around each nipple) also enlarge and become darker. Little bumps on the areola (called *Montgomery glands*) become more prominent as they enlarge to produce more lubricant in preparation for breastfeeding.

You may need to urinate frequently because of pressure of the enlarging uterus on your bladder. In addition, vaginal secretions increase. Because the changes, although dramatic in nature, have been minuscule in size (the top of the uterus barely reaches above your pubic bone), you feel more different than you look.

Emotions

Along with the physical changes, the early months of pregnancy are often filled with emotional ups and downs. The thought of motherhood may at times be pleasing to you, at other times not. You may cry easily. It is sometimes puzzling that you can be so happy about the pregnancy and yet feel so blue. Mood swings seem more pronounced and may be difficult for you and your partner to understand.

Finding out that you are pregnant may bring about a mixture of emotions in you and your partner: pride in your ability to produce a child, fear of losing your independence, apprehension about changes in your relationship, hesitancy to focus on the baby if awaiting results of genetic testing, doubts about your ability to parent, and happiness about becoming parents. Sharing your thoughts and feelings with each other can help you work through this time of transition.

Second Trimester Changes for Mother and Baby

The Fifteenth through Twenty-Seventh Weeks of Pregnancy

Unborn Baby

The fifteenth week of pregnancy marks the beginning of the 'development' period, when the already formed organs and structures of the foetus enlarge and mature. During the second trimester, head hair, eyelashes and eyebrows appear. Fine, downy hair called *lanugo* develops on the arms, legs and back of the foetus. Fingernails and toenails appear. At about eighteen weeks, the foetus has developed all the different movements seen in a newborn. The heartbeat is strong enough by eighteen to twenty weeks that it can be heard with an ordinary stethoscope.

By the end of the twenty-fourth week, the foetus is about 30 centimetres long (23 centimetres crown to rump) and weighs about 675 grams. Hearing begins around this time. *Meconium,* a collection of digestive enzymes and residue from swallowed amniotic fluid, forms in the intestines but is not usually expelled until after birth. The foetal skin is wrinkled and covered with a creamy protective coating called *vernix caseosa*. During this period, you will probably feel the foetus move (called *quickening*). At first, you may feel a light tapping or fluttering sensation that reminds you of gas bubbles, or the gentle movements of the small foetus may go unnoticed until activity becomes more vigorous. Although still very immature, some babies born at this point do survive.

Placenta and Uterus

Your uterus expands into your abdominal cavity in response to the enlarging foetus, placenta and increased amniotic fluid. By twenty weeks of pregnancy, the top of your uterus reaches your navel, and by the end of the second trimester, it is above your waist. During prenatal appointments, your caregiver measures the height of your uterus to check that the foetus is growing adequately and to confirm the length of your pregnancy. Although foetal size and the amount of amniotic fluid can differ, the length of your pregnancy can be approximated by measuring the distance in centimetres between your pubic bone and the top of the uterus (the *fundus*).

Though often unnoticed, your uterus contracts periodically throughout pregnancy. These non-painful contractions (called *Braxton-Hicks contractions*) make your uterus hard for about a minute or so. They are different from labour contractions and are a normal part of pregnancy. (For more on preterm labour, see page 60.)

Expectant Mother

During these middle months of pregnancy, you probably feel physically well, and your nausea and fatigue probably disappear or decline. Your breasts may not increase much in size during the second trimester, but *colostrum* (a yellowish fluid produced before breast milk) is usually present in the milk glands by the middle of pregnancy. (See the discussion in Chapter 15 about preparation for breastfeeding.)

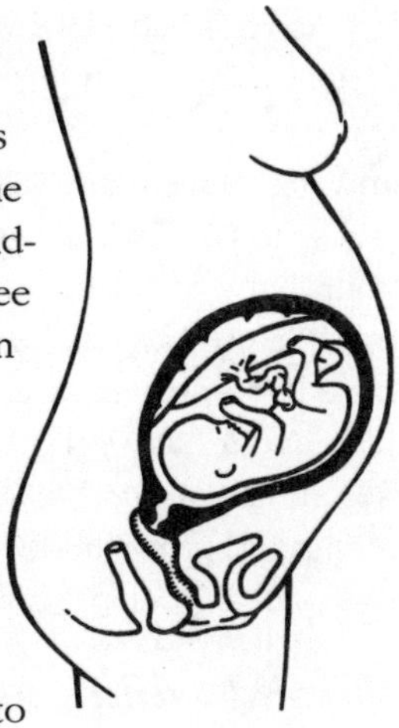

Second trimester

Just as your nipples and areola get darker during pregnancy due to hormonal changes, other skin areas also become more pigmented. A dark line *(linea nigra)* between the pubic bone and the navel appears in some women. *Chloasma,* the mask of pregnancy, may appear as darkening of the skin around your eyes and nose. Chloasma usually disappears after the birth of your baby, but not immediately.

Emotions

The physical changes of advancing pregnancy bring varying psychological responses. Some women enjoy how they look and feel, while others consider themselves unattractive, inconvenienced and restricted. A heightened sense of growth and creativity may make you more sensitive; a kind word, a beautiful sunset, a touching photograph or a needy child may elicit unusually strong emotions. You may recall more of your dreams than you did before pregnancy; you may also become introspective at this time and find yourself examining your thoughts and feelings. In the middle months, you may want to start preparing for parenthood by reading books about child care or preparing the nursery and layette. (See page 388.)

During the second trimester, your pregnancy usually becomes more real for your family and friends. Your partner can feel the baby move when he or she places a hand on your abdomen or when you are in close physical contact. This contact with the developing baby enhances your partner's feelings of involvement and interest in the pregnancy and the baby. Like you, your partner may have a variety of thoughts and feelings about your changing appearance. (See pages 39–42 on sex during pregnancy and the expectant father or partner.)

Third Trimester Changes for Mother and Baby

The Twenty-Eighth through Thirty-Eighth Weeks of Pregnancy

Unborn Baby

The third trimester is the 'growth' period for the foetus. Babies born during this period are usually able to survive, although their chances for both survival and an easier transition to independent life improve as they get closer to their due date. In late pregnancy, antibodies pass through the placenta to the foetus, providing short-term resistance to the diseases to which you are immune. The baby born prematurely has received less of this protection than the full-term baby and is thus more prone to infections after birth and in early infancy. (For more information on prematurity, see pages 409–410.)

During the last three months of pregnancy, the foetal features are refined: the fingernails reach the fingertips and may even need cutting at birth, the hair on the head grows, the lanugo almost disappears, fat is deposited under the skin and buds for the permanent teeth are laid down behind the primary teeth buds.

You can learn much about your baby at this time. The foetus has periods of sleep and wakefulness and responds to bright light. Loud external noises may elicit a reaction and stir her into action. The baby hears and becomes familiar with your voice and after birth will prefer your voice to a stranger's voice. Of course, the baby hears other sounds as well: your digestion, the circulation of blood within your uterus, your heartbeat and other external sounds such as music and your partner's voice. The baby shows a clear preference for such familiar voices and sounds after birth. These familiar sounds or similar ones (like the rhythmic sloshing sounds of a dishwasher or washing machine or the droning of a vacuum cleaner) often soothe a fussy newborn.

At some point during the last trimester, your baby assumes a favourite position, usually head down. During prenatal visits, your doctor or midwife manually palpates your abdomen to determine which position the foetus has adopted. The procedure used is known as *Leopold's manoeuvres*.

As your baby continues to grow and gain weight, her activity diminishes since there is less room for her to move. You may feel arm and leg movements rather than whole body shifts. If you feel a series of rhythmic jolts, your baby probably has the hiccups. You most likely notice the hiccups, which may have been present since the second trimester, when your baby gets bigger and the amniotic fluid diminishes. The foetus gains about 1600 grams and grows about 14 centimetres during this part of your pregnancy.

Placenta and Uterus

The placenta and membranes are part of the complex and intricate foetal-maternal-placental system. In late pregnancy, changes within this system help prepare you physically and psychologically to give birth and to nourish and nurture your infant. They also help prepare your baby for birth and survival outside the uterus. The elaborate process leading to and including birth is only partly understood. Here we can barely touch on some of the known steps that bring all the vital elements to readiness for birth. (See pages 209–211 for more details.)

The placenta and the foetus both begin producing *cortico-releasing hormone (CRH)* that increases placental oestrogen production in late pregnancy. With this increase in the ratio of oestrogen to progesterone, the uterus becomes more sensitive to *oxytocin* (a hormone that causes contractions of the uterus). You will probably begin to notice more contractions now. The hormone interaction also seems to trigger release of *prostaglandins,* which soften the cervix and influence the onset of labour.

Amniotic fluid volume decreases in the last weeks of pregnancy, from about 1.7 litres at about seven months to about 1 litres at term. Though there is less amniotic fluid, the umbilical cord is protected because foetal blood flows at about 6.5 kilometres an hour, keeping the cord firm, almost like a garden hose full of water.

Expectant Mother

During the third trimester, your uterus expands to a level just below your breastbone. The high levels of progesterone and crowding by the uterus may cause indigestion and heartburn. You may also experience shortness of breath or soreness in your lower ribs as your uterus presses on your diaphragm and ribs. Varicose veins in the legs, haemorrhoids and swollen ankles sometimes develop due to the increased pressure within your abdomen, the decreased blood return from your lower limbs and the effect of progesterone relaxing the walls of the blood vessels. As pelvic ligaments relax in preparation for birth and as the increasing weight of the uterus and foetus changes your centre of gravity, backaches are more common. (For ways to alleviate backaches, see pages 134–136.)

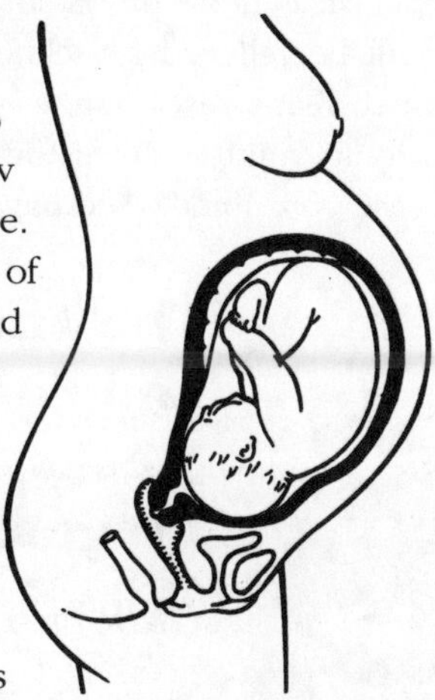

Third trimester

During the final months of pregnancy, you may develop small red elevations called *vascular spiders* on the skin of your upper body. Also during this time, you may develop stretch marks on your abdomen, thighs or breasts. These marks, called *striae gravidarum,* are reddish during pregnancy and become glistening white lines after the birth. Many women attempt to prevent these stretch marks by applying various lotions or oils to their skin, but there is no evidence that these products are effective. About half of women in these final months develop striae whether they use such lotions or not.

Emotions

Near the end of the third trimester, you will probably start looking forward to the end of the pregnancy, the relief from the physical discomforts and the long-awaited joy of having the baby. You may become more introspective and find yourself thinking more and perhaps worrying about labour, birth and the baby. By taking childbirth education classes, you and your partner can learn more and worry less about labour and birth and can also discover ways to cope with the stresses of late pregnancy.

You may feel protective of the developing baby and try to avoid exposing yourself to things that might threaten her wellbeing. You may also feel more vulnerable and more dependent on your partner and others. As you anticipate the responsibilities of parenthood, you may think more of your own parents and how they parented you. Adjustments in your sexual relationship continue as your abdomen enlarges and you become less agile. Keep the lines of communication open between you and your partner as your sexual feelings, needs and desires change. (See pages 39–40 for more about your sexual relationship during pregnancy.)

You and your partner may worry from time to time about your health or your baby's wellbeing. Thoughts of death or injury may come up. This is not surprising, because pregnancy and birth do carry certain potential risks. These risks can be greatly diminished, however, with good self-care and early and consistent prenatal care. Currently in Australia maternal death is extremely rare. Fewer than ten women per one hundred thousand die around the time of birth. Infant mortality has declined in Australia, and now fewer than eight babies per one thousand die. If you find yourself worrying or dreaming about death or harm to you or your baby, share these fears with someone who will be supportive—your partner, a relative, you caregiver, a childbirth educator or an empathetic friend. You might be tempted to avoid telling anyone about such fears, perhaps thinking that talking about them might somehow make them more real or likely to happen. It is more probable, however, that you will be relieved to acknowledge and share such fears. Also, thinking through how you would want such misfortunes handled may ease your mind. (See pages 305–307.)

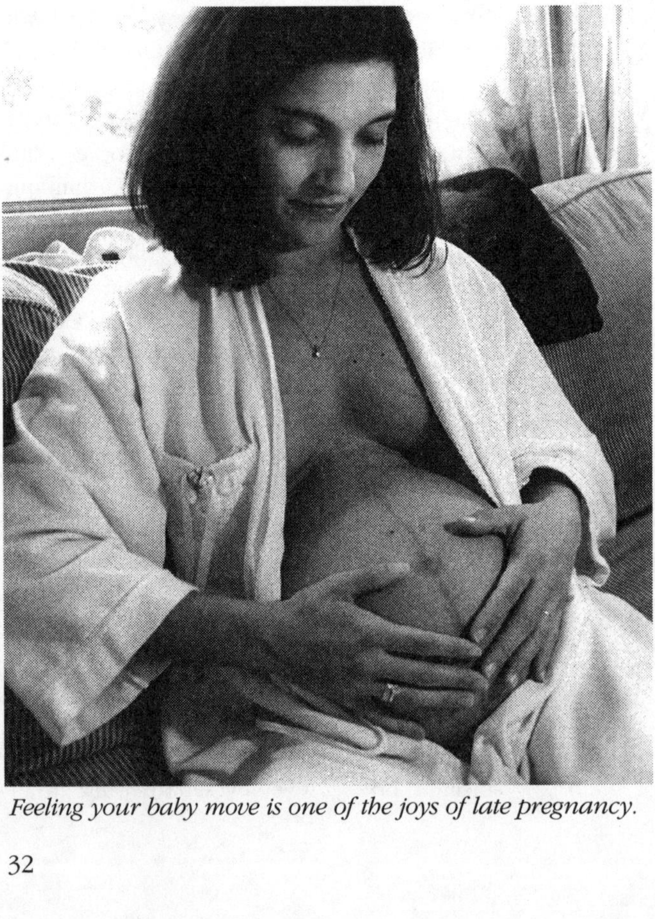

Photograph by Marilyn Nolt

Feeling your baby move is one of the joys of late pregnancy.

The Thirty-Ninth and Fortieth Weeks of Pregnancy

Unborn Baby

During these last weeks, the foetal organs continue to mature to prepare your baby for life outside your uterus. The foetus also adds fat and gains about 1 pound. At birth, the average baby weighs 3–3.5 kilograms although normal weight for a full-term baby can vary from 2.5 to 4.5 kilograms. Newborns average 50 centimetres in length, but a range of 45–55 centimetres is normal. During the pregnancy, the weight of the fertilised egg has increased six billion times! In the next twenty years, your child's weight will increase to only about twenty times the birth weight.

Placenta and Uterus

The mature placenta is flat and round, 15–20 centimetres in diameter, and 2.5 centimetres thick; it weighs about one-seventh of the foetus's weight. The size and weight of the placenta vary in proportion to the size and weight of the baby.

If you look at your placenta right after the birth, you can expect to see the following: the side of the placenta that was implanted in the uterine wall (the maternal side) is rough and appears bloody; it is divided into lobes called *cotyledons*. As the placenta aged, hard gritty areas (calcium deposits) began to appear as whitish spots on either side. The foetal side of the placenta is smooth, pale and shiny and is covered by the amniotic membrane. The amniotic and chorionic membranes extend from the edge of the placenta to form the sac (bag of waters) that contained the amniotic fluid and foetus. Branches of the blood vessels from the umbilical cord can be seen on the foetal side of the placenta, spreading out from the cord and entering the placenta at various places.

At term, the average cord length is 50–55 centimetres, but anywhere from 30–80 centimetres is considered normal. The moist, white cord has a twisted or spiral appearance; two arteries and one vein are contained within it. At birth, as your baby breathes, his circulation pattern begins to change, sealing off the blood flow to his navel and re-routing more blood to his lungs.

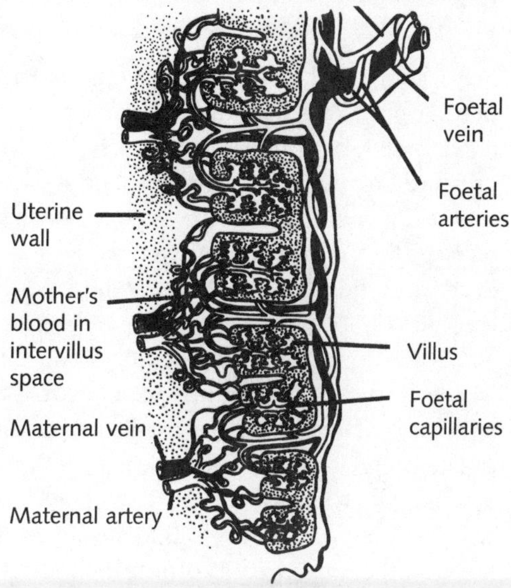

Cross section of placenta

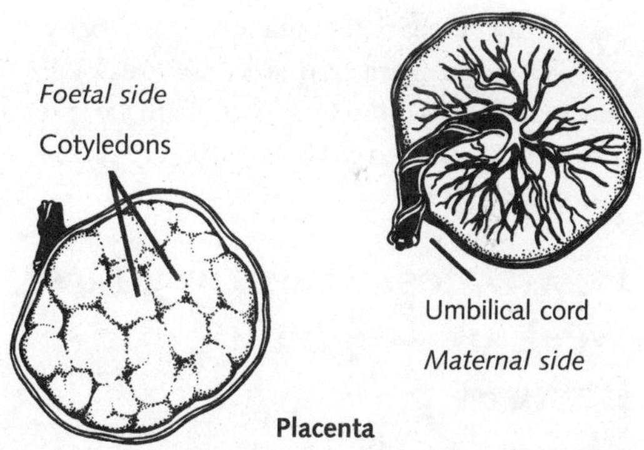

Placenta

Towards the end of your pregnancy, your uterine contractions become even more obvious and frequent. These pre-labour contractions serve the useful purposes of enhancing circulation in your uterus, pressing the baby lower in your pelvis and against your cervix, and working with prostaglandins to *ripen* (soften) and *efface* (thin) your cervix.

Expectant Mother

About two weeks before the birth, your profile may change as the foetus descends into the pelvic cavity. This noticeable descent is called *engagement*, or lightening. You may feel less pressure on your diaphragm and find it easier to breathe and eat as the foetus becomes engaged in the pelvis. However, as the foetal head descends, it presses on your bladder, causing you to urinate even more frequently.

You may find yourself looking forward to labour and the end of pregnancy. Anxiety, light sleep, fatigue and the usual discomforts of late pregnancy add to this desire. At times, you may feel as though you have been and will be pregnant forever. But at the same time, all the customary late pregnancy activities (more frequent visits to your physician or midwife; your childbirth preparation classes; baby showers; and preparation of the baby's clothing, equipment and sleeping area) help you realise that pregnancy will soon be over and a new stage in your life—parenthood—will begin.

Post-Dates: The Forty-First Week of Pregnancy and Beyond

Unborn Baby

The average length of pregnancy is forty weeks, but many pregnancies last longer. Some post-date pregnancies are cases of mistaken due dates; others involve foetuses who are not quite ready to be born at forty weeks and need more time to grow and mature. Occasionally, the foetus is ready to be born, but for unexplained reasons, labour does not begin on time. In this case, the foetus may become post-mature and may not receive sufficient nourishment and oxygen from the aging placenta. To determine if the post-date baby is post-mature, tests of foetal wellbeing and placental function are performed. (See Chapter 3 for information on these tests.) A baby is considered post-mature if the following characteristics are present: absence of lanugo; little vernix; long fingernails and toenails; loose, pale, dry, peeling or cracked skin; and unusual alertness. In addition, the amniotic fluid may be low in volume (reflecting an aging placenta) or stained with meconium (reflecting a full bowel). True post-maturity is rare even in babies born two weeks or more after their due dates.

Placenta

In many post-date pregnancies, the placenta continues to support the growth and well-being of the foetus, and labour almost always begins by forty-three weeks. In true post-maturity, placental function declines, the amniotic fluid volume drops and the foetus may be stressed. Under these circumstances, the foetus really needs to be delivered.

Expectant Mother

Physically, you may continue feeling much as you have been during late pregnancy. Emotionally, however, you may find the waiting frustrating, worrisome or depressing. The longer the wait, the more difficult it becomes. You may want to try ways to start labour. Talk with your caregiver to help you understand your options. (See pages 260–263 for advantages and disadvantages of induction.)

Special Considerations in Pregnancy

Age of the Mother

Statistics indicate that the most favourable age for a woman to bear children is between twenty and the mid-thirties. Fewer problems arise during this period than during the early teens, the late thirties or the forties. Despite this, however, the birth rate for first-time mothers in their thirties and forties is higher than ever. While younger and older women may face more pregnancy risks, a healthy pregnant woman of any age is very likely to have a healthy baby.

Teen Pregnancy

If you are a teenager and pregnant, you have a special set of strengths and needs. Your young body is probably strong. Your chances for a healthy pregnancy are good, especially if you take good care of yourself by eating well, starting visits to the doctor or midwife early in pregnancy, and staying away from drugs, alcohol and tobacco.

Teenagers usually give birth well since their bodies are in good condition. Because you are young, your uterus is probably strong and your ligaments and tissues are stretchy. This may not mean a quick or painless labour, but you may not need medical interventions to help the labour along.

Let your love for your baby guide you in making decisions about taking care of yourself, going to school, dealing with your parents and your baby's father, and deciding whether to keep or relinquish your baby. You can get help from your doctor or the social work department attached to a hospital, pregnancy counselling organisations or childbirth education organisations, all of which can be found in your phone book. (Also see Recommended Resources, page 487, for books on teen pregnancy and parenting.)

First Pregnancy after Age Thirty-Five

Women today have many reasons for delaying their first pregnancy until they are beyond age thirty-five: career or education priorities, financial considerations, infertility, lack of a partner and postponement of parenthood until the 'biological clock' says it is now or never. Waiting until mid-career before having children is the norm today among well-educated or professional women for whom parenthood is only one of many appealing choices. You have probably heard that the pregnant woman over age thirty-five is at greater risk of medical complications than a younger woman. That is true, although the reasons are not clear. Age in itself is not a disease, like diabetes or heart disease, but older women seem to be more likely than younger women to develop the problems that caregivers watch for in every pregnant woman: high blood pressure, gestational diabetes, foetal growth problems or inherited disorders, placental problems, fibroids, labour complications and others.

Why are older women at greater risk?

Perhaps because the longer a woman lives, the more likely she is to have been exposed to poor health practices, accidents, illnesses or environmental influences. If, however, you have enjoyed good health over the years and have taken care of yourself, your age is less of a risk factor.

A stressful lifestyle or job, commonplace for women in this age group, may also increase the likelihood of pregnancy complications such as high blood pressure or preterm labour. A demanding job, added to the full-time job of growing a baby, may be too much. You may find it necessary or desirable to reduce the stress of your job and take more time to rest and relax.

Older women are more likely than younger women to carry a baby with a genetic disorder such as Down syndrome, which causes mental retardation and physical abnormalities. This condition can be detected with amniocentesis or chorionic villus sampling. (See pages 81–82.) Women over age thirty-five are offered one of these tests in early pregnancy. If Down syndrome or another genetic disorder is discovered, you may choose to have an abortion or prepare yourself for life with a special-needs child.

As an older pregnant woman, your attitudes towards childbearing may be affected by your age and experiences. If you have a history of infertility or miscarriage, you are more likely to be vulnerable to the suggestion that you are 'high-risk' or 'unhealthy'. You may seek assurances that the baby will be normal and healthy through extensive testing and procedures designed to detect and treat problems. Some women find the testing stressful in itself, especially because the tests are not always accurate and cannot detect every possible problem. (For discussion of pregnancy complications and the relevant tests and treatments, see Chapter 3.) As for labour complications, it is true that the caesarean rate for women over thirty-five is higher than average, but the reasons are not clear. It may be the increased rate of pregnancy complications, like placenta previa, that usually require a caesarean birth. Or sometimes, depending on the medical staff, it may be that problems arising in the older woman's labour are more likely to be treated by a caesarean than the same problems in a younger woman's labour.[1]

If you are pregnant and thirty-five or over, what should you do to help improve the possibilities of a good outcome and emotional satisfaction? Really, you should do no more and no less than any pregnant woman having a baby. Take good care of yourself, reduce stress, get good prenatal care with a competent and caring physician or midwife, consider your options regarding the tests and procedures available, and deal with problems if and when they arise. Take childbirth classes to learn what to expect, how to work with your partner in making decisions and how to help yourselves deal with the stresses of labour.

Although problems will arise in some women—and you might be one—the problems are almost always treatable or manageable. And even though you may be older than other pregnant women, you can still expect a healthy outcome.

When You Are Pregnant Again

We usually refer to a woman expecting her second (or more) baby as a *multipara*, or multip. As a multip, you may find this pregnancy not as emotionally exhilarating as the first. Pregnancy is no longer new and may have lost some of its lustre. For this reason and because of the older child's needs for care, you may focus less on this pregnancy than the first.

Although each pregnancy is different, second pregnancies share some predictable differences from the first. You can expect to feel the baby's movements about one month earlier, because you will recognise the sensation sooner. Because your abdominal muscles tend to relax more easily in a subsequent pregnancy, your abdomen may enlarge sooner so that the pregnancy becomes noticeable earlier. Your pelvic ligaments may soften sooner this time. You may also feel you are carrying the baby lower. Braxton-Hicks contractions may be more noticeable and numerous, especially towards the end of pregnancy. While you may not be delighted at these earlier discomforts and physical changes, it might be reassuring to realise that pregnancy changes take place more readily in a body that has done it before.

You may feel less emotionally involved in this pregnancy than you were the last. Your attention shifts from thoughts about the foetus to thoughts about integrating a new baby into the family. This is partly because you have a clearer picture of yourself this time as a mother of a newborn. Your partner may also be less involved and less attentive to you during this pregnancy, which could be due to his or her added experience and diminished fears about your health and your baby's health.

Should you participate in childbirth preparation classes this time? Even if you attended excellent classes with your first

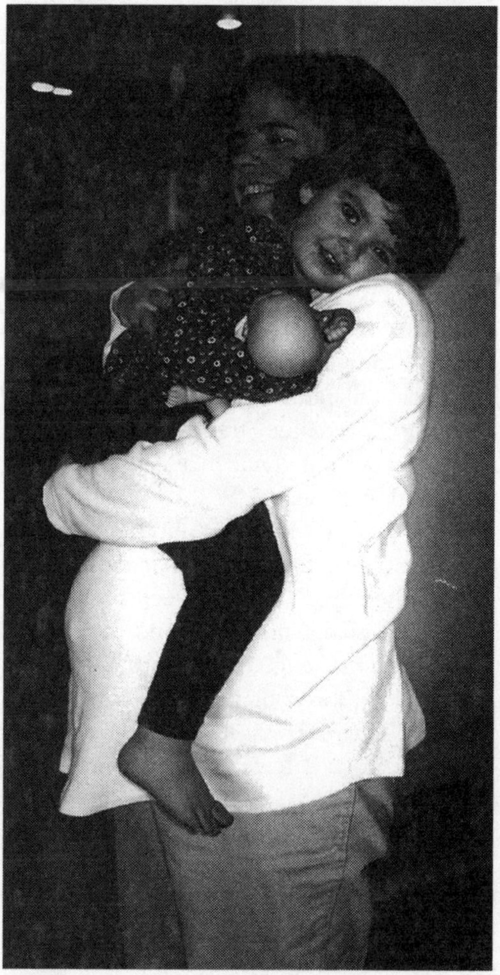

There is always room for the older child.

pregnancy, there are some good reasons to attend classes again, particularly refresher classes designed for your needs. Besides reviewing labour and a variety of coping techniques, refresher classes prepare you for how this labour may differ from the first. They offer ideas on preparing siblings and managing the household with more than one child. They also give you time to focus on this baby and may enhance your emotional attachment.

Anxiety about the upcoming labour is not uncommon among multiparas. If you had a straightforward and positive birth experience before, you may wonder if you will have another one. If your previous birth was difficult or disappointing, you may be burdened with worries that these problems will arise again. These normal doubts are worth talking about with your partner, caregiver or childbirth educator. Much can be done to overcome these self-doubts, to increase your self-confidence and to improve your birth experience.

Many second-time mothers worry whether they can possibly have enough love for another child. You may feel that all your love goes to the first child and the second will be short-changed. Or you may wonder if your love for your first will lessen when the new baby arrives. It helps to remember that you do not have a limited amount of love to share. You do not run out of love. Just as the flame of a candle can light other candles without putting out the first flame, you will find you can spread love without using it up.

Expecting Multiples: Twins, Triplets or More

Any pregnancy in which the woman carries more than one baby is called a *multiple pregnancy*. Multiple pregnancies occur in about one in every eighty pregnancies. When compared with rates among people of European descent, multiple pregnancies are less frequent among people of Asian descent and more frequent among people of African descent. Older women, those with twins in the family, women who are large or very tall, multiparas, and women using fertility drugs or procedures also have an increased likelihood of a multiple pregnancy.

Fraternal twins are produced by the fertilisation of two eggs by two sperm, making the twins only as similar as non-twin siblings would be if they were the same age. Identical twins occur when one sperm fertilises one egg, which later divides into two developing babies. One out of every three sets of twins is identical. Triplets, quadruplets or quintuplets are even rarer.

A multiple pregnancy may be suspected if two or more foetal heartbeats are heard, if you have a family history of multiple births, if you have rapid weight gain or if your uterus grows faster than normal. If a multiple pregnancy is suspected, an ultrasound scan will be ordered to confirm it. Although ultrasound can detect more than 95 percent of multiple pregnancies by the early part of the second trimester, some still remain undetected until birth.

Expecting multiples can be both exciting and stressful. Supporting the growth of more than one baby places extra demands on your body. You may be encouraged to increase the number of calories in your diet, and you may need to rest more because of discomfort, fatigue and the increased possibility of premature labour. Most problems for newborn twins, triplets or more occur in those born prematurely. Since birth with multiples may be more complicated, you may need the care of an obstetrician instead of or in addition to your midwife or general practitioner. Besides the increased medical attention, you can also expect more attention from your friends and relatives.

Books and support groups are available to help parents of multiples cope with their unique emotional and practical problems. The Australian Multiple Birth Association in NSW (phone 02 9875 2404) is a self-help group that provides information and support. Also, your childbirth educator may be able to connect you with other parents of twins from previous classes.

Sex during Pregnancy

What happens to your sexual relationship during pregnancy? Will you or your partner feel differently about making love? Is intercourse safe? Is orgasm safe?

For most women and their partners, pregnancy brings changes in the sexual relationship, but these changes are not the same for everyone. While one woman may feel ripe, beautiful and sexual, another may feel clumsy and fat. While one woman may feel secure and loved by a caring and considerate partner, another may be alone or in a difficult relationship. One woman may be concerned about her health or the baby's, while another feels robust and wonderful. One partner may feel anxious about the woman's health or turned off by her changing appearance, while another relishes the entire process.

Your own and your partner's feelings

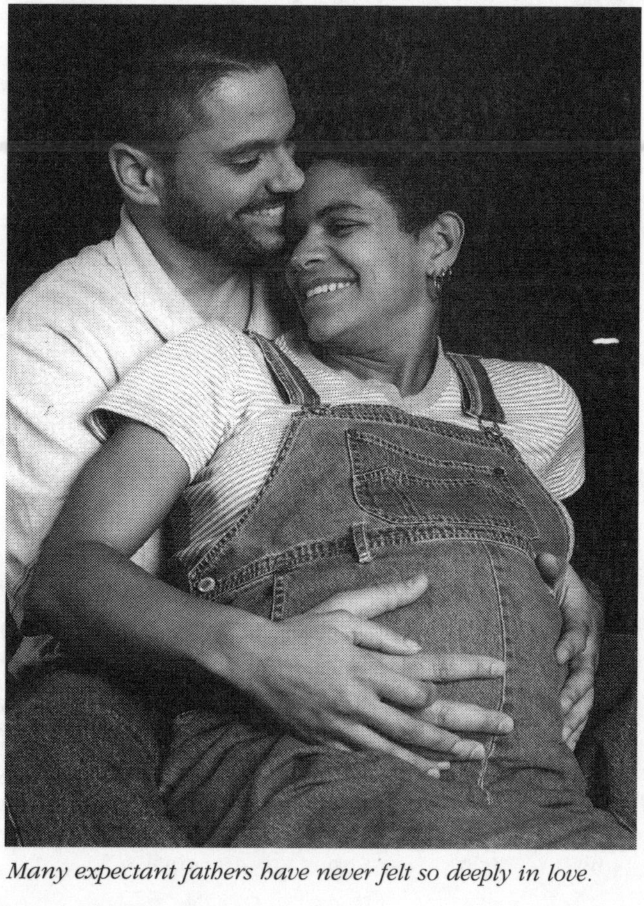

Many expectant fathers have never felt so deeply in love.

about pregnancy and its associated changes will undoubtedly influence your sexual relationship. So will bodily changes such as nausea, fatigue, weight gain, breast tenderness, changes in pelvic circulation and hormonal changes. As these physical factors fluctuate, so may your sexual feelings. The kinds of things that excite and please you may also fluctuate. At times you may feel more desire than usual; at other times, less or none. Your partner may or may not understand and accept your changing sexuality. Pregnancy can create tensions between the two of you, so open communication is important at this time.

What about safety? Reports or rumours of associations between intercourse or orgasm and vaginal bleeding, infection, miscarriage or preterm labour are scary. In addition, you may have questions about whether deep entry of the penis into your vagina and your partner's weight on top of your abdomen can endanger the baby.

Intercourse or orgasm may cause problems if you are at risk for a miscarriage or preterm labour, if you have had vaginal bleeding during pregnancy, if you have continuing or painful cramps after intercourse, or if you have a new sexual partner who has a sexually transmitted disease. If you are at risk, you should avoid intercourse. The only other warning usually given is that your partner should not blow air into your vagina, since this can cause an *air embolus* (an air bubble in the bloodstream), which is a very serious complication.

If you are not at risk for miscarriage or preterm labour, most medical caregivers recommend sexual activity as desired by both partners. Uterine contractions are a normal part of orgasm and do not pose a problem for a healthy foetus. Gentle, shallower penetration and the use of positions that avoid placing your partner's weight on your abdomen help prevent discomfort and alleviate the worry you may feel about the baby. Remember that the baby is protected by the cushioning effect of the amniotic fluid and by the seal provided by the amniotic sac and cervical mucus.

Pregnancy can be a time to explore new ways to please each other sexually; it can also be a time to more openly express your needs and desires to each other.

The Expectant Father

Waiting for fatherhood is a unique emotional experience—less understood, but no less significant than waiting for motherhood—yet fathers' needs and concerns are often not addressed. Many have never felt so important yet so ignored, so committed yet so abandoned, so deeply in love and sexual yet so afraid of sex, and so creative yet so drained of energy. Paying attention to these new feelings and sharing them with their pregnant partner or close friends will help men through this rich but challenging time. Counselling or discussions with others in similar circumstances are also helpful. When expectant fathers get together and share their feelings and concerns, several themes come up:[2]

Responsibility. Many men feel that they are leaving freedom behind. Their happy-go-lucky days are almost over, and it is time to be a responsible and mature provider and parent. The role of wage earner becomes more pressing. The pregnant mother's more vulnerable state and increased emotional needs may make a father feel overwhelmed with duties and responsibilities he is not quite ready to accept. He may at times yearn for the good old days when he was relatively independent. Sometimes getting away for an afternoon or a day helps relieve the pressure.

Life and death. Pregnancy and the impending birth of a child often prompt thoughts about the biological life cycle and immortality. Continuing the family for another generation is a source of pride and fulfilment. Many expectant fathers fear the death or injury of their partner and/or unborn child. Some even worry about their own death. These concerns may lead a man to buy life insurance, change jobs from one that involves physical danger to a safer one, or become more protective of his partner. He may urge her to use a seat belt or to avoid potentially risky activities or exposure to illness. He may encourage the use of any obstetrical test or popular remedy that claims to improve the chances of a healthy outcome and so on. As long as the protectiveness is reasonable and not overdone, it is probably constructive and appreciated by the expectant mother.

Displacement. An expectant father sometimes feels left out as the pregnant mother focuses inwards and becomes more preoccupied with the baby, especially if she also turns more to others for some emotional support. He may feel she is less available to him emotionally, physically and sexually, while he, at the same time, is expected to give more than ever in their relationship. To complicate it all, he may also feel guilty for any resentment or lack of enthusiasm about the pregnancy. It may help to discuss these feelings with a friend who has experienced this, but it is also very important to explain these feelings to the expectant mother, who may be unaware of what he is feeling.

Anxiety about his role during labour and birth. 'How will I perform during labour? What about seeing blood? Will I faint or get sick? Can I handle it?' Every expectant father questions himself in this way—some more than others. Childbirth preparation classes, films, books and discussions with other fathers are all very helpful in building confidence and helping to prepare him for his role in childbirth. It is also a good idea to consider having another support person at the birth to help both the father and the labouring woman. A friend, relative or a midwife can help the couple with comfort measures and also offer perspective and advice.

Sympathetic physical discomforts. Many men experience physical symptoms during their partner's pregnancy. This is sometimes called the Couvade (Fathering) Syndrome. Weight gain, food cravings, abdominal bloating, nausea, vomiting, backaches, toothaches, loss of appetite or abdominal cramps may be among the symptoms which reflect sympathy for and identification with the pregnant woman, or perhaps some anxiety. If an expectant father becomes preoccupied with pregnancy-like symptoms, counselling may be needed.

If You Have No Partner

If you are pregnant and without a partner, you face a different set of challenges.

Although there are thousands of single parents in Australia, society offers them little support. You may notice that people show a variety of reactions to your pregnancy (from happiness to hostility) when they learn you are single.

In a sense, you are taking on a role usually shared by two people. The parenting role is hard work, and there may be times when you doubt whether you can or want to do it. You may feel lonely or vulnerable at times and wish for a reliable partner. At other times, however, you may be relieved that you are not burdened with an incompatible partner. This is a time to reach out to others for help and emotional support.

If Your Partner Is Not the Baby's Biological Father

If your partner is not the father of your baby, you both may encounter new and different challenges as you go through the pregnancy and become parents. If your partner is a new lover or a lesbian lover, his or her role is less defined by society than the role of husband/father. If your baby was conceived by artificial insemination due to your male partner's infertility, your partner may have had to make some difficult emotional adjustments.

The lack of a biological tie may cause your partner to feel less involved in the pregnancy—that it is 'your' pregnancy rather than 'our' pregnancy—or to question his or her role in decision-making and support. If the biological father is also involved, your partner's role can be even less clear.

You and your partner need to anticipate that your relationship with each other and with the baby may be challenged by misplaced or unrealistic expectations and assumptions made by relatives, friends, acquaintances, society and yourselves. Honest and open discussion, coupled with extra patience and a willingness to try different, non-traditional solutions, will help.

If You Have a History of Childhood Trauma

As we learn more about how early childhood experiences can influence adults, we discover that early trauma sometimes causes unexpected reactions during pregnancy, birth or post partum. Anyone who has been abused during childhood knows that the effects continue long after the abuse stops. Physical, sexual and/or psychological abuse by an older, more powerful person teaches the child victim some long-lasting and damaging lessons about herself and others. For example, many women (and men) who were hurt by trusted adults have difficulty trusting others, especially strangers (for example, doctors or midwives) who expect to be trusted and who have authority to influence decision-making. A victim of sexual abuse may find vaginal exams, nakedness or the prospect of a baby coming through her vagina extremely disturbing or even intolerable. The loss of control over her body that inevitably occurs in labour may trigger responses in a woman similar to those she had as a child when she was helpless to stop painful things that were done to her. The thought of giving another human being, even her baby, total access to her breasts, even for feeding, may cause feelings similar to ones in earlier times when she could not keep her abusers away from her body.

Because so many women (estimates range from 20 to 40 percent) have been sexually, physically or emotionally abused in childhood, it is not surprising that many victims (though not all) experience some of the after-effects mentioned above. The extent of later problems for abuse survivors varies and is influenced by many factors, including the ages at which the abuse occurred, how long it went on, the nature of the abuse, and the presence or absence of other loving and trustworthy adults in the child's life. Psychotherapy and emotional support promote healing and help the victim find new ways to deal with old abuse issues.

If you are an abuse survivor and are aware of some of these (or other) abuse-related concerns, it might help to discuss these with your caregiver or another knowledgeable health professional. Some doctors, midwives and childbirth educators are more aware than others about the later impact of child abuse on the childbearing woman. If your caregiver seems empathetic and non-judgmental, you might disclose your abuse history and explain how you think it is affecting your feelings about your body, your baby, the upcoming labour, your relationships with important people in your life or other matters. A good childbirth educator, midwife, birth counsellor, maternity social worker or nurse may be able to help you address any abuse-related worries. These people may also help you communicate your concerns in a birth plan that will help your caregivers care for you in a way that is sensitive to your needs and that will increase your chances for a safe, satisfying childbirth and post partum.

Travel during Pregnancy

Being pregnant should not interfere with your need or desire to travel. If you are aware of a few precautions, safety tips and comfort measures, you can increase your enjoyment when travelling by car, plane, train, boat or bus.

When planning a trip during your pregnancy, tell your caregiver your destination and mode of travel. Find out his or her usual suggestions for travel and any specific precautions that are needed for your pregnancy. Some caregivers do not recommend travel in the last month of pregnancy or at any time for women who have high-risk pregnancies.

If planning to fly or take a cruise, especially in late pregnancy, talk with your travel agency to find out if there are specific limitations on certain airlines or cruise ships. Some carriers limit travel in the week before your due date on domestic flights, and many have restrictions for longer travel time on international trips. All pregnant women should avoid flying in small planes without pressurised cabins at altitudes above 7000 feet, as this might affect the oxygen available to the foetus.

Long trips by car, bus, plane or train can be difficult for pregnant women because lack of movement can decrease circulation and increase swelling in the legs. You can avoid some of these problems by stretching out as much as possible, by getting up or out frequently to walk around and by doing some simple exercises while in your seat. (Suggested exercises to increase circulation to your legs and to your arms and hands are described on pages 135–137. Positions and movements to decrease back discomfort can be found on pages 134–136.)

Whenever you travel by car or aeroplane, you should always wear your seat belt. Some women worry that the belt will injure the foetus if a collision occurs. In fact, you and the unborn baby are safer when you are wearing a seat belt. The foetus is protected inside the uterus by the cushioning effect of the amniotic fluid and by your muscles and pelvic bones. In a car, seat belts with both shoulder and lap belts are safest and most comfortable. Fasten the belt snugly across your shoulders and low on your hips. The lap belt should fit below the bulge of your abdomen. Sometimes a soft cloth or pad between the lap belt and your body will provide comfort during the trip or, in the case of impact, during a car crash. In an aeroplane, buckle the belt low under the bulge like you would with the lap belt in a car.

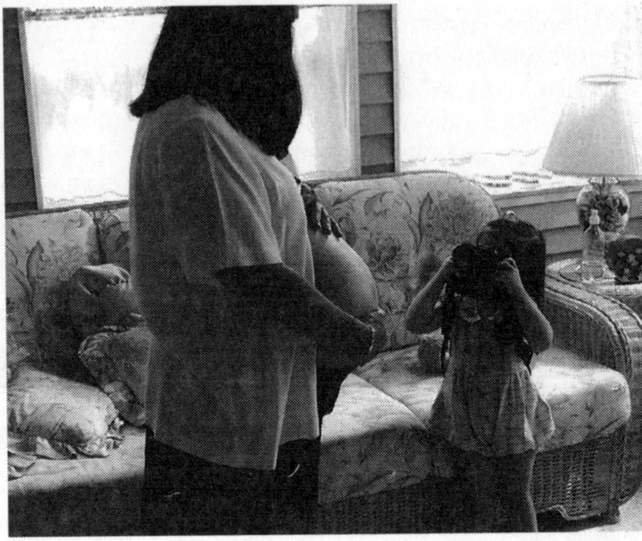

Photograph by Marilyn Nolt

The little photographer practises before taking a trip.

Most women can travel safely during pregnancy, though sometimes the discomforts of pregnancy go with you. Morning sickness may be increased when combined with motion. Fatigue may increase with long days of sightseeing or long business meetings. Your need for good food and plenty of fluids may be not be met when you are not following your normal routines. Remember the methods that enhance your comfort and health at home and try to find ways to fit them into your busy days when you are travelling.

Calendar of Pregnancy: First Trimester

Gestational Age	Six Weeks	Ten Weeks	Fourteen Weeks
Unborn baby	• About 2.5 mm long • Beginning development of spinal cord, nervous system, gastrointestinal system, hear, and lungs • Amniotic sac envelops the preliminary tissues of entire body • Is called a blastocyst from five days to two weeks, then called an embryo	• About 2.5 cm long • Face is forming with rudimentary eyes, ears, mouth and teeth buds • Arms and legs are beginning to move • Fingerprints are present • Brain is forming • Foetal heartbeat may be detectable with ultrasound • External genitals beginning • Is called an embryo	• About 8 cm long • Weighs about 2.8 g • Can move arms, legs, fingers and toes • Can smile, frown, suck and swallow • Sex is distinguishable • Bone cells begin to appear • Can urinate • Is called a foetus
Placental and uterine changes	• Uterus is enlarging • Uterine lining is thick, with increased blood supply • Implantation of ovum, usually in upper back portion of uterus • Placenta and umbilical cord are forming • Human chorionic gonadotropin (hCG), produced by chorionic villi (which becomes placenta), is present in mother's blood and urine and is used for pregnancy test	• Uterus is size of tennis ball • Umbilical cord has definite shape • Amniotic fluid cushions foetus, maintains even temperature and allows easy movement	• Uterus is size of grapefruit and is just above pubic bone • Amniotic fluid fills uterine cavity and is continually replaced • Placenta is small but complete, with full exchange of nutrients and waste products • Placenta is now major source of oestrogen and progesterone

First Trimester Changes (You may experience some or all of these)

Common physical changes in mother	• No menstrual periods • Fullness, bloating, or ache in pelvis or lower abdomen • Constipation • Nausea and vomiting (morning sickness) • Fatigue and sleepiness • Occasional feelings of faintness	• Frequent urination • Breast changes: fullness, tenderness, tingling of nipples, darkened areolas • Aversions to some foods and odours • Metallic taste • Increased salivation • Increased vaginal secretions • Weight loss or gain up to 2.3 Kg
Common emotional changes in mother	• Anxiety or hope while awaiting pregnancy confirmation and results of genetic testing • Focus on body changes and foetal development	• Mood swings • Greater interest in meaning of motherhood • Fear of miscarriage
Common emotions of father/partner	• Difficulty acknowledging pregnancy	• Sympathetic physical changes: weight gain, nausea • Fascination with foetal heartbeat
Common changes for both	• Concern about mood swings and fatigue • Questioning of parenting roles and priorities • Changes in sexual relationship • Fear that sexual intercourse harms foetus • Ambivalence towards pregnancy (joy and excitement vs resentment and anxiety)	• Examination of feelings towards own parents • Financial concerns • Concern over wellbeing of baby

Calendar of Pregnancy: Second Trimester

Gestational Age	Nineteen Weeks	Twenty-Three Weeks	Twenty-Seven Weeks
Unborn baby	• About 13–15 cm long • Weighs about 115 g • Heartbeat is strong • Skin is thin, transparent • Downy hair (lanugo) covers body • Fingernails and toenails are forming • Has coordinated movements; is able to roll over in amniotic fluid	• About 25–30 cm long (15–20 cm crown to rump) • Weighs 230–450 g • Heartbeat is audible with ordinary stethoscope • Hiccups • Hair, eyelashes, eyebrows are present	• About 28–36 cm long (23–25 cm crown to rump) • Weighs 450–900 g • Skin is wrinkled and covered with protective coating (vernix caseosa) • Eyes are open at about 26 weeks • Begins to hear • Meconium is collecting in bowel • Has strong grip
Placental and uterine changes	• Uterus is 8 cm above pubic bone • Placenta performs nutritional, respiratory, excretory and most endocrine functions for foetus • Amniotic fluid volume increases	• Uterus is at level of navel • About 1–1.7 L of amniotic fluid • Placenta is fully developed and covers about half the inner surface of uterus	• Uterus is above level of navel • Placental growth is complete; placenta covers less of inner surface of uterus as uterus grows • Uterus contracts periodically (Braxton-Hicks contractions), which may not be noticed by mother

Second Trimester Changes (You may experience some or all of these)

Common physical changes in mother	• Sense of physical wellbeing, increased energy • Noticing foetal movement • Increased appetite • Disappearance of nausea • Constipation • Food cravings or non-food cravings (pica) • Groin pain from round-ligament contractions • Less tenderness in breasts	• Skin changes: linea nigra, mask of pregnancy (chloasma) • Nasal congestion • Bleeding gums or nose • Relaxation of pelvic joints • Leg cramps • Weight gain averaging 360–450 g per week
Common emotional changes in mother	• Greater feelings of dependency • Acceptance of pregnancy • Increased interest in babies and parenting • Introspectiveness • More daydreaming and dreaming at night	• Developing sense of growth and creativity • Varying feelings about changing appearance
Common emotions of father/partner	• Greater involvement in pregnancy • Varying feelings about partner's changing appearance	• Feelings of closeness to the baby • Evaluation of readiness and ability to be a parent
Common changes for both	• Changes in sexual desire and activity • More enjoyment of pregnancy	• Increasing interest in and awareness of parenting styles

Calendar of Pregnancy: Third Trimester

Gestational Age	Thirty-One Weeks	Thirty-Five Weeks	Thirty-Nine Weeks
Unborn baby	• About 36–43 cm long (28–30 cm crown to rump) • Weighs 1.1–1.8 Kg • Is adding body fat • Is very active • Rudimentary breathing movements are present • Responds to sound	• About 42–46 cm long (30–33 cm crown to rump) • Weighs 1.8–2.7 Kg • Has periods of sleep and wakefulness • May assume birth position • Bones of head are soft and flexible • Iron is being stored in liver	• About 48 cm long (33–36 cm crown to rump) • Weighs 2.7–3 Kg • Skin is less wrinkled • Lanugo is mostly gone • Vernix caseosa is thick • Is less active • Is rapidly gaining antibodies from mother • Foetus may be engaged in pelvis
Placental and uterine changes	• Uterus is three finger-breadths above navel	• Uterus is just below breast-bone and ribs • Uterine contractions are more frequent	• When foetus engages, uterus returns to same height as at 34 weeks • Uterine contractions are more frequent due to increased sensitivity to oxytocin • Cervix is softening (ripening) and thinning (effacing) • Amniotic fluid volume is decreasing • Efficiency of placenta may be decreasing • Hormone changes: decreasing progesterone levels, increasing oestrogen and prostaglandin levels

Third Trimester Changes (You may continue to notice some second trimester changes as well as some or all of these)		
Common physical changes in mother	• More noticeable Braxton-Hicks contractions • Increased colostrum production • Heartburn or indigestion • Shortness of breath (diminishes with engagement/lightening) • Soreness in lower ribs • Urinary urgency and frequency • Tingling or numbness in hands • Stretch marks, abdominal itching • Increased perspiration	• Increased feelings of body warmth • Backache • Changes in balance • Light sleep or insomnia • Vascular spiders • Haemorrhoids • Varicose veins • Swollen ankles • Anaemia • Total weight gain of 11–16 Kg
Common emotional changes in mother	• Excitement over preparations for baby • Focus on labour and birth, anxiety about the unknown • Variety of feelings about body image • Feelings of clumsiness • Difficulty in focusing attention	• Increased dependency on others • Desire for protection • Decreased sexual interest • Enjoyment of increased attention from family and friends
Common emotions of father/partner	• Protectiveness towards family • Anticipation of parenthood	• Longing for independence • Anxiety over support role in labour
Common changes for both	• Continuing changes in sexual relationship • Fear of harm to foetus during sexual intercourse • Excitement about baby's arrival • Eagerness for pregnancy to end	• Fears and concerns about pain of labour and birth, health of mother and baby, and responsibilities of being parents

Calendar of Pregnancy: Term and Post Partum

	Term (forty weeks)	Post Partum (first week or two)
Baby	• About 50 cm long (about 36 cm crown to rump) • Weighs about 3–3.4 Kg • Fingernails may protrude beyond fingers • Arms and legs are in flexed position • Body fat is ample • Lungs are mature	• Newborn needs sleep, milk, suckling, warmth and comfort (touching and cuddling) • Enjoys looking at and listening to parents
Placental and uterine changes	• Pre-labour contractions occur • Placenta is 15–20cm in diameter, 2.5 cm thick and about 450 g • Umbilical cord is 30–80 cm long (usually 50–56 cm); is moist, white, and twisted or spiral-shaped in appearance	• Uterus is at height of navel right after birth and almost back to pre-pregnant size by 10–20 days post partum
Common physical changes in mother	*Pre-labour signs:* • Vague backache • Menstrual-like cramps • Soft bowel movements • Nesting urge • Blood-tinged mucus from vagina • Uterine contractions • Leaking of amniotic fluid (See Chapter 9 for signs of labour)	• Afterpains, especially in multiparas • Increased urination and perspiration • Vaginal bleeding (lochia) • Enlargement/engorgement of breasts • Fatigue • Constipation and haemorrhoids • Perineal discomfort or pain • Incision pain after caesarean birth • Initial weight loss of 4.5–6.8 Kg (See Chapter 13 for more on post partum)
Common emotional changes in mother	• Predictions of what labour and birth will be like • Fear of childbirth pain • Doubts about performance during labour and birth	• Emotional ups and downs • Variety of feelings towards the baby (fascination, love, protectiveness, anxiety, frustration, anger)
Common emotions of father/partner	• Fear for health of mother and baby during childbirth • Questioning ability to cope or perform during childbirth	• Engrossment with baby • Protectiveness of family • Feelings of being displaced by baby • Uncertainty over role and responsibilities
Common changes for both	• Emotional preparation for birth • Feelings of anticipation, exhilaration, excitement and apprehension—all at the same time	• Constant care of baby • Falling in love with baby (bonding/attachment) • Trial and error in parenting techniques • Fatigue-induced impatience • Strengthened or strained relationship with partner • Learning ways to cope with fussiness and crying • Utilising resources (family, friends and community services)

Chapter 3

Prenatal Care and Pregnancy Complications

Though pregnancy and childbirth are usually normal, healthy events in a woman's life, they can be enhanced by the expertise of maternity care providers. This chapter discusses the range of maternity care available to most women today and includes routine prenatal screening tests and the diagnostic tests that might be needed. In addition, possible pregnancy complications are described. It may be helpful to remind yourself as you read this chapter that with good prenatal care you may be able to avoid or minimise adverse outcomes from most of these pregnancy complications.

Preparing for Pregnancy

Ideally, prenatal care begins long before pregnancy. If possible, do not wait until you are pregnant to make needed life changes or seek medical care aimed at having a healthy pregnancy. Here are ten steps that will improve your chances of having a healthy baby:

1. Make an appointment with a maternity care provider to discuss your current state of health and your plans for pregnancy. Make a dental appointment and have your teeth checked and cleaned.

2. Learn about the family health history of both you and your partner, if possible. Find out if there are any special risks for you or your future baby. If desired, meet with a genetic counsellor.

3. Stop smoking, drinking alcohol and using recreational drugs. (See page 107.)

4. Eat well and try to achieve your appropriate weight. Start taking a daily prenatal vitamin or a multivitamin. Make sure it contains a sufficient amount of folic acid. (See pages 91 and 103.)

5. Update your immunisations. Ask to be checked for immunity to rubella (German

measles). Get vaccines for measles, mumps, rubella, chicken pox, diphtheria, tetanus and polio as needed. Note that some immunisations, such as rubella and chicken pox, should be given at least three months before you are pregnant. Try to avoid exposure to contagious illnesses. Wash your hands carefully before eating, do not eat undercooked meat and avoid handling cat litter. (See pages 63 and 119.)

6. If you have a chronic illness—such as diabetes, depression, anaemia, epilepsy, multiple sclerosis, systemic lupus erythematosus, inflammatory bowel disease, high blood pressure or cardiac disease—work with your doctor to stabilise it as much as possible.

7. Talk with your caregiver about continuing the use of prescription medications. Stop taking oral contraceptives several months before getting pregnant. If you use medications known to be harmful in pregnancy, try to avoid them or find safer substitutes. (See pages 112–117.)

8. Avoid exposure to toxic chemicals and substances. Evaluate your home, workplace and environment to identify and eliminate potential toxins.

9. Remember that the father's health and lifestyle influence fertility. He should evaluate these factors and make improvements as needed.

10. Maintain good health and adopt a healthy lifestyle. Exercise regularly, get adequate sleep, reduce stress and work towards stabilising relationships.

Prenatal Care

Prenatal care comprises a variety of exams and evaluations to ensure your wellbeing and the health of your baby. Your doctor, midwife or other staff provide this care. They are interested not only in medical aspects of your pregnancy but also in your health history, your current life situation and any concerns you may have. Once you suspect or know you are pregnant, schedule a visit with your doctor or midwife. It sometimes takes several weeks to get an appointment, so call early.

At your first or second prenatal visit, it is typical to have a complete physical examination, a number of tests and an interview about your own and your family's medical histories. At each prenatal appointment, your caregiver checks on your health and the growth and wellbeing of your baby. In mid-pregnancy, your appointments are scheduled monthly. Towards the end, they are scheduled every two weeks and then every week. Some caregivers schedule very short appointments; others schedule longer visits. While most of the tests can be carried out very quickly, the value of more time lies in building a relationship with your caregiver, discussing personal matters, and exploring other important concerns and questions. Some caregivers schedule periodic longer appointments for such discussions. If you need a longer appointment, request it in advance. You may use these longer visits to work with your care provider in planning your birth experience. (See Chapter 7 for more on birth plans.)

At some or all appointments during pregnancy, your partner should accompany you to become familiar with your caregiver and discuss the partner's role at the birth. Also, try to meet the other doctors or midwives in the practice, since one of them might be on call when you are in labour. If this is not possible, a written birth plan is a good way to introduce yourself and communicate your specific birth preferences to unfamiliar care providers.

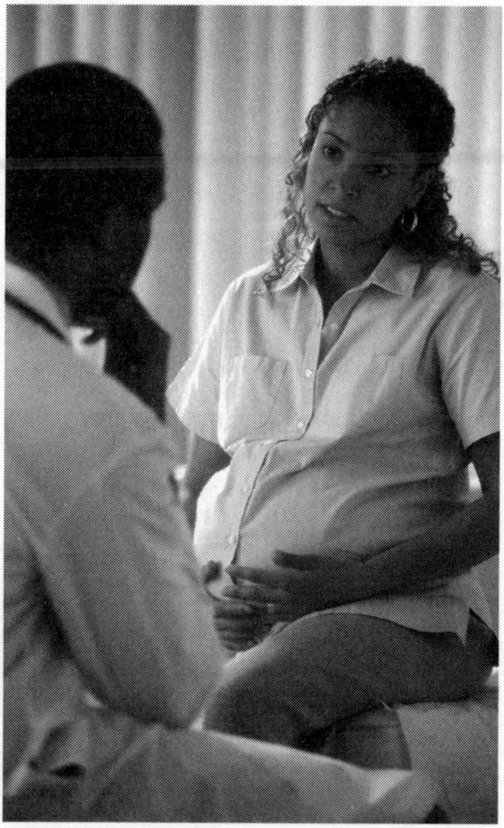

© Jose Pelaez/Corbis Stock Market

At prenatal appointments, be sure to ask any important questions.

Medical and Family History

As part of the interview about your medical histories, you and your partner will be asked about your personal histories. The information you provide helps your doctor or midwife individualise your care. Topics to discuss include the following:

- Medical illnesses that seem to have been passed down from generation to generation; babies that have been born with birth defects, mental retardation, blindness or deafness; stillbirths or many pregnancy losses
- Information about your ethnic background and specific traditions and rituals that are important to you during pregnancy, at the time of birth and during the hours and days following childbirth
- Past experiences that might influence your responses to medical care or procedures, such as negative feelings about a previous hospitalisation, health care provider or illness
- History of past sexual abuse, domestic violence or any other significant mistreatment
- Any thoughts, feelings, memories or experiences that should be shared to ensure that you receive the best care during this important time in your life

Prenatal Tests

Throughout pregnancy, you will be offered routine screening tests and/or diagnostic tests to detect a variety of foetal or maternal problems. (See the 'Prenatal Examinations and Tests' chart at the end of this chapter, beginning on page 78.) It is important to know the difference between screening and diagnostic tests.

A *screening test* is a relatively quick and easy way to determine whether you or your baby is at higher risk than the general population for a particular condition. If your results are positive, it does not mean you have the condition; it means only that you may have it and you need further testing. If additional testing determines you do not have the condition, your screening test is said to have had a 'false positive' reading. If your screening test results are negative, it means you have a low chance of having the condition and do not need further testing. To be included in standard practice, screening tests must have a very low 'false negative' rate; that is, they must be unlikely to miss someone who has the condition.

Diagnostic tests are usually more specific and more reliable in identifying those women who actually have a pregnancy complication or a foetus with a problem. However, because they may not be 100 percent accurate, several tests may be done to confirm a diagnosis. Diagnostic tests are often more invasive, more expensive and usually have more side effects than routine screening tests of pregnancy. Due to these factors, most care providers use diagnostic tests only if indicated by a positive screening test or other factors.

Prenatal tests are reassuring when the results indicate a normal pregnancy or a healthy foetus. But if the results are uncertain or if they indicate a problem, you may face some difficult choices and considerable anxiety. (For example, an amniocentesis may indicate a baby with Down syndrome and the family would be asked how they feel about a therapeutic abortion.) When such tests are suggested by your care provider, answers to the following questions will help you make an informed decision as to whether or not to have the test. These key questions are particularly important if the test carries potential risks.

- What is the purpose of the test?
- Is it a screening test or a diagnostic test?
- How is it done?
- How reliable or accurate are its results?
- Are there risks or drawbacks for either mother or foetus?
- How will the information gained influence the management of my pregnancy?
- What steps follow a negative or positive result?
- How much does it cost? Is it covered fully or in part by my insurance policy or Medicare?
- What are the consequences of not having it done?
- Are there other ways to get similar information? (Ask the above questions about any alternatives.)

With today's advancing medical technology, the ability to detect or diagnose prenatal problems is improving; however, the ability to treat or cure these problems is not nearly as advanced. Nevertheless, with good prenatal care, including screening and diagnostic tests, the chances of having a favourable pregnancy and birth outcome are greatly increased.

If your physician or midwife suspects a pregnancy complication, or if more information is needed on the size, age or condition of the unborn baby, he or she will schedule the needed tests. Two of these tests deserve further discussion: ultrasound, because it offers so much information that caregivers often perform it routinely; and foetal movement counting, because it is a screening test you can perform yourself.

Ultrasound

Few pregnant women today go through pregnancy without having tests using ultrasound. In pregnancy, ultrasound is used in different ways for different purposes. *Doppler ultrasound,* to monitor the foetal heartbeat, uses continuous transmission of sound waves to detect foetal heart wall motion. (See page 258 for more information on monitoring the foetal heart rate.) *Diagnostic ultrasound,* to 'see' inside the uterus, uses intermittent transmission of sound waves, which are transmitted into the body less than 1 percent of the time during the test. The rest of the time the equipment is receiving the sound waves echoing back. The echoes indicate differences in tissue density and are converted into a video image that shows the foetal skeleton and organs, amniotic fluid, umbilical cord, placenta and maternal structures. (See the chart on page 85 for a description of the tests that use diagnostic ultrasound.)

With the help of ultrasound, caregivers gain extensive information about the foetus and the intrauterine environment. They rely heavily on it to make clinical decisions. Accuracy, however, varies depending on the quality of the equipment used, the skill and experience of the technician and doctor, and the purpose of the ultrasound test. Some tests are less reliable than others. (For example, estimation of gestational age and foetal weight is less accurate late in pregnancy.)

Expectant parents like ultrasound for their own reasons. Seeing the baby inside is exciting—his face, fingers and toes; his heart beating; and his body wriggling. Many parents have been inspired by this first sight of the baby to take special care to ensure a safe arrival. Studies of diagnostic ultrasound have found no evidence of harmful effects, and researchers conclude that wise use of ultrasound outweighs the possible risks. However, because of the possibility that high exposure could cause harmful side effects, routine or frequent ultrasound scans (done without a medical reason or simply for curiosity) are not recommended.

Foetal Movement Counting

Keeping track of your baby's movements for a short time each day during late pregnancy gives you and your caregiver valuable information about your baby's health and wellbeing. Babies who are doing well in the uterus have several active, wakeful periods during the day. They also have quiet periods, as if sleeping, characterised by a lack of activity. Even though healthy babies may reduce their activity slightly towards the end of pregnancy, they do not slow down markedly unless they have a problem. If your baby becomes less active, you should notify your caregiver, who can test further and take action (for example, early delivery) if necessary. Some caregivers ask only those women with high-risk pregnancies to do foetal movement counting, while others suggest that all pregnant women do it. Since this is a test that you do yourself, you can decide to do it on your own. The following directions tell you how.

The most accurate way to keep track of your baby's activity is to set aside a period of time each day to focus on the baby and actually count the number of times he moves. What is a movement? Foetal movements may be short (a kick or a wiggle) or long (a continuous squirming motion). Count it as one movement when it ends with a clear, if brief, pause. Hiccups should not be counted. Many methods of foetal movement counting have been proposed and found to be beneficial. One method involves daily foetal movement counting for an hour and recording the number on a chart. A simpler method is described as follows:

The Count-to-Ten Method

Beginning at twenty-eight weeks of pregnancy or anytime thereafter, count foetal movements each day during roughly the same time period. Don't worry if you miss a day now and then. Pick a time when the baby is normally active. After the evening meal is a convenient time for most people. Find a comfortable position and avoid doing anything that might distract you. The method consists of timing how long it takes for your baby to move ten times. The length of time it takes varies among individual babies. The important thing is not how your baby compares with others, but whether he is slowing down compared to his usual pattern as recorded on a chart like the one below.

If your baby does not move at all during the time you set aside, he may be asleep. Try waking him with a loud noise, or wait

Foetal Movement Count

Date	Starting Time	Record of Movements	Time of 10th Movement	Total Time
24/8	7:30pm	𝍸 𝍸	7:43pm	23 min
25/8	6:00pm	𝍸 𝍸	6:15 pm	15 min
26/8	6:30pm	𝍸 𝍸	6:35pm	5 min
27/8	7:00pm	𝍸 𝍸	7:25pm	25 min
28/8	7:15pm	𝍸 𝍸	7:33pm	18 min
29/8	6:30pm	𝍸 𝍸	6:47pm	17 min
30/8	9:00pm	𝍸 𝍸	10:05pm	65 min

until you feel him move and then begin timing how long it takes for him to move ten times. Report to your caregiver if your baby clearly takes a longer time to reach ten movements or if your baby does not have an active period within twelve hours.

Complications during Pregnancy

Unfortunately, not every pregnancy is free of complications. Early recognition and treatment greatly improve the chances of a good outcome, and early recognition is more likely if you are knowledgeable and observant and report any problems or concerns to your doctor or midwife. (See page 57 for the warning signs of pregnancy complications.) Optimal prenatal care depends on cooperation between the expectant parents and their caregiver.

Chronic Conditions

A woman who already has a chronic condition or illness may or may not experience problems in her pregnancy. Existing conditions that may affect your medical care during pregnancy or birth include diabetes; high blood pressure; heart disease; sickle cell anaemia; lung disorders such as asthma; kidney disease; epilepsy; gastrointestinal illnesses such as eating disorders, absorption problems and PKU; auto-immune disorders (in which the immune system harms instead of protects the body) such as rheumatoid arthritis, systemic lupus erythematosus and antiphospholipid syndrome; hormonal diseases such as thyroid or pituitary disorders; and physical disabilities. To determine how your condition may affect you, ask your caregiver. He or she will help you know what to expect during your pregnancy, in labour and in the months following the birth. Remember, you improve your chances of a healthy baby by working towards controlling the symptoms of your chronic illness before pregnancy. Once pregnant, work with your family doctor or specialist as well as your maternity caregiver to create a plan to maintain your health and work towards a good pregnancy outcome. Having a chronic health problem can be challenging during pregnancy, but with good medical care, most women have healthy babies.

Ectopic or Tubal Pregnancy

Ectopic pregnancy occurs when the fertilised ovum implants itself outside the uterus, usually in the wall of a fallopian tube. The most common symptom of an ectopic pregnancy is sudden, severe abdominal pain in early pregnancy (usually in the first eight weeks). Sometimes there is vaginal bleeding. Treatment usually involves surgery and termination of the pregnancy. An untreated tubal pregnancy is a serious threat to a woman's future fertility because of the risk of damage to the fallopian tubes or a possible threat to her life if blood loss is severe.

Vaginal Bleeding

There are several causes of *bleeding during pregnancy;* however, many times a specific cause is not known. Some women experience spotting when the fertilised egg implants in the uterus or at the time of an expected menstrual period. For half of the women who have vaginal bleeding in early pregnancy, the bleeding stops and they have no further complications. Sometimes, however, vaginal bleeding during early pregnancy is serious. It could indicate an ectopic pregnancy or a possible miscarriage. Call your caregiver with any bleeding during early pregnancy so he or she can determine if you need immediate medical attention.

In late pregnancy, fairly heavy vaginal bleeding may occur due to a separation of the placenta from the uterine wall (placenta praevia or placental abruption). If you see slight spotting in late pregnancy, it may be a sign of labour. If you are less than thirty-seven weeks pregnant, call your caregiver, as it may be preterm labour. (For more information on any of these conditions, read the appropriate sections in this chapter.)

Miscarriage

A *miscarriage* (or spontaneous abortion) is the unexpected death and delivery of the embryo or foetus before the twentieth week of pregnancy. Although the specific cause of most miscarriages cannot be determined, some are due to chromosomal abnormalities that interfere with normal development, and others are caused by acute infection, uterine abnormalities, placental circulation problems or rarely a severe physical injury.

The signs of a possible miscarriage include vaginal bleeding and intermittent abdominal pain. The pain often begins in the lower back and is later felt as abdominal cramping. Only rarely can a miscarriage be stopped. If you have any vaginal bleeding in early pregnancy or suspect you are having a miscarriage, call your caregiver for advice on what to do. You may be advised to rest and wait to see if the bleeding stops, or to go to the medical centre for confirmation and support. Sometimes the caregiver discovers that the foetus has died before the miscarriage begins. Besides the shock of such a discovery, waiting for the miscarriage can be extremely stressful and you may want an immediate end to the pregnancy. Because the procedures used for ending a pregnancy involve risks, discuss all the options with your caregiver first. However it is managed, attempt to have supportive people with you when it happens.

If you have a miscarriage, you will probably feel some degree of shock, grief and depression, even when the pregnancy has not been visible to others. These feelings tend to be more pronounced if you have needed special help to become pregnant or if you have previously miscarried. After a miscarriage, you and your partner may need extra rest and support. You may find that talking about your loss eases the pain. Seek out family and friends who can understand and comfort you. Support groups and books on pregnancy loss are helpful at this difficult time. (You may also find some of the information in the section on 'When a Baby Dies or Is Seriously Ill' on page 305 useful.)

Most women who have one or more miscarriages go on to have normal and healthy

Warning Signs of Pregnancy Complications

During your pregnancy, report any of the following warning signs to your doctor or midwife. Your caregiver may ask you to report other pertinent signs and symptoms and any pain that concerns you.

Warning Signs	Possible Problems
Vaginal bleeding (even a small amount)	Miscarriage (page 56); placenta praevia (page 58); placental abruption (page 59); preterm labour (page 60)
Abdominal pain	Ectopic pregnancy (page 55); miscarriage (page 56); placental abruption (page 59); preterm labour contractions (page 60)
Continuing, intermittent abdominal tightening (contractions) or cramping	Preterm labour (page 60)
Constant, painful firmness of the abdomen, with or without vaginal bleeding	Placental abruption (page 59)
Leaking or gushing of fluid from the vagina	Rupture of the membranes (page 220)
Sudden puffiness or swelling of the hands, feet or face	Pregnancy-induced hypertension or pre-eclampsia (pages 74–75)
Severe, persistent headache	Pregnancy-induced hypertension or pre-eclampsia (pages 74–75)
Disturbance of vision (spots, flashes, blurring or blind spots)	Pregnancy-induced hypertension or pre-eclampsia (pages 74–75)
Severe and persistent dizziness, light-headedness	Pregnancy-induced hypertension or pre-eclampsia (pages 74–75); supine hypotension (page 126)
Noticeable reduction or change in foetal activity	Foetal distress as determined by foetal movement counting (page 53)
Painful, reddened area in leg, or pain in leg when standing or walking	Venous thrombosis (inflammation and blood clots in the vein) (page 59)
Severe pain in pubic area and hips, with impairment of leg movements	Strain or separation of pubic symphysis joint
Pain or burning sensation when urinating	Urinary tract infection (page 63); sexually transmitted disease (STD) (page 63)
Irritating vaginal discharge, genital sores or itching	Vaginal infection or STD (page 63)
Fever (temperature over 38°C, taken orally)	Infection (page 63)
Persistent nausea or vomiting	Hyperemesis gravidarum (page 58); infection (page 63)

pregnancies in the future. To increase your chances of a healthy pregnancy, talk with your caregiver about planning your next pregnancy and maintain your health by following the ten pre-pregnancy suggestions at the beginning of this chapter. You may also want to seek counselling and support during your next pregnancy, as this can be a very stressful time.

Severe Nausea and Vomiting (Hyperemesis Gravidarum)

Hyperemesis gravidarum is a rare condition characterised by persistent, excessive nausea and vomiting (far more than the 'morning sickness' of early pregnancy, described on page 95). The condition may involve weight loss, dehydration and changes in blood chemistry. Treatment includes the usual methods to control morning sickness, plus medications to relieve nausea and vomiting, and, if necessary, medications to treat infection and intravenous (IV) nourishment to restore the balance of body fluids.

High Body Temperature (Fever)

A *high body temperature* (an oral temperature over 38°C) over a period of three to four days may harm your baby, especially in early pregnancy. Consult your doctor or midwife to help determine the cause of your fever. Do not take any fever reducing medication unless you have spoken with your caregiver. To lower your temperature, drink plenty of liquids and take a lukewarm bath or shower. Also, be aware that hot tubs and saunas may raise your body temperature to a level that can be dangerous in early pregnancy. (See page 118.)

Fibroids

Fibroids (leiomyomas, myomas) are non-malignant tumours of the uterine wall that are present in 20–30 percent of women. A small percentage of these women experience symptoms such as excessive menstrual bleeding or pelvic pain. Most pregnancies are unaffected by uterine fibroids and proceed well without any problems for mother or baby. If you have fibroids, your caregiver will probably watch your pregnancy more closely for signs of preterm labour and may use ultrasound to look for possible changes in the fibroids or an effect on foetal growth. Fibroids may grow or shrink during pregnancy. Sometimes they do both. When they are associated with abdominal pain, treatment may include bed rest, ice packs or heat, and pain medications appropriate for pregnancy.

Fibroids sometimes complicate childbirth, depending on their number, size and location. Their presence increases the risk of problems with the baby going into a head-down position for birth or with slow labour progress. Occasionally, previous uterine surgery for fibroid removal (myomectomy) makes a caesarean delivery necessary.

Placenta Praevia

Placenta praevia is an infrequent condition in which the placenta lies over (or partially over) the cervix. Some women learn from an early pregnancy ultrasound that the placenta is 'low-lying'. In many cases, this will not develop into placenta praevia because as the uterus grows in pregnancy, the placenta attachment site rises away from the cervix. Placenta praevia is the diagnosis only if the placenta reaches or is over the cervix. An ultrasound later in your pregnancy will determine the placenta's current location. If you do not have placenta previa at fourteen weeks of pregnancy, you do not have to worry about developing it later.

The most common symptom of placenta praevia is painless vaginal bleeding in the last trimester of pregnancy. The bleeding is usually intermittent, ranging from light to heavy with occasional periods of no bleeding. As with any bleeding from the vagina, notify your physician or midwife immediately. An ultrasound can determine the cause of bleeding. Treatment might involve hospitalisation or bed rest and close medical observation of mother and foetus. An elective caesarean delivery is usually performed before labour begins to decrease the risk of excessive bleeding.

Placental Abruption

With *placental abruption*, the placenta partially or almost completely separates from the uterine wall before birth. This condition (sometimes called *abruptio placenta*) most often occurs in the third trimester or during labour. Although it usually happens for no apparent reason, the risk is greater in women with high blood pressure and in those who smoke, drink heavily, use cocaine or have suffered severe physical trauma. Any or all of the following symptoms may occur: vaginal bleeding, continuous severe abdominal pain, tenderness of the abdomen to touch and constant firmness of the uterus. Sometimes, if the blood collects high in the uterus, there is no vaginal bleeding.

Besides the danger of haemorrhage to the mother, extensive separation of the placenta can deprive the baby of adequate oxygen. Ultrasound may help determine the amount of separation and the degree of damage to the placental circulation. Treatment depends on the amount of bleeding and the estimation of separation. When the abruption is small and the foetus remains healthy, bed rest and close medical observation may be the only treatment. Otherwise, a caesarean delivery is performed.

Venous Thrombosis

Venous thrombosis, a rare disorder of pregnancy or post partum, is characterised by inflammation of a vein in the leg or pelvis and development of blood clots that adhere to the wall of the blood vessel. If the condition develops in a surface vein, it causes swelling, tenderness and redness over the affected vein. With deep vein thrombosis, there is leg or pelvic pain, heaviness, tenderness and/or swelling. Fever is sometimes present.

Because of the risk of the blood clots travelling to vital organs such as the lungs, signs of venous thrombosis should be reported immediately to your caregiver. Treatment consists of bed rest, hot packs to the affected area and special support hose. If a deep vein thrombosis is suspected, you might be hospitalised and given heparin, an anticoagulant, to prevent further clot formation. Treatment may then continue at home. If the pain is severe, pain medication may be prescribed.

Preterm Labour

Approximately 6–10 percent of births are *preterm*—that is, they occur before the thirty-seventh week of pregnancy. Preterm babies tend to have more health problems after birth because they are immature and underdeveloped. (See page 409.) Therefore, one of the major goals of maternity care is to prevent preterm labour and birth. The medical profession has attempted to identify those who are most likely to have preterm labour and recognises the need for more reliable methods of predicting it. A significant breakthrough in the 1990s revealed that asymptomatic or subclinical infections (those without obvious symptoms in the mother) sometimes cause preterm labour. If these infections are detected and treated early, the preterm birth rate can be reduced by as much as 10–30 percent.[1] In addition, early detection of preterm labour may be enhanced by two tests. One is an expensive test that analyses vaginal and cervical secretions for foetal fibronectin. Fibronectin (a protein produced by the foetal membranes) increases in labour and may be used as an indicator of true preterm labour, as opposed to the normal contractions of late pregnancy. The other test is to measure the length of the cervix by internal ultrasound. These tests are currently not performed routinely but reserved for women with signs of preterm labour or a history of a previous pregnancy complicated by preterm delivery.

In most preterm births, the mothers have one or more of the following risk factors. It is important to note, however, that many women with these risk factors do not go into preterm labour. Also, preterm labour often occurs in women who have no known risk factors.

Risk Factors

If you have any of these risk factors, you are more likely than others to go into preterm labour:

- Multiple pregnancy (being pregnant with more than one baby)
- Previous preterm labour or birth
- Uterine variations caused by fibroids, an abnormally shaped uterus or conisation of the cervix (removal of a cone of tissue)
- Being a DES daughter (Your mother took diethylstilbestrol [DES] when she was pregnant with you)
- Bleeding during this pregnancy (placenta praevia or other causes)
- Abdominal surgery during this pregnancy
- Current or chronic infection in the vagina or uterus
- Current or chronic urinary tract infection (bladder or kidney)
- Infection of the membranes (amniotic and chorionic)
- Being underweight or obese
- Heavy smoking
- Drug abuse
- Age under eighteen or over thirty-five years
- Poor nutrition before or during pregnancy
- Maternal disease such as hypertension
- Foetal disease such as birth defects
- Constant emotional stress (domestic violence, severe poverty or other stresses)
- High degree of physical stress (heavy lifting, long periods of standing or long work hours)

Symptoms

All pregnant women should know the symptoms of preterm labour because some women with none of the above risk factors go into preterm labour. Since these symptoms are often similar to normal pregnancy sensations, watch for slight differences or changes. If you have two or more of these symptoms, call your doctor or midwife immediately and let your caregiver help you decide if you are in preterm labour.

- Uterine contractions that are frequent and regular—at least one every fifteen minutes or less, or four contractions in one hour. Contractions come in waves as the uterus alternately tightens and softens. They do not have to be painful. (See below for directions on checking for contractions.)
- Menstrual-like cramps causing intermittent or continuous discomfort in the lower abdomen
- Dull lower backache that is not influenced by position change
- Pressure in the lower abdomen or thighs that may come and go (pelvic heaviness)
- Intestinal cramping with or without diarrhoea or loose stools
- Sudden increase or change in vaginal discharge (more mucousy, watery or blood-tinged)
- General feeling that something is not right

When *checking for contractions*, it is important to know what is common and usual for your uterus during pregnancy. Contractions that are irregular in length and occur at variable intervals are normal in pregnancy. So do not panic if you feel them. It is the combination of persistent, fairly regular contractions with some of the other symptoms that indicates labour.

Before checking for contractions, first empty your bladder and drink two tall glasses of water. Then sit with your feet up or lie down on your side and relax. Place your fingertips gently but firmly on your abdomen at the top of your uterus to tell if there are regular episodes of hardness. Time them for one hour. (See page 221.) Note the length and frequency of your contractions. If you have four or more during the hour while you are lying down, call your doctor, being sure to mention the measures you have already taken.

A diagnosis of preterm labour is made if cervical changes (effacement and dilation) are discovered during a vaginal exam. While it is important to be aware of the above symptoms, remember that more than 90 percent of expectant mothers do not go into preterm labour.

Treatment

If your caregiver determines that you are in preterm labour, the following measures may be used to try to stop the contractions and prevent a premature birth:

1. Adequate fluid intake. Initially, you may be asked to drink several glasses of water and observe your contractions for an hour or two to see if they stop. Sometimes, an increased fluid volume can stop preterm labour contractions. Keep well hydrated by drinking at least eight glasses of water or fluid each day. If you are hospitalised, you may be given fluids intravenously.

2. Bed rest. Rest may help decrease uterine irritability. Your caregiver may recommend that you reduce your physical activity. This may range from complete bed rest to a slight decrease in your activity level. You may want to spend some time resting in a tub filled with warm (not hot) water. The relaxing effects of warm water may reduce uterine activity.

3. Monitoring uterine contractions. If you are hospitalised, you will have uterine monitoring and electronic foetal monitoring (EFM). At home you will be asked to continue checking for contractions and to watch for other symptoms of labour. Home monitoring of your uterus with a portable electronic contraction monitor (tocodynamometer or 'toko') similar to one used in the hospital is sometimes used to transmit information via phone lines to your caregiver. Because home uterine activity monitoring is expensive and has not been found to reduce the rate of preterm birth, its use is declining. (See page 258.)

4. Surgical purse-string suturing (cervical cerclage) of an incompetent cervix. The medical term *incompetent cervix* indicates a cervix that shortens and opens in mid-pregnancy without preterm labour contractions. An incompetent cervix may occur in a pregnant woman whose cervix has been weakened by conisation, surgery or trauma. Cervical cerclage may be done in early pregnancy as a preventive measure or in mid-pregnancy if cervical changes occur. The sutures are re-moved in late pregnancy before labour begins.

5. Restriction of sexual activity. Orgasm causes the uterus to contract and semen contains prostaglandins, which could promote preterm labour. However, sexual activity has not been found to be the sole cause of preterm labour and need not be restricted for women not at risk for preterm labour.

6. Avoidance of nipple stimulation from caressing or with attempts to prepare nipples for breastfeeding.

7. Medication to stop or slow labour (tocolytics). Possible drugs include salbutamol, ibuprofen, nifedipine and indomethacin. (See page 298.) The route of administration depends on the chosen drug and the severity of symptoms. They may be given intravenously, orally or by subcutaneous injection. Most of these drugs have side effects that discourage their use unless medically indicated. Also, although tocolytics have been found to postpone delivery for up to seven days, it is not clear that they actually improve outcomes for the baby.

8. Antibiotic or other treatment for infection, if indicated.

Once you reach thirty-six to thirty-seven weeks, the treatment will probably be stopped and your pregnancy will be allowed to follow its own course. If the treatment is unsuccessful in stopping the contractions or in preventing dilation of the cervix, your caregiver may want you to give birth in a hospital with a newborn intensive care unit (NICU). The decision about where you receive care is based on the services your hospital can offer, the degree of prematurity and the kind of care your caregiver thinks your baby will need after birth. You may have an amniocentesis to determine the baby's lung maturity. (See page 81.) If you are between twenty-four and thirty-four weeks gestation, you will probably receive corticosteroids in labour to help reduce the risk of respiratory distress syndrome (breathing problems) and intracranial bleeding (brain haemorrhage) in the newborn baby.[3] (See page 301 for more information on corticosteroids and page 409 for more on premature babies.)

Infections

Although the risk is low for getting a serious infection during pregnancy, *infectious diseases*—including STDs and other common and uncommon illnesses—can complicate your pregnancy or harm your baby. The percentage of babies who are affected and the seriousness of the infection depend on the particular organism, whether you have antibodies to the organism, whether the disease is treatable and when during pregnancy you came down with the illness. If you have had multiple sexual partners, you are at greater risk of having an STD that might endanger your baby. If you now have or ever have had symptoms of an STD—such as genital sores, abnormal vaginal discharge or discomfort or difficulty with urination—tell your caregiver so you can be tested and treated, if necessary.

The chart beginning on page 64 presents information on some infections that could harm your baby or affect the uterine environment and increase the risk of preterm labour. One of these infections, however—group B streptococcus (GBS)—needs further explanation. Medical professionals are currently debating the testing and treatment protocols for pregnant women with GBS. Some caregivers prefer to screen all their pregnant patients at thirty-five to thirty-seven weeks and to treat those who are strep 'carriers' during labour or treat their babies immediately after birth. If their client goes into labour before the test is done, she would be treated with an appropriate antibiotic. Other caregivers prefer not to test routinely, but to treat those pregnant women who are considered at risk for GBS disease. These risk factors include:

- A previous baby who had invasive GBS disease
- A urinary tract infection, due to GBS, during this pregnancy
- Labour or ruptured membranes before thirty-seven weeks gestation
- Labour not beginning within eighteen hours after rupture of membranes
- Fever in labour with a temperature of 38°C or higher

The goal for both protocols is to reduce newborn GBS disease, which is the most common cause of life-threatening infection in newborn babies. If you have questions about your caregiver's testing or treatment protocols, talk with him or her. There are many issues to consider when choosing a test or treatment, such as cost, overuse of antibiotics and routine versus indicated use. In the future, neither protocol may be needed as a vaccine may be available to help a woman produce antibodies to protect her baby during pregnancy, at birth and in early infancy.

Infections during Pregnancy

Infection	Signs and Symptoms	Mode*	Pregnancy Complications	Treatment	Comments
Bacterial vaginosis (BV) Common vaginal infection caused by imbalance of normal bacteria Diagnosed by laboratory tests of vaginal secretions	• Thin, milky-white or grayish vaginal discharge that often has strong fishy odour • Possible vaginal itching or burning • Sometimes asymptomatic (no symptoms)	A	**Mother:** Increased risk of: • Preterm labour • Premature rupture of membranes (PROM) • Infection of membranes (chorioamnionitis) • Post-partum or post-caesarean uterine infection (endometritis) **Baby:** None other than effects of prematurity	**For pregnant woman:** Antibiotic vaginal gel in early pregnancy, or oral antibiotics after 12 weeks gestation	Treatment of sexual partners has not been shown to affect re-infection rate. Screening and treatment is recommended in second trimester of next pregnancy of women with history of BV and preterm birth in prior pregnancy.
Chicken pox (varicella zoster) Viral infection, usually mild if acquired in childhood, more serious in adults Diagnosed by presence of chicken pox blisters on skin	• Itchy red rash with fluid-filled blisters all over body • Cold symptoms and low-grade fever before rash appears • Headache, swollen glands in neck, fever and fatigue • Pneumonia (rare) • Encephalitis (rare)	T B P	**Mother:** Effects of having chicken pox Possibility of pneumonia, especially in third trimester **Baby:** Small risk of developing numerous birth defects in first 20 weeks gestation If mother has infection from 5 days before birth to 2 days after, chance that severe case could cause neonatal death	**For pregnant woman:** Treat symptoms; if pneumonia develops, hospitalisation and antiviral drugs **For foetus:** None other than prevention **For newborn baby:** Treat with varicella zoster immune globulin (VZIG) to prevent or reduce severity of infection	Low risk, since most adults are immune because they had the disease or were vaccinated Vaccine gives limited immunity, not lifelong immunity, as does having the disease. If vaccination is recommended, have it at least three months before becoming pregnant.

* Mode of transmission

Infections during Pregnancy

Infection	Signs and Symptoms	Mode*	Pregnancy Complications	Treatment	Comments
Chlamydia trachomatis Common bacterial STD Diagnosed by culture of vaginal secretions	• Range from none to vaginal discharge, painful urination and pelvic pain • Symptoms of post-partum uterine infection include vaginal discharge, pelvic pain and fever	A B	**Mother:** Increased risk of: • Preterm labour • Premature rupture of membranes • Post-partum uterine infection **Baby:** Infection in newborn's eyes and lungs	**For pregnant woman:** Oral antibiotics; treat sexual partner to prevent re-infection **For newborn baby:** Antibiotics, if mother was not treated	Routine eye treatment with erythromycin ointment soon after birth usually prevents chlamydial infection in baby's eyes. Women at risk for STD are screened more often.
Cytomegalovirus (CMV) Fairly common viral infection that can recur Spread by close contact with infected person through blood, saliva, urine, breast-feeding or sex Diagnosed by blood test	• Flu-like symptoms such as fever, sore throat, swollen lymph glands and fatigue	T B P	**Mother:** None other than effects of the disease **Baby:** About 10 percent of babies whose mothers have their first (primary) CMV infection in the first trimester are affected and have increased risk of jaundice, deafness, eye problems, mental retardation or death.	**For pregnant woman:** Treat symptoms **For foetus:** None other than prevention Termination of pregnancy, if desired	Most women have had CMV and are at low risk during pregnancy. Recurrent CMV infection can produce foetal problems, but less severe than with primary infection.

* Mode of transmission

(T) Trans-placental
Infecting organisms cross from mother's blood to foetus's blood via the placenta, causing infection in baby.

(A) Ascending
Infecting organisms (present in the vagina or cervix) migrate upwards into the uterus to infect membranes, amniotic fluid or baby. Baby is at greater risk after membranes rupture.

(B) At Birth
During vaginal birth, baby comes in contact with maternal lesions, infecting organisms in maternal blood or vaginal secretions. During caesarean birth, baby comes in contact with infecting organisms in maternal blood.

(P) Post Partum
Baby acquires infection through breast milk, physical contact with mother or from others who have the infection.

Infections during Pregnancy

Infection	Signs and Symptoms	Mode*	Pregnancy Complications	Treatment	Comments
Fifth disease (parvovirus B19) Mild, highly contagious disease caused by airborne virus Diagnosed by blood test	• Distinctive rash on cheeks (like a slapped cheek) that later spreads to backs of arms and legs • Possible fever, headache, sore throat or joint pain	T	**Mother:** None other than effects of the disease **Baby:** Most exposed foetuses are unaffected. If infected, a few may develop anaemia and heart failure, which may result in miscarriage or stillbirth.	**For pregnant woman:** Treat symptoms **For foetus:** Cordocentesis and intrauterine blood transfusion are available in a limited number of medical centres.	Origin of name: This disease was the fifth disease discovered that causes a skin rash and fever in children. About 50 percent of expectant mothers have been exposed before pregnancy and are immune. Ultrasound scans may be recommended to detect foetal problems.
Genital warts (human papillomavirus, HPV) Also called condyloma, common viral STD Diagnosed by presence of warts or test of secretions from cervix	• Warts in and around cervix, vagina and rectum • May cause minor symptoms such as itching, or none at all	Unknown	**Mother:** Depends on severity of disease and location of warts **Baby:** If affected by HPV, may develop laryngeal papillomatosis later in teen years. This throat infection has occurred in children delivered both vaginally and by caesarean. Route of transmission is unknown.	**For pregnant woman:** Surgical removal of warts involving cryotherapy ('freezing' with chemicals) or topical medication. Most medications are not recommended in pregnancy. Caesarean delivery is performed if warts obstruct vaginal opening or if they might bleed severely at birth.	Treatment of extensive growth is recommended to reduce risk of cervical or vaginal cancer developing later. Sexual partners are probably infected, even if they do not show visible signs of warts (subclinical HPV). Treatment of subclinical HPV is not recommended. About 20–30 percent of genital warts go away on their own.

* Mode of transmission

Infections during Pregnancy

Infection	Signs and Symptoms	Mode*	Pregnancy Complications	Treatment	Comments
Gonorrhea *(Neisseria gonorrhea)* Common bacterial STD Diagnosed by culture of vaginal secretions	• May include lower abdominal pain, vaginal discharge, painful urination or no symptoms at all	A B	**Mother:** None other than usual discomforts of infection **Baby:** If mother was not treated during pregnancy, baby is at high risk for eye infection that can cause blindness.	**For pregnant woman:** Oral antibiotics **For newborn baby:** Routine antibiotic eye treatment in first hour after birth	Chlamydia (see above) often accompanies gonorrhoea. Eye treatment is given to all babies because screening in early pregnancy misses infections acquired later in pregnancy.
Group B streptococcus (GBS) Presence of GBS bacteria (called colonisation) in vagina and/or rectum Woman who is colonised called a 'GBS carrier' Diagnosed by culture of mother's vaginal and rectal secretions or urine, or of baby's blood, spinal fluid or urine	• Though GBS is present in genital tract, bowel, bladder or kidney, carriers usually show no sign of infection. • Infection (GBS disease) occurs if bacterial count rises. Signs of infection include fever, pain, frequent urination, preterm labour and general feeling of being sick.	A B P	**Mother:** Possible infection of uterus, amniotic fluid, bladder or incision sites; increased risk of: • Premature rupture of membranes • Preterm labour • Caesarean birth for those with prolonged rupture of membranes **Baby:** About 1–2 percent of newborns whose mothers are colonised develop GBS disease and could have: • Neonatal sepsis (a blood infection) • Meningitis (infection of the fluid surrounding the brain and spinal cord) and/or brain damage • Newborn pneumonia • Death	**For pregnant woman:** With signs of GBS disease, treat with oral antibiotics Intravenous (IV) antibiotics during labour to mother who is colonised or to mother with risk factors who is thought to be infected **For foetus:** Antibiotics for infected mother in pregnancy reduce risk of infection. **For newborn baby:** IV antibiotics, if mother was not treated	GBS is not the same as Group A strep, the type that causes strep throat. About 10–30 percent of pregnant women are 'GBS carriers'. Screening culture of vaginal and rectal swabs usually done at 35–37 weeks to predict colonisation with GBS at time of birth. See page 63 for more information.

* Mode of transmission

Infections during Pregnancy

Infection	Signs and Symptoms	Mode*	Pregnancy Complications	Treatment	Comments
Hepatitis B (HBV) Viral STD; also spread by other contact with infected blood Diagnosed by blood test	• At time of infection, may or may not have symptoms of acute illness (nausea, vomiting, fever, extreme fatigue or jaundice) but could become a chronic HBV carrier	B	**Mother:** None other than effects of infection **Baby:** High risk of becoming a chronic carrier of HBV	**For pregnant woman:** Hepatitis B immune globulin (HBIG) and HBV vaccine within fourteen days of exposure can prevent infection. **For newborn baby:** HBIG and HBV vaccine in first hours after birth, if mother is carrier	About 6–10 percent of infected adults become chronic carriers, and most untreated infected newborns become carriers. HBV carriers are at high risk for developing chronic liver disease and liver cancer later in life.
Hepatitis C (HCV) Viral disease spread by contact with infected blood Diagnosed by blood test	• Many do not have symptoms. A few have nausea, fatigue, fever and headaches. Jaundice is rare.	B	**Mother:** None other than effects of disease **Baby:** Slight (about 5 percent) risk of becoming a chronic HCV carrier	**For pregnant woman:** Injections of interferon not recommended during pregnancy. **For newborn baby:** Treatment of children is under investigation.	Vaccine is not yet available. Treatment with interferon does not cure most infected people. High risk that carrier will develop liver damage later in life

* Mode of transmission

(T) Trans-placental
Infecting organisms cross from mother's blood to foetus's blood via the placenta, causing infection in baby.

(A) Ascending
Infecting organisms (present in the vagina or cervix) migrate upwards into the uterus to infect membranes, amniotic fluid or baby. Baby is at greater risk after membranes rupture.

(B) At Birth
During vaginal birth, baby comes in contact with maternal lesions, infecting organisms in maternal blood or vaginal secretions. During caesarean birth, baby comes in contact with infecting organisms in maternal blood.

(P) Post Partum
Baby acquires infection through breast milk, physical contact with mother or from others who have the infection.

Infections during Pregnancy

Infection	Signs and Symptoms	Mode*	Pregnancy Complications	Treatment	Comments
Herpes simplex virus (HSV) Common viral STD spread during times of viral shedding Diagnosed by culture of mother's vaginal secretions or lesions, or of baby's secretions or lesions	• Some have blisters or sores in the genital area only once, while others have periodic outbreaks. • Viral shedding occurs during first episode and at other times, whether there are symptoms or not (asymptomatic shedding).	B P	**Mother:** None other than usual discomforts of infection **Baby:** Infection of skin, eyes and central nervous system. Can cause death. Risk of transmission appears highest during mother's first episode. Risk of transmission is low (about 3 percent) among women with a recurrent outbreak.	**For pregnant woman:** Antiviral drugs (acyclovir and others) reduce symptoms but do not cure the disease. **For newborn baby:** Antiviral drug may be given if mother had primary herpes near term and if baby has neonatal herpes.	During herpes outbreak, a caesarean may be done to reduce risk of infection. It is important that all pregnant women who do not have HSV avoid sexual contact in late pregnancy with partners who have or might have HSV.
Human immunodeficiency virus (HIV) Viral STD; also spread by other contact with infected blood Causes AIDS Diagnosed by blood test	• Slow weight gain or weight loss, recurrent infections, fever, skin rash and pneumonitis	T B P	**Mother:** Most adults with AIDS have a shortened lifespan. **Baby:** Infected newborns usually die within several years.	**For pregnant woman:** Treat symptoms and take medications to treat foetus **For foetus:** Oral antiviral drugs (ZDV or AZT or others) to mother during pregnancy and intravenously during labour **For newborn baby:** For six weeks after birth, antiviral medication in syrup form	Pregnancy has little or no effect on the progression of the disease in the expectant mother. Expect to be offered a screening blood test in early pregnancy Treatment greatly reduces risk of passing virus to baby during pregnancy or at birth. Babies can be infected by breastfeeding.

* Mode of transmission

Infections during Pregnancy

Infection	Signs and Symptoms	Mode*	Pregnancy Complications	Treatment	Comments
Listeriosis *(Listeria monocytogenes)* Rare food-borne illness caused by bacteria found in soil, water, meats and dairy products Diagnosed by blood test	• Mild flu-like symptoms with fever, muscle aches, nausea and vomiting	T A	**Mother:** Pregnant women about 20 times more likely to get listeriosis than other healthy adults. Risk of preterm labour **Baby:** An infection soon after birth causing respiratory and feeding difficulties Possible stillbirth	**For pregnant woman:** Oral antibiotics **For foetus:** Antibiotics given to mother during pregnancy often prevent infection in foetus or newborn. **For newborn baby:** Antibiotics	Risk of infection can be reduced by: • Washing knives and cutting boards • Cooking all meat products (including hot dogs) • Washing vegetables • Avoiding raw milk and soft cheeses such as Camembert and Brie
Lyme disease Bacterial infection caused by bite from infected tick Diagnosed by blood test	• First sign is large red sore that may look like bull's-eye at the site of tick bite. Skin rash may develop later. • Without treatment, sore heals but infection continues, causing problems in the heart, joints or nervous system.	T	**Mother:** Discomforts of infection and possible health problems later **Baby:** If bacteria passes through placenta during pregnancy, associated with: • Miscarriage • Stillbirth • Birth defects	**For pregnant woman:** Oral antibiotics, if symptoms of Lyme disease develop **For foetus:** Treat infected mother during pregnancy to prevent problems for baby	Prevention strategies include avoiding areas inhabited by ticks or animals that harbour ticks, checking for ticks if exposed and removing them if discovered.

* Mode of transmission

(T) Trans-placental
Infecting organisms cross from mother's blood to foetus's blood via the placenta, causing infection in baby.

(A) Ascending
Infecting organisms (present in the vagina or cervix) migrate upwards into the uterus to infect membranes, amniotic fluid or baby. Baby is at greater risk after membranes rupture.

(B) At Birth
During vaginal birth, baby comes in contact with maternal lesions, infecting organisms in maternal blood or vaginal secretions. During caesarean birth, baby comes in contact with infecting organisms in maternal blood.

(P) Post Partum
Baby acquires infection through breast milk, physical contact with mother or from others who have the infection.

Infections during Pregnancy

Infection	Signs and Symptoms	Mode*	Pregnancy Complications	Treatment	Comments
Mumps (Paramyxovirus) Viral infection, rare today since most adults have been vaccinated as children Diagnosed by presence of symptoms, especially swollen glands	• Fever, swollen neck glands (especially salivary glands under ears), diarrhoea and a general feeling of being sick	T	**Mother:** Possible preterm labour **Baby:** Risk of miscarriage if infected during first trimester	**For pregnant woman:** Treat symptoms **For foetus:** None other than prevention	If not immune, avoid contact with anyone with mumps Immunisation soon after birth is recommended.
Rubella (German measles) Viral infection, rare in adults who have been vaccinated Diagnosed by blood test	• Fever, swollen lymph glands and rash that appears about 2–3 days after other symptoms	T	**Mother:** None other than discomforts of infection **Baby:** If infected in first half of pregnancy, possible congenital rubella syndrome: • Vision problems • Heart defects • Deafness • Mental retardation	**For pregnant woman:** Treat symptoms **For foetus:** None other than prevention	If not immune, avoid contact with people with measles. Immunisation during pregnancy is not recommended, as it may cause an infection in foetus. Immunisation soon after birth is recommended. Risk to foetus depends on stage of development at time of infection.

* Mode of transmission

(T) Trans-placental
Infecting organisms cross from mother's blood to foetus's blood via the placenta, causing infection in baby.

(A) Ascending
Infecting organisms (present in the vagina or cervix) migrate upwards into the uterus to infect membranes, amniotic fluid or baby. Baby is at greater risk after membranes rupture.

(B) At Birth
During vaginal birth, baby comes in contact with maternal lesions, infecting organisms in maternal blood or vaginal secretions. During caesarean birth, baby comes in contact with infecting organisms in maternal blood.

(P) Post Partum
Baby acquires infection through breast milk, physical contact with mother or from others who have the infection.

Infections during Pregnancy

Infection	Signs and Symptoms	Mode*	Pregnancy Complications	Treatment	Comments
Syphilis *(Treponema pallidum)* Bacterial STD Diagnosed by blood test	• Small painless sore or ulcer in genital area within 2 months of exposure • Illness (6 weeks after ulcer heals) with rash, fever, headache and swollen glands • If untreated, can cause problems in the eyes, heart, nervous system, skin and bones	T B	**Mother:** Possible preterm labour **Baby:** Problems in the eyes, heart, nervous system, skin and bones Possible stillbirth	**For pregnant woman:** Oral antibiotics (penicillin) **For foetus:** Treat infected mother during pregnancy **For newborn baby:** Antibiotics, if mother not treated	Expect screening blood test in early pregnancy Early treatment and follow-up testing help reduce development of problems for baby.
Toxoplasmosis *(Toxoplasma gondii)* Protozoan infection caused by organism found in raw meats, faeces of outdoor cats and in root vegetables from contaminated soil Diagnosed by blood test	• Mild infection with cold-like symptoms, or no apparent illness at all in adults	T	**Mother:** None other than discomfort of infection **Baby:** Possible congenital malformations or foetal death Risk of severe problems is greatest if mother has primary infection in first half of pregnancy.	**For pregnant woman:** Treat symptoms **For foetus:** Treatment of mother with antibiotics may reduce severity of foetal problems.	Most women who own cats have been exposed, had the infection and have developed immunity. To avoid exposure, cook meats well, wash vegetables thoroughly, avoid soil where cats defaecate, wash your hands after handling cats and have someone else clean the litter box.

* Mode of transmission

Infections during Pregnancy

Infection	Signs and Symptoms	Mode*	Pregnancy Complications	Treatment	Comments
Trichomoniasis *(Trichomonas vaginalis)* Common STD caused by protozoan Diagnosed by examination of vaginal secretions	• Vaginal irritation with foul-smelling yellow-green discharge • Sometimes no symptoms	A	**Mother:** Increased risk for: • Premature rupture of membranes • Preterm labour **Baby:** None other than effects of prematurity	**For pregnant woman:** Oral antibiotic (Metrondazole) after first trimester	Sexual partner should be treated.
Yeast (candida, monilia) Fungal infection of vagina, skin or nipples of mother, or of mouth and nappy area of baby Diagnosed by presence of signs or symptoms, or by microscopic exam of infected tissue	• Itchy and painful rash of vagina, nipples or moist areas of skin • Sometimes pain without rash • White patches in baby's mouth or nappy rash	B P	**Mother:** None other than discomfort of infection **Baby:** Yeast may cause sore mouth (thrush), upset gastrointestinal tract and nappy rash.	**For pregnant woman or new mother:** Antifungal cream, oral medication or natural remedies **For newborn baby:** Oral antifungal medication in liquid form	Prior use of antibiotics increases chance of having yeast infection. Yeast infection is not serious for mother or baby, though it may be difficult to treat. Extreme nipple pain in nursing mother may be only symptom.

* Mode of transmission

(T) Trans-placental
Infecting organisms cross from mother's blood to foetus's blood via the placenta, causing infection in baby.

(A) Ascending
Infecting organisms (present in the vagina or cervix) migrate upwards into the uterus to infect membranes, amniotic fluid or baby. Baby is at greater risk after membranes rupture.

(B) At Birth
During vaginal birth, baby comes in contact with maternal lesions, infecting organisms in maternal blood or vaginal secretions. During caesarean birth, baby comes in contact with infecting organisms in maternal blood.

(P) Post Partum
Baby acquires infection through breast milk, physical contact with mother or from others who have the infection.

Diabetes Mellitus and Gestational Diabetes

Diabetes, a glucose intolerance that affects about 2–3 percent of pregnancies, presents special problems for the pregnant woman and her baby. *Diabetes mellitus* occurs when a person's body has a problem making or utilising insulin, a hormone that enables the body to use glucose (sugar) as an energy source. Without the help of insulin, the blood glucose level rises dramatically. A woman who has diabetes mellitus before pregnancy (pre-gestational diabetes) needs the care of a specialist when she is considering getting pregnant. She may need to adjust her insulin injection schedule or begin taking it for the first time to help control her blood glucose levels. She will need to balance her insulin dosage with her diet and activity level. Intensive management of diabetes during pregnancy may reduce the risks of problems for the baby, such as an overly large baby, hypoglycaemia (low blood sugar), newborn jaundice, delayed lung development and possible birth defects. Chances for a healthy baby are improved if an expectant mother has tight control of blood glucose levels before and during pregnancy.

Gestational diabetes is a type of diabetes that develops or is first recognised in pregnancy. Gestational diabetes is not caused by diminished insulin production. Rather, it is related to normal changes in glucose metabolism that promote foetal growth. Human placental lactogen (HPL), a pregnancy hormone, diminishes the effect of insulin, thus freeing up more glucose for foetal growth. In some women, their response to HPL is out of balance, leading to excessively high blood glucose levels. Early detection and appropriate treatment of gestational diabetes can help prevent problems similar to those for a woman with pre-gestational diabetes.

Urine tests to screen for sugar and ketones may or may not be done in early pregnancy, but most women have a blood glucose screening test between twenty-four and twenty-eight weeks gestation. If this blood screening test is positive (indicating high blood glucose), a two-hour glucose tolerance test (GTT) will usually be scheduled. (See page 80.) Some feel that gestational diabetes is over-diagnosed and recommend that a woman have two GTTs before making a final diagnosis. If you have gestational diabetes, treatment usually consists of a special diet, regular exercise and, in some cases, insulin injections. You will probably be taught how to regularly check your blood glucose levels. Labour may be induced near term if excessive growth of the baby is suspected or if placental circulation appears affected by the diabetes. After the birth, your blood sugar levels usually return to normal, though some women continue to have abnormal GTT results and half develop diabetes later in life.

Pre-eclampsia

Elevated blood pressure in the last half of pregnancy accompanied by oedema (excessive fluid retention and swelling) in the hands, feet or face and the presence of protein in the urine is called *pre-eclampsia*. Previously it was called toxaemia. Currently, pre-eclampsia is considered a group of symptoms that is now included in the diagnosis of pregnancy-induced hypertension (PIH). (See below for more details.)

High Blood Pressure and Pregnancy-Induced Hypertension (PIH)

High blood pressure (hypertension), defined as a blood pressure higher than 140/90 for at least two readings, has the potential of causing serious problems in pregnancy. With a sustained elevated blood pressure, a pregnant woman is at increased risk for such complications as reduced placental blood flow to the baby, placental abruption and possible damage to her internal organs. Both chronic hypertension (high blood pressure present before pregnancy) and pregnancy-induced hypertension (PIH) have the potential of causing these problems. PIH (high blood pressure that develops after the twentieth week of pregnancy) affects 6–8 percent of expectant mothers in Australia.

Your blood pressure may vary according to your activity level, emotional state and body position. It is usually lower when you are at rest, free of emotional stress and lying down. Your blood pressure normally drops during the middle trimester of pregnancy and then returns to your first trimester levels in the last part of your pregnancy. Blood pressure readings may differ, depending on the type and quality of equipment used and the skills of the person taking your blood pressure.[4] Since your caregiver depends on these readings, if there is a wide variation, it is reasonable to request that the same person with the same equipment check each time.

The terms used to describe the complications associated with pregnancy-induced hypertension include pre-eclampsia; *eclampsia,* which indicates a seizure has occurred; and the HELLP (haemolysis, elevated liver enzymes, low platelets) syndrome, which indicates blood and liver complications. Currently, the term *pregnancy-induced hypertension* or *PIH* may be used to refer to any or all of the above problems.

PIH is a multi-organ condition with mild to severe symptoms. Mild PIH is characterised by blood pressure over 140/90 that is accompanied by oedema, especially in the hands and face, a rapid weight gain and presence of protein in the urine. Severe PIH is characterised by any or all of the following signs or symptoms: a blood pressure over 160/110, headaches, blurred vision, spots before the eyes, pain in the upper abdomen, decreased urine output, increased knee and ankle reflexes, and changes in blood chemistry that indicate problems with the liver, kidney and blood platelet levels. In the most severe cases, seizures, coma or even death of mother and baby can occur. Prevention of these tragic complications is the rationale for aggressive treatment of PIH.

Currently, the treatment for mild PIH includes bed rest (preferably on your side), periodic blood pressure checks and close medical supervision to watch for the signs and symptoms of severe disease. Although the supine (back-lying) position can lower your blood pressure in pregnancy, it is not good because the supine position also reduces blood return to your heart. Side-lying, however, safely lowers your blood pressure while improving the blood flow back to your heart and then to your internal organs (including the uterus and placenta, thus increasing nutrients and oxygen to your baby). Sometimes, medications are given to lower blood pressure or decrease the risk of intra-uterine foetal growth retardation. With severe PIH, you may be hospitalised and given drugs, such as magnesium sulphate, to decrease the risk of seizures. (See page 302 for more on these medications.)

Although the causes of PIH are not yet understood, studies indicate that it is more likely to occur in women who are first-time mothers, those with twin pregnancies, teenagers, women over thirty-five, obese women, those with poor diets and women in highly stressful living conditions. In addition, expectant mothers with a personal or family history of kidney or vascular disease, chronic hypertension, diabetes mellitus or a past pregnancy complicated by PIH are more likely to develop PIH.

Researchers are looking for ways to differentiate women with PIH who are at risk for severe disease from those who have no serious problems. They are also seeking better ways to prevent PIH and for effective medications and methods to treat it.

If signs of severe PIH persist after treatment, labour may be induced or a caesarean birth planned. A return to normal blood pressure usually takes place within days or weeks after the birth of the baby. With early diagnosis and treatment, complications from PIH are generally minimal and a healthy pregnancy outcome can be expected. Occasionally, prematurity of the baby results when the severity of PIH requires induction of labour and early delivery.

Rh Incompatibility

Each person inherits specific blood characteristics, one of which is the presence or absence of a particular antigen known as the Rh (Rhesus) factor. About 85 percent of the population is Rh positive, which means they have the Rh factor in their blood. If you do not have the Rh factor, you are said to be Rh negative. A woman who is Rh negative will receive special care during pregnancy.

If you are Rh negative and the baby's father is Rh positive, your baby may be Rh positive. If so, you and your baby are said to be Rh incompatible. In this case, there is a risk that the baby's positive Rh factor will cross through the placenta into your bloodstream. You would then become sensitised to the foreign Rh factor and begin to produce antibodies against it. Because your antibodies are produced slowly, the first Rh-incompatible pregnancy is usually unaffected. However, a problem can arise in the next or future pregnancies if the baby is Rh positive. Without preventive treatment, your antibodies against the Rh-positive factor will cross the placenta and destroy some of your unborn baby's red blood cells, resulting in mild to severe anaemia in the baby (erythroblastosis foetalis).

Sensitisation of the mother can usually be prevented by giving her injections of Rh immune globulin (Rhogam). Rhogam will soon be routinely given to pregnant Rh-negative mothers at twenty-eight weeks gestation. Rhogam is also given after a miscarriage or abortion, with any invasive procedure (such as amniocentesis), or if indicated by an episode of uterine bleeding or trauma.

Because the effects of each dose of Rhogam last about twelve weeks, a dose given at twenty-eight weeks gestation lasts until term. After birth, if the baby is found to be Rh positive, the mother will again be given Rhogam.

Even though sensitisation is extremely rare due to the wide use of Rhogam, if you are Rh negative, your blood will be drawn and tested for the presence of antibodies at specific times throughout your pregnancy. If you are in the small minority of women who have unknowingly become sensitised and your number of antibodies has increased, tests are done to discover how seriously your foetus has been affected. Treatment possibilities include early delivery of the baby or, in severe cases, intrauterine blood transfusions to the baby using a procedure known as cordocentesis. (See page 83.) If seriously affected by Rh incompatibility, a newborn infant will be given an exchange transfusion. Fortunately, the appropriate use of Rhogam has greatly reduced the need for these lifesaving procedures.

Prenatal Examinations and Tests

I. Routine Examinations and Screening Tests

The following examinations and tests are usually done during pregnancy. Some caregivers do not perform all the tests listed.

Routine Exam/Test	Purpose	Comments
Pelvic (vaginal) examination	*First or second prenatal visit:* • To confirm pregnancy and estimate size of uterus • To estimate size and shape of pelvis • To obtain vaginal secretions to detect infectious organisms • To screen for cervical cancer (Pap smear) *Late pregnancy:* • To assess the cervix and station (descent) of baby • To obtain vaginal secretions to detect infection or infectious organisms	• See page 63 for a discussion of infections during pregnancy. • Exam may cause dark brown or reddish vaginal discharge. • Numerous exams of cervix may increase risk of infection or premature rupture of membranes.
Urine test	*First prenatal visit:* • To confirm pregnancy • To screen for urinary tract bacteria *Each prenatal visit:* • To screen for sugar and ketones, which might indicate diabetes • To screen for protein, which might indicate pre-eclampsia or infection *As indicated:* • To detect bacteria or other infectious organisms • To diagnose a urinary tract infection	• See pages 74 and 84 about early screening test for gestational diabetes. • See page 74 about pre-eclampsia and page 63 about infections. • Infectious organisms can be present in the urinary tract without causing infection. • Early treatment could decrease the risk of preterm labour.
Blood test	*First or second prenatal visit or later, if indicated:* • To confirm pregnancy • To determine blood type and Rh factor or screen for antibodies in Rh-negative mother • To test for anaemia (haematocrit and haemoglobin) • To test for infectious organisms or antibodies against them (syphilis, hepatitis B virus, human immunodeficiency virus [HIV], rubella [German measles]) • To evaluate status of blood glucose levels in women with diabetes mellitus	• See page 76 for a discussion of Rh incompatibility. • See page 91 for information on iron treatment for anaemia. • See page 63 for information about infections during pregnancy. • Some tests may be repeated. • Other screening tests (glucose and multiple marker) also involve using blood samples. See page 80.

Prenatal Examinations and Tests

Routine Exam/Test	Purpose	Comments
Blood pressure check	*Each prenatal visit:* • To screen for high blood pressure, which might indicate pregnancy-induced hypertension (PIH)	• See page 75 for a discussion of PIH. • Blood pressure readings are often different when different types of monitoring devices are used (electronic versus auscultation monitor) or if different people are doing the monitoring.
Maternal weight check	*Each prenatal visit:* • To detect sudden weight gain that could be due to pre-eclampsia (which is now called PIH) • To help monitor mother's nutritional status	• See page 75 for information on PIH. • See page 93 for a discussion of nutrition and weight gain in pregnancy.
Abdominal examination	*Each prenatal visit:* • To measure the growth of the uterus (fundal height), which indicates foetal growth and gestational age *Each visit in last weeks of pregnancy:* • To estimate size and position of the foetus (Leopold's manoeuvres) • To estimate amniotic fluid volume • To detect breech presentation	• If problem is suspected, an ultrasound scan (pages 53 and 85) is usually recommended. • See page 295 for more information on breech presentation.
Listening to foetal heart tones (FHT) The foetal heartbeat is heard through the mother's abdomen with a foetal stethoscope or a Doppler.	*Each prenatal visit after FHT can be heard (about 10–12 weeks):* • To check that the foetus is living • To check the heart rate for foetal wellbeing	• With Doppler, FHT can be heard at about 9–12 weeks; with a foetal stethoscope, at about 18–20 weeks gestation. • Hearing the FHT increases the expectant parents' feelings of attachment to their baby and makes the baby seem more real.
Breast exam	*Once or more during pregnancy:* • To assess condition of the breasts for breastfeeding • To screen for breast cancer	• See pages 427 and 429 for a discussion of conditions that influence breastfeeding. • Breast self-exams (page 369) should continue to be performed regularly throughout pregnancy.
Dental exam	*Once or twice during pregnancy:* • To check for tooth decay and repair, if necessary • To clean teeth, which may prevent gum disease • To check for infection of the gums (gingivitis)	• Gum tenderness and bleeding is fairly common in pregnancy. • Gingivitis may worsen during pregnancy or appear for the first time (due to hormonal changes, more bacterial growth, and gum sensitivity). • Gingivitis has been associated with preterm labour. • Tell your dentist that you are pregnant, as some drugs are not given in pregnancy (for example, no nitrous oxide in first half of pregnancy).

Prenatal Examinations and Tests

Routine Exam/Test	Purpose	Comments
Multiple marker screening A test that measures maternal blood levels of two to five of the following substances: 1. Pregnancy associated plasma protein A (PAPPA), a substance produced by the placenta 2. Alpha-foetoprotein (AFP), a substance produced by the foetal liver 3. Human chorionic gonadotropin (hCG), a hormone produced by the placenta 4. Oestriol (E3), a by-product of oestrogen metabolism, affected by foetal and placental function 5. Dimeric inhibin A, a substance produced in the ovaries Test results are usually available in one week.	*At 11–14 weeks gestation:* • To screen for low levels of PAPPA and high levels of hCG, which may be associated with Down Syndrome. These tests are performed in conjunction with a nuchal translucency ultrasound *At 14–20 weeks gestation:* • To screen for low levels of AFP and oestriol combined with high levels of hCG and dimeric inhibin A, which could indicate Down Syndrome or other potential adverse pregnancy outcomes • To screen for high levels of AFP, which could indicate an open neural tube defect (spina bifida, anencephaly) or an increased risk of other foetal abnormalities or death	• Sometimes called triple screen, triple marker, double screen, quadruple screen or maternal serum AFP screen. The name may or may not indicate the number of substances tested. • If test results are outside the normal range, then further testing may include a repeat blood test to confirm findings, ultrasound, genetic counselling and amniocentesis. • AFP test accuracy is questionable if the due date is unclear. • Pregnancies with twins or multiples show a higher AFP level, and insulin-dependent diabetics usually show a lower AFP level than normal for a specific gestational age. • As a screening test, it may miss some Down syndrome pregnancies and miss some cases of other conditions. • There is a high rate of false positives. (The test indicates a problem when there is none.) • Useful for those not wanting invasive testing, although it does not detect the many other possible inherited disorders that can be detected by amniocentesis or chorionic villus sampling. • The test helps parents make decisions about pregnancy or birth. (They could terminate the pregnancy, plan a caesarean if spina bifida is detected or prepare for a child with a disability.)
Glucose screening A blood sample is taken from the mother one hour after she drinks a sugary (glucose) drink or eats a special carbohydrate meal or snack.	*At 24–28 weeks gestation:* • To screen for gestational diabetes, which, if untreated, may cause problems for mother and baby	• If the mother's blood sugar is elevated, a two-hour glucose tolerance test (GTT) is usually planned. • Many women with an elevated blood sugar in the screening test will be found to have normal blood sugar levels in the GTT. • See page 74 for a discussion of gestational diabetes.
Group B streptococcus (GBS) screening Vaginal and rectal secretions are cultured in a laboratory to determine the degree of colonisation.	*At 35–37 weeks gestation:* • To screen for presence of GBS and identify women who are GBS carriers	• Not all caregivers screen for GBS. Some only treat women who show signs of high risk of GBS colonisation at the time of labour. See pages 63 and 67 for more on GBS.

Prenatal Examinations and Tests

II. Diagnostic Tests

The following tests might be done if a screening test indicates a potential problem. Tests are listed in alphabetical order, not by frequency of use or when they are done during pregnancy.

Diagnostic Test	Purpose	Comments
Amniocentesis Using ultrasound for guidance, the doctor passes a needle through the abdomen and uterus into the amniotic sac, withdraws fluid, and sends it to a lab for the appropriate examination. Amniocentesis can be performed when there is an adequate amount of fluid. The amniotic fluid is processed or treated differently, depending on the test being done. To identify chromosomal abnormalities, foetal cells are separated from the amniotic fluid and given time (about two weeks) to multiply, which provides enough cells to allow analysis. For other tests, the fluid can be checked quickly for the presence of various substances that reveal specific information about your unborn baby.	*In early to mid pregnancy:* • Provides information on particular birth defects, metabolic disorders and chromosomal or genetic diseases • May detect Down syndrome, sickle cell anaemia, neural tube defects and many other disorders • Performed to evaluate foetus if results from particular screening tests indicate a problem • Helps you make a decision about continuing or terminating a pregnancy	• Usually done at 15–16 weeks, though could be done anytime after 13 weeks gestation • Slightly increases risk of miscarriage; one in two hundred have a miscarriage that they would not have had without test. • Used for metabolic and genetic disorders only if family history indicates a risk • Requires injection of Rhogam if mother is Rh negative • Is invasive and carries a slight risk of intrauterine infection or intra-amniotic bleeding • Length of time required to obtain results (about 2 weeks) may be stressful. • Termination of pregnancy (abortion), if desired, might not be performed until 15–20 weeks gestation. (Later abortions are riskier and may be more stressful than earlier abortions.) • Is expensive, although health insurance covers costs for women over thirty-five and those with medical indications
	In late pregnancy (often in last trimester): • Provides vital information on foetal lung maturity when early delivery is being considered for the health of mother or baby • Reveals severity of Rh disease or other suspected blood disorders and helps determine if treatment of baby will be necessary	• May cause premature labour • Slight risk of injury to foetus, placenta or cord • May cause intrauterine infection • Slight risk of intrauterine bleeding

Prenatal Examinations and Tests

Diagnostic Test	Purpose	Comments
Biophysical profile (BPP) This test evaluates foetal bio-physical functions and has five components. A non-stress test (NST) checks: 1. The foetal heart rate's response to movement An ultrasound scan helps assess: 2. Foetal movement and activity 3. Foetal muscle tone 4. Foetal breathing movements 5. Amniotic fluid volume (AFV) Each component is scored with 0, 1 or 2 points, so the highest possible total is 10 points. Foetal bio-physical profiles take about one hour or less.	• Estimates foetal wellbeing in the latter weeks of pregnancy • Used to determine if a high-risk or a post-date pregnancy could safely continue or if labour should be induced	• Is a fairly good predictor of foetal condition when scores are high (6–10) or low (0–2) • Intermediate scores (3–5) are difficult to interpret, and repeat testing is done. • Sometimes, variations of the biophysical profile are performed (for example, evaluating only the NST and AFV, or evaluation of only the four components from the ultrasound). • Sometimes the NST and ultrasound are done in two separate locations.
Chorionic villus sampling (CVS) Using ultrasound for guidance, the doctor passes a slim catheter through the opening of the cervix (trans-cervical CVS) or a needle through the abdomen and uterus (trans-abdominal CVS), placing it on the chorionic membrane, which covers the foetus. Tiny pieces of the chorionic villi are suctioned into a syringe and sent to a laboratory for analysis. The procedure takes about 15–20 minutes. Chorionic villus sampling is usually performed between 10 and 12 weeks gestation, and results are available in a week or two.	• Provides information about chromosomal abnormalities (same as that obtained from mid-trimester amniocentesis, except for spina bifida) • Provides information at an earlier gestational age than amniocentesis, allowing for earlier decision about termination of pregnancy • Provides a sample large enough to take advantage of molecular genetics technology such as DNA analysis (done if indicated by family history)	• Not as widely used as amniocentesis • Risk of miscarriage is about 1 percent above those not having test (miscarriage rate is normally as high as 4 percent at this stage of pregnancy). • May cause maternal spotting and cramping, amniotic fluid leakage or infection • Not available in all medical centres • Requires injection of Rhogam if mother is Rh negative • Often requires mother to have a full bladder, which may be uncomfortable • Reasons not to do a trans-cervical CVS include genital herpes, inflammation of cervix or cervical myoma. • Small risk for foetal limb defects if CVS done before 10 weeks gestation

Prenatal Examinations and Tests

Diagnostic Test	Purpose	Comments
Contraction stress test (CST) or oxytocin challenge test (OCT) This test shows how the foetal heart rate (FHR) responds to uterine contractions. Contractions are induced until the mother has three contractions in 10 minutes. Then, while the uterus continues contracting at that rate, an external electronic foetal monitor measures the FHR. Test results are 'reassuring' if FHR remains normal during contractions. The test is 'non-reassuring' or 'ominous' if the FHR indicates foetal distress. It sometimes takes several hours to complete the test.	• Used to predict whether the foetus can withstand stress of labour contractions • Used to decide if high-risk pregnancy can continue, if labour should be induced or if a caesarean birth is indicated • Estimates placental function and foetal reserves	• Usually not done unless non-stress test indicates a problem with foetal wellbeing • May cause preterm labour • Difficult to interpret results • Produces occasional false results, which could lead to unnecessary intervention • Considered reliable only during the last weeks of pregnancy
Cordocentesis or percutaneous umbilical blood sampling (PUBS) During cordocentesis, the doctor, guided by ultrasound, passes a needle through the mother's abdomen and uterus into the umbilical cord, allowing foetal blood to be withdrawn for testing. Cordocentesis can be performed after 16–18 weeks gestation. The procedure takes about 10 minutes.	• Assesses foetal blood characteristics, such as red blood cell count, to detect anaemia and level of oxygen • May be used to give a blood transfusion, administer medications or monitor effectiveness of drug treatment for foetus • Can diagnose Rh incompatibility, sickle cell disease, suspected foetal infection, haemophilia and other conditions, but rarely used for these purposes	• Not a commonly used procedure • Under special circumstances, may be used instead of amniocentesis, with quicker results (within 48–72 hours) • Requires greater technical skill than amniocentesis on part of doctor and is only available at large prenatal diagnostic centres • Is invasive, with higher rate of foetal loss than with amniocentesis • Potential complications include bleeding from umbilical cord, infection, preterm labour, premature rupture of membranes, placental abruption, blood clot in cord and transient irregular foetal heart rate.
Doppler blood flow studies A Doppler ultrasound unit placed on the woman's abdomen obtains information about the rate of blood flow (velocity) in the umbilical artery, the foetal blood vessels and/or the uterine artery of the mother. This information is recorded as velocity waveforms that show the differences in blood flow during and between heartbeats (reported as the 'systolic/diastolic ratio').	• Provides information about condition of utero-placental and/or foetal circulation • Used to identify a foetus at risk due to foetal-placental blood flow problems (intrauterine growth retardation, pregnancy-induced hypertension and others)	• Not commonly used; full range of applications still being explored • Is non-invasive • Ability to predict maternal and foetal disease and/or outcome is unclear. • Not available in all medical centres

Prenatal Examinations and Tests

Diagnostic Test	Purpose	Comments
Foetal movement counts During late pregnancy, the woman counts and records her baby's movements during a brief period each day. (See page 53 for a description of foetal movement counting.) This formal foetal movement counting is a more reliable predictor of outcome than reliance on the mother's impressions of foetal activity.	• Helps assess wellbeing of foetus • Helps mother learn about her baby	• Is non-invasive, free and relatively simple • Can be done by the mother herself, at her convenience, in her own home • Requires more time and work by expectant mother • May raise mother's anxiety over her baby's wellbeing
Glucose tolerance test (GTT) A glucose tolerance test is a blood test that evaluates the body's ability to handle a large dose of sugar or glucose. The technician draws blood before the mother drinks a sugary drink and then again at one hour, two hours and three hours afterwards.	• Used to diagnose gestational diabetes if a screening test indicates this possibility	• A special high-carbohydrate meal or snack could possibly be used if the glucose drink is not tolerated. • Normally, blood glucose levels remain stable; however, with diabetes, two or more of the readings are elevated. • See page 74 for more on gestational diabetes.
Magnetic resonance imaging (MRI) Images are obtained with a superconductive magnet that moves over the skin of the mother above the area that is to be visualised. A number of multi-slice images projected onto a video screen show the different levels (or planes) of the maternal or foetal organs or vessels being evaluated.	• Allows a detailed look at several layers (multi-planar) of an internal organ of the unborn baby • Estimates size and volume of anatomical structures and maturity of foetal organs (for example, for lung maturity) • Helps assess maternal internal organs and blood vessels (for example, to detect deep vein thrombosis)	• Not commonly used; costly, not readily available and used only if medically indicated • Allows non-invasive evaluation of internal organs, blood vessels and blood flow without use of dyes or ionising radiation • Echo-planar imaging (a form of MRI) helps overcome imaging problems due to movement of the foetus, because a shorter time (less than 10 seconds) is needed for each picture in the imaging sequence than with traditional MRI. • Not recommend by FDA for the first trimester of pregnancy. No reported harmful effects of its use in pregnancy have been found to date.

Prenatal Examinations and Tests

Diagnostic Test	Purpose	Comments
Non-stress test (NST) This non-invasive test indicates how the foetal heart rate (FHR) responds when the foetus moves. The FHR is recorded for 20–30 minutes with an external electronic foetal monitor, and the woman indicates each time she feels the baby move. If there is no spontaneous foetal movement, the baby may be asleep. The examiner may push on the woman's abdomen or sound a loud noise near her abdomen to stimulate the baby to move. An increase of 15 beats above the baseline heart rate for 15 seconds (while the foetus is moving) is normal and a sign of foetal wellbeing and is called a 'reactive test'.	• Used to predict foetal wellbeing • Used to determine if a high-risk pregnancy can safely continue or if further testing is desirable	• Can be done in caregiver's office, clinic, hospital or at home • Considered reliable only during the last weeks of pregnancy (after 30 weeks gestation) • Occasionally produces false results • In many cases when NST is non-reactive, further testing shows a healthy foetus.
Ultrasound (sonography) High-frequency sound waves are sent through a transmitter (called a transducer or probe) into the woman's uterus via the abdomen or the vagina. These waves echo back from various structures of the foetus, the placenta and the mother's internal organs to form a picture on a video screen. An ultrasound scan takes about 10–30 minutes to get an entire image of the foetus and other structures. It can be performed at any time during the pregnancy. The timing depends on the reason for testing.	• Confirms pregnancy and pregnancy with multiples • Helps estimate the age of foetus by measuring various landmarks such as the skull, femur or crown-rump length • Helps estimate foetal growth and weight • Helps locate foetal organs and structures for inspection, measurement, diagnosis or treatment • Helps assess the position and condition of the placenta and cord • Detects how foetus is lying in uterus, showing presentation and position • Helps assess amniotic fluid volume to detect polyhydramnios (too much fluid) or oligohydramnios (too little fluid) • Helps evaluate foetal characteristics and amniotic fluid volume for a bio-physical profile • Helps confirm diagnosis if other testing shows a possible problem • Measures length of cervix to determine effacement	• Adds expense to prenatal care • Can determine whether the pregnancy is uterine or ectopic • Accuracy varies depending on the quality of equipment, skill of person interpreting results and gestational age of foetus. • Can detect structural defects such as spina bifida and heart defects • Can screen for some chromosomal defects, such as Down syndrome, that have associated structural components • Gives immediate results • Vaginal ultrasound may be better for detecting some problems such as placenta praevia and ectopic pregnancy. • Appears safe; should only be used if medically indicated • The technician performing the ultrasound usually does not give information. A physician reports the results either to the woman or to her regular caregiver. • May provide estimate of baby's gender. (Accuracy depends on age of foetus, foetal position and quality of testing.)

Prenatal Examinations and Tests

Diagnostic Test	Purpose	Comments
Vaginal/cervical smear At any time during pregnancy, secretions from the mother's vagina or cervical area can be obtained with a swab or suction bulb and then examined with a microscope or cultured in a laboratory.	• Detects organisms that cause infections (bacteria, virus, fungus or protozoa) • Determines if premature rupture of membranes has occurred • May be used to evaluate the lipid content of amniotic fluid with premature rupture of membranes to determine foetal lung maturity • Used to measure the level of foetal fibronectin, which may help identify those at risk for preterm labour	• See page 63 about infections in pregnancy and childbirth. • Carries a very slight risk of introducing an infection • Amniotic fluid is less acidic (lower pH) than urine and it has a fern-like appearance under the microscope. • See page 60 about preterm labour.
X-ray Ionising radiation is used to take an internal picture of the mother and the foetus.	• Helps estimate size and shape of mother's pelvis (pelvimetry) • Helps discover foetal position and presentation and number of babies	• Rarely used in pregnant women today • Poor predictor of 'fit' of baby when used for pelvimetry • Early prenatal exposure to radiation has been associated with leukemia and genetic mutations in babies. • Should be done only after the first trimester

Chapter 4

Nutrition in Pregnancy

The quality of the foods you eat before and during pregnancy affects your baby's health as much as or more than any other single factor. Therefore, you should know how to provide the best nourishment for yourself and your unborn child.

It is never too late in pregnancy to improve your eating habits. Your baby will benefit whenever you make any needed changes, even in late pregnancy. In fact, your baby's requirements for iron, protein and calcium are greatest in the last eight to twelve weeks of pregnancy. Permanent improvements in your diet will give your children other long-term benefits, since they will grow up with better eating habits and will feed their own families better.

Over the years, there has been much misunderstanding of what constitutes good nutrition during pregnancy. Such matters as weight gain, calorie intake, the use of salt, what foods to eat and avoid and vitamin supplementation were poorly understood. As a result, women were given erroneous information. Although there is still much to learn, nutritional information today is based on more solid research and a better understanding of the physiology of pregnancy.

Good Nutrition during Pregnancy

During pregnancy, you supply all the nutrients for your developing baby, who will weigh an average of 3–3.4 kilogram at birth. Your baby's life-support system (the placenta, uterus, membranes, fluid and maternal blood supply) grows during pregnancy, developing as necessary to meet her increasing needs. Your body also prepares to nourish your baby after birth by storing some of the nutrients she will receive in your breast milk. These added demands require that you nourish yourself adequately; otherwise, your pregnancy may deplete you and deprive

Sample Daily Menu during Pregnancy*

Breakfast

- wholegrain cereal (e.g. muesli, wheat biscuit)
- milk (fat-reduced)
- toast (wholemeal)
- margarine (thin spread of polyunsaturated or monounsaturated)
- fresh fruit or unsweetened fruit juice (fruit contains more fibre)

Lunch

- sandwich or roll (wholemeal bread) with fillings of lean meat, fish or cottage cheese
- salad
- fruit
- milk or yoghurt (fat-reduced)

Dinner

- lean red meat, chicken, fish or bean dish
- salad or cooked vegetables (green and yellow)
- fruit
- milk pudding or fat-reduced yoghurt, ice-cream occasionally

Snacks (options for completing the number of servings recommended on the Food Pyramid)

- water
- milk (fat-reduced)
- yoghurt (fat-reduced)
- fresh or dried fruit
- raw vegetables

*See 'Food Pyramid Groups and Servings' for other food choices (page 90).

your baby of important nutrients.

Which foods (and how much of them) should you eat to ensure the best possible pregnancy outcome? Why are these foods important? How much weight should you gain while pregnant? What about salt, fluid retention, special diets, heartburn, nausea and vomiting? A discussion of these questions, some practical advice, and an opportunity to evaluate your own diet are provided in this chapter.

In the last two trimesters of your pregnancy, you will need about 300 calories per day more than you did before pregnancy. For the average woman, this amounts to approximately 2100–2500 calories per day. These added calories should be in the form of high-protein, high-calcium and iron-rich foods. Three hundred calories are really not all that much—2 tall glasses of milk, a bowl of hearty soup, a serving of meat or 3 tablespoons of peanut butter. Avoid adding calories to your diet with high-calorie foods lacking in nutrition, such as chips, cake, biscuits, sweets and soft drinks.

Basically, a good daily pregnancy diet is a varied diet that includes plenty of fresh fruits and vegetables, whole grains, dairy products, protein foods (meat, fish, nuts, eggs and legumes), some fat (margarine, oil or butter) and about 2 litres of liquids per day.

Food Pyramid

The Food Pyramid was developed by the United States Department of Agriculture (USDA) to provide a visual display of the current dietary recommendations known to promote health. Six food groups make up the pyramid, with the food groups that

Food Pyramid: A Guide to Daily Food Choices

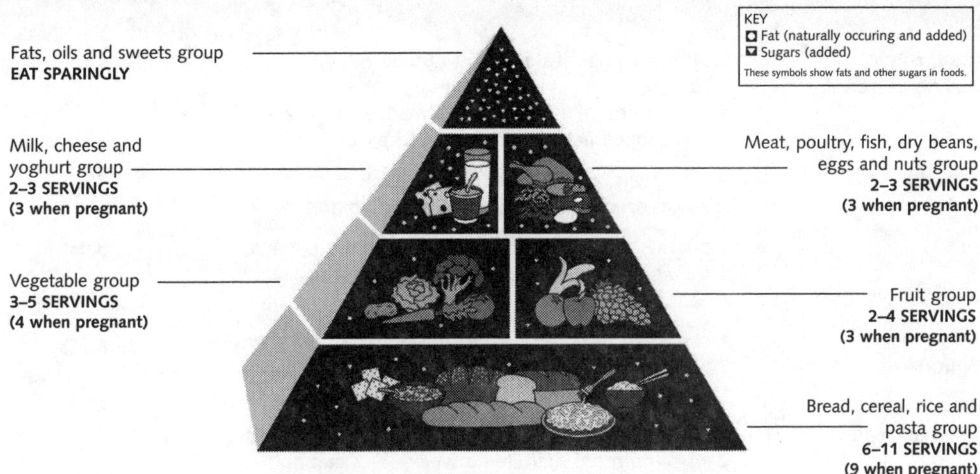
KEY
Fat (naturally occuring and added)
Sugars (added)
These symbols show fats and other sugars in foods.
Fats, oils and sweets group
EAT SPARINGLY
Milk, cheese and yoghurt group
2–3 SERVINGS
(3 when pregnant)
Meat, poultry, fish, dry beans, eggs and nuts group
2–3 SERVINGS
(3 when pregnant)
Vegetable group
3–5 SERVINGS
(4 when pregnant)
Fruit group
2–4 SERVINGS
(3 when pregnant)
Bread, cereal, rice and pasta group
6–11 SERVINGS
(9 when pregnant)

Source: Adapted from the USDA Food Guide Pyramid booklet.

should be most heavily consumed at the foundation and foods that should be consumed sparingly at the top of the pyramid. Intake at a moderate calorie level, using the pyramid as a guide, does meet a pregnant woman's nutritional requirements. Serving recommendations at this moderate calorie level for a pregnant woman are shown in the Food Pyramid charts above and on the next page. In addition to the foods listed in the pyramid, water and fluids are an essential part of the daily diet.[1]

Dietary preferences are greatly influenced by ethnic or cultural background. As you check the 'Food Pyramid Groups and Servings' chart, you will notice that no matter what your preferences, the foods suggested provide you with many choices.

Nutrients

The chart that begins on page 101 presents a brief summary of nutrients (calories, liquids, protein, vitamins and minerals) along with their functions and sources. Recently, the Institute of Medicine adopted a new approach to nutrient recommendations. New Dietary Reference Intakes (DRIs) have been established for most nutrients, expanding and replacing the previous Recommended Daily Allowances (RDAs). The accompanying chart reflects these changes. Certain nutrients are particularly important during pregnancy and deserve special mention.

Food Pyramid Groups and Servings

Food Group	One Serving Equals:	Recommended Daily Servings
Bread, cereal, rice and pasta	1 slice of whoelmeal bread, 1 cup porridge, 1 cup breakfast cereal, 2 weetbix, 4–5 crispbreads, 1 pocket pita bread, 2 rice cakes, ½ cup cooked rice, 1 cup uncooked pasta	9
Vegetable	½ cup green or yellow vegetables (such as corn, pumpkin, spinach, broccoli, carrots, lettuce and potato)	4
Fruit	1 orange, 1 apple, 1 peach, ½ grapefruit, 1 banana, 1 tomato, ⅛ section rock melon, ¼ section papaya, a handful of grapes, 1 kiwifruit, 1 plum	3
Milk, cheese, yoghurt	1 cup milk, 1½ cups cottage cheese, 30 g hard cheese, 220 g carton yoghurt	3
Meat, poultry, fish, dry beans, eggs and nuts	100 g lean red meat meat or chicken, 120 g fish, 1 cup cooked beans (4–5 tablespoons dried beans), 2 eggs (no more than 3–4 a week), ½–⅔ cup nuts	3
Fats, oils and sweets	Eat sparingly. If you are trying to reduce caloric intake, avoid these foods as much as possible.	

Source: Adapted from the Nutrition Australia booklet 'Nutrition for Pregnancy' and the USDA Food Guide Pyramid booklet.

Protein

All cells are formed from protein. Since pregnancy involves the rapid growth of the foetus, placenta, uterus, breasts and the volume of blood and amniotic fluid, your protein requirement increases by about 14 grams over your normal requirement. (See page 101.) Keep in mind that prenatal vitamin and mineral supplements supply no protein. Food is your only source of protein, as protein supplements are not recommended in pregnancy. Be sure that any meat, poultry or fish you eat is well cooked to avoid food-borne illness. In addition, check with your caregiver or local public health department to learn about possible toxins in your sources of meat or fish.

Calcium

Calcium promotes the mineralisation of the foetal skeleton and teeth. The foetus requires approximately 66 percent more calcium during the third trimester (when his teeth are forming and skeletal growth is most rapid) than earlier in his development. Calcium is also stored in the mother's bones as a reserve for production of breast milk. High caffeine intake can interfere with one's ability to use calcium. (See page 108.)

Iron

Iron is required for the production of haemoglobin (the oxygen-carrying protein in the blood). Since blood volume increases by 50 percent during pregnancy, haemoglobin and the other constituents of blood need to increase accordingly. In addition, during the last six weeks of pregnancy, the foetus stores enough iron in his liver to supplement his needs for the first three to six months of life. This is necessary because the main food during that period—breast milk or formula—only partially fulfils an infant's iron requirements. Since a healthy person absorbs only 10–20 percent of the iron ingested, the Institute of Medicine recommends a daily supplement of 30–60 milligrams of iron during pregnancy to ensure absorption of the iron needed each day.[2]

Although necessary for good nutrition, iron supplements upset the digestive tract in many people. The side effects—nausea, heartburn, diarrhoea or constipation—are related to the *amount* of elemental iron given and individual reactions, not to the *type* of preparation. In other words, whether you are taking ferrous sulphate, ferrous fumerate or ferrous gluconate is less important than how much iron you take at a time. To relieve the unpleasant side effects, you may be advised to decrease each dose of iron or take food along with the tablets. Foods rich in vitamin C (citrus fruits, tomatoes) enhance iron absorption, while some antacids interfere with it. Check with your caregiver.

The easiest and most effective way to take iron is to eat a variety of iron-rich foods such as red meats, poultry (especially dark meat), dried fruits, prune juice, dried peas, beans, lentils, oysters, almonds, walnuts and blackstrap molasses.

Essential Fatty Acids

Essential fatty acids in the diet provide lifelong health benefits for everyone. Some essential fatty acids are found in vegetables and plants; others can be found in oily fish. When consumed by the mother during pregnancy and lactation, essential fatty acids contribute to the healthy neurological development of the baby.

Since the amount of essential fatty acids found in fish is much larger than the amount in vegetables, the best advice based on research is to consume oily fish (such as salmon) before, during and after pregnancy. If you do not eat fish, consult your care provider for other ways to get fatty acids. Breast milk (unlike formula) naturally contains essential fatty acids. Breast milk is the best source of long-chain polyunsaturated fatty acids for infants.[3]

Vitamins

Vitamins are essential to most life functions. (See the chart on pages 101–104.) Vitamins are classified by their solubility: water-soluble (vita-mins C and B complex) and fat-soluble (vitamins A, D, E and K). The water-soluble vitamins can be lost in cooking. Vege-tables high in these vitamins should be eaten raw or briefly cooked in small amounts of water, stir-fried or steamed.

Folic acid is a water-soluble vitamin in the B complex. Folic acid is essential for the baby's normal growth from conception on and is especially important in early pregnancy. Since folic acid intakes from food are often low, a daily supplement of 400 micrograms (0.4 milligram) is recommended for all women of childbearing age.

The only way to make sure you get all the vitamins and minerals you need is to eat a varied, high-quality diet. While most pregnant women take a prenatal vitamin as a supplement to their diet, it is not a good idea to depend solely on vitamin or mineral supplements to make up for a poor diet. There are other nutrients present in food about which we still know very little. They may be present only in trace amounts, and their functions are not yet fully understood. Because vitamin manufacturers do not include them in their preparations, food is your only source.

Fluid Balance

Salt

For years, pregnant women were told to eliminate or restrict their use of salt. The rationale for this policy was based on the tendency of the pregnant woman to retain fluid, which was assumed to cause pre-eclampsia. (See Chapter 3 for a discussion of pre-eclampsia.) It is now known that gradual, moderate water retention in pregnancy is not only normal, it is necessary to ensure an adequate volume of blood and amniotic fluid. The abnormal, sudden increase in fluid retention seen in pre-eclampsia is not due to excessive salt intake but rather to the impaired functioning of the liver and kidneys, which normally regulate protein, electrolyte and fluid balance. Adequate salt intake during pregnancy is now known to be important in maintaining fluid balance. The wise pregnant woman does as any well-nourished person does; she salts her food to taste.

Fluids

As stated earlier, water and other fluids are essential elements of a balanced diet. Fluid retention, a normal part of a healthy pregnancy, ensures the increase in blood and amniotic fluid volume. As a pregnant woman, you need to retain more fluid for two reasons:

- Your blood volume increases by 50 percent or more (from approximately 3 to 4 litres).
- Towards the end of pregnancy, your baby is immersed in about 1 litre of amniotic fluid, which is replaced every three hours. Fluid is also retained in your tissues, shifting across blood vessel walls, to help maintain a healthy balance of fluids. It is estimated that tissue fluid volume increases by 2–3.5 litres during pregnancy.

During pregnancy, try to drink at least 2 litres of liquids (water, milk and fruit juice) a day. This is difficult if you are not in the habit of drinking enough fluids. It may be helpful to fill a 1-litre container with water, put it in the refrigerator at home (or take a 1-litre bottle of water to work), and drink from it throughout the day, making sure it is empty by bedtime. In addition, plan to have a glass of milk or other liquid with each meal and at snack times. You can easily develop this habit with a little conscientious effort.

Weight Gain

How much weight should you gain during pregnancy? No single amount is appropriate for every pregnant woman. Proper weight gain depends on many variables: your pre-pregnancy weight and stature, the size of your baby and placenta, the quality of your diet before and during pregnancy, your ethnic background and your number of previous pregnancies.[4] Until the early 1970s, most Australian obstetricians placed great emphasis on limiting weight gain to between 6.5 and 8 kilograms, believing this range would result in easier labours and less post-partum obesity. It was assumed that the foetus always managed to extract the necessary nutrients from the mother. This may have been the advice your mother received when she was pregnant with you. Research now shows that a weight gain of 9–16 kilograms results in more full-term pregnancies and healthier babies.

If your pre-pregnancy weight was below normal, it may be wise for you to gain more weight than a woman who is of normal weight or overweight. If your baby is large (over 3.6 kilograms) the chances are that your placenta is also larger than average. In this case, it stands to reason that you will gain more weight than if your baby and placenta are of average or small size.

If the quality of your diet is normally excellent and you and your baby are of average size, you will probably gain between 9 and 16 kilograms. If, on the other hand, you are well-nourished but overweight, you may gain less weight. Excessively large weight gains may increase the risk of delivery complications and increase the difficulty of returning to your normal weight after the baby is born.

The point to keep in mind is that your weight gain is less important than the quality of your diet. If you eat consistently well and in appropriate quantities, and if you maintain an active lifestyle that includes moderate exercise, you can trust that the amount of weight you gain is right for you.

You may be weighed at each prenatal visit. Weight gain is typically slow early in pregnancy and increases rapidly as the baby grows and the placental system develops to meet her requirements. A maternal weight gain of 1–2 kilograms by the end of the first trimester is fairly typical. Of course, other amounts are common, too. A sudden, excessive gain or drop in weight can be a sign of illness or other problems, or it may be a sign that during the last week you ate more or less.

If you gain 12.3 kilograms and have a 3.4 kilogram baby, where does the rest of the weight go? The list below shows approximately how the weight is distributed during pregnancy.

Average Weight Gain Distribution during Pregnancy

Baby	3.4 kg
Placenta	450 g
Uterus	900 g
Amniotic fluid	900 g
Breasts	450 g
Blood volume	1.1 kg
Fat	2.3 kg
Tissue fluid	2.8 kg
Total	**12.3 kg**

Most women accept the weight they put on during pregnancy, especially when they realise that most of it is lost either during birth or shortly thereafter. But what about that extra 2.3 kilograms or more of fat? Since it may take weeks or months before that disappears, many weight-conscious women dislike putting on fat during pregnancy. Consider the following:

- It is not possible to gain only the weight necessary for the baby and placenta, and avoid adding the fat. The fat is not the last 2.3 kilograms of weight you gain, so it cannot be avoided if you stop gaining weight at 10 kilograms instead of 12.3 kilograms. In fact, fat is produced gradually along with the other components of the weight gain. Trying to avoid the fat may deprive you or your baby of essential nutrients.
- Most women are able to lose their extra weight gradually over a period of several months after the baby is born—that is, if they maintain sensible eating habits and exercise adequately. Breastfeeding promotes the loss of these extra pounds because calories are required for milk production. The stored fat provides some of these calories; the rest come from additional calories consumed by the breastfeeding mother. The usual recommendation for a breastfeeding woman is to add 500 calories per day above the requirement for a non-pregnant woman.

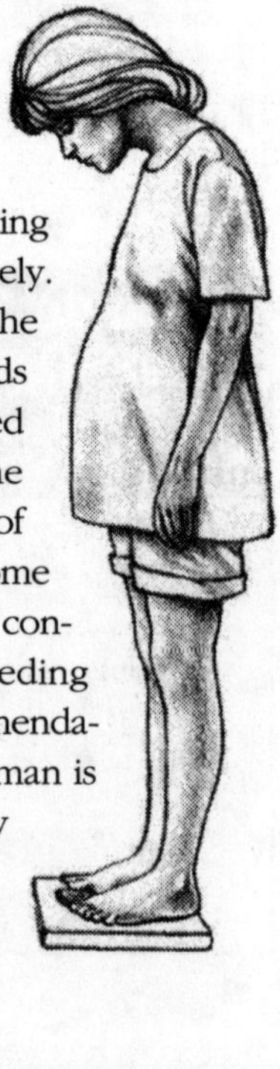

This should be individualised as described on page 441 in Chapter 15.

The key point is that pregnancy is not a time to lose weight or overeat. It is a time to concentrate on a high-quality diet.

In summary: by gaining an appropriate amount of weight, eating a well-balanced diet, using salt as desired, drinking a generous amount of liquids, and supplementing your diet with a prenatal vitamin and mineral supplement that includes iron and folic acid, you are following the nutritional guidelines most likely to produce a healthy baby and mother.

Food Additives

Aspartame: A Sugar Substitute

The sugar substitute aspartame (marketed as NutraSweet or Equal) is present in numerous products including diet drinks, chewing gum, desserts and vitamins. Aspartame is a combination of two amino acids, phenylalanine and aspartic acid, both of which are known to be toxic at high levels. Unlike other artificial sweeteners, aspartame has never been found to increase the risk of cancer, and there are no reports associating birth defects with the use of aspartame in pregnancy. But, even though the Food and Drug Administration (FDA) has established a safe upper limit of aspartame for adults (3.4 grams of aspartame per day for a 68-kilogram adult, which is equivalent to fifteen 375-millilitres cans of soft drink), it has not addressed the issue of safe levels for pregnant women and their unborn babies. Even if such levels were known, food companies usually do not list the amount of aspartame in food products. This makes it difficult to determine how much you take in and even more difficult to determine whether a safe level for the foetus has been exceeded. In addition, aspartame does not contribute to good nutrition, as does milk or juice. Probably the best advice is to limit or avoid aspartame during pregnancy. Few people really need artificial sweeteners. Sparkling water sweetened with a dash of fruit juice may be just as satisfying as diet soft drinks.

Olestra: A Fat Substitute

Olestra, a fat substitute, has been approved by the FDA for use in certain snack foods such as chips and crackers. Olestra is made of a non-absorbable mixture of sucrose (a type of sugar) and fatty acid. It does not add fat calories to the food, but it does sometimes cause abdominal cramping and loose stools. It also prevents the absorption of fat-soluble vitamins (A, D, E and K) and other nutrients such as carotenoids (found in carrots, sweet potatoes and green leafy vegetables). In an effort to counteract this effect, vitamins A, D, E and K have been added to products containing olestra. This is of questionable benefit. Olestra has not been shown to be harmful to pregnant women. (For more information, call The Dietitians Association of Australia on 02 6282 9798.)

Common Concerns

Several nutrition-related problems commonly arise during pregnancy due to normal changes in hormone production and the increased size and weight of the uterus. The following pages discuss these problems, their causes and their treatments.

Nausea and Vomiting

As noted earlier, nausea and vomiting are sometimes referred to as morning sickness (although for many women it is not restricted to the morning). Pregnant women frequently feel nauseated and may vomit when they have not eaten for several hours or when they smell certain odours such as cigar smoke, a stuffy room or certain foods being cooked. Although the trigger may vary from woman to woman, the problem is common.

With today's emphasis on good nutrition, you may worry about your baby's health if nausea and vomiting are a problem. Studies indicate, however, that women who are healthy when they conceive have sufficient reserves to supply the growing embryo and foetus, even if they are unable to eat well for the first several months.[5]

Be assured that nausea is neither abnormal nor a sign of unconscious rejection of the baby, as is sometimes thought. The cause is probably related to the body's increased production of twenty-six hormones, plus the manufacture of at least four other hormones produced only during pregnancy. Some of these hormones, when present in large quantities, may cause nausea until the body adjusts.

Treatment

- Try modifying your eating habits. You may find it helpful to eat several (five or six) small meals a day to avoid an empty stomach and to help maintain a stable blood sugar level. Include some protein in each of these meals. Eating crackers, a bagel or toast whenever you feel queasy is also helpful. To prevent morning sickness, try leaving bland food, such as crackers, by your bed at night and eating some of this food just before you get up. Trust your food preferences. What sounds good to eat will probably be best tolerated.
- Try increasing your intake of foods rich in vitamin B_6 (pyridoxine), such as whole grains and cereals, wheat germ, nuts, seeds, legumes and corn. Vitamin B_6 supplements, as prescribed by a caregiver, can effectively reduce nausea for some women.[6] Large amounts of vitamin B_6, however, have been associated with toxic effects. It is wise to discuss safe amounts with your caregiver, a nutritionist or another health professional.
- Some women find acupressure wristbands (Sea-Bands) to be an effective way to treat nausea. These can be purchased from boating stores or travel agencies.
- Ginger is sometimes recommended to treat nausea. You can eat ginger in foods or drink ginger tea or a natural ale. Supplements of dried, powdered ginger root are not recommended in pregnancy, as one of the compounds they contain has been linked to cell mutation.
- Know that the nausea and vomiting will usually pass within three to four months.
- Try to maintain a sense of humour. For some women, throwing up becomes as much a part of their morning routine as brushing their teeth and combing their hair. Their attitude has much to do with how well they cope with this condition.
- On very rare occasions, nausea and vomiting are severe and a woman actually becomes dehydrated, loses a great deal of weight and is unable to retain any food. This condition (called hyperemesis

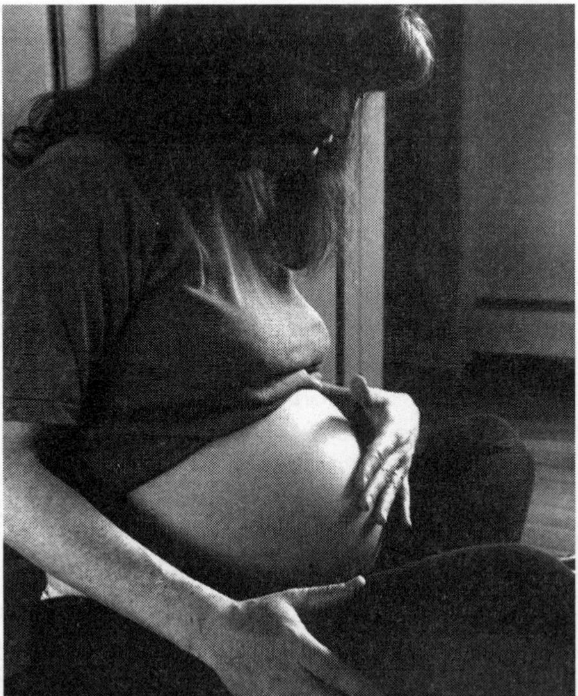

Photograph by Marilyn Nolt

Your body knows how to nourish and grow a baby.

gravidarum) may require medication or even hospitalisation if the nausea and vomiting endanger the health of the mother and/or baby.

- Medications are available to help control severe nausea and vomiting. However, these medications cross the placenta to the foetus and their safety to the unborn baby has not been established. Therefore, weigh the risks of the nausea and vomiting against the potential risks of the medications. It is wise to try the non-medical forms of treatment first and to think twice before requesting medication.

Heartburn

Heartburn (a feeling of fullness accompanied by the burping up of stomach acid) is a common complaint in late pregnancy. Heartburn is caused by a combination of increased pressure from the growing uterus and the hormonal effects that relax the muscular opening at the top of the stomach and cause the stomach to empty more slowly. Fatty foods, foods that produce gas and large meals may make the heartburn worse.

Treatment

- Avoid fatty food and foods that produce gas or heartburn.
- Eat several small meals rather than a few large meals. Some women find that eating slowly and not eating just before bedtime also help reduce heartburn.
- Semi-sitting rather than lying flat in bed may decrease discomfort.
- Antacids or other drugs are sometimes used to control heartburn, but they should be used only if necessary. Consult your caregiver for recommendations for safe antacids and to learn about possible undesirable side effects.

Constipation

During pregnancy, the movement of food through the intestines is slowed. This allows for greater absorption of nutrients and water, but also sometimes causes constipation. Pressure from the growing uterus on the large intestine magnifies the problem. Some iron supplements may also aggravate this common condition.

Treatment

- Drink plenty of fluids and eat high-fibre foods such as fruits and vegetables, whole grains, bran and prune juice. They encourage elimination.
- Exercise regularly. Exercise, such as walking, is an often neglected but effective aid to regularity.
- If proper diet and exercise do not prevent constipation, you can try over-the-counter high-fibre products containing psyllium seed. Such products are safe and effective in adding soft bulk to the stool. Intestinal stimulants (laxatives) should be avoided.
- If you are taking an iron supplement, ask your caregiver about the possibility of changing to an iron supplement that might be less constipating.

Prevention of constipation helps to alleviate the discomfort of haemorrhoids, another common problem during pregnancy.

Food Cravings and Pica

Pregnant women frequently find themselves craving specific food in large quantities. Sometimes, foods they otherwise rarely eat are especially desired, such as hot peppers or other hot or spicy foods, one flavour of ice cream, potatoes or other foods. Although we do not understand such cravings, they are probably harmless unless they interfere with good nutrition. Cravings for non-food items are also common during pregnancy.

Eating non-foods in response to a craving is called *pica*. Pregnant women have reported craving and eating ice, baking soda, baking powder, cornflour, dirt, clay, cigarette ashes and other non-food substances.[8] Women have also described cravings to smell substances such as gasoline, fingernail polish remover, bleach, ammonia, pine oil disinfectant and body powder.

Along with these unusual cravings comes a need to keep the craving secret. Many women feel confused and isolated because of their behaviour. They worry about the effect these substances have on their developing baby. Many women are reluctant to share their cravings and concerns with their health care provider. Worry or shame about the cravings even causes some women to avoid prenatal care.

Eating non-food products and smelling substances like gasoline are associated with symptoms such as constipation, bowel obstruction, elevated blood pressure and anaemia. If you have non-food cravings, seek the help of a health care provider, childbirth educator or counsellor with whom you feel comfortable. Show your provider this section of this book (including the reference). He or she can help you find out if your craving presents a danger to you or your baby. Your provider can also help you find ways to cope with the craving and to avoid those harmful substances.

Nutrition-related Birth Defects

Folic acid supplements taken before conception and during early pregnancy have been shown to dramatically reduce the incidence of neural tube defects and oro-facial clefts (cleft lip and cleft palate). *Neural tube defects* are due to incomplete prenatal development of the structures of the central nervous system (the brain and the spinal cord). These defects cause conditions such as anencephaly, encephalocele and spina bifida.[9]

Neural tube defects occur in one of every one thousand births. When women take 0.4 milligram (400 micrograms) of folic acid as a supplement beginning at least one month before conception and continuing at least until the third month of pregnancy, there is a 72 percent reduction in the incidence of neural tube defects. Women who have had a child with a neural tube defect are advised to take 4 milligrams of folic acid at least one month before conception and during the first three months of pregnancy. Taking this amount of folic acid reduces the risk of recurrence by five times.

Another group of researchers found that women who took a multivitamin containing folic acid during the period from one month before pregnancy through two months after conception had 25–50 percent fewer infants with clefts in the lip or palate.[10] Since at least 40 percent of all pregnancies are unplanned, it is recommended that all women capable of becoming pregnant should take 0.4 milligram of folic acid daily throughout their reproductive years. Check your food labels as many cereals and bread are fortified with folic acid.

Vitamin A, taken in amounts above the recommended daily allowance in the first seven weeks of gestation, is associated with a higher incidence of defects of the cranial-neural-crest tissue. These defects include cranio-facial anomalies, defects in the central nervous system (not including neural tube defects) and defects of the thymus gland and heart. When pregnant women took more than 10,000 IU (more than double the recommended amount) of vitamin A, one in every fifty-seven infants of these mothers had a malformation attributable to the supplement.[11]

Special Circumstances

Good nutrition in pregnancy is always an important concern, but in some circumstances you need to be even more aware of the foods you eat. If your pregnancy is a 'special pregnancy' or if you are on a special diet, your nutritional demands will be greater than normal.

If you are in one or more of the following categories, seek nutritional counselling and be particularly conscientious about eating nutritious foods. Nutritional counselling is available from your midwife, your physician or a nutritionist. These professionals can help you plan your diet in a practical and beneficial way.

Special Pregnancies

Multiple Pregnancy

If you are carrying two or more babies, you need to consume more calories and more nutrients. (For further information on nutrition in multiple pregnancies, see the Recommended Resources.)

Adolescent Pregnancy

If you are a teenager, you are still growing and have greater-than-adult requirements for most nutrients. You need to eat particularly well when pregnant to maintain your own growth while nourishing your foetus.

Pregnancies Close Together

Sometimes, a pregnancy depletes your reserves of certain nutrients such as calcium and iron. If you have sufficient time between pregnancies to replenish those reserves, no nutritional deficiency occurs. However, if your pregnancies are very close together, your reserves may be depleted and you may need extra calories and nutrients. The length of time needed between pregnancies to correct deficiencies depends, of course, on your overall nutritional status and the quality of your diet. Talk with your midwife or physician about your individual dietary needs.

Special Diets

Vegetarian Diet

If you are a vegetarian, you can, with knowledge and careful planning, adequately nourish yourself and your unborn baby, especially if you include milk and eggs in your diet. Your major concerns are these: the need to take in sufficient calories, the need to choose a variety of protein-rich foods to obtain all the essential proteins each day, and, for vegans, the need to supplement vitamin B_{12}, which is found mostly in animal protein. (See Recommended Resources for references on vegetarian diets.) The information in this chapter applies to both the vegetarian and the meat eater.

Milk Intolerance

If you cannot tolerate milk, explore other ways to get enough calcium. Try cultured forms of milk—such as cheese, yoghurt and acidophilus milk—which are often well tolerated by people who are upset by milk. Another option is to drink low-lactose milk, which contains lactase (an enzyme that helps convert the lactose in milk into a more digestible sugar). If you simply do not like the taste of milk, try cooking with dry-powdered milk or eating cream soups and cheeses. These alternatives will give you the benefits of milk without its taste. If your diet does not usually contain dairy products, you will need other foods rich in calcium. If you are not meeting your needs through your diet, however, you may need calcium supplements. Consult your physician or midwife if this is a problem for you.

Food Allergies

If you have significant food allergies, you may need a nutritionist to help you plan a healthful pregnancy diet. Sometimes, the elimination of problem foods leads to an inadequate diet, so you will need careful guidance.

Anorexia and Bulimia

If you have been anorexic or are struggling with bulimia, it may be more difficult for you to accept the weight gain and body changes that occur with pregnancy. In addition, you may be at risk for a poor pregnancy outcome. Nutritional and psychological counselling may be beneficial for your wellbeing and the health of your baby. Many urban areas have anorexia and bulimia support groups that may be helpful as well.

Medical Problems

If you are pregnant and have a medical problem such as diabetes, anaemia, or heart or lung disease, you will need special nutritional guidance and close prenatal observation and management. It is beyond the scope of this book to cover such medical problems that may exist during pregnancy, except to emphasise the necessity of thorough prenatal care. Be sure you understand and follow the instructions you are given for any medical problems.

Nutrients, Vitamins, and Minerals

Key Nutrient and Daily Recommendation	Important Functions	Major Sources	Comments
Calories N: 2,200 P: 2200 (1st trimester) P: 2500 (2nd & 3rd trimesters) L: 2700	• Provide energy for tissue building and increased metabolic requirements	Carbohydrates, fats, proteins	Caloric requirements vary depending on your stage of pregnancy, size, activity level, pre-pregnant weight and how well nourished you are.
Water and other liquids N: 4 cups P: 8+ cups L: 8+ cups	• Carry nutrients to cells and carry waste products away • Provide fluid for increased blood, tissue and amniotic fluid volume • Help regulate body temperature • Aids digestion	Water, juices, milk	Liquid is often neglected, but it is an important nutrient.
Protein (RDA*) N: 46–50 g P: 60 g L: 65 g	• Builds and repairs tissues • Helps build blood, amniotic fluid and placenta • Helps form antibodies	Meat, fish, poultry, eggs, milk, cheese, dried beans and peas, peanut butter, nuts, whole grains, cereals	Foetal requirements increase by about ⅓ in late pregnancy during the baby's growth period.
Minerals			
Calcium (DRI†) N: 1000–1300 mg P & L: <18 yrs: 1300 mg 19–50 yrs: 1000 mg	• Helps build bones and teeth • Important in blood clotting	Milk, cheese, whole grains, vegetables, egg yolk, canned fish (with bones), ice cream	Foetal requirements increase in late pregnancy. Absorption increases in pregnancy.
Phosphorus (DRI) N: 700–1250 mg P & L: <18 yrs: 1250 mg 19–50 yrs: 700 mg	• Helps build bones and teeth	Milk, cheese, lean meats	Calcium and phosphorus exist in a constant ratio in the blood. An excess of phosphorus limits the use of calcium.

KEY:

N: non-pregnant
P: pregnant
L: lactating (first 6 months)

g: grams
mg: milligrams
mcg: micrograms
IU: International Units

Nutrients, Vitamins, and Minerals

Key Nutrient and Daily Recommendation	Important Functions	Major Sources	Comments
Iron (DRI) N: 15–18 mg P: 27 mg L: 9–10 mg	• Combines with protein to make haemoglobin • Provides iron for foetal storage	Liver, red meats, egg yolk, whole grains, leafy vegetables, nuts, legumes, dried fruits, prunes, prune and apple juice	Foetal requirements increase tenfold in last 6 weeks of pregnancy. Daily supplement of 30 mg of iron is recommended by the Institute of Medicine. 60–120 mg is recommended for anaemia.
Zinc (DRI) N: 8 mg P: 11–13 mg L: 12–14 mg	• Component of insulin • Important in growth of skeleton and nervous system	Meat, liver, eggs, seafood (especially oysters)	Deficiency has been associated with poor foetal growth and development.
Iodine (DRI) N: 150 mcg P: 220 mcg L: 290 mcg	• Helps control the rate of body's energy use • Important in thyroxine production	Seafoods, iodised salt	Deficiency may cause goitre in mother and developmental disorders in infants.
Magnesium (DRI) N: 310–360 mg P: <18 yrs: 400 mg 19–30 yrs: 350 mg 31–50 yrs: 360 mg L: <18 yrs: 360 mg 19–30 yrs: 310 mg 31–60 yrs: 320 mg	• Helps energy, protein and cell metabolism • Enzyme activator • Helps tissue growth and muscle action	Nuts, cocoa, green vegetables, whole grains, dried beans and peas	Most is stored in bones. Deficiency may cause neuromuscular dysfunction.
Fat-Soluble Vitamins			
Vitamin A (DRI) N: 700 mcg RE[‡] P: <18 yrs: 750 mcg 19–50 yrs: 770 mcg L: <18 yrs: 1200 mcg 19–50 yrs: 1300 mcg *Note:* 800 mcg RE is equivalent to 5000 International Units (IU).	• Helps bone and tissue growth and development • Essential in development of enamel-forming cells in gum tissue • Helps maintain health of skin and mucous membranes • Helps protect against infection	Butter, whole and fortified milk, deeply coloured vegetables, eggs, fish oils, liver	Toxic to foetus in excessive amounts. It can be toxic to mother above 25,000 IU. It loses its potency when exposed to light. It can be converted from beta-carotene in the body.

KEY:
N: non-pregnant
P: pregnant
L: lactating (first 6 months)
g: grams
mg: milligrams
mcg: micrograms
IU: International Units

Nutrients, Vitamins, and Minerals

Key Nutrient and Daily Recommendation	Important Functions	Major Sources	Comments
Vitamin D (DRI) N: 5 mcg P: 5 mcg L: 5 mcg	• Aids absorption of calcium from the blood • Needed for mineralisation of bones and teeth	Fortified milk, fish liver oils, fatty fish, egg yolks	Toxic to foetus in excessive amounts. It is manufactured by the body with adequate sunlight on the skin.
Vitamin E (DRI) N: 15 mg ∞-TE[§] P: 15 mg ∞-TE L: 19 mg ∞-TE	• Needed for tissue growth • Protects cell wall integrity	Vegetable oils, cereals, meat, eggs, milk, nuts, seeds	Enhances absorption of vitamin A. It is an antioxidant.
Vitamin K (DRI) N: 75–90 mcg P: <18 yrs: 75 mcg 19–50 yrs: 90 mcg L: <18 yrs: 75 mcg 19–50 yrs: 90 mcg	• Essential for the synthesis of blood clotting factors	Leafy green vegetables	Produced in the body by intestinal flora
Water-Soluble Vitamins			
Folic acid (folate) (DRI) N: 400 mcg P: 600 mcg L: 500 mcg	• Participates in DNA and RNA synthesis in rapidly growing cells • Essential in haemoglobin synthesis • Needed for synthesis of amino acids	Leafy green vegetables, yeast and enriched flour, grains, cereals	Supplement of 400 micrograms per day is recommended for all women of childbearing age to prevent neural tube defects in babies. During pregnancy, plan to get the extra 200 mcg from foods. Deficiency leads to anaemia. Can be destroyed in cooking and storage. Oral contraceptives may reduce blood level of folic acid.
Thiamin (B_1) (DRI) N: 1.0–1.1 mg P: 1.4 mg L: 1.4 mg	• Helps convert food to energy • Plays a role in initiating nerve impulses	Pork, yeast, organ meats, whole and fortified grain products, legumes, seeds, nuts	Essential for conversion of carbohydrates into energy in the muscular and nervous systems
Riboflavin (B_2) (DRI) N: 1.0–1.1 mg P: 1.4 mg L: 1.6 mg	• Essential for energy and protein metabolism	Milk products, lean meat, whole and fortified grains, leafy greens	Oral contraceptives may reduce serum concentration of riboflavin.
Niacin (B_3) (DRI) N: 14 mg P: 18 mg L: 17 mg	• Helps release energy from carbohydrates • Needed for protein metabolism • Aids production of lipids, hormones and red blood cells	Meats, peanuts, beans, peas, fortified cereals, whole grains	Stable; only small amounts are lost in food preparation.

Nutrients, Vitamins, and Minerals

Key Nutrient and Daily Recommendation	Important Functions	Major Sources	Comments
Vitamin B_6 (Pyridoxine) (DRI) N: 1.2–1.5 mg P: 1.9 mg L: 2.0 mg	• Important in amino acid metabolism and protein synthesis • Required for foetal growth	Chicken, fish, organ meats, pork, eggs, unprocessed cereals, oats, soybeans, brown rice, nuts, seeds, legumes	Excessive amounts may reduce milk supply in lactating women. May help reduce nausea in early pregnancy.
Vitamin B_{12} (Cobalamin) (DRI) N: 2.4 mcg P: 2.6 mcg L: 2.8 mcg	• Aids folate function • Essential in protein metabolism • Important in formation of red blood cells • Maintains nerve fibres	Organ meats, milk products, clams, oysters, eggs	Deficiency leads to anaemia and central nervous system damage. Is manufactured by micro-organisms in the intestinal tract. Oral contraceptives may reduce serum concentration.
Pantothenic acid (DRI) N: 5 mg P: 6 mg L: 7 mg	• Helps convert food into energy • Aids production of lipids, hormones and neuro-transmitters	Meats, whole grains, legumes	
Biotin (DRI) N: 25–30 mcg P: 30 mcg L: 35 mcg	• Aids energy metabolism • Synthesises and breaks down fatty acids	Egg yolks, soybeans, yeast	
Vitamin C (DRI) N: 65–75 mg P: <18 yrs: 80 mg 19–50 yrs: 85 mg L: <18 yrs: 115 mg 19–50 yrs: 120 mg	• Helps tissue formation and prevents cell damage • Is 'cement' substance in connective and vascular tissue • Promotes iron absorption	Citrus fruits, peppers, green vegetables, tomatoes, berries, melons, potatoes, fortified cereals	Large supplemental doses in pregnancy may create a larger-than-normal need in infant. Benefits of large doses in preventing colds have not been confirmed. Is an antioxidant.

KEY:

N:	non-pregnant	g:	grams
P:	pregnant	mg:	milligrams
L:	lactating (first 6 months)	mcg:	micrograms
		IU:	International Units

*RDA: Recommended Dietary Allowances. The average daily intake level that is sufficient to meet the nutrient requirement of nearly all healthy individuals (97–98 percent) in a group.

†DRI: Dietary Reference Intakes. In January 2000, the Institute of Medicine established DRIs to replace the previous categories of Recommended Dietary Allowances (RDA) and Adequate Intakes (AI). For nutrients that have not yet been updated, RDA is used.

‡RE: Retinol equivalent. Note: 800 mcg RE equals 5000 International Units (IU).

§∞-TE: Alpha tocopherol (the most active form of vitamin E).

Sources: Food and Nutrition Board Institute of Medicine. *Dietary Reference Intakes for Thiamin, Riboflavin, Niacin, Vitamin B_6, Folate, Vitamin B_{12}, Pantothenic acid, Biotin and Choline*. Washington D.C.: National Academy Press, 1998.

Food and Nutrition Board Institute of Medicine. *Dietary Reference Intakes for Calcium, Phosphorus, Magnesium, Vitamin D and Fluoride*. Washington D.C.: National Academy Press, 1998.

E.R. Monsen, 'Dietary Reference Intakes for the Antioxidant Nutrients: Vitamin C, Vitamin E, Selenium and Carotenoids', *Journal of the American Dietetic Association* 100 (June 2000): 637–40.

P. Trumbo et al., 'Dietary Reference Intakes: Vitamin A, Vitamin K, Arsenic, Boron, Chromium, Copper, Iodine, Iron, Manganese, Molybdenum, Nickel, Silicon, Vanadium, and Zinc', *Journal of the American Dietetic Association* 101 (3) (March 2001): 294–301.

Diet Diary

Photocopy this chart and use it to record what and when you eat. Opposite each food group, indicate how many servings you eat on each day. If you eat a serving of the food at breakfast, use the letter B; if at lunch, L; if at dinner, D; and if as a snack, S. Compare your diet with the recommendations. Try checking yourself several times during your pregnancy, especially if you find you need to change some of your eating habits.

Food Group	Number of Recommended Daily Servings*	Sample Day	Day 1	Day 2	Day 3	Changes to Make
Bread, cereal, rice and pasta	9	BB, LLL DD, SS				
Vegetable	4	LL, DDDD				
Fruit	3	BB, L, D				
Milk, cheese and yoghurt	3	B, L, D, S				
Meat, poultry, fish, dry beans, eggs and nuts	3	LL, D				
Fats, oils and sweets	Eat sparingly	B, L, DD				
Water/liquids	8+ cups	BB, LL, D, SSS				

*See the 'Food Pyramid Groups and Servings' chart for a description of serving sizes (page 90).

Chapter 5

Drugs, Medications and Environmental Hazards in Pregnancy

In recent years, studies have examined the effects of various drugs and environmental agents on the unborn baby. Until the 1960s, it was assumed that the placenta protected the foetus. Now we know that most drugs and other potentially harmful substances cross the placenta freely. Some cause birth defects; some cause other harmful effects such as slow growth, mental or developmental retardation, or problems in organ development. Some medications may be harmless; others may be beneficial to the foetus. At the least, their effects on the foetus are similar to and (because of the foetus's small size and rapid growth and development) possibly greater than their effect on the mother. The best course to follow when considering the use of a medication is to weigh the possible risks against the possible benefits. Your caregiver can help you with this. If the benefits clearly outweigh the risks, then use the medication; if not, look for alternative treatment.

Are all drugs bad? What about social or 'recreational' drugs such as tobacco and alcohol? What about caffeine and herbs? What about the medicines the mother has been using? What is an environmental hazard? This chapter reviews what is known about the answers to these questions, provides some guidelines on what to avoid, and suggests some substitutes for common social drugs and medications.

Social and Street Drugs

If you are pregnant, be very cautious about using any drug. No drug has been proven safe for all foetuses under all circumstances. Though some drugs are thought to be safe or at least have not been proven to be harmful, others are known to harm the foetus. This section discusses drugs used for social or recreational purposes.

Caffeine

Coffee, tea, colas and other soft drinks (read the labels) contain significant amounts of caffeine. Several over-the-counter drugs include caffeine along with other agents. Chocolate contains a small amount of caffeine. How harmful is caffeine? Researchers have investigated associations between normal to heavy caffeine intake (up to eight cups of coffee per day) and various outcomes such as birth defects, miscarriage, foetal growth retardation and child development in preschool years. No clear associations were found. Associations between coffee drinking during pregnancy and miscarriage or poor foetal growth have been observed in numerous studies, but in many cases confounding effects of maternal cigarette smoking and other factors were present.[1]

Some effects of caffeine may concern you as a parent. Foetal and newborn heartbeat irregularities have been reported among women who drank large amounts of caffeine during pregnancy, but these cardiac problems resolved after caffeine intake was stopped. Caffeine increases urinary excretion of calcium and decreases the amount available for you and your baby. Pregnant women eliminate caffeine from their bodies more slowly than non-pregnant women. This means that its effects on both mother and foetus last longer. Caffeine also causes an increased production of 'stress' hormones—epinephrine (adrenaline) and norepinephrine (noradrenaline). These hormones constrict peripheral blood vessels, including those in the uterus, and cause a temporary decrease in the amount of oxygen and other nutrients available to the foetus. The more caffeine you take in, the more the foetus is affected in this way.[2] Caffeine readily crosses the placenta and enters the foetal bloodstream. If the baby has caffeine in his circulation at birth, it takes a much longer time to clear his system than it would take for an adult.[3] Considering its potentially undesirable if not harmful effects, it seems wise to reduce or avoid caffeine intake during pregnancy.

Alcohol

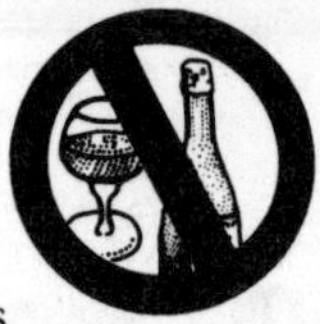

Alcohol has a direct toxic effect on the developing foetus.[4] Alcohol quickly crosses the placenta and enters the foetus's blood in the same concentration as in the mother's blood. Babies born of alcoholic mothers are at substantial risk for foetal alcohol syndrome (FAS)—a cluster of defects and disabilities that includes growth deficiencies, mental retardation, developmental delays, behaviour problems and characteristic facial abnormalities. FAS occurs in about 6 percent of children of women who drink heavily during pregnancy. Heavy drinking has been defined as taking more than 90 millilitres of absolute alcohol daily. This is equivalent to six mixed drinks, six cans of beer or six glasses of wine. Lesser amounts of alcohol (more than two drinks a day or a single drunken episode in early pregnancy) have been associated with alcohol-related birth defects (ARBD). These are less severe than FAS but still have some of the lasting harmful effects. Maternal alcohol use during pregnancy has been associated with an increased risk of miscarriage, stillbirth and various forms of childhood cancer.[5]

If you are pregnant, it is recommended that you give up drinking—the earlier the better. While drinking in early pregnancy is more likely to be associated with birth defects, drinking later in pregnancy is more likely to be associated with smaller foetal size and lower birth weight. Stopping at any time, therefore, will allow your baby the opportunity to catch up in growth before birth.

Questions about Alcohol

- *What if I have drunk too much during my pregnancy because I did not know the dangers of alcohol or did not know that I was pregnant?* It would be difficult for you not to be concerned about the health of your baby. You will need to talk to your caregiver to assess your personal risk, but a few points may be helpful here. Whenever you stop drinking, it will be helpful. Also, the foetus is remarkably strong and resilient. Consider the high percentage of healthy babies born to mothers who drank alcohol, took drugs or medicines, or had health problems during pregnancy. Of course, you should not depend on the strength of the foetus and deliberately abuse drugs.
- *What if I drink only occasionally, and then only lightly or moderately?* Current studies show that moderate drinking (less than two mixed drinks, two glasses of wine or two beers per day) has little or no effect on the risk of having a baby with alcohol-related birth defects. We know, however, that the baby receives alcohol when you drink, and that no safe level of maternal alcohol intake has been established. FAS and ARBD are known to occur in children whose mothers consumed alcohol throughout pregnancy. But the effects of moderate drinking, binge drinking or occasional drinking during pregnancy are less clear. In addition, blood alcohol levels vary widely depending on physical size, the amount of food eaten while drinking and the amount of time between drinks. The critical issue is that alcohol-related birth defects are dose related. This means that below a threshold level of alcohol, birth defects do not occur. The problem remains, as previously stated, that we do not know what the 'safe' level is. There-fore, it is best not to drink any alcohol as soon as you know you are pregnant.

It has also been shown that women commonly develop an aversion to alcohol (and to smoking and caffeine) during pregnancy. Many women cut down on their use of alcohol simply because it loses its appeal. Perhaps our bodies are trying to tell us something! In any situation where you might drink alcohol, you might substitute, for example, mineral water with a twist of lemon, fruit or vegetable juice, or some other non-alcoholic beverage.

Tobacco

Tobacco smoking has been widely studied for its effects on the unborn baby. The evidence strongly suggests that if you are pregnant and you smoke, you should stop or cut down as much as possible and as soon as possible—before pregnancy begins, if you can.

Cigarette smoke contains many substances that are harmful to both you and your child: tars, nicotine, carbon monoxide, lead and others. Compared to nonsmokers, pregnant women who smoke give birth to babies of smaller average size. This low birth weight is primarily due to foetal growth retardation and not to prematurity. preterm birth, perinatal death, placental abnormalities and other pregnancy complications have also been associated with cigarette smoking during pregnancy. These conditions are directly proportional to the amount of smoking. The more you smoke, the greater your chance of having these problems.[6] A few studies have noted an association between smoking in pregnancy and sudden infant death syndrome (SIDS). At this time, the link is unclear, since maternal smoking often occurs with other factors that could influence the risk of SIDS.

Smoking may also produce harmful long-term effects on the child. The incidence of respiratory problems is higher in children whose mothers smoked in pregnancy and in households where adults smoke. In one very large study that compared the children of smokers with those of nonsmokers, the children of smokers were an average of 1 centimetre shorter and three to five months behind the children of nonsmokers in intellectual ability. (The study accounted for associated social and biological factors.)[7]

What if you do not smoke, but your friends, family or coworkers smoke in your presence? Passive smoking (breathing in other people's smoke) can be uncomfortable to you and possibly harmful to your foetus, depending on how smoky the area is and how much time you spend in it. You may choose to avoid smoky areas and ask friends, colleagues and family members not to smoke near you.

Marijuana

Most studies of infants of women who smoked marijuana lack detailed information about the amount, timing and frequency of foetal exposure. It is clear, however, that smoking marijuana affects the foetus at least as much as it does the mother. The amounts of tar and nicotine in marijuana are considerably greater than in tobacco cigarettes, because no effort is being made to reduce these substances in marijuana. Carbon monoxide, which is present in all smoke, including marijuana smoke, significantly reduces the blood's capacity to carry oxygen. There is some evidence that foetal growth retardation occurs more commonly in pregnancies in which the expectant mother uses both alcohol and marijuana. There may also be a link between prenatal marijuana use and behavioural problems in the child. In summary, marijuana smoking during pregnancy poses some health problems for both mother and infant.

Cocaine

Cocaine, a widely abused recreational drug, is a central nervous system (CNS) stimulant and a local vasoconstrictor. Crack is a very potent form of cocaine. It is the constriction (or narrowing) of the blood vessels that appears to cause the complications associated with maternal cocaine use in pregnancy. These complications include placental abruption; intrauterine stroke, heart attack or growth retardation; preterm birth; and specific birth defects. The degree to which these complications are caused or aggravated by alcohol, cigarette smoking or other illegal drugs used along with cocaine is still unknown. Newborns sometimes suffer withdrawal symptoms (constant high-pitched crying, hyperactivity, poor suckling) that may last for weeks or months. Some studies indicate a possible association between cocaine use during pregnancy and sudden infant death syndrome (SIDS). It is clear that you should avoid using any form of this dangerous drug, especially during pregnancy and lactation.

Amphetamines and Methamphetamine

Methamphetamine is the most potent of the amphetamine group and has become a popular recreational drug. Amphetamines are central nervous system stimulants and their use by pregnant women increases the risk of premature birth. Newborn problems associated with maternal amphetamine use include rapid heart and respiratory rates and altered newborn behavioural patterns.[8] Methamphetamine abuse in pregnancy has been linked to low birth weight and possible intracranial bleeding in the newborn baby. Long-term intellectual and behavioural problems for the baby are difficult to determine because most women who take these drugs also abuse alcohol and other drugs.

Methadone

A pregnant woman may take methadone in an attempt to regulate her addiction to narcotics such as heroin and prescription pain medications. Therapeutic doses monitored by caregivers are unlikely to cause significant problems for the foetus. The newborn baby, however, is born addicted to methadone and will often experience withdrawal symptoms if the drug is suddenly removed. A baby can be helped to come off methadone by gradually reducing the drug given to him or to his breastfeeding mother, since a baby receives methadone through breast milk.

Herbs (Tinctures, Teas, Capsules)

Hundreds of herbs are available commercially. Traditional healers use them for various curative or restorative purposes. It is not possible to comment on the safety or value of herbs for the foetus since there has been little scientific scrutiny and little is known about the active ingredients that produce the benefits. It is known, however, that some herbs can produce undesirable side effects in some adults.[9] For instance, teas made from juniper berries, buckthorn bark, senna leaves, duck roots and aloe can irritate the stomach and intestinal tract, sometimes severely. People allergic to ragweed and related plants may develop unusual allergic symptoms after drinking chamomile tea. If used in large quantities, licorice root (a popular tea ingredient) is associated with water retention and loss of potassium. Blue cohosh, sometimes used to start labour, has been associated with elevated blood pressure and irritation of mucous membranes.

Sassafras root contains safrole, known to cause liver cancer in rats. The Food and Drug Administration (FDA) has stated that safrole cannot be considered safe for human use. Ginseng contains small amounts of oestrogen, and there have been reports of swollen and painful breasts after taking it in large quantities. Various combinations of herbs are used during pregnancy to tone the uterus and during labour to nourish the labouring woman's body.[10] The ingredients in these herbal preparations almost certainly reach the foetus and affect the baby at least as much as they do the mother. Because dosages vary and little is known about the risks and benefits of most herbs, you should avoid them while pregnant or use them with caution and only under the guidance of an expert, as you would any medication.

Medications

Medications such as pain relievers, sedatives and tranquillisers, antihistamines, decongestants, cough suppressants, antacids and anti-emetics (for control of nausea and vomiting) are used by many women during pregnancy. Many are self-prescribed. These drugs do not treat or cure an illness; they relieve symptoms like pain, headache, nervousness, sleeplessness, runny nose, cough, heartburn and nausea. Other medications such as antibiotics, insulin, antidepressants and steroids either cure or control an illness, and their benefits are surely greater than those drugs that merely relieve symptoms. Even so, a medication should be used only when the benefits clearly outweigh the potential hazards.

Some conditions are risky enough to mother and child to require treatment. Conditions such as epilepsy, pneumonia, asthma, strep throat, high fever, arthritis, diabetes, hypertension and heart disease may require treatment with strong medications even during pregnancy. Under these circumstances, non-treatment would be far more harmful to mother and foetus than treatment. If you needed medications for a serious chronic condition before you became pregnant, you should review your treatment with your maternity caregiver and with the doctor who prescribed the medication. In deciding whether to use medication, consider the seriousness and risks of the condition, the benefit to be gained from the medication, and the possible risks of the medication for your unborn baby. You may also want to discuss other available treatments and their benefits and risks.

Particular mention should be made of a few medications that are widely used, are generally considered harmless or are of special concern to pregnant women.

Drugs to Reduce Pain (Analgesics) or Fever

Aspirin

Brand names include Disprin. Even one tablet of aspirin (325 milligrams) reduces the body's ability to clot blood and prolongs bleeding time.[11] There is greater concern over aspirin taken towards the end of pregnancy, because normal maternal bleeding after birth may be increased and prolonged. In addition, aspirin is metabolised more slowly by newborn babies than by adults, and the blood level of aspirin in the foetus/baby is often higher than in the mother who has taken the drug.

Maternal aspirin use within a week of delivery has been associated with increased intracranial haemorrhage in premature and low-birth-weight infants. Frequent, high-dose use of aspirin in late pregnancy interferes with prostaglandin production and may delay the onset of labour and increase the length of labour. You are better off avoiding aspirin during pregnancy unless it is specifically prescribed by your doctor or midwife and its benefits outweigh its risks.

Paracetamol

Brand names include Panadol and Panamax. Paracetamol is less potentially harmful than aspirin. No adverse foetal effects have been reported with moderate use. It does not increase maternal, foetal or newborn bleeding as aspirin does. However, paracetamol overdose in pregnancy increases the risk of birth defects and foetal deaths. Liver and kidney problems can occur in infants born to women who take toxic doses of paracetamol in late pregnancy. If you normally tolerate paracetamol, it is preferable to use it (in moderation) rather than aspirin if you really need a pain or fever medication during pregnancy. Generally speaking, it is wise to use non-medical forms of treatment before resorting to medications. (See 'Home Remedies' on page 115.)

Ibuprofen

Brand names include Brufen. Ibuprofen is used for relief of pain, fever and inflammation. Like aspirin, it interferes with prostaglandin production and may postpone the onset of labour and increase post-partum bleeding. It can decrease the effect of antihypertensive drugs and possibly affect heart function in the foetus. Ibuprofen has been used as a medication to stop contractions in women with premature labour, but these same women have developed oligohydramnios (low volume of amniotic fluid). You are better off not using ibuprofen during pregnancy unless it is specifically prescribed by your caregiver, who has considered these risks.

Other Analgesics

New over-the-counter pain relievers continue to be created. Some non-steroidal anti-inflammatory drugs (NSAID)—such as naproxen (Aleve) and ketoprofen (Actron)—act like ibuprofen, have similar benefits and side effects, and should be avoided in pregnancy. Remember to check with your caregiver before taking any medicines while you are pregnant.

Drugs to Treat Migraine Headaches

Some drugs used for migraine pain relief should be avoided in pregnancy; others should be used with caution. The ergot derivatives (such as ergotamine and dihydroergotamine) can decrease blood flow to the uterus and placenta and have been associated with preterm labour contractions when used in late pregnancy. The newer triptan drugs (such as sumatriptan, zolmitriptan and naratriptan) that show great promise for migraine relief have not been well studied in pregnancy. However, the evidence on sumatriptan (Imitrex) suggests that it is unlikely to increase the risk of birth defects when used in therapeutic doses during pregnancy.[12]

Non-drug therapies such as relaxation skills, massage, ice packs and biofeedback are your best choices for treatment of migraines in pregnancy. If these are not effective, your doctor may prescribe drugs such as paracetamol or narcotics for pain, calcium channel or beta-blocking agents for their cerebral-vascular effects, and metoclopromide for nausea. Fortunately, many women who have a history of migraine headaches note that pregnancy reduces the frequency of headaches. However, in rare cases migraines may appear for the first time during pregnancy.

Drugs to Relieve Symptoms of a Cold

Always read the labels when considering taking any cold medications. Some contain a single ingredient, while others have numerous components. Discuss any medication use with your caregiver while you are pregnant. Nasal decongestants such as phenylpropanolamine or ephedrine are common components of cold remedies and are unlikely to increase the risk of birth defects. There are insufficient studies, however, to say that there is no risk to the foetus. Recent studies have shown an association between phenylpropanolamine and an increased risk of stroke in adults. Studies on phenylephrine, another decongestant, have shown inconsistent results about the association between its use and birth defects. Phenylephrine should be avoided in pregnancy.

Two widely used drugs in cough medications appear safe for use in pregnancy. Studies on guaifenesin, an expectorant, and dextromethorphan, a cough suppressant, have shown no association with birth defects in exposed infants. Though use of codeine in cough syrup has not been proven to cause birth defects, its use in pregnancy is not recommended if other cough controlling methods are available and effective.

Drugs to Treat Allergies and Asthma

Many of the medications commonly used for severe allergies and asthma can be used during pregnancy, if used with your caregiver's knowledge. Maternal use of oral corticosteroids has been associated with an increased risk of pregnancy-induced hypertension (PIH) and newborn jaundice, but these complications may have been related to poorly controlled asthma. In fact, if untreated, severe asthma in pregnancy puts you at greater risk than medication use. Severe asthma has been associated with adverse outcomes such as maternal haemorrhage, preterm labour and placental problems.

For relief of allergy symptoms, try to use topical agents or inhalers since they are absorbed minimally into your system and tend to have fewer side effects. For allergic symptoms of the nose and eyes, preferred agents include drops or sprays with cromones or antihistamines. For asthma, inhaled steroids are preferred.

Drugs to Treat Nausea and Vomiting

Many medications used to treat nausea and vomiting during pregnancy (NVP) are a type of antihistamine and are generally considered safe if used in therapeutic doses.

Drugs to Treat Depression and Other Mood Disorders

Studies of prenatal use of drugs for treatment of mood disorders show that some drugs can be used in pregnancy and others should not be prescribed. If you require medication, you should work with your caregiver who is treating your mood disorder, as well as your maternity caregiver, to assure coordination of care. By working together, you will be better able to weigh the risks of medications and the benefits of treating your illness during pregnancy.

Drugs to Treat Seizure Disorders

Use of anticonvulsants during pregnancy needs to be weighed with the risks of non-treatment and the loss of seizure control. The risk of birth defects in infants of epileptic mothers taking phenytoin (Dilantin) during pregnancy is twice as great as the frequency of such malformations in the general population. The risk of defects with chronic use of phenobarbital is much less, but addiction in the newborn is a concern. Another point to consider is that epilepsy itself is associated with an increased risk of birth defects. Women with seizure disorders need to consult their doctors before pregnancy to plan the best way to treat their disease.

Potentially Dangerous Medications

Isotretinoin (Roacutane), an oral drug used to treat severe acne, is known to cause foetal defects or death. To avoid these severe problems in pregnancy, women taking isotretinoin are told to stop taking it before conception. The use of a similar drug, tretinoin, which is applied to the skin, appears to have little or no effect on the rate of birth defects. Isotretinoin is a vitamin A congener, but this does not mean that taking vitamin A in prenatal vitamins in recommended doses is dangerous. (See page 102 for more on vitamin A in pregnancy.)

Other medications that are known to harm the growing foetus include radioactive isotopes, thalidomide and some chemotherapy drugs used for treating cancer. Others will undoubtedly be discovered in the future. What can you do? When considering any treatment or test, remember to tell all medical staff that you are pregnant so that the risks and benefits can be evaluated.

Home Remedies

Taking any medication (whether over-the-counter or prescription) during pregnancy should be done with caution and with your caregiver's knowledge and consideration. If possible, try some of the home remedies listed below to help you feel better without the potential problems of medications that go into your bloodstream and cross through the placenta to your unborn baby. These alternatives to the medical treatment of common ailments may be helpful, but if any of your discomforts persist or seem harmful to your wellbeing, consult your doctor or midwife for further treatment.

Headache

Instead of using medications for pain relief (analgesics), try a warm, relaxing bath, a massage, tension-reducing exercises such as shoulder circling and relaxation techniques. (See pages 181–185.) Hot packs or cold packs on the back of the neck or shoulders and cold packs on the forehead also help relieve headaches for many people. Try increasing the amount of sleep you get and arrange for more rest and relaxation time in your daily routine. Hunger can cause headaches, so don't miss a meal. Remember that a severe, persistent headache is one of the warning signs of pregnancy complications and should be reported to your doctor or midwife.

Cold, Hay Fever, Runny Nose and Cough

A cool-mist vaporiser, saline nose drops (available from the pharmacy or made at home by mixing 1 cup of warm water, ⅛ teaspoon of salt and a small pinch of soda), inhaling menthol vapours, sleep and rest, plenty of liquids, and a mixture of honey and lemon juice are safe and as effective at curing a cold as decongestants, analgesics and cough syrups. Drugs treat only the symptoms of a cold and do nothing to cure or shorten it.

Nausea, Vomiting and Heartburn

There are several non-medicinal treatments for these common discomforts of pregnancy. (See the discussion on pages 95–97 in Chapter 4.)

Backaches

Backaches are a common problem for pregnant women. Try to prevent upper and lower back pain by maintaining good posture, using good body mechanics, and doing exercises to strengthen the abdominal muscles and to decrease the curve in the lower back. (See Chapter 6 for suggestions on posture, exercises and comfort measures.) You can treat a backache with rest, massage and use of hot or cold packs. Avoid aspirin and muscle relaxants unless the condition is severe, and check with your caregiver before taking these drugs.

Sleeplessness

Sleeplessness is especially common in late pregnancy, when you have more periods of light sleep or have difficulty moving around in bed and finding a comfortable sleep position. (See pages 125–126 for sleep positions and pillow placement.) Try taking a brisk walk each day (but not just before bedtime) to help release tension that might keep you from sleeping. At bedtime, try a warm bath, a glass of warm milk, a massage or soothing music. If you find yourself wide-awake in the middle of the night, try reading (a dull book is more likely to help you get back to sleep) or using the relaxation techniques described in Chapter 8.

Harmful Environmental Agents

Pregnant women (and young children) should avoid the following environmental agents or hazards.

Herbicides and Insecticides

Weed- and insect-killing sprays are widely used along roadsides, in farming areas and in residential communities. Their presence in the atmosphere and on food has been associated with both miscarriage and birth defects. While numerous chemicals are used against weeds and insects, their safety for the unborn and young child has not been established. Some have already been banned because they are known to be harmful. While you are pregnant, avoid frequent, long-term exposure to herbicides and insecticides. Also, wash fruits and vegetables well to help remove pesticides and other chemicals.

Radiation

During pregnancy, you should avoid x-rays (or ionising radiation) for medical and dental diagnosis, and you should not work in areas where radiation levels may be high. This is especially important during your first trimester, since radiation interferes with cell division and organ development. The adverse effects of radiation are dose related. Diagnostic x-rays use much less radiation than radiotherapy, which is used to treat cancer. The overall risk of malformations in infants exposed to one diagnostic x-ray (1 rad) during the first four months of pregnancy is so small that it is not considered a risk factor by medical professionals.

In the past, x-rays were used in late pregnancy to assess the relationship between the size of the baby's head and the size of the mother's pelvis (x-ray pelvimetry), to find out if there were twins and to determine foetal presentation. Today, x-rays are rarely used, because ultrasound, which is safer, is used for the same purposes. If diagnostic x-rays are suggested, ask your physician if the needed information could be gained from safer alternatives—such as ultrasound, magnetic resonance imaging (MRI) or a CT scan—that involve significantly lower doses of radiation. Like any potentially risky procedure or medication, x-rays should not be done routinely or if there is reasonable doubt about the benefits. Fortunately, most x-rays can be avoided or postponed until after the birth.

Video Display or Computer Terminals

Video display or computer terminals (VDTs) have been investigated as a potential hazard to the unborn child due to concerns that heavy VDT use may be a source of radiation exposure. Ionising radiation (or x-ray), which causes the most harm to foetal cells and increases the chance of cancer and birth defects, is not emitted in any meaningful amount from VDTs.[13] The amount of non-ionising radiation (radio waves, microwaves, infrared and visible light) emitted from VDTs is very small and consists of frequencies that have not been shown to be harmful to the growing foetus.

While an association between miscarriage and VDT use is unlikely, there are some other possible side effects (unrelated to radiation exposure) resulting from prolonged time and repetitive activity at a computer terminal: fatigue, muscle strain, headache, carpal tunnel syndrome and eyestrain. These side effects, of course, can also occur in non-pregnant women. It makes sense to vary your work responsibilities so that you are not constantly in front of a VDT. Take occasional breaks away from the VDT and request that your workstation be as comfortable and free from glare and radiation exposure (even very low frequency radiation) as possible.

Electric Blankets

Like all other electrical household appliances, electric blankets emit low-frequency electromagnetic energy. However, because of prolonged exposure and close proximity to the body, they are of some concern. Recently, low-emission electric blankets that reduce the magnetic field exposure have been marketed.

Very few studies have looked at the effects of electric blankets on reproductive health, but those that have been done are inconclusive about the association between miscarriage and electric blanket use in pregnancy. Until further research is done, you would be wise to avoid exposure to electric blankets during pregnancy and possibly before conception.

Saunas and Hot Tubs

During the first half of pregnancy, prolonged exposure to extreme heat, such as that found in saunas or hot tubs, may raise the mother's body temperature, creating a fever that impairs foetal development. The high temperature may cause birth defects or even foetal death if the exposure occurs repeatedly, for extended periods, or at a crucial time in foetal development.[14] If you find saunas or hot tubs relaxing and beneficial, you would be wise to keep your temperature below the level of a fever. You can take your oral temperature while you are in the hot tub or sauna. When your normal body temperature rises ½ degree or more, it is time to get out and cool down. Ten minutes in a sauna or hot tub seems to be a reasonable limit since it does not seem to cause the body temperature to rise. If you become uncomfortably hot in a sauna or hot tub, even if you have been there for only a short time, get out or reduce the temperature of the sauna or hot tub water. When in a hot tub, holding your shoulders and arms out of the water will help promote heat loss and maintain a safe body temperature. Tub baths are usually not a problem because you are not fully submerged in the water.

Hair-Care Products

Many expectant mothers want to know what hair-care products they can use during pregnancy. There is no direct evidence that personal use of hair dyes or permanent wave solutions is harmful in pregnancy. Some animal studies indicate toxic effects of oxidative hair dyes (found in some permanent and semi-permanent dyes), but no human studies show an increased risk for their non-occupational use. Temporary hair rinses, which coat the hair shaft and easily wash off, and henna, a natural semi-permanent vegetable dye, do not contain oxidative agents. To limit your exposure when dyeing your hair or giving yourself a home permanent, you can wear gloves and avoid leaving the solutions on your head for extended periods of time.

Toxoplasmosis

Toxoplasmosis is a mild infection caused by the parasite *Toxoplasma gondii*. Infected individuals have cold-like symptoms or no apparent illness at all and eventually develop immunity, which prevents further infection. However, a primary (first-time) infection during pregnancy can be very serious for the unborn baby, sometimes causing congenital malformations or foetal death. If you are worried, you may have a blood test before you are pregnant to determine if you have antibodies from a previous infection and therefore would not develop toxoplasmosis during pregnancy.

Cats are the common carriers of toxoplasmosis, especially outdoor cats that eat raw meat such as rats and mice. The toxoplasmosis organism passes from the cat in its faeces and lives for up to a year. Transmission of the parasite (from your hands to your mouth) may occur after handling cats, emptying cat litter boxes or working in soil where a cat has buried its faeces. You may also acquire the disease by eating raw or undercooked meat or unwashed root vegetables. To avoid getting toxoplasmosis and passing it on to your unborn baby, be sure to cook your meat, wash vegetables thoroughly, wash your hands after handling cats, have someone else clean the cat litter box and avoid soil where cats defecate. If diagnosed with a primary infection in pregnancy, maternal treat-ment with antibiotics can reduce the severity of complications for the unborn baby.

Other Infectious Diseases

Lyme disease, German measles, chicken pox, fifth disease (parvovirus B19), listeriosis, hepatitis and sexually transmitted diseases (STDs) are examples of infectious diseases that may harm the foetus or newborn. (See pages 63–73 for a discussion of infections.)

Occupational and Recreational Hazards

Scientific studies have shown that exposure to certain chemicals in the workplace can cause severe pregnancy problems such as spontaneous abortion, congenital malformations or preterm birth. The agents associated with adverse pregnancy outcomes in human studies include anaesthetic agents, cytotoxic drugs, ethylene oxide, lead, methyl mercury, organic solvents, polybrominated biphenyls (PBBs), and polychlorinated biphenyls (PCBs).[15]

Recreational activities ranging from arts and crafts to furniture refinishing to auto mechanics are enjoyed by millions of people. Many hobbies pose no threat to the pregnant woman, but some involve use of the same toxic products listed above that are dangers in the workplace. If you plan to continue a hobby during pregnancy, you would be wise to obtain specific information about the product ingredients that you will be using. You could call the manufacturer or a poison control centre or get the Safety Data Sheets from a retail store that sells the product.

Preparation for parenthood often includes home repair and painting. Fortunately, many of the hazardous agents in industrial and art paints have been removed from products for household use. The pigments and fillers in house paint, when brushed or rolled onto surfaces, probably pose no health risk to the home renovator. Spray painting, however, is discouraged. Potentially dangerous paint ingredients include ethylene glycol, ethers, mercury, formaldehyde-releasing bromids and hydrocarbon solvents. Remember to read labels and get information about the ingredients in your painting supplies. Other protective measures that you could use when painting include having effective ventilation in the painting area and wearing gloves. For prolonged, high-dose exposure, a respirator could be used, but having someone else paint seems a wiser choice. Removal of lead-based paint, which is often found in older homes, should be done by professionals who can safely handle the toxic paint chips and dust without harm to you or other household members.

Drugs, Environmental Hazards and the Father

At this time, there is little known about how drugs, environmental hazards or other influences affect the reproductive capability of the male. Evidence is growing, however, that the man's health and wellbeing are more important than previously suspected in producing a healthy baby. Consider the following:

- One report concluded that there was a decrease in sperm density and motility among smokers.[16] Another study of infertility found that men who smoke more than twenty cigarettes a day and drink more than four cups of coffee a day have a decrease in sperm motility and more dead sperm than nonsmoking, non-coffee drinking males.[17]

- The age of the father seems to be important for normal foetal development. Just as the mother's age at conception has been found to be significant as a risk factor for Down syndrome, the father's age can be a risk factor for other congenital disorders such as dwarfism (achondroplasia). These disorders (called 'autosomal dominant mutations') are still rare; however, they are more likely in children born to fathers over forty.

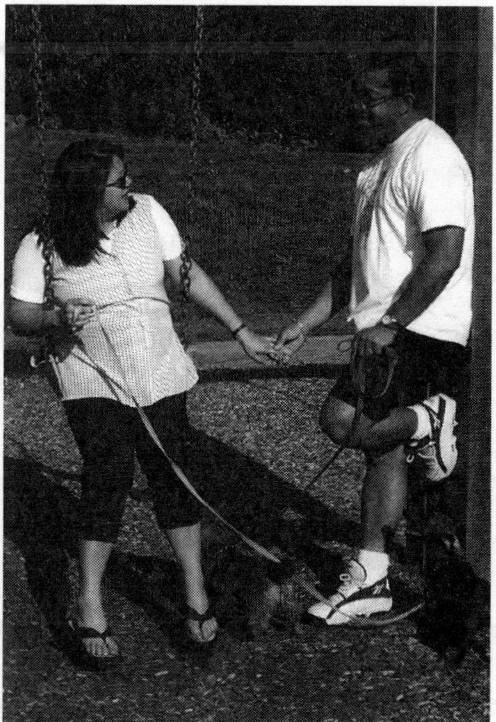

Photograph by Jan Dowers

Pursue the pleasures that are good for you and the baby.

- A man's exposure to herbicides, pesticides and solvents before conception is suspected, but not proven, to cause genetic mutations and birth defects in his offspring.

Other than a few reports on how certain drugs may alter the reproductive potential of men, the direct contribution by the father to his unborn infant's health is poorly understood. However, the indirect contribution of the partner, whether male or female, is of great significance. Both before and during pregnancy, a woman is much more likely to control her use of drugs, tobacco and alcohol if her partner also controls his or her use of these agents. If the woman is supported in her concern for a positive pregnancy outcome and joined in making any change she has to make, she is much more likely to be successful.

Conclusion

After reading this chapter, you may wonder if there are any pleasures left for the pregnant woman or expectant couple! Concentrate on the pleasures that have not been taken away: exercise, sports, dancing, outdoor recreation, good food, massage, love and sex, music, art, movies, reading, TV and—perhaps best of all—the experience of growing a baby.

Chapter 6

Exercise and Comfort

Exercise and general fitness during pregnancy and afterward deserve special attention. As your body grows and you gain weight, regular exercise helps maintain health and comfort. Even beginning a fitness program in mid-pregnancy may provide benefits. Appropriate exercise tones and strengthens the muscles most affected by pregnancy, including those in the pelvic floor, the abdomen and the lower back. Exercise also helps maintain good respiration, circulation and posture. Prenatal exercise and physical fitness ease some of the discomforts of pregnancy, help prepare your body for labour and promote emotional wellbeing.[1]

Although being physically fit does not guarantee an easy labour, it may give you more stamina to cope with a long, hard labour. One study found that women who exercised moderately and regularly during the last trimester perceived their labours as less painful than women who did not exercise. Furthermore, the exercising women produced higher levels of endorphins (the body's natural pain-relieving substances).

A major benefit of prenatal exercise comes after birth. Recovering your energy level, strength and pre-pregnant size is easier when you maintain good physical condition during pregnancy and in the weeks following birth. Many of the common discomforts of normal pregnancy can be eased not only by exercise, but also by improving your posture and body mechanics (in other words, the way you move your body as you lift heavy objects, rise to standing and even roll over in bed).

This chapter suggests ways to improve your posture and perform everyday tasks comfortably, provides specific exercises for the parts of your body most affected by pregnancy and birth, and includes a discussion of sports and aerobic exercise. You will also find explanations for some common discomforts of pregnancy, along with ways to relieve them.

Posture and Movement in Pregnancy

Good posture and body mechanics are the cornerstones of a comfortable pregnancy. As you gain weight and your body changes shape, you must adjust your posture to maintain balance and you must learn new ways to perform everyday activities to reduce strain, fatigue, and common aches and pains. In fact, the following guidelines are useful whether you are pregnant or not, and they are especially important in the first few months after your baby is born.

Good Posture

Stand tall with your

Head: high

Chin: level, not jutting out

Shoulders: relaxed, down and back

Abdominal muscles: firm, working to straighten spine

Back: slightly curved (avoid sway-back)

Buttocks: tucked under

Hips: level

Knees: relaxed, not locked

Feet: supporting body weight evenly on both feet

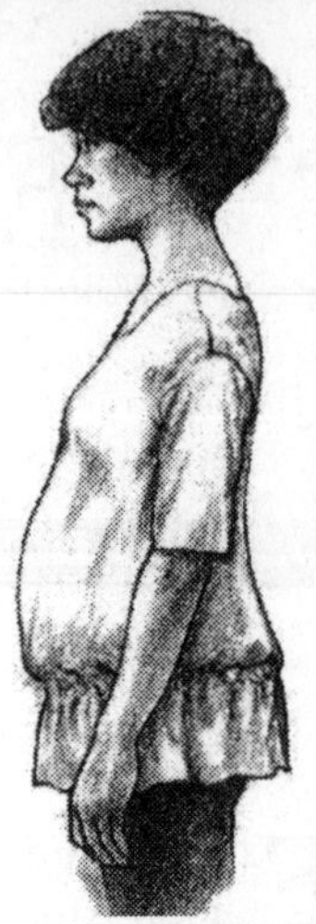

Posture

You can improve your posture by standing as tall as possible and by keeping your chin level. Imagine a string attached to the crown of your head, pulling it towards the ceiling. If you hold your head high, the rest of your body usually aligns itself properly.

Check the following list for signs of good posture. Watch yourself in windows and mirrors to increase your awareness of your posture, and ask a friend or your partner to observe you.

Poor posture often causes backache because your abdominal muscles are relaxed, the curve of your back is exaggerated, and the small muscles of your lower back shorten and tighten to maintain your balance and alignment. This continuous shortening and tightening of the back muscles may cause lower back pain.

During pregnancy, your centre of gravity shifts as your baby and uterus grow, and it takes special effort to maintain good posture. Flat or low-heel shoes help. Exercises to maintain abdominal muscle tone and strength and to stretch lower back muscles are also beneficial. (See pelvic tilt exercises on page 132.)

Standing

Whenever possible, avoid standing for long periods of time during late pregnancy. Standing still may slow the return of blood from your legs to your heart and head, which can make you feel light-headed. If you must stand for long periods, use your leg muscles to stimulate the blood flow from your legs to your heart. Shift your weight from leg to leg, 'march' in place from time to time, rotate your ankles in small circles and rock back and forth from your toes to your heels. Be fidgety; avoid standing still in one spot.

To help prevent backache while standing, place one foot on a low stool or opened drawer. After a while, shift to the other foot. This helps flatten your back and reduces the strain on your lower back muscles.

Sitting

During late pregnancy, try to avoid prolonged sitting, since this also slows the return of blood from your legs. To improve the circulation in your legs while sitting, do not cross your legs at the knees for long periods, and frequently move and rotate your feet at the ankles. Also, sit with your feet up and your calves supported. On a long car trip, stop hourly to get out and move around. In the car, shift your position frequently and move your legs about.

As your uterus enlarges, you will find a straight-back chair more comfortable (and easier to get out of!) than a low, deep one. A small, firm pillow in the small of your back and a low stool under your feet will provide additional comfort for your back. To avoid back strain when you get up, first move to the edge of the chair and use your leg muscles to raise your body.

Lifting

Joints and ligaments soften and relax from the effects of hormones during pregnancy. This makes you more likely to injure your back if you lift heavy objects the wrong way. You can safely lift light objects if you do so properly.

To lift or pick up an object or a toddler, use your strong thigh muscles instead of the short, weaker muscles of your lower back. Remember to bend at the knees when lifting, not at the waist. Follow these guidelines for picking up anything, even a piece of paper:

1. Get as close to the object as possible.

2. With your feet shoulder width apart, lower yourself by bending both knees (squatting), keeping your back upright.

3. Grasp the object and hold it close to your body. Try to avoid twisting at your waist.

4. As you rise, try to avoid strain on your perineum by contracting your pelvic floor muscles and blowing out rather than holding your breath. Straighten your legs and lift the object. Remember to keep your back upright.

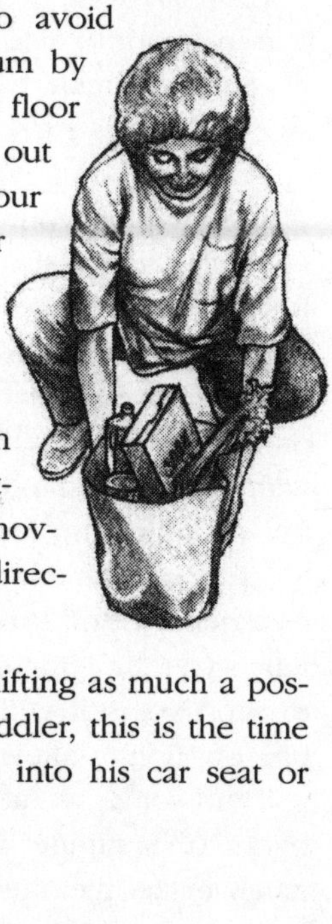

5. When moving with the object, avoid twisting at your waist by moving your feet in the direction you plan to go.

6. Try to avoid heavy lifting as much a possible. If you have a toddler, this is the time to teach him to climb into his car seat or onto your lap.

Lying Down

As your pregnancy progresses, it becomes more difficult to lie down comfortably for very long. Pillows help. When you are lying on your side, put a pillow between your knees and a pillow or two under your head so that your head is well supported. In late

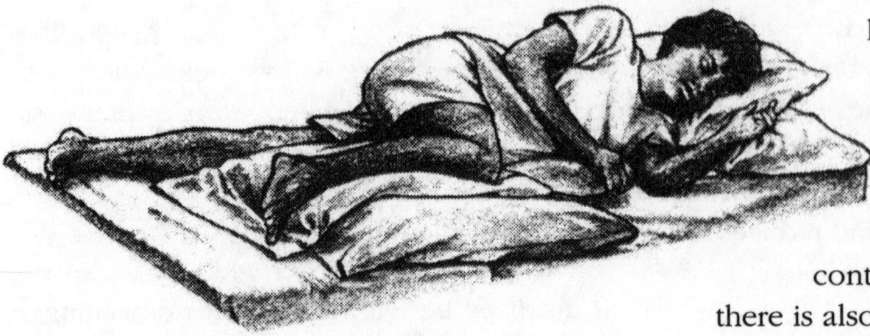

pregnancy, you may need a small pillow or a wedge-shaped pad to prop your abdomen and support your uterus. Long body pillows are popular with pregnant women for support in front or back.

Some women find side-lying comfortable if they lean towards the front of their body. Try it. Put your lower arm behind you. Straighten your lower leg. Bend your upper leg and rest it on a firm, fat pillow. Bend your upper arm, bringing your hand towards your face. (You will need only a flat pillow for your head.) Another position is on your back but tilted towards one side with pillows or the long body pillow under one shoulder, hip and leg.

Towards the end of pregnancy, you may experience heartburn or shortness of breath when you are lying down. Lie on your side or prop yourself with pillows to a semi-sitting position to alleviate these problems.

For some women, lying flat on their backs (the supine position) in late pregnancy makes them feel dizzy, short of breath or light-headed. This condition, called *supine hypotension* (a drop in blood pressure while lying on your back), is caused by pressure on the large abdominal vein (the inferior vena cava) located between the spine and the uterus. This vein carries blood from your legs to your heart, and when the heavy uterus presses on it, the blood returning to your heart may be reduced. This sometimes causes a drop in blood pressure and light-headedness. If this continues for many minutes, there is also a reduction in blood flow to the placenta and in oxygen for the foetus. If you feel light-headed while lying on your back, simply roll over to your side or sit up. The side-lying position is recommended to avoid supine hypotension.

Getting Up

Getting up from the floor or out of bed becomes more difficult as pregnancy advances. The usual 'jackknife' style of getting up (a sudden, jerking sit-up) may strain your abdominal and lower back muscles. To avoid this strain when getting out of bed, roll onto your side, put your legs over the edge of the bed, then push yourself to a sitting position and stand up. To get up from lying on the floor in late pregnancy:

1. Roll onto your side and bend your hips and knees. Using your arms, push your upper body up.

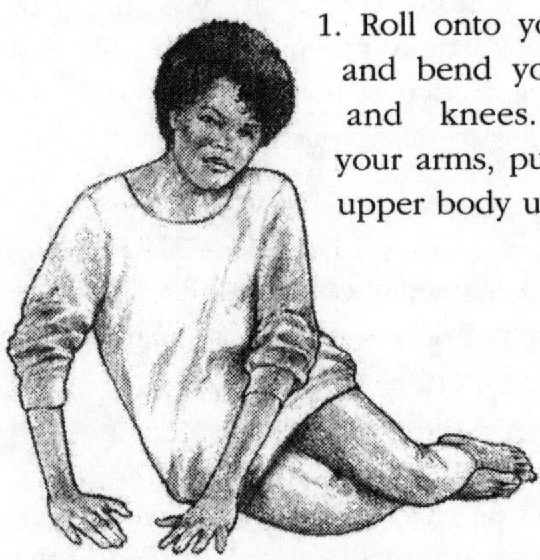

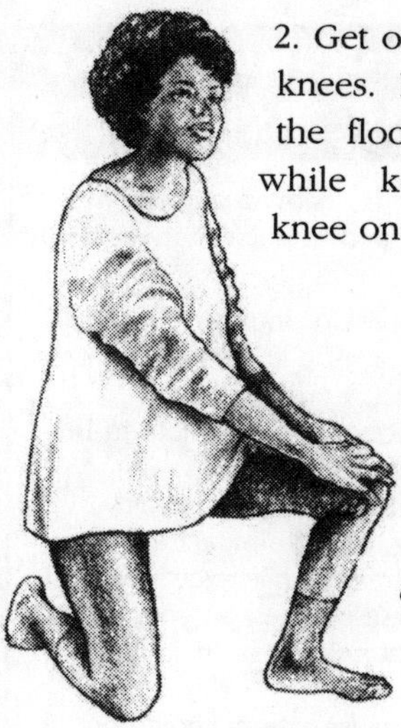

2. Get onto your hands and knees. Place one foot on the floor in front of you, while keeping the other knee on the floor.

3. Stand up using your leg muscles. Use your knee or another stable object for balance.

Exercise in Pregnancy

The amount and type of exercise that is best for you during pregnancy depends on your general health, the course of your pregnancy, your fitness and your usual activity level. Physical changes during pregnancy directly affect your tolerance for exercise. Hormonal changes cause your ligaments to relax and your joints to become more mobile. Your centre of gravity shifts because of the enlargement of your abdomen. Your heart rate speeds up because of changes in your cardiovascular system, and your body temperature and metabolic rate are higher.

Regular, moderate exercise during pregnancy maintains muscle tone, strength and endurance. Exercise also protects against back pain and has a positive effect on your energy level, mood and self-image. If you do not have pregnancy complications—such as pain with exercise, pregnancy-induced hypertension (PIH) or preterm labour—you can continue to exercise. To ensure that a fitness program is appropriate for you, check with your doctor or midwife before starting or continuing to exercise during pregnancy.

Sports

Pregnancy is not a time to take up vigorous sports, such as softball, tennis or skating, that require good balance or sudden jerky movements. If you are already skilled and active in those or other demanding sports, however, you may continue playing as long as you feel comfortable. In other words, as long as your pregnancy remains normal, you may safely continue a recreational sport or activity in which you feel competent, including tennis, swimming, cross-country skiing, jogging or cycling. However, you should avoid potentially dangerous activities such as skydiving, scuba diving, springboard diving, surfing or rock climbing. In late pregnancy, you should probably restrict participation in downhill skiing, water-skiing and horseback riding. Talk with your caregiver if you have questions about a particular athletic activity during pregnancy.

Aerobic Exercise

The goal of aerobic exercise is to improve heart and lung performance. Aerobic exercise programs for expectant mothers should include at least five minutes of warm-up (slow, smooth movements and stretching); a period of sustained, vigorous aerobic exercise lasting approximately fifteen minutes;

and at least five minutes of cool-down consisting of mild activity while your heart rate returns to normal. Exercises for strength and flexibility are sometimes added in the cool-down period.

Guidelines for aerobic exercise during pregnancy are based on your age, health and fitness level. If you begin an aerobic program, start slowly and gently. The American College of Obstetricians and Gynaecologists (ACOG) recommends that you take your pulse during peak activity and reduce your exercise intensity if your pulse rate exceeds your target heart rate range. Your range can be found by subtracting your age from 220 and multiplying the result by 60 percent and by 80 percent. The formula is (220 – age) x 60% to (220 – age) x 80% = your target heart rate range.[2] With a pulse rate in this range, you can improve or maintain your fitness without risking overexertion, no matter how accustomed you are to regular exercise. If you already exercise regularly, you will need more intense activity to raise your heart rate to your target heart range; if you do not exercise regularly, mild exertion will elevate your heart rate to this level. As pregnancy advances, it usually takes less activity to raise your heart rate to your target zone.

In addition to taking your pulse, you may want to use the 'talk test': the exercise is too vigorous if you are gasping and unable to continue speaking aloud. Slow your activity to a level that allows you to talk comfortably.

Avoid exhausting exercise, which may adversely affect you or your baby. Stop exercising if you experience pain, headache, nausea, severe breathlessness, dizziness, vaginal bleeding or continuing strong uterine contractions. You can let your body be your guide if you listen to it carefully.

General Guidelines for Safe, Effective Exercise

During exercise sessions, follow the guidelines below to avoid injury and to obtain the most benefit:

- Exercise regularly, three or four times a week. Always include a warm-up and cool-down.
- For land exercise, use a firm surface.
- Wear supportive footwear appropriate to the type of land exercise.
- Exercise with smooth movements; avoid bouncing or jerking, or high-impact exercises.
- Do not hold your breath while exercising; doing so can increase pressure on your pelvic floor and abdominal muscles or make you feel dizzy.
- Keep track of your pulse rate (it should not exceed the number of beats per minute at the top of your target heart rate range) or use the talk test. (See left.)
- Stop the exercise if you feel pain. Your body might be telling you that muscles, joints or ligaments are being strained.
- To avoid strain and fatigue, start with the easiest position, then try others as your muscles strengthen. Start with a few repetitions, gradually increasing the number. Towards the end of pregnancy, you may need to decrease your level of exercise.
- Consider your calorie and liquid intake. You need to eat enough to meet the caloric needs of pregnancy. Liquids should be taken before, during and after exercise to replace body fluids lost through perspiration and respiration. You can take a water bottle along with you.
- Avoid vigorous land exercise in hot, humid weather or when you are ill and have a fever. Your body temperature should not exceed 38°C.
- Check with your doctor or midwife if you have questions about exercise.

What kind of aerobic exercise is best for pregnant women? Generally speaking, low-impact exercise (exercise that does not involve jumping, bouncing or leaving the ground) is preferable because it is easier on your joints. Examples of low-impact activities include brisk walking, cross-country skiing, cycling, swimming and low-impact aerobic exercises (in or out of water). Swimming and low-impact aerobic exercise provide more total body involvement than the others listed above. Swimming and water exercise offer still other benefits. They cause the lowest impact possible because of the buoyancy provided by the water. Standing or sitting up to your shoulders in deep water has the added advantage of reducing swelling (oedema) by moving tissue fluid back into your circulation (and eventually out through urination). As you become heavier and less comfortable, non-weight-bearing exercise such as swimming or cycling is preferable.[3]

Conditioning Exercises

The conditioning exercises described in this section are designed to keep the muscles most affected by pregnancy (the pelvic floor and abdominal muscles) in good condition during pregnancy, to help you to use your muscles effectively during birth and to speed your post-partum recovery. These exercises should be added to your general fitness activities.

Conditioning the Pelvic Floor Muscles

The pelvic floor (or perineal) muscles are attached to the insides of the pelvic bones and act like a hammock to support your abdominal and pelvic organs. During pregnancy, these muscles may sag in response to the increased weight of your uterus and the relaxing effect of the hormones produced by your body. Regular exercise of the pelvic floor muscles maintains tone and improves circulation, which can reduce the heavy, throbbing feeling that you might experience during pregnancy or post partum. Since the pelvic floor muscles are stretched during birth and their condition is of lifelong importance, regular exercise of the pelvic floor is essential during pregnancy and throughout your lifetime.

The pelvic floor muscles form a figure-eight pattern around the urethra, vagina and anus. During childbirth, the circle of muscles around the vagina stretches to allow the birth of the baby. When they are in good tone, they are elastic, which means they can stretch but also return to their original length. Birth is quicker, more comfortable and easier if these muscles are in good tone and if you

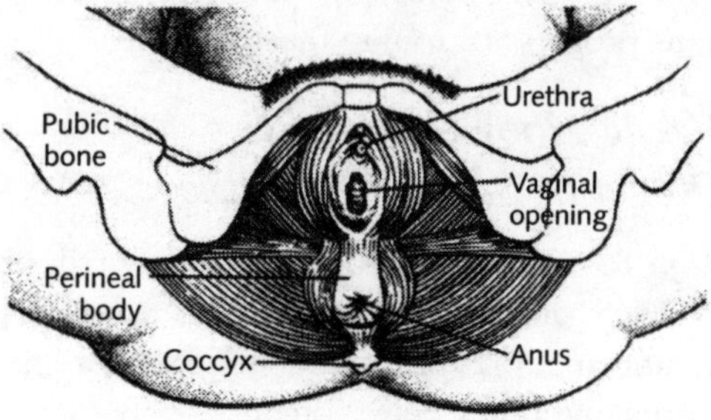

Pelvic floor muscles

relax them rather than tighten them as the baby is being born. Pelvic floor exercises during pregnancy (along with perineal massage, described on page 203) will help prepare you to relax these muscles during the second stage of labour.

Regular exercise of these muscles during pregnancy and for the rest of your life has other benefits. It may enhance sexual enjoyment for you and your partner and may prevent problems with incontinence (leaking urine) during pregnancy or later in life. If incontinence remains a problem even with exercise, consult your caregiver for a referral to a professional who specialises in non-surgical treatment of incontinence.[4]

To check the strength of your pelvic floor muscles, try this exercise while you are urinating. Partially empty your bladder, then stop the flow. If you cannot, it is a sign of weakness, but do not despair. These muscles respond quickly to exercise. You may also check by inserting one or two fingers in the vagina and tightening your pelvic floor muscles around them. You should feel some tightening of the muscles on your fingers. If you do not feel the tightening, it is a sign of weakness. During intercourse, check by tightening your pelvic floor muscles around your partner's penis; he can help evaluate your progress of toning these muscles.

Pelvic Floor Contraction (Kegel or Super Kegel Exercise)

Aim: To maintain the tone of the pelvic floor muscles, improve circulation to the perineum and provide better support for the uterus and other pelvic organs.

Starting position: Assume any position (sitting, standing or lying down).

Exercise: Concentrate on the muscles of your urethra and vaginal opening—not the muscles of your buttocks, thighs or abdomen. Without holding your breath, contract or tighten the pelvic floor muscles as you would to stop the flow of urine. You will feel tension and a slight lifting of the pelvic floor. Hold as tightly as you can for ten seconds. At first you will probably notice the contraction diminishing or fading, even though you have not deliberately let go. Simply tighten the muscles whenever you feel this letting go, again and again, until ten seconds have passed, then relax and rest for at least ten seconds. When you are able to hold the contraction for ten seconds, work up to holding it for twenty seconds or more. This longer hold is called a Super Kegel. If at first you are unable to maintain the tightening effort for ten seconds, begin with three or five seconds and gradually work up to ten, then twenty.

Repetition: Try to do at least ten Super Kegels spread throughout the day. For example, do one or two while washing your hands after using the toilet.

Pelvic Floor Bulging

Aim: To practice and prepare for the second stage of labour—pushing the baby out. You should bulge the pelvic floor (not contract it) as the baby is coming out. This exercise is only needed during pregnancy. Make sure your bladder is empty when practising this one!

Starting position: Get into a tailor-sitting position (sitting cross-legged), or any of the birthing positions. (See Chapter 9, pages 227–229.)

Exercise: Consciously relax the pelvic floor muscles. Hold your breath and bear down or strain gently as you do when you are having a bowel movement, letting the perineal muscles relax further and bulge outward. Do not bear down hard or strain forcefully. Putting your hand over your perineum will help you feel this bulge. Hold for three to five seconds.

Stop bearing down. Breathe in, contract your pelvic floor, then relax and rest. Once you have learned to do this while holding your breath, try doing it while letting air out. You will find that you do not have to hold your breath to bulge your perineum.

Repetition: Repeat once or twice a week.

Mobilising the Pelvic Joints

Squatting

Aim: To gain flexibility of the pelvic joints, stretch the muscles of the inner thighs and Achilles tendons, and increase comfort with squatting (a position you may use to assist the birth of the baby).

Starting position: Stand with your feet comfortably apart (approximately 60 centimetres) and your heels on the floor. Squat, dropping your buttocks down towards the floor. Keep your weight evenly on your heels and toes to allow for greater stability and more of a curve of the lower back. If you have trouble maintaining your balance, squat with support by holding your partner's hands, a stable piece of furniture or the doorknobs on either side of a door. Your partner can also support you from behind by sitting on a chair as you squat and lean back between his or her knees with your arms over the knees.

If your feet roll inwards or if you cannot squat with your heels flat, it is because of short or tight Achilles tendons. Try spreading your feet further apart, wearing shoes with moderate heels, elevating each heel with a 2.5- to 5-centimetre book, or squatting with support. Many hospital birthing beds come equipped with squatting bars, which can be attached to the bed to give you something solid to hold onto while squatting. (See the illustration on page 228.) When you take a hospital tour, you may want to ask if a squatting bar is available.

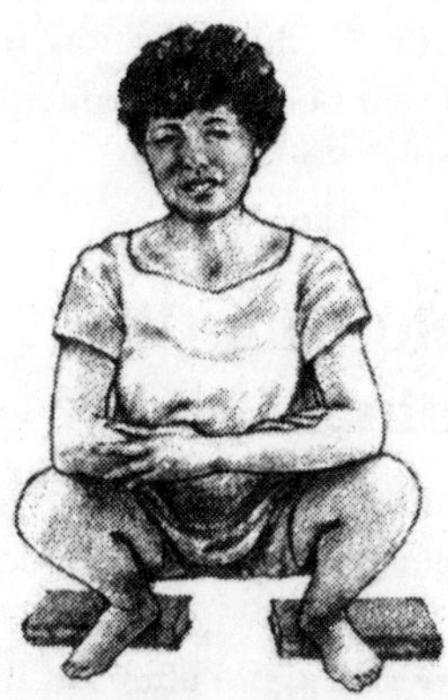

Caution: If you have hip, knee or ankle problems, consult your caregiver before trying this exercise. If the squatting position causes pain anywhere in your legs or pubic area, try squatting and leaning back with support. If support does not help, discontinue this exercise. If you cannot squat, you can stretch the muscles of the inner thighs by trying tailor-sitting (page 134) with the soles of your feet touching. Bringing your heels closer to your body increases the stretch.

Exercise: Slowly squat with your weight on your heels and toes, not just your toes. Do not bounce. Stay down for at least thirty seconds, then rise slowly.

Repetition: Repeat ten times daily. Progress to squatting for one and a half minutes at a time.

If you find it difficult to rise from a squat without using your hands to help, you should add an exercise to increase the strength in your thigh and buttock muscles. Try wall-sitting: stand with your back resting on a wall and your feet about 30 centimetres away from the wall. Partially bend your knees so that they are directly above your feet. Remain in that position for up to a minute. As you become stronger, bend your knees more. Repeat five to ten times throughout the day.

Conditioning the Abdominal Muscles

Keeping your abdominal muscles strong helps you maintain good posture, avoid backache, push your baby out more easily and hasten recovery of your figure after the birth.

There are four layers of abdominal muscles that support the contents of the abdomen. These layers work together with other trunk muscles to bend your body forward or sideways, rotate your trunk, tilt your pelvis and help with breathing. Because your growing uterus stretches these muscles, many abdominal exercises done by non-pregnant women are potentially risky for pregnant women, especially in late pregnancy. To avoid back and abdominal muscle strain in late pregnancy, do not do double leg lifts, sit-ups or sit-backs (page 141). An exercise that conditions these muscles without causing excessive strain is described below.

Pelvic Tilt

Aim: To strengthen your abdominal muscles, improve posture and relieve backache. The pelvic tilt can be performed in various positions: lying on your back, on your hands and knees, or standing. The back-lying position may be easier when learning this exercise but may cause light-headedness in late pregnancy. After learning the pelvic tilt, use the other positions until after the baby is born.

Repetition: Do ten pelvic tilt exercises each day.

Pelvic Tilt on Your Back

Starting position: Lie on your back with your knees bent and your feet flat on the floor.

Exercise: Flatten the small of your back onto the floor by contracting your abdominal muscles. Do not push with your feet or tighten your buttocks to tilt the pelvis. Hold the abdominal muscle contraction for a count of five as you exhale. Relax for five to ten seconds, then repeat.

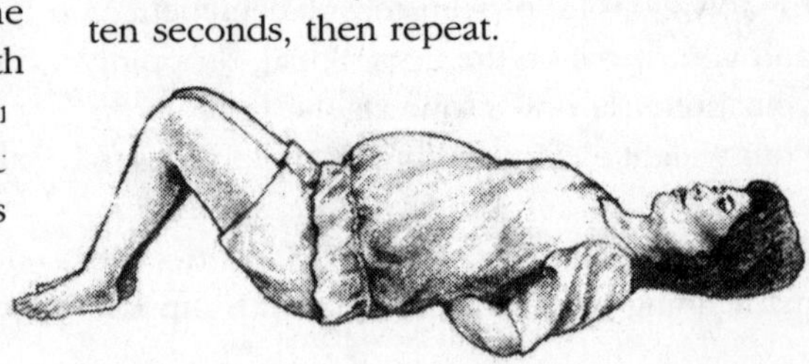

Note: To check that you are doing the exercise correctly, place your hand beneath the small of your back as you tilt your pelvis. You will press your back onto your hand. If you feel light-headed while lying on your back, roll over. Use the back-lying position only in early pregnancy or while learning the pelvic tilt. In late pregnancy, use the other positions described below.

Pelvic Tilt on Hands and Knees

Starting position: Get on your hands and knees. Keep your back straight—not hollowed, swayed or arched—and your knees comfortably apart.

Exercise: Tighten your abdominal muscles to arch your lower back. (Imagine a frightened dog who tucks her tail between her legs.) Hold for a slow count of five. Relax and return your back to the starting position. Do not sag. If desired, repeat after waiting five to ten seconds.

Pelvic Tilt when Standing

Starting position: Stand leaning against a wall. Have your buttocks and shoulders touching the wall, your feet apart and 30–40 centimetres away from the wall, and your knees slightly bent.

Exercise: Breathe in. As you exhale, press your lower back against the wall by contracting the muscles of your abdomen. Imagine

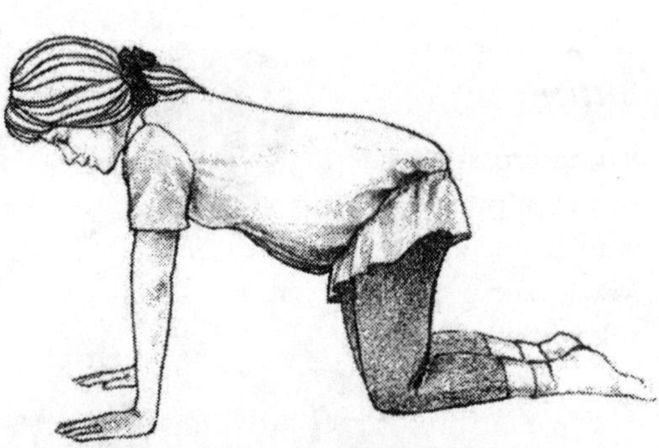

Relaxed (no pelvic tilt)

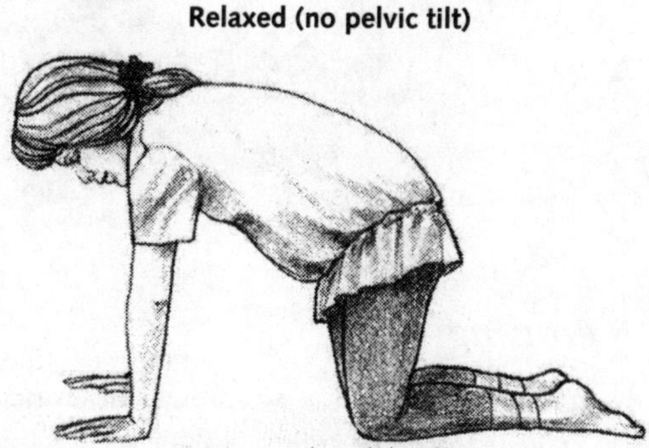

Contracted (pelvic tilt)

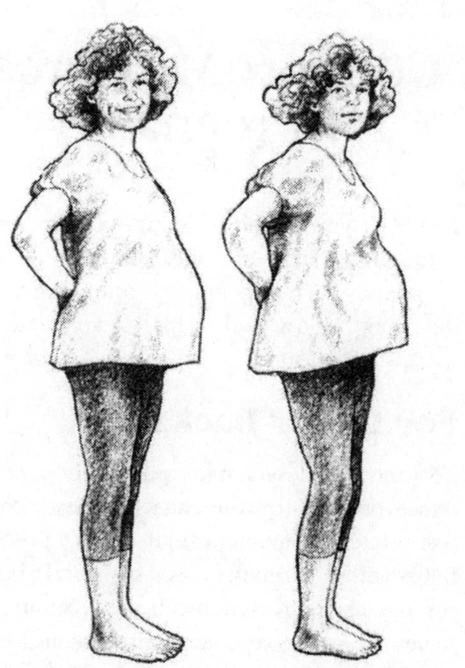

Relaxed (no pelvic tilt) **Contracted (pelvic tilt)**

that your abdominal muscles are hugging your baby within your uterus. Hold for a slow count of five without holding your breath. Relax. Wait five to ten seconds and repeat, if desired. To check yourself, put your hand between the wall and the small of your back. As you tilt your pelvis, you should feel your back press against your hand.

After you have mastered the pelvic tilt leaning against a wall, try it while standing upright. To check, put your hands on your hips. You will feel your hip bones move as you tilt your pelvis and raise your pubic bone upwards. By using a partial pelvic tilt (flattening your back and raising your pubic bone in front) when standing, you can maintain good posture and help relieve or even prevent backache.

Comfort Measures for Pregnancy

Even if you stand and move properly, aches and pains are still common during pregnancy. The positions and exercises described below can help relieve some of these discomforts.

For Lower Backache

Treatment of lower back pain during pregnancy depends on the cause of the discomfort. Increased awareness of correct posture helps most women. Use of good body mechanics decreases mechanical strain on joints, ligaments and tendons that are softened and relaxed by hormonal changes. Positions and exercises that reduce swayback and/or increase abdominal muscle tone, described below, also may prevent or relieve lower back pain. A heating pad, hot water bottle, or a warm bath or shower helps relieve pain from muscular tension. A massage by your partner or a professional may work wonders on a sore back. If your back pain is severe or if these measures do not help, ask your caregiver for a referral to a physical therapist who can diagnose the problem and treat it with cold packs, heat, hydrotherapy, massage, techniques that mobilise joints and an exercise program for your specific problem. Your caregiver or therapist might recommend a special garment that provides additional support to the abdomen and lower back.

Cross-legged Sitting

Sitting cross-legged is a comfortable way to keep the lower back relaxed.

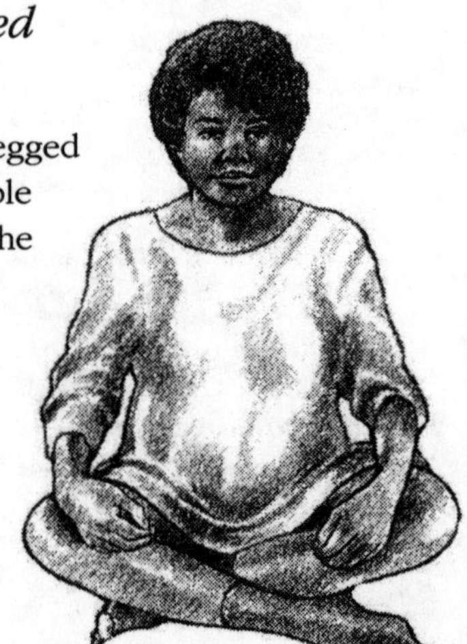

Squatting

Many women find that squatting (described on page 131) helps relieve lower backache.

Pelvic Tilt on Hands and Knees

This exercise (described on page 133) relieves lower back pain by stretching the lower back muscles and strengthening the abdominal muscles.

Knee-to-Shoulder Exercise

Starting position: Lie on your back with your knees bent and your feet flat on the floor.

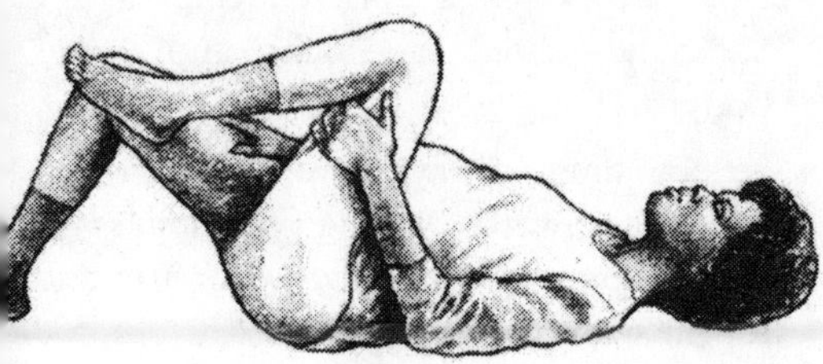

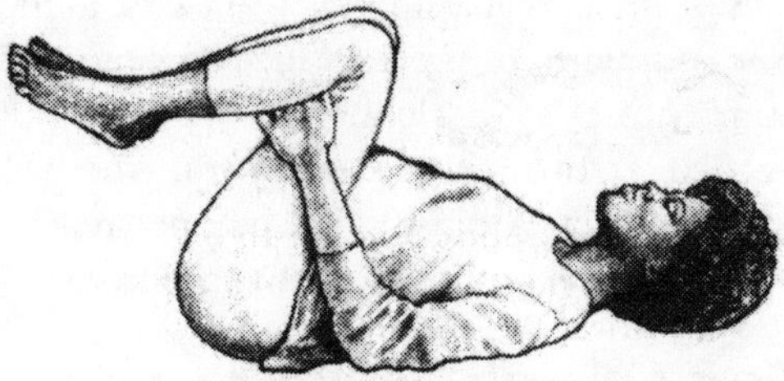

Exercise: Draw one knee up towards your chest and hold it behind your thigh with one hand. Bring your other knee up and hold it, keeping your knees apart to avoid pressure on your abdomen. Keeping your head on the floor, gently pull your knees towards your shoulders until you feel a slight stretch in the lower part of your back. Hold for a slow count of five. Release the pull without letting go of your knees. Repeat the pull-hold-release five times. Lower one foot, then the other.

Note: In late pregnancy, you may wish to raise and pull only one leg at a time. Roll onto your side as soon as you finish the exercise. If this exercise causes light-headedness, do not do it.

For Upper Backache

To prevent or relieve an upper backache, try reducing tension in your shoulders, neck and jaw. Several times a day, take a deep breath and drop your shoulders and jaw. (You can do it without opening your mouth.) The relaxation exercises and massage and acupressure techniques described in the next chapter for use in labour can also help with upper backache during pregnancy. In addition, the exercises below will help increase circulation, stretch tense muscles and decrease your backache.

Shoulder Circling

Starting position: Stand or sit with your back straight, arms relaxed and chin level.

Exercise: Raise your shoulders towards your ears, then slowly roll them forward, down, back and up again. Think of making large circles with your shoulders. Feel the release of tension. Finish with your shoulders back and down in a relaxed position. Do five rotations, then repeat, reversing the direction.

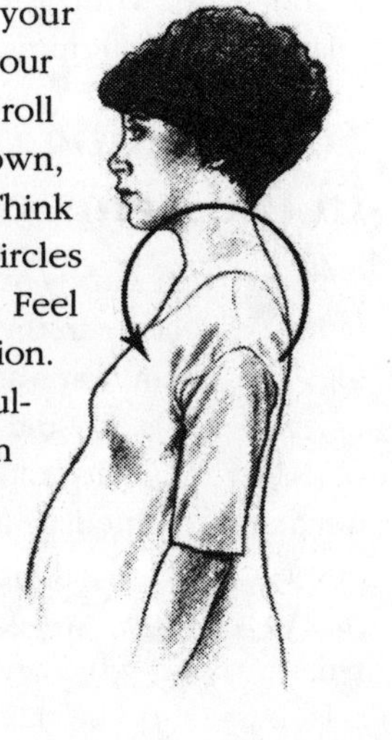

Upper Body Stretch

Starting position: Sit cross-legged or stand with your arms straight and extended in front of you.

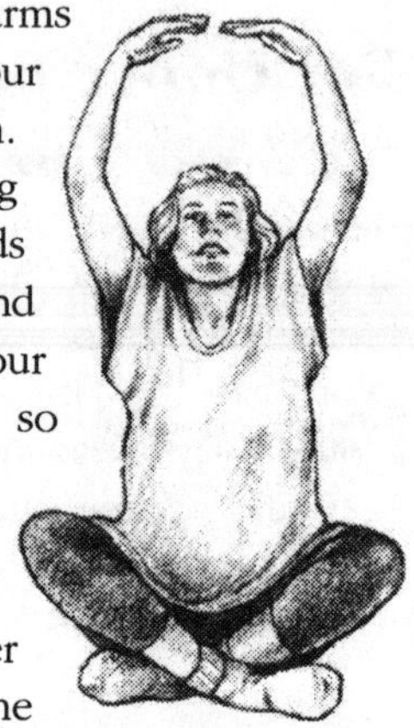

Exercise: Cross your arms at the elbows; feel your upper back stretch. While slowly breathing in, raise your hands towards the ceiling and gradually uncross your arms. Reach upwards so you feel the stretch in your entire upper body.

Exhale as you lower your arms out to the sides and behind you with palms up. Feel the stretch across your chest and upper arms. With your arms down and behind you, stretch further by pressing your arms back with five gentle pulsing motions. Exhale with each stretch, making a 'who' sound. Drop your arms to your sides and relax without slumping. Repeat five times.

For Tingling or Numbness in the Arms or Hands

Some women's arms or hands tingle and feel numb, especially in the morning after sleeping. These symptoms are caused by pressure of excess tissue fluid on the nerves and blood in the arms and wrists. If the symptoms are confined to the hands, the condition is called 'carpal tunnel syndrome', referring to a narrow passage on the inside of the wrist through which nerves and blood vessels pass into the hand. If the symptoms involve the entire arm, the condition is called 'thoracic outlet syndrome', referring to the space through which nerves and blood vessels pass to the arm.

If you have tingling, pain or numbness in your arms or hands, try the following to prevent or treat the problem:

- Use positions and pillows to support you on your side without lying on your arm. (See page 126.)
- Do the exercises for relieving upper backache—shoulder circling and upper body stretch.
- Several times a day, raise one arm and stretch it upwards. Wiggle your fingers for a slow count of five. Lower your arm and repeat with the other.

If carpal tunnel syndrome is severe, use a wrist splint at night. It holds your wrist in the best position to prevent the tingling and numbness. Use it during the day, too, if needed. Your caregiver can tell you where to get the splint. A wrist splint will not relieve the symptoms of thoracic outlet syndrome.

For Aching Legs or Swollen Ankles

If you are bothered by aching legs, swollen feet and ankles, or varicose veins, do the following to promote better circulation:

- Walk. Do not stand still. Walking, swimming or using an exercise bike several times a week may help.
- When you are sitting, rotate your feet at the ankles and do not cross your legs at the knees. Rock in a rocking chair when you plan to sit for a while. This helps exercise the muscles in your legs and feet.

- When you are resting during the day, lie on your side or elevate your feet. (Sit with your feet up, for example.)
- Do the pelvic tilt exercise on your hands and knees. (See page 133.) This position reduces the weight of the uterus on the blood vessels in the pelvis and abdomen. The rocking movements promote blood flow.
- Exercise or simply rest in water for an hour every other day. (A large tub, pool or lake is better than a regular bathroom tub.) The weight of the water pressing your swollen tissues reduces the swelling and promotes urination to reduce excess fluid. The benefits last for approximately forty-eight hours after one hour in water. If you use a hot tub, the water temperature should not be warmer than normal body temperature.
- Wear support stockings. Put them on before you get out of bed, since this is when there is the least amount of swelling.

For Leg and Foot Cramps

Cramps in the calves or feet commonly occur in late pregnancy when you are resting or asleep. Cramps are caused by fatigue in calf muscles, pressure on the nerves to the legs, impaired circulation or a mineral imbalance in the blood. This imbalance can result from too little calcium or magnesium or from too much phosphorus, which is found in foods such as processed meats, snack foods and soft drinks. Even with a good diet, mineral supplements and activities to promote circulation in the legs, you may still get cramps. To prevent leg and foot cramps, avoid pointing your toes or standing on your tiptoes. Right before going to bed, try exercises that stretch your legs. The techniques described below to relieve cramps are based on the fact that a muscle cramp disappears when the muscle is slowly stretched.

Relieving Leg Cramps

To relieve a cramp in the calf, straighten your knee and bend your foot up, bringing your toes towards your shin. Here are two ways of doing this:

- Stand with your weight on the cramped leg. Keep your knee straight and your heel on the floor, then lean forward to stretch the calf muscle.
- When a leg cramp is severe, you may need help. While sitting on a chair or bed, have your partner hold your knee straight with one hand and, while gripping your heel with the other, use his or her forearm to gently press your foot and toes towards your face. When the cramp is gone, do not point your toes or it will return.

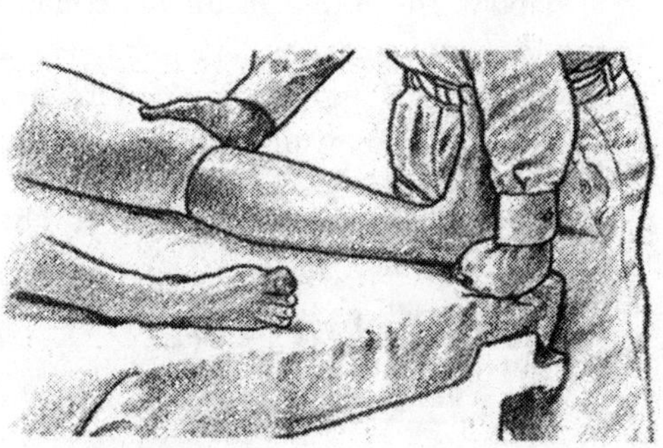

Relieving Foot Cramps

A cramp in the foot tightens the muscles of the arch and curls the toes. To relieve the cramp, stretch out your toes and the bottom of your foot by pulling your toes up towards your shin. To prevent cramping, do not curl your toes.

For Sudden Groin Pain

You may sometimes feel a sudden pain in your lower abdomen or groin (on one or both sides) when you stand up quickly or when you sneeze, cough or laugh while lying down with straight legs or standing. The pain is caused by sudden stretching of one or both of the round ligaments of the uterus. These two ligaments, which connect the front sides of the uterus to each groin, contract and relax like muscles, yet much more slowly.

Any movement that suddenly stretches these ligaments makes them rapidly contract and causes pain. You can avoid this pain by moving slowly, allowing the ligaments to stretch gradually. If you anticipate a sneeze or expect to cough, bend or flex your hips to reduce the pull on these ligaments.

In labour, the round ligaments contract when the uterus contracts. This is beneficial because they pull the uterus forward and align it and the baby with the birth canal for the most efficient and effective action.

Post-partum Exercise

The exercises described here (including some that you practised during pregnancy) will help you recover your former shape and muscle strength during post partum. After birth, two areas of your body need special attention—your abdominal muscles and your pelvic floor. You can see that your abdomen is not as flat as it was. After months of stretching, it needs toning and conditioning. At the same time, the pelvic floor muscles need exercise to increase circulation, to reduce swelling and promote healing in the perineum, and to restore vaginal and rectal muscle tone. The pelvic floor muscles need support while you exercise your abdominal muscles, so when you are doing abdominal exercises, first contract the pelvic floor muscles. When both these muscle groups are in good condition, they form an internal girdle of muscle support for your entire body.

With your doctor's or midwife's approval, you can start doing the Kegel exercise, pelvic tilt and leg sliding (one leg only) described below as early as one hour after delivery (though we doubt you will be thinking much about exercise that soon). If you have had a caesarean birth, however, you should check with your caregiver before starting to exercise. Next, begin taking walks. Besides being an excellent conditioning exercise, it is easy to take the baby along. Getting out of the house and walking can lift your spirits and calm a fussy baby. After a few weeks of walking and these gentle conditioning exercises, many new mothers want to resume more vigorous exercise. Check with your caregiver first. If you find exercising on your own difficult, consider joining a post-partum exercise class (check the yellow pages or call your hospital or local recreation or fitness centre) or use one of the excellent videotapes on post-partum exercise.

Checking for Separation of the Rectus Muscles

Before you begin any abdominal muscle exercise (other than the pelvic tilt), check for separation (or diastasis) of the rectus muscles—the muscles that run up and down from your chest to your pubic bone. Like a zipper opening under stress, the connective tissue between these muscles may have responded to stretching during pregnancy by separating painlessly and without bleeding. This separation protects the muscles from stretching excessively. It is normal but requires some special attention to help close the separation.

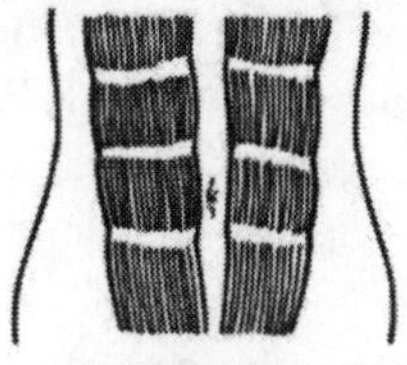

Normal

To test for separation of the rectus muscles, lie on your back with your knees bent. Press the fingers of one hand into the area just above your navel. Slowly raise your head and shoulders off the bed or floor. The rectus muscles will tense, allowing you to detect any gap. A slight gap (2.5 centimetres or less—the width of one or two fingers placed side by side) indicates normal muscle weakness after pregnancy. An extreme gap between the muscles (2.5–8 centimetres—three or four fingers wide) indicates that you need some preliminary work before you begin strenuous abdominal exercises. Strenuous exercise in the presence of a wide separation only increases the separation and defeats the purpose of the exercise. Use the head-lift to decrease this separation. After the gap has narrowed to the width of one or two fingers, proceed to the leg sliding, sit-back and central/diagonal lift exercises. (See page 141.)

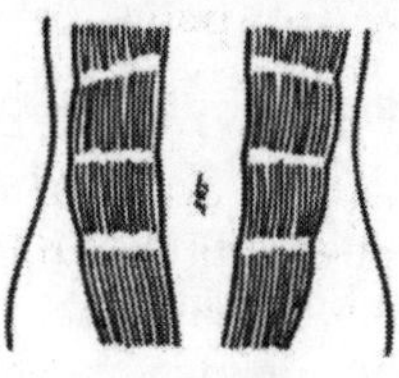

Separated

Head-Lift Exercise

Aim: To help close a separation of the rectus muscles and support them during exercise.

Exercise: Lie on your back with your knees bent. Cross your hands over your abdomen, placing them on either side of your waist. Breathe in. As you exhale, raise your head and shoulder blades off the floor or bed. At the same time, pull the rectus muscles towards the mid-line with your hands. Hold for a slow count of five. Slowly lower your head back down. Rest for at least ten seconds. Repeat about ten times daily.

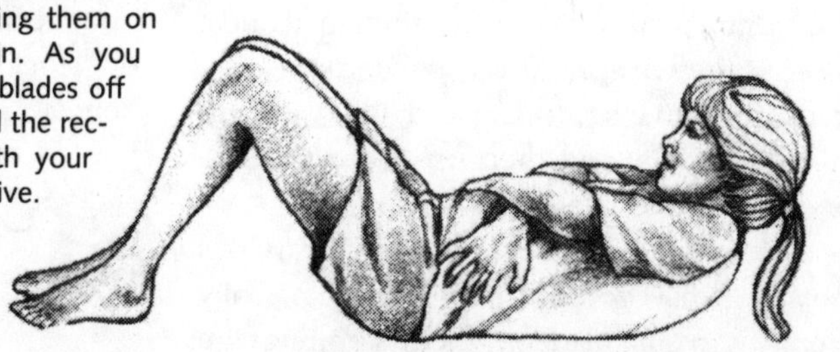

Exercises during Post Partum

After the birth of your baby, you may think you do not have time to exercise. Luckily, these exercises can be done while you go about your daily tasks. For example, each time you change a nappy you can contract the pelvic floor muscles or do several pelvic tilts. Before a feeding you can do wide arm circles. Once every day or two, sit on the floor and perform the exercises that are done in this position. You can also combine baby play with the last four exercises in this chapter. Do not overdo it. If you experience any pain, are very fatigued or have a large increase in vaginal bleeding, discontinue that exercise for a while. You practised many of the following exercises when you were pregnant. Refer to the pages indicated to review the complete descriptions.

Pelvic Floor Contraction or Kegel Exercise (page 129)

Starting right after birth, gently tighten and then relax the muscles of your perineum. You can perform this exercise when you are lying down, sitting or standing. You may not feel the contractions of these muscles at first, but if you did this exercise before delivery, you will know how to do it now. Start by doing two to three short contractions each hour or whenever you think about it, then progress to five contractions several times a day. At first, you may only be able to hold the contraction for two to three seconds. After a few days, hold the pelvic floor contraction for five seconds. Gradually work up to ten seconds, and then up to twenty seconds (the Super Kegel).

To test your progress, occasionally try this exercise while you are urinating by partially emptying your bladder, then stopping the flow. Do not be discouraged if you cannot do this at first. The Kegel exercise improves the strength of your pelvic floor muscles.

Pelvic Tilt (page 132)

The pelvic tilt exercise will help tone and strengthen your abdominal muscles and relieve backache. Soon after the birth, lie flat in bed or on the floor with your knees bent. Tighten your abdominal muscles to tilt your pelvis, and press your lower back into the bed for a count of two or three. Increase gradually to a count of ten. After a few days, do pelvic tilts while standing, sitting or on hands and knees. Remember to contract your pelvic floor muscles before doing abdominal muscle exercises.

Note: Check for separation of the rectus abdominal muscles (page 139) before doing the next exercises. If present, do the head lift exercise to diminish the separation before doing leg sliding, sit-back or central/diagonal lift exercises.

Leg Sliding

Aim: To help strengthen the lower abdominal muscles. Start with one leg and work up to sliding both legs.

Starting position: Lie on your back with your knees bent and your feet flat on the floor. Your feet will slide better if you wear socks or stockings. Place one or both hands beneath the small of your back.

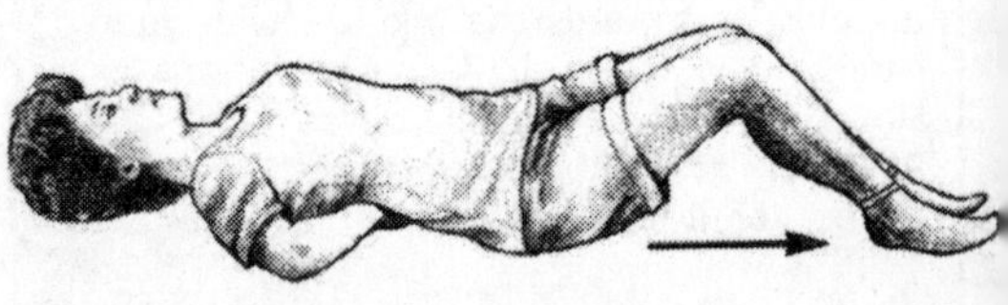

Exercise: Press your lower back to the floor by tightening your abdominal muscles, as in the pelvic tilt. Hold the pelvic tilt and slowly slide one foot along the floor, away from your body, extending your leg. If you feel your lower back begin to come up off your hands and the floor, stop sliding your leg and bring it back to the starting position.

Repetition: Repeat the exercise five times per day.

When you feel that your abdominal muscle tone has improved, begin sliding both legs. Remember to extend your legs only as far as you can without your lower back rising off your hands. If that happens, bring your legs back to the starting position, one at a time. As your abdominal muscles become stronger, you will be able to extend your legs completely and still keep your lower back flat.

Sit-Back

Aim: A week or two after the birth, begin this exercise, which strengthens the abdominal muscles. This and the central/diagonal lift (described next) are safer and more effective than sit-ups, which require jerking movements and can unduly strain the abdomen and lower back. The sit-back is smooth and safe because it is tailored to your strength and because you do not have to overcome the force of gravity at the beginning of the exercise.

Starting position: Sit with your knees bent, feet flat on the floor and arms stretched out in front of you.

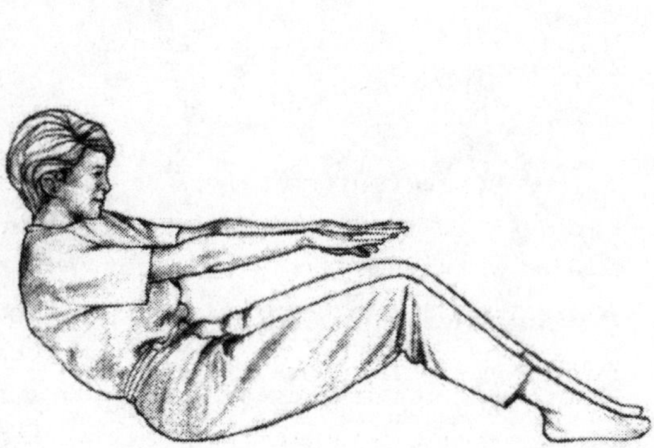

Exercise: Lean back, but only as far as you can without feeling weak or losing control of the position. In other words, when you begin to feel unsteady or weak, you have found your limit. Sit back up. Gradually increase the distance you lean back as you build strength. Soon you will be able to lean all the way down to the floor. Folding your arms across your chest makes the exercise more difficult. Later, try it with your hands clasped behind your head.

Central/Diagonal Lift

Aim: To strengthen your abdominal muscles.

The central lift. *Starting position:* Lie on your back with your knees bent and your feet flat on the floor.

Exercise: Breathe in, tilt your pelvis and keep your lower back pressed towards the floor. While breathing out, raise your head and shoulders from the floor, reaching your outstretched arms towards your knees. Move smoothly and keep your waist on the floor. When your shoulders are raised about 20 centimetres, hold the lift for a slow count of five. Relax and gently lie back. Do not use sudden jerky movements.

Repetition: Repeat about five times daily.

The diagonal lift. *Starting position:* Lie on your back with your knees bent and your feet flat on the floor.

Exercise: By rotating your upper body to the left or right as you raise your head and shoulders, you can strengthen different abdominal muscles (the oblique muscles). Remember to begin by breathing in and tilting your pelvis.

While breathing out, raise your upper body diagonally by rotating to the left, and reach towards the outside of your left knee. Hold for a slow count of five. Repeat, rotating towards your right side.

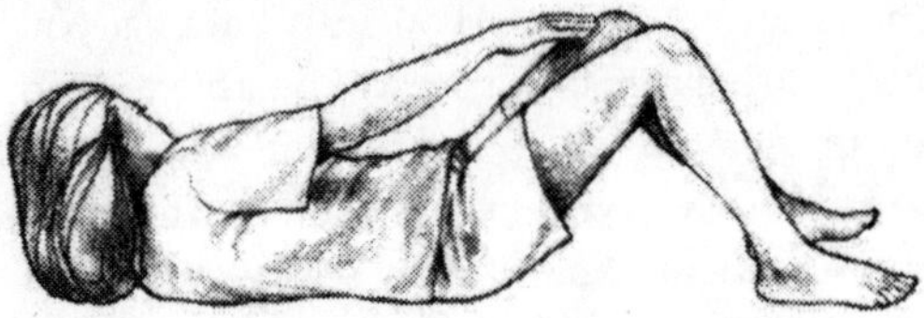

Repetition: Do the exercise five times daily on each side.

Your movements in the central and diagonal lifts should always be smooth, not jerky. As you strengthen your abdominal muscles, you can progress to more challenging central and diagonal lifts by folding your arms across your chest and later clasping your hands behind your head. Gradually increase the number of repetitions from five to ten per day.

Wide Arm Circles

Aim: To help increase circulation in the chest and upper back and to relieve tension in the neck and shoulders.

Starting position: Stand, kneel or sit with your arms straight and extended to the side.

Exercise: Move both arms in large, wide circles, first in one direction, then in the other. Try this exercise without a bra on. Do five to ten rotations in each direction, once to several times a day or once before each feeding.

Shoulder Circling

This exercise relieves tension in the shoulders. (See page 135 for directions.)

Relaxation and Slow Breathing

Because the post-partum period is stressful, it is wise to use the same relaxation techniques you found helpful during pregnancy and childbirth. Try five minutes of slow breathing (page 193) and passive relaxation (page 181) or the relaxation countdown (page 183) during a hectic day, and see how it relaxes and refreshes you. These techniques are also useful for afterpains, which occur during breastfeeding and at other times, especially in women who have had more than one child.

Exercising with Your Baby

Shaping up can be fun for both you and your baby. These exercises, which combine conditioning for you with play for your baby, are designed as all-around toners for the abdomen, back, arms, legs and buttocks.

Up, Up and Away (Arm Toning)

Starting position: Lie on your back with your knees bent and feet flat. Place your baby face-down on your chest, holding him under his arms.

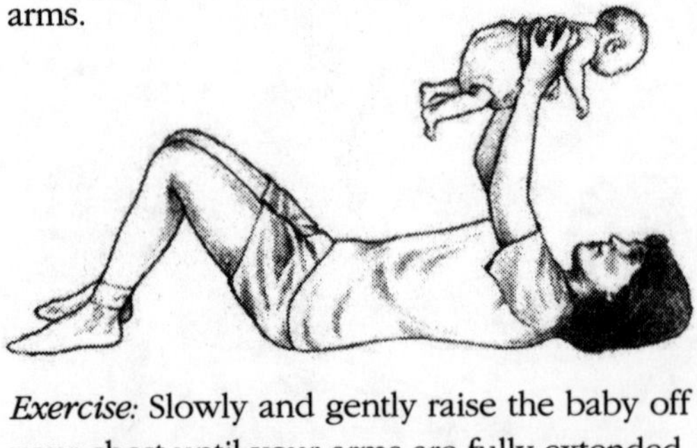

Exercise: Slowly and gently raise the baby off your chest until your arms are fully extended. Gently lower the baby back onto your chest.

Repetition: Repeat five times.

The Twist (Hip Walking)

Starting position: Sit on the floor with your legs extended. Hold your baby on your thighs, with his head and shoulders cradled in your hands.

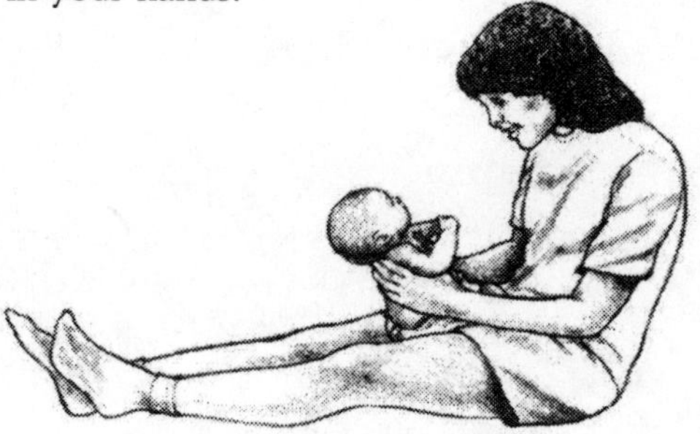

Exercise: 'Walk' forward on your buttocks, twisting as you go. Then 'walk' backwards.

Repetition: Repeat five times.

Rocking (Central Lift)

Starting position: Lie on your back with your hips and knees bent and your lower legs parallel to the floor. Place your baby facedown on your shins, with his eyes peeking over your knees. Hold him under the arms.

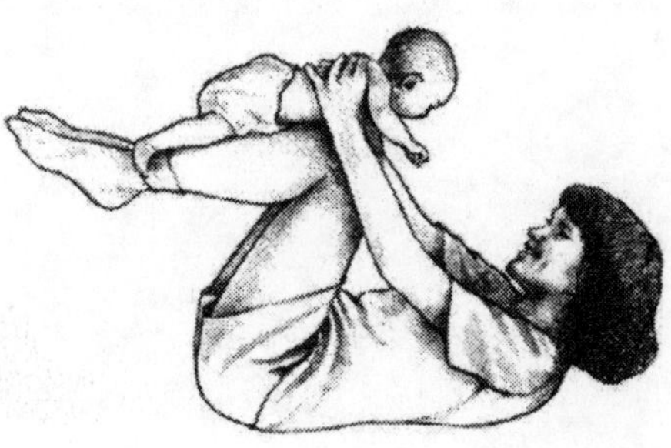

Exercise: Tuck your chin, slowly raise your head and shoulders and rock forward. (This is like a gentle central lift.) Then gently rock back, lowering your head to the floor. Avoid holding your breath.

Repetition: Repeat five times.

Rolling (Sit-Back)

Starting Position: Sitting on the floor with knees bent and feet flat on the floor, hold your baby against your chest or rest the baby on your thighs.

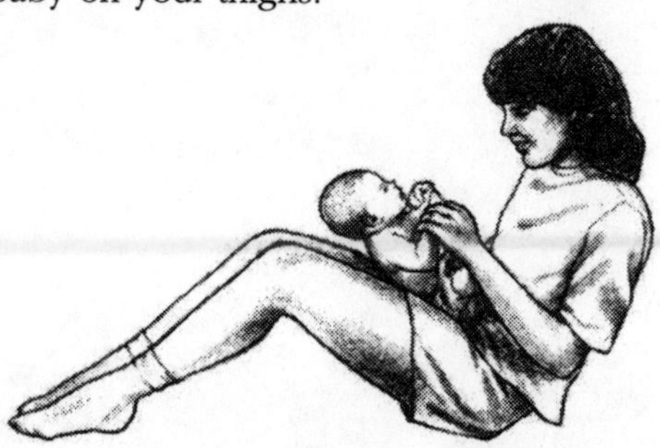

Exercise: Gently lean back as you would in the sit-back exercise (page 141). Roll back about halfway, then return to an upright position.

Repetition: Work gradually up to five repetitions.

Chapter 7

Planning for Birth and Post Partum

Modern maternity care is group care. Your doctor or midwife is almost surely a member of a group of caregivers who share 'call'. In other words, each member is scheduled to be on duty for births and other clinical care at specific times only. The caregiver on call covers not only his or her patients, but those of other caregivers in the group. Your caregiver is assisted by a staff of nurses who work shifts in the hospital's maternity department. This system is designed to ensure that the people responsible for your care are well rested.

Even though many professionals are involved in your care, the system is quite efficient, as long as communication is good among all members of the team. When nursing shifts change in a hospital, nurses finishing their shift often communicate personally with those coming on duty about the clinical status of each patient and other important factors. Nurses also communicate with physicians or midwives in person or by phone whenever necessary.

The medical chart, however, is the major means of communication among caregivers. At each prenatal visit and frequently during your labour and post partum, specific physical and psycho-social findings are recorded in your chart. It becomes a permanent record that is available whenever you need medical or maternity care in the future. Although most caregivers think of the medical chart as a means of communicating with one another, you can have access to your records and obtain a copy, if you wish. When requesting a copy from your hospital or caregiver's office, you will be asked to sign a release form and may need to pay a photocopying fee.

Despite the communication channels that exist within a group of caregivers, you may have problems with the lack of continuous care by one person throughout your pregnancy and at your birth. Your important personal preferences and needs may not be recorded or may not show up clearly in your chart, even though you have discussed them with one or more of your caregivers. If you have preferences for non-routine maternity care options, or if you have specific fears or concerns you would like your caregivers to consider, you need to communicate them efficiently and effectively. When your maternity caregivers understand and respect your preferences, you are more likely to feel satisfied and well cared for than if your desires and concerns are not recognised.[1] How can you communicate such information to those involved in your care? We suggest that you use a birth plan.

The Birth Plan

A birth plan is essentially a letter written to your caregivers and nurses that describes your concerns, fears, wishes, and how you and your partner would like your labour and birth to be managed and why. Some people prefer the terms *preference list, wish list* or *goal sheet*. Whatever you choose to call it, a birth plan is your chance to tell the medical staff about yourself and your priorities and needs. It is not a contract and does not attempt to dictate your caregivers' or nurses' actions. Rather, it is an expression of your preferences in areas of care in which different acceptable approaches exist. There are several advantages to birth plans.

Advantages to you. Preparing a birth plan requires that you look ahead to the birth. It encourages you to reflect and imagine how you will best cope with the unpredictability, stress and pain that are part of childbirth. It requires that you discover, think about and discuss the available options. It helps both of you clarify your needs and preferences. It helps you and your partner work together. The birth plan is also an excellent vehicle for discussion with your caregiver. By enhancing communication and clarifying your expectations of one another, working with a birth plan can build trust and understanding among all members of the childbirth team. Throughout labour and birth, the birth plan frees you from having to explain and re-explain your wishes and expectations, especially if you have an unfamiliar caregiver and when there is a change of nursing staff.

Advantages to your doctor or midwife. Working with you on a birth plan helps your doctor or midwife understand your goals and expectations and allows her or him to assist you in refining them to a realistic plan that is satisfactory to all involved. Reviewing your birth plan during pregnancy allows your caregiver to identify areas of misunderstanding or disagreement and gives you time to work out a suitable compromise. The birth plan is not a binding legal agreement (even if signed or initialled by your caregiver), nor is it a promise or guarantee that circumstances will not require a change in plan. A carefully considered birth plan includes preferences for situations when problems arise.

Advantages to the nursing staff. At the hospital, the birth plan helps nurses become acquainted with you and helps them individualise your care. When you enter the hospital in labour, you will probably be a stranger to the nurses. The birth plan gives them important information about you, especially your concerns and care preferences, which were selected when you were calm and able to think clearly. Studies show that women often feel disappointment, anger or even depression if their desires and expectations about their birth experiences are not met.[2] If the nurses know what is important to you, they are more able to meet your needs and to help you fulfil your wishes.

The success of a birth plan depends on you being realistic, informed, flexible and able to communicate. It also requires your caregivers to welcome your participation and individualise your maternity care to meet your needs.

Getting Started with Your Birth Plan

If you decide to prepare a birth plan, tell your caregiver. This may be a new idea for some doctors or midwives. Others, especially those who are accustomed to making most of the decisions, may be uncomfortable with birth plans. You may need to explain why you are preparing a birth plan, emphasising that you want it to enhance cooperation and trust between yourself, your caregiver and the nurses. Explain that it will help you know what to expect under both normal and abnormal circumstances.

Reactions of doctors and midwives vary. Some feel the birth plan is an essential element in your care. They ask you to prepare one and sometimes supply you with a form to fill out. Others believe birth plans are unnecessary, because no decision will be made during labour without your consent. Some caregivers may not realise how helpful it is for you to know *in advance* whether your desires for care are realistic and acceptable. Also, they may not realise how stressful it can be to explain your wishes to each doctor, midwife or nurse while you are in labour dealing with your contractions. If your caregiver is opposed to a birth plan, then you have gained valuable insight (your caregiver does not want to know what is important to you) and you can act on it. You can give up your birth plan and do what your caregiver requires, you can negotiate, or you can try to find another caregiver. At the very least, you have clarified your relationship and will not be confused or surprised in labour.

If your doctor or midwife supports the idea of a birth plan, then you have an excellent opportunity to discuss and plan how your labour and birth will be managed. This builds a sense of cooperation and trust between you, which continues through the birth experience and adds greatly to everyone's satisfaction. The feelings of trust and understanding are perhaps most reassuring if problems arise during labour and you have to adjust to changes in the plan.

Step by Step: Preparing Your Birth Plan

Preparation of your birth plan is best done gradually over several weeks. There are a number of steps to complete in order to come up with the most meaningful and helpful birth plan:

1. Decide what basic approach to maternity care you prefer.

2. Learn about specific options available to you when everything goes normally. Also, find out what happens when the unexpected occurs. Select the options you prefer.

3. Make a rough draft of your plan and discuss it with your caregiver.

4. Using what you learned in the first three steps, prepare a brief final birth plan that summarises your wishes, needs and priorities.

Step 1: Your Preferred Approach to Maternity Care

Ask yourself, 'Of the following two basic approaches to maternity care, which is closer to my way of thinking about birth'?

A) I will feel more secure if I can participate fully in my labour, making decisions about and using self-help measures to handle my pain and promote labour progress. Unless there is a medical reason to do otherwise, I prefer to rely on myself and my support team, with the advice and encouragement of my expert caregiver and nurses. My partner and I are reading, practising self-help measures and attending childbirth classes to prepare for this experience. (This is called the 'self-reliant approach'.)

B) I will feel more secure if I rely on my expert caregivers to use their judgment in managing my labour and relieving my pain. I feel more comfortable relying on appropriate technological and medical resources than on my own knowledge and ability to handle pain. I will do whatever is asked of me, but I would like to be kept informed about what to expect and about the reasons behind any clinical decisions. I am not spending much time outside of childbirth classes preparing for childbirth. (This is called the 'caregiver-reliant approach'.)

If neither of these basic approaches quite reflects your point of view, try to explain how you would like to participate and what role you would like the caregivers and nurses to play. The 'Worksheet for Preparing Your Birth Plan' (pages 160–165) may help you clarify your preferences.

Step 2: Learn about Options and Identify Preferences

Once you determine your preferred approach, you and your partner should learn about options available within that approach. This step may seem quite overwhelming at first, because there may be numerous options. There are many sources of help: this book (see the worksheet on pages 160–165 and check the index for pages where most of these options are discussed), other books (see Recommended Resources), caregivers, friends, childbirth education classes and hospital tours. The 'Worksheet for Preparing Your Birth Plan' (page 160) lists common practices during labour, birth and post partum, along with options for handling each. Some practices you may welcome; others you may want to avoid. You will see that some options are more compatible with the self-reliant approach, while others are more compatible with the caregiver-reliant approach. As you learn about options and imagine yourself in labour, you may discover that the options you prefer do not reflect the approach you selected in Step 1.

This process may help you clarify your values. It may also reveal any basic differences of opinion between you and your partner. It is desirable to discover and resolve these differences ahead of time. If this step is too time-consuming or too complex, or if it is simply too much work to learn about all these options, you can skip Step 2 and base your plan on your instinctive preferences and on what you learn in childbirth classes.

Step 3: Prepare a Rough Draft and Discuss It with Your Caregiver

Once you have completed Steps 1 and 2, make two enlarged photocopies of the Birth Plan form (page 166) or enter items from the form into your computer. Prepare a rough draft on one copy of the form or on your computer. When preparing to discuss your draft with your caregiver, you may need to schedule a longer appointment or several shorter appointments. During these appointments, you will learn whether your caregiver supports your wishes and how compatible your wishes are with your caregiver's and the hospital's usual practices. If you discover that some of your preferred options are not available to you, find out alternatives by asking questions on the hospital tour, in childbirth class or during another prenatal care appointment.

Until you have discussed your birth plan with your caregiver, you cannot have a meaningful final draft. Birth plans are not one-sided documents. They are collaborative and include input from three of the important players in the birth drama—you, your partner and your caregiver. Unfortunately, it is not usually possible to get direct input from the nursing staff before labour.

Step 4: Prepare the Final Draft

The last step in preparing your birth plan is to revise your rough draft into a final draft. Use your second photocopy or make changes on your computer. Incorporate what you discussed with your caregiver and others. Once the final draft is complete, make copies for yourself, your partner, your caregiver and the midwives. Make a backup copy in case one is misplaced, and be sure to have yours with you in labour.

The Birth Plan form (page 166) allows you to summarise your preferences and other important personal information about yourself, your partner and your baby. Notice that the form limits the amount of space for each topic. There are good reasons for this: (1) Your most important preferences stand out clearly; (2) A lengthy birth plan is time-consuming for the busy midwife or caregiver who can grasp the gist of your preferred approach and personal needs in relatively few words; (3) You do not need to (nor should you) produce a list of procedures that are and are not acceptable to you. If circumstances change, some 'unacceptable' procedures may become necessary and 'acceptable', especially if problems develop in your pregnancy, labour or delivery. For example, induction of labour at forty weeks 'for convenience' may be relatively unacceptable to you, while induction at forty-two weeks or earlier 'for health reasons' may become acceptable.

If you think about it, you may realise that a lengthy, detailed list of dos and don'ts for the caregiver or midwives is bound to distress or even anger the people who are entrusted with the care of you and your baby. You certainly do not want to put up barriers to good communication and a good relationship. Read it over, putting yourself in your caregiver's place. From your caregiver's point of view, is your birth plan friendly, respectful and flexible (indicating your awareness that labour is not always normal or predictable)? Does your tone promote mutual trust and collaboration? If so, your caregiver should respond in the same spirit. A brief yet complete birth plan is easy for your caregiver and nurses to read and understand. Also, by starting with a rough draft, you are making it clear that you are not rigid and that you desire input from your caregivers.

Components of the Birth Plan

Your birth plan should contain the following: an introduction; your most important wishes, issues, fears or concerns; a general description of your preferences for managing labour pain; and sections on each stage of normal labour and birth, unexpected events (labour complications, caesarean birth, a premature or sick baby, the death of the baby) and post-partum (after birth) care in the hospital for you and your baby.

This book discusses most of the routine practices you may encounter. Use it as background for your birth plan and for talking with your caregivers. In addition, because routine practices vary from area to area, your childbirth educator may be a helpful resource as you prepare your birth plan, especially if she or he is familiar with the options available in your community. Your childbirth educator may also help you with wording or other aspects of your birth plan.

The Introduction

The introduction is a paragraph about you and your partner, why you chose your caregiver and place for birth, and why your birth plan is important to you. For example, you may want to tell the staff if your pregnancy has been healthy and pleasant or if you have had difficulties such as infertility, previous miscarriage, or emotional or physical problems during this or a previous pregnancy. You may share information about cultural or religious preferences, special personal needs or strong feelings about having a natural or a medicated birth.

If you are a newcomer to Australia, you may find the childbirth and baby care customs quite different from your native country. Your family, especially your mother or mother-in-law, may be surprised or disturbed by some Australian customs, methods and advice. If so, it may help if you explain some of your country's customs and ask if your care can be similar to and reflect your native customs.

Also, you may provide the names and give any helpful information about your partner or others who will be present. Do they have any physical, social or emotional problems that, if known, would help the staff take better care of you? Will there be a less conventional combination of family members present, such as adoptive parents, lesbian co-parents or children? Are there any stressful family dynamics? Are there people you do not want to be present at the birth? The midwives can help you more effectively if they have this kind of information. You may also state that you will appreciate the expertise, help and support of the nursing staff in carrying out your birth plan.

Important Wishes, Issues, Fears and Concerns

This paragraph is optional. You may have no particular fears or concerns, but if you do, this is your opportunity to disclose them to the staff. For example, you may worry about your baby's wellbeing. You may fear hospitals or medical procedures. You may be uncomfortable with or distrustful of nurses and doctors or midwives. You may worry about the pain of labour and how you may behave or cope. You may have issues with modesty. You may fear losing control. You may find vaginal exams, blood taking or other procedures very stressful.

Sometimes, negative previous experiences play a role in these fears. Previous pregnancy losses or traumatic births, negative experiences with doctors or hospitals, growing up in a dysfunctional, abusive or neglectful family—all these experiences and more may influence your feelings as you anticipate birth.

By disclosing your feelings and (if appropriate) some of the reasons, you can help the staff provide sensitive care and take your special needs into account. (See pages 42–43 for further discussion of how early childhood experiences sometimes influence a woman's later childbearing, and pages 331–333 for more on previous disappointing or traumatic birth experiences associated with a previous caesarean birth.)

Preferences for Managing Labour Pain

After becoming familiar with both the non-medical and medical measures for pain relief (see Chapters 8 and 12), describe your preferences in this section. The midwives need to know if you prefer a natural birth and, if so, which comfort measures and support people you will rely on. If you prefer to use pain medications, the midwives need to know if you want to try to delay them until labour is well established, or if you want them as early in labour as allowed. Do you want narcotics, an epidural or other medications? Many women state that as long as labour is progressing normally and they are coping, they prefer to avoid or minimise pain medications. However, if complications arise or the pain is

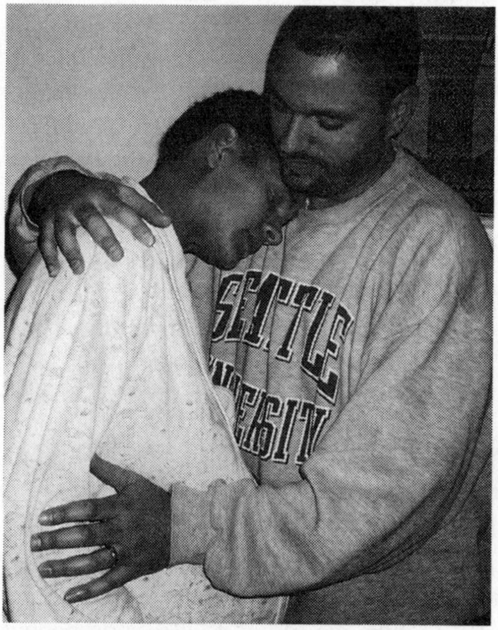

Photograph by Katie McCullough

For your birth plan, think about the role your partner will play.

too great, they like to keep the option of pain medications open. Some women ask the midwives not to offer pain medications, stating that they will ask for them when needed. State your preferences as clearly as you can, even though you cannot know how much pain you will have or how long labour will last.

Preferences for Normal Labour and Birth

First Stage, Second Stage and Third Stage

When labour and birth proceed normally, few interventions are necessary for medical safety. Some interventions may be used, however, for other reasons. Sometimes, for example, caregivers induce labour or start giving intravenous (IV) fluids, even when there is no problem, in the belief that it is better to use them before rather than after a problem arises. Other routine interventions—such as the back-lying position for birth, the use of stirrups and taking the baby from the mother for testing and observation—exist for the convenience of the staff or caregiver. Still others—such as the use of antibiotics for the baby's eyes and newborn screening for PKU, hypothyroidism and other conditions—are preventive and required by State law.

Some practices—such as enemas, shaving the perineum and draping the mother's body and legs during birth—are less common today but continue in some areas. Such procedures became routine at a time when they were believed to be beneficial, but they are now known to be of little or no benefit and may even be harmful. Some procedures—such as epidural, caesarean and circumcision—require your informed consent. This means that your signed consent is recorded in your chart after your caregiver has explained the procedure, its benefits and risks, and the risks and benefits of alternatives (including not doing it).

Part of your preparation involves finding out which routines you are likely to encounter (along with the reasoning behind them). Childbirth classes, the hospital tour and your caregiver can help you find out which routines are used in first stage, second stage and third stage. As you prepare this section of your birth plan, mention only the preferences that matter to you. You do not have to express an opinion on everything. Better yet, summarise your preferences with a blanket statement such as, 'I prefer to avoid routine interventions and procedures and want to discuss any that are being considered'. Or, you may want to say, 'I am comfortable relying on my caregiver to make decisions about interventions and procedures'.

Preferences for Unexpected Labour Events

This section will be most helpful if something unforeseen occurs. If problems arise before, during or after labour, your preferences for a normal labour and birth may have to be modified. Consider this possibility, recognising that some problems are more serious than others and may require that you rely more on your caregiver's judgment and on medications and interventions to ensure the safety of you and your baby. Be sure to ask the key questions about your care (page 52) to help you understand the problem, how serious it is and what your options are. Of course, in the rare emergency situation, the need for immediate action may mean there is little or no time for explanations or discussion. Under most circumstances, however, there is time for you to become informed, ask questions and participate in the decision.

You will find that when unexpected problems arise, a good outcome requires more reliance on your caregiver's judgment and actions. Your participation in the form of cooperation, willingness to accept suggestions from your midwife or caregiver, and ability to be flexible will help ensure a healthy outcome and satisfaction with your birth. For example, a birth plan for a caesarean birth can help you retain some of the priorities of your original birth plan. Though an unexpected caesarean can be a disappointment, you will feel better about the experience if you have thought about this possibility, know your options and express your preferences. (Information in Chapter 11 will help you with a caesarean birth plan.)

Preferences for Healthy Baby Care for the First Days

This section describes how you want your baby cared for during the first few days after birth. There are as many differences in the way healthy newborns are cared for as there are differences in every other aspect of maternity care. Generally, the healthy newborn needs little more than access to her mother's breast and parents' arms, a warm environment, nappies and clothing. Particular observations, tests and procedures are done routinely to discover serious congenital disorders or to prevent potentially serious illnesses. When considering the options listed in the chart on page 164, balance concerns for your baby's comfort and wellbeing with the potential benefits and risks of each procedure. Some routines and procedures once considered beneficial are now known to be unnecessary or even harmful. For example, feeding sugar water or formula to the breastfed baby is now considered unnecessary by lactation specialists. Circumcision, although sometimes chosen by parents for personal or religious reasons, is now recognised as having little medical benefit.

Preferences for Unexpected Events for Newborn Baby

Although almost all babies are born healthy, there is a slim possibility that your baby might have a problem. This possibility worries most expectant parents to some degree. You know that prematurity, illness, birth defects or even death sometimes occur. It is helpful to consider in advance how you would want these misfortunes handled. Otherwise, you will have to make decisions when you are upset and unable to think clearly. Your birth plan can reflect your consideration of such possibilities, so that the staff can care for you and your baby with knowledge of your preferences. (See pages 164–165 for further discussion.)

Preferences for Post Partum in the Hospital for New Mother

This section describes your wishes and needs for your one- to three-day hospital stay after the birth. Think about your preferences concerning visitors. Do you want friends and relatives to visit, or do you prefer to get more rest and focus more on your baby? Think about your educational needs and make a list of the major items you want to learn while in the hospital. Do you want help with breast-feeding, nappy changing, dressing or bathing the baby? Do you want to know more about your infant's cues for hunger and for over-stimulation, and what to expect of your baby for the next few days at home (sleeping, feeding, bladder and bowel patterns, and so on)? Since your length of stay is very limited, plan carefully how you will use it. For women who have had a caesarean birth and for some of those with extensive episiotomies or lacerations, pain control needs to be considered. (The discussion on pages 357–358 can help with your decision about post-partum pain relief.) Also, include your preferences for follow-up care for the first days when you return home. Find out what care is available to you and your baby and what you will need to do to set up an appointment for any services.

As you can see, preparing a birth plan requires time, thought and information gathering. When you are finished, you should have a fairly complete picture of what you can expect in terms of your care during childbirth and immediately afterward. Not only will you and your caregivers have made a general plan for managing your

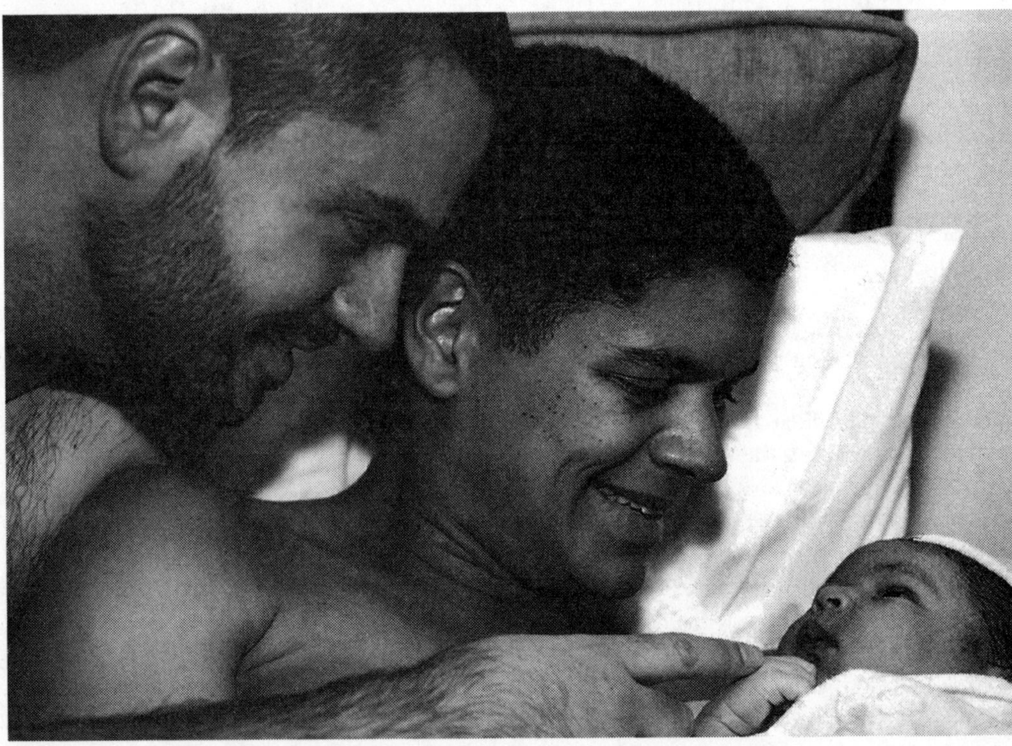

Photograph by Katie McCullough

One thing you cannot plan for—being totally engrossed with your baby.

uncomplicated, normal labour and birth, but you will also know how unexpected variations and complications are likely to be handled. The decisions you make in advance when you are calm and able to concentrate will help guide you and your caregivers during situations when you need to devote all your mental and physical energies to coping with childbirth.

After the Birth: Your Post-partum Plan

A post-partum plan is as important as a birth plan, though in a different way. The purpose of a birth plan is to help your maternity care professionals understand your needs and priorities during and immediately after birth. Once you arrive home, however, you need a different kind of plan to help make sure your needs and your baby's are met.

The amount of hands-on experience a new mother can expect to gain before leaving the hospital has steadily declined over the last forty years. In 1960, it was common for a mother and her newborn to stay in the hospital for seven days after childbirth. Today, most hospitals discharge mother and baby within two to four days after birth. Even after a caesarean, a mother can expect to be home after five days. Many parents report that they suddenly find themselves at home, with their charming and needy baby, and hardly any idea of what to expect and what to do.

You and your baby will continue to need professional health care, and daily demands on your time will increase greatly. Most likely, you will resume your usual responsibilities while, at the same time, you are learning to feed, nurture and care for your baby. For most new parents, the first weeks are more challenging and stressful than expected. Assistance from family, friends and other professionals can help.

Decisions to Make for the Post-partum Period

You can ease the transition into the first days of parenthood by identifying some of your post-partum needs in advance and planning for how they will be met. As with the birth plan, decisions about the post-partum period also require information gathering, discussion and introspection.

Choosing a Health Care Provider for Your Baby

This is one of the most important decisions during the post-partum period. It can be a great relief to have chosen your baby's health care provider before the birth, so that you know the schedule of routine baby (preventive) visits and have someone to call whenever you have a concern. There are several types of health care providers for children. Each has its own advantages.

Paediatricians specialise in children's health care. Their offices and waiting rooms are geared for children. Paediatricians have completed medical school and a paediatric residency. They have more training in child development and childhood illness than the following practitioners.

General practitioners provide care for the entire family. They refer seriously ill children to doctors with specialty training. They have spent several months in paediatrics as part of their medical school and residency training. If your pregnancy care was provided by a family doctor, it may be a natural transition to have the same doctor care for your baby.

Naturopaths and other alternative practitioners provide well-child care and emphasise non-medical treatment of illness. Their education varies but may consist of four years of training after secondary school. They usually provide care for the entire family. They refer seriously ill children to medical doctors.

Choosing Your Child's Health Care Setting

The cost of your child's health care varies depending on your health insurance coverage and on the setting you choose. Usually, most of your baby's visits in the first year are routine-child visits in which your health care provider checks the healthy baby and gives immunisations. If you have a choice of health plans, you may want to compare their coverage of routine-child visits.

Private care is more expensive than health centre care, but may be more personalised and convenient. Many health care plans cover most or part of private-care costs and include a list of approved practitioners from which to choose. Some plans do not pay for routine-child visits but have almost full coverage if your child is ill.

Community health centres usually cost less, but there may be more waiting time. If associated with a medical school, the staff may change frequently. The caregivers are doctors or nurse practitioners rotating through phases of their advanced training. They are supervised by fully trained professionals. Such centres usually also provide social services and other services helpful to low-income families.

Baby health centres (associated with the public health department or community health centres) offer free or low-cost check-ups and immunisations, but usually do not provide care for sick children.

Prenatal Interview

After determining which health care providers and settings are available, you may wish to get opinions and recommendations from your family and friends, doctor or midwife, your childbirth educator or a local hospital. In narrowing down which providers to contact, consider the convenience of their locations and office hours. If possible, make a prenatal interview appointment with one or more of the practitioners to ask questions and get to know them. You may be able to do this before your baby is born. Check your health insurance plan to determine if such appointments are covered and, if they are not, find out what (if anything) the interview appointment will cost before you make it. At the appointment, ask for information and the caregiver's opinion or advice on some of the following topics. (Information may also be obtained from the caregiver's receptionist.)

- Breastfeeding or formula feeding
- Availability of lactation consultants or other resources for breastfeeding mothers

- Circumcision, if your baby is a boy
- Access to the caregiver for telephone consultation, and names and qualifications of other personnel who answer calls
- Immunisations
- The use of home remedies or alternative therapies versus antibiotics and other medicines for minor ailments and common illnesses (colds, ear infections, colic or viruses)
- Arrangements for backup caregivers when he or she is not available
- Names of hospitals where the caregiver has privileges
- Availability of the caregiver to examine newborn baby soon after birth
- Limits on the caregiver's practice and referral plans, if needed

During the interview, pay as much attention to *how* your questions are answered as to *what* is said. You should be able to sense if this person is competent, caring and considerate. Try to find someone whose style and philosophy are compatible with yours. You should feel you can trust the health care of your child to this person.

Other Things to Think About before Your Baby Is Born

For more information about these issues and concerns, see the chapters and page numbers suggested.

- Think about visitors after the birth. Whom will you want and not want to see? How can you restrict visitors when you are tired and frazzled?
- Learn about classes, support groups, books and resources you could use to help you in the first weeks after birth. Make a list of helpful phone numbers. (See the table on page 159.)
- Will your baby be breastfed or formula-fed? (Chapter 15 provides information about each method.)
- Make a list of areas in which you are likely to need assistance, such as transportation, housework, meal preparation, shopping and child care for older children. Ask friends and relatives for help.
- Who will help you at home after the birth? You will need rest and help with household tasks. If this is your first baby, you may need advice and instruction on newborn care and feeding. Your partner may take time off, your parents or a relative may visit, friends may offer to help out, or you may hire a mother's helper for a few hours each day. A mother's helper may be an agency employee, a student or an independent contractor who cleans and cooks but who does not necessarily know about baby care and new family adjustment. Ask your childbirth educator or caregiver for referrals.
- If you are feeling overwhelmed, extremely sad or depressed after the baby is born, whom can you call? Make a list of family, friends and counsellors who can help if these feelings persist. (See Chapter 13.)
- What equipment, supplies and preparations are needed for the baby, such as a car seat, crib, room, clothes, linens, toiletries and so on? (See Chapter 14.)
- Will you use cloth or disposable nappies or both? If you use cloth nappies, will you

use a nappy service?

- Will you work outside the home after the baby is born? If so, when will you start? Who will provide child care when you and your partner are at work? Can you and your partner share some or all of the child care?
- Will you return to part-time or full-time employment? Will you continue to breast-feed while working? Is there a private, comfortable place at work where you can pump your breast milk? (See page 451.)
- How will your financial situation change? If you reduce your work hours or if you are not employed, plan and follow a budget, if necessary, to avoid excessive spending and to ensure that expenses can be met.

Develop your post-partum plan from the answers to these questions and from information you have gathered about what you need after the baby arrives. Your post-partum plan is for your personal use. You do not need to create a formal document as you did with your birth plan. Having the phone numbers of helpful people and agencies may be all you need in a post-partum plan. Make your list of post-partum resources before the baby is born.

Your Personal Post-partum Resource List

You will thank yourself many times over if you take the time to prepare a list of names and phone numbers of people who can help you after the birth. Fill in the following list with names and numbers and make copies for you and your partner. Place them on your refrigerator door, in your purse and near your phone.

Personal Post-partum Resource List

(Make your list of helpful people and phone numbers before the baby is born.)

Resource/Service	Name	Telephone
Start Using before the Birth:		
Doctor/midwife		
Childbirth educator		
Hospital maternity unit		
Health care information line		
Medical insurance provider		
Start Using after the Birth:		
Baby's health care provider		
Breastfeeding counsellor		
Breast pump rental service		
Nappy service		
Friend or family helpers		
Child care, babysitters		
Support groups		
Emergency Services:		
Police, fire, medical		000
Help line		
Other:		

Worksheet for Preparing Your Birth Plan

This optional worksheet is for your use as you prepare your birth plan. It is not intended to be used as a birth plan itself. Make a check by the items that are important to you. These may be items that elicit strong positive or negative feelings in you or your partner. Put a question mark by items you are unsure about, and plan to learn more about those options. The page numbers following each topic tell you where to find general information in this book about that topic.

This worksheet may help you clarify your preferred approach to maternity care. You may discover that you want to participate in decision-making and self-help comfort measures for pain relief (self-reliant approach) or that you prefer to rely more on your caregiver and nurses for these things (caregiver-reliant approach). You may find that you prefer a combination of these two approaches.

Once you have completed this worksheet, write a short description of the roles you envision for yourself, your partner and your caregivers (the approach you prefer). Then prepare a draft of your birth plan to discuss with your caregiver.

Options for Normal Labour and Birth

First Stage

Presence of partner/others (pages 175–178 and 467–471)

__ Partner

__ Friends or relatives

__ Children (during labour and/or at birth)

Positions for labour (pages 227–228)

__ Freedom to change positions, stand and/or walk around

__ Postural aids (birth ball, tub, beanbag chair or other)

Vaginal exams (pages 215–216)

__ Only at mother's request or if needed for clinical decision

__ Frequency of exams

__ Number of different examiners

Monitoring foetal heart rate (pages 258–259)

__ Auscultation with foetoscope or stethoscope

__ Auscultation with Doppler (ultrasound stethoscope)

__ Intermittent external electronic foetal monitoring

__ Continuous with telemetry

__ Continuous electronic monitoring (internal or external)

Food/fluids (page 191)

__ Eat and drink as desired

__ Water, juice, iceblocks

__ Ice only

__ Saline (or Heparin) lock

__ IV fluids

Pain relief (pages 181–199 and Chapter 12)

__ Emotional support from partner, friends and staff

__ Relaxation, breathing and comfort measures

__ Bath, whirlpool or shower

__ Medications (narcotics) and/or anaesthesia (epidural or other)

Worksheet for Preparing Your Birth Plan

Options for Normal Labour and Birth

Second Stage (pushing and birth of baby)

Position for pushing and for birth (pages 227–229)	Promoting descent and delivery (pages 235–237)
__ Mother's choice of positions __ Caregiver's choice of positions	__ Gravity-enhancing positions __ Prolonged pushing on command __ Episiotomy __ Forceps or vacuum extractor
Expulsion techniques (pages 199–203) __ Spontaneous bearing down __ Directed pushing __ Prolonged breath-holding and straining	**Covering the perineal area (pages 238–242)** __ Undraped, mother may touch baby during birth __ Drapes around vagina and on abdomen and legs
Bed/equipment for pushing and for birth (pages 227–229) __ Choice of birth stool, beanbag, bathtub (water birth), floor or bed __ Birthing bed __ Delivery table with or without stirrups	**Episiotomy (care of perineum at birth) (pages 240 and 291–293)** __ Measures to help maintain intact perineum and to avoid a tear (warm compresses, pressure, controlled pushing, positions) __ No episiotomy (willing to risk having a tear) __ Decision left to caregiver __ Anaesthesia before episiotomy __ Anaesthesia after birth for stitches

Third Stage and First Hours after Birth

Cord cutting (pages 243–244)	Maintaining uterine muscle tone (pages 245–246)
__ Partner cuts cord __ Caregiver cuts cord __ Clamp and cut immediately __ Clamp and cut after cord stops pulsating	__ Breastfeed baby __ Fundal massage by nurse or mother __ Medication to contract uterus
Immediate care of baby (pages 243–247) __ In parents' arms for observation and Apgar score __ In mother's bed for observation and Apgar score __ Near parents in bassinet or isolette __ In mother's room for observation, weighing and first bath __ In nursery for observation, weighing and first bath	**Warmth of baby (pages 246–247)** __ Baby skin-to-skin with mother, with blanket or heater over both __ Wrapped in heated blanket, held by parent __ In heated bassinet in mother's room __ In special heated unit in nursery

Worksheet for Preparing Your Birth Plan

Options for Normal Labour and Birth

Third Stage and First Hours after Birth (continued)

Airway (page 242)

__ Suction only if necessary
__ Suction with bulb syringe almost immediately

Vitamin K (page 389)

__ Oral doses
__ By injection soon after birth

Eye care (page 290)

__ At end of first hour of life
__ Use of non-irritating antibiotic agent
__ Refusal of eye care

Cord care collection (depends on availability) (pages 244–245)

__ Not planned
__ Public cord blood bank donation
__ Private or family cord blood collection and storage

Options for Unexpected Labour Events

(If problems develop before or during labour, you have to let go of some of your preferred options, because more interventions may be necessary for safety. Consider these options, as they may be available even under such circumstances.)

Induction; Prolonged or Complicated Labour

Induction (pages 260–274)

__ Avoid induction
__ At woman's or caregiver's convenience
__ Self-induction methods
__ Stripping membranes
__ Cervical dilators
__ Artificial rupture of membranes
__ Pre-induction agents (prostaglandins)
__ Induction agents (Syntocinon)

Maternal exhaustion (pages 230–235)

__ Rest, relaxation skills
__ Bath, dim lights, privacy
__ Narcotics or sedatives for sleep
__ Epidural anaesthesia

Prolonged active labour (pages 283–290)

__ Walk, change positions, take a bath
__ Nipple stimulation
__ Artificial rupture of membranes
__ Medication (Oxgiocin)

Prolonged second stage (pages 290–293)

__ Time spent before interventions
__ Rest from pushing
__ Change positions
__ Directed pushing
__ Oxytocin
__ Vacuum extractor, forceps and/or episiotomy

Worksheet for Preparing Your Birth Plan

Options for Unexpected Labour Events

Induction; Prolonged or Complicated Labour (continued)	
Suspected foetal distress (Chapters 10 and 11) __ Mother changes position, uses oxygen __ Foetal scalp stimulation to evaluate foetal well-being __ Amnio-infusion __ Continuous electronic foetal monitoring, internal scalp electrode __ Caesarean delivery	**Prolonged third stage (page 293)** __ Placental separation encouraged by breast stimulation, suckling __ Upright position __ Hastened with fundal massage __ Hastened with medication __ Manual extraction of placenta
Caesarean Birth	
Timing of planned caesarean (page 321) __ After labour begins __ Scheduled before labour begins	**Participation by mother (page 323)** __ Mother watches delivery of baby (window in screen or screen lowered) __ Anaesthesiologist or obstetrician explains events during surgery __ No description of events during surgery
Anaesthesia (page 323) __ Regional anaesthesia (spinal or epidural) __ Regional anaesthesia with or without premedication __ General anaesthesia	**Post-operative medications (page 327)** __ Only at mother's request __ Medications to mother for anxiety, trembling or nausea at anaesthesiologist's discretion
Presence of partner/others (page 323) __ More than one supportive person present __ Father or partner only __ Partner seated at mother's head __ Partner stands and watches or photographs surgery and birth __ Partner not present	**Contact between baby and mother/parents (pages 325–327)** __ Held by partner soon after birth, where mother can touch and see __ Baby held by mother during surgical repair of incisions __ Baby taken to nursery for routine observation __ If baby goes immediately to nursery or intensive care: partner goes with baby or remains with mother; or, if there are two labour partners, one partner goes with baby and another partner remains with mother.

Worksheet for Preparing Your Birth Plan

Options for Healthy Baby Care for First Days

First feedings (pages 241 and 462)
__ Breastfeeding within first hour
__ Breastfeeding, but could be delayed
__ Infant formula
__ Feeding on cues from baby
__ Feedings scheduled by hospital staff
__ Supplemental feedings to breastfed baby (water, glucose water, formula)
__ Supplement (if used) given to breastfed baby by parents or nurse

Circumcision (pages 402–404)
__ None
__ Immediately (within two days of age)
__ Delayed (within two weeks of age)
__ With one or both parents present to comfort baby
__ With local anaesthesia
__ No anaesthesia
__ At religious ceremony

Contact between baby and mother/parents (pages 246–247)
__ 24-hour rooming-in
__ Daytime rooming-in
__ For feedings only, in nursery at other times

Newborn exam (pages 246–247)
__ Performed by baby's caregiver
__ Performed by hospital caregiver
__ Performed in presence of parents
__ Performed in nursery away from parents

Immunisations on first day or two (page 415)
__ None
__ Hepatitis B

Options for Unexpected Events for Newborn Baby

(If problems develop after the birth, you will need to have a plan for these events.)

Premature or Sick Baby

Contact between baby and mother/parents (pages 303, 306, and 409–410)
__ Parents visit baby in special care nursery (as desired)
__ Kangaroo care for premature baby
__ Parents feed and care for baby as much as possible
__ If baby is in different hospital than mother, partner goes with baby

Feeding when baby is able to swallow food (pages 409 and 452–455)
__ Mother breastfeeds baby, if possible
__ Mother pumps breast milk and feeds baby by tube or bottle
__ Formula feeding by parents
__ Formula feeding by nurse

Contact with support group (pages 306 and 410)
__ Initiated by parents, nurses or support group
__ No contact desired

Medications and procedures (pages 303 and 306)
__ Parent involvement in decision-making and procedures
__ Availability of staff for updates to parents

Worksheet for Preparing Your Birth Plan

Options for Unexpected Events for Newborn Baby

Stillbirth or Death of Baby (These choices are highly personal and may not be desirable for all parents.)

Medication for mother before, during or after childbirth (page 305) __ None __ At mother's request __ At caregiver's suggestion	**Mother's participation (pages 305–307)** __ Use of labour coping techniques (with or without pain medication) __ Involved in decision-making __ Labour management left to hospital staff
Mother's recovery and support (pages 305–307) __ Recovery on maternity unit __ Recovery in room separate from maternity unit __ Early discharge __ Spiritual and grief counselling __ Later contact with parent support group __ Amount of supportive care from outside sources	**Memories of baby (pages 305–306)** __ Obtain mementos (photographs, locks of hair, foot- and handprint, silhouettes, baby's blanket) __ No mementos __ Name baby
Contact with baby after death (pages 305–306) __ See and hold baby after death __ No contact with stillborn baby	**Care of baby after death (pages 305–306)** __ Spiritual services (baptism, memorial service, funeral) __ Autopsy __ Burial or cremation

Options for Post Partum in Hospital for New Mother

Infant feeding (pages 423–425) __ Breastfeeding __ Formula feeding	**Controlling pain (pages 357–358 and 362–367)** __ Use of self-help techniques before use of medications __ Medications
Visits by family and friends (pages 153–154) __ Unlimited visitation desired __ Limit who will visit __ Limit when visitors can come into room __ Hours or amount of time limited by hospital	**Dietary preferences (page 100)** __ General diet __ Vegetarian __ Kosher __ Food allergies and sensitivities __ Other
Educational needs (pages 153–154) __ Breastfeeding __ Infant feeding __ Baby care __ Post-partum care for new mother __ Other	**Plans for follow-up from hospital staff after discharge (page 154)** __ Availability for centre or home visit with mother-baby nurse __ Availability of lactation help and support __ Availability of phone call to/from hospital nurse __ Amount of follow-up care desired by parents

Birth Plan

Name: ______________________________ Due date: ____________

Primary caregiver: ______________________ Birth setting: ______________

My support people will be: ______________________, ______________________
(name) (relationship/role)

______________________, ______________________
(name) (relationship/role)

We realise that our birth plan is neither a contract nor a guarantee of an uncomplicated labour. Our purpose is to introduce ourselves and to help you understand our preferences.

Introducing ourselves:

Important wishes, issues, fears or concerns regarding mother or baby:

Preferences for managing labour pain:

Preferences for Normal Labour and Birth:

First stage of labour (positions, movement, comfort measures, and food and beverages):

Second stage (positioning and pushing efforts):

Third stage and first hours after birth (for mother and baby):

Preferences for Unexpected Events:

Induction and prolonged or complicated labour:

Caesarean birth:

Premature or sick baby:

Stillbirth or death of baby:

Preferences for Post Partum in Hospital for New Mother:

I plan to: ❑ Breastfeed ❑ Formula feed

Concerns and questions:

Feelings about visitors:

Controlling pain:

Educational needs:

Follow-up after discharge:

Newborn Care Plan

Newborn care preferences
for the baby of: ______________________________

Baby's name: ______________________________

Baby's doctor: ______________________________

Infant feeding: ❑ Breast milk ❑ Formula

Newborn concerns, issues, wishes and/or fears:

My previous experience with newborns:

Preferences regarding newborn examinations and procedures (immunisation, circumcision, contact with baby and routine procedures):

Preferences for unexpected problems for the baby:

Educational needs (infant care, feeding and so on):

Source: Adapted from the form prepared by Carla Reinke, RN, MSN, CNM, for use at the Virginia Mason Medical Centre, Seattle, Washington.

Chapter 8

Coping with Childbirth Pain

During pregnancy, you and your partner will want to prepare yourselves physically, emotionally and intellectually for the extraordinary experience of having a baby. During labour, you can help yourself immensely by using relaxation techniques, patterned breathing, and a variety of other comfort measures and body positions. This chapter includes complete descriptions of these techniques, guidelines for adapting them and a practice guide (a step-by-step approach to childbirth preparation found on pages 206–207).

Though these techniques do not lead to a pain-free childbirth, they can help keep the pain and stress manageable in most labours. They also promote labour progress and give you a greater sense of personal mastery during the experience. In addition to the support you will have from your partner and others, these techniques and your adaptations of them are your resources for coping with labour. You may use them instead of, or along with, pain medications and other interventions. When you use these techniques and participate fully, the birth of your child can be rewarding exciting and fulfilling—an experience to remember with satisfaction, pride and joy.

Historical Overview

Since the 1920s, the efforts of many outstanding individuals have led to the development of the methods now used to enhance relaxation, reduce stress, relieve labour pain, promote labour progress and strengthen early parent-infant bonds.

Grantly *Dick-Read,* a British physician, actively studied and promoted natural childbirth from the 1920s until the 1950s. He taught his obstetrical patients that when a woman is afraid of labour, she becomes tense and thereby increases her pain. The more pain she feels, the more frightened she becomes, and the cycle is perpetuated and intensified. To interrupt this vicious cycle, he advocated education, relaxation and controlled abdominal breathing.

In the 1950s, Dr. Fernand *Lamaze,* a French physician, developed his psychoprophylactic method, which he adapted from methods used by Soviet physicians. It is based on the theories of conditioned response developed by Ivan Pavlov. *Psychoprophylaxis,* which literally means 'mind prevention', involves the use of distraction techniques during contractions to decrease the perception of pain or discomfort. These techniques include various patterns of controlled chest breathing, a light massage of the abdomen (called *effleurage*) and visual concentration on an object (called a *focal point*). Elisabeth Bing, a physical therapist, and Marjorie Karmel, an expectant mother, both of whom were trained by Dr. Lamaze in France, introduced and popularised the Lamaze method in the United States. They helped found the American Society for Psychoprophylaxis in Obstetrics (ASPO), now called Lamaze International. Lamaze International promotes the Lamaze method through teacher training and certification and through education of parents and professionals. The Lamaze method has evolved over the years to incorporate more flexibility and now offers a great variety of coping techniques.

In the 1950s and 1960s, Robert *Bradley,* an American physician, promoted and refined Dick-Read's methods. Bradley's major contribution, however, was to encourage husbands to participate as labour coaches. His idea of involvement at birth by the husband, father or other loved ones eventually became the norm in most North American hospitals, and childbirth education began to include expectant couples rather than women only. Bradley founded the American Academy of Husband-Coached Childbirth (AAHCC) to train teachers and promote the Bradley method.

Since the 1960s, Sheila *Kitzinger,* British anthropologist and childbirth educator, has influenced childbirth preparation all over the world with her psycho-sexual approach. She described childbirth as a highly personal, sexual and social event. Kitzinger's methods emphasise body awareness, innovative relaxation techniques and special breathing patterns.

During the 1960s, the voice of the consumer in maternity care was given a great boost by the formation of the International Childbirth Education Association (ICEA), whose members promote the concepts of family-centred maternity care and 'freedom of choice based on knowledge of alternatives'. The ICEA certifies teachers but, unlike Lamaze International and the AAHCC, does not promote a particular method of childbirth preparation.

In the 1970s, the childbirth movement began to examine and criticise conventional obstetrical practices and emphasise more natural physiological and psychological approaches. The various methods of childbirth education began incorporating the teachings and research findings of various leaders and experts in maternity care. These included such ideas as the mother moving out of the bed during labour and the use of upright positions to enhance labour progress (Roberto Caldeyro-Barcia and others); more spontaneous pushing techniques for birth (Kitzinger, Caldeyro-Barcia, Joyce Roberts, Penny Simkin and Elizabeth Noble); greater contact between parents and newborn (Marshall Klaus and John Kennell); gentler handling of the newborn (T. Berry Brazelton and Frederic Leboyer); and a recognition of the obstetrical and psychological impact of support during labour, a home-like environment and freedom for the mother to behave spontaneously (Michel Odent, Gayle Peterson, Klaus, Kennell, Niles Newton and many more). In the late 1970s, consumer interest in home birth, midwifery and patients' rights began to grow.

The 1980s ushered in home-like birthing environments, including out-of-hospital birth centres and more attractive birthing rooms in hospitals. Also, the midwifery profession began to grow rapidly in response to consumer demand. Scientific research found many conventional maternity care practices to be ineffective, expensive or even harmful. All this set the stage for change. The Pre- and Perinatal Psychology Association of North America (now called the Association of Pre- and Perinatal Psychology and Health) was founded by Thomas Verny and David Chamberlain. This association brought together interested persons from a variety of professions to improve the understanding and care of the foetus and newborn. In an effort to improve the health of the world's youngest citizens, the United Nations and the World Health Organisation adopted the Baby-Friendly Initiative. (See Recommended Resources and Appendix II.) The aim of this initiative was to increase the number of women choosing to breastfeed and to introduce other measures to improve infant health in both developed and developing nations.

Also in the 1980s, childbirth education from independent childbirth educators declined as hospitals began offering their own childbirth classes. In hospital classes, the emphasis shifted from natural and prepared childbirth to an endorsement of the maternity care practices and philosophy of each sponsoring hospital.

In the 1990s, some common obstetrical practices—such as routine episiotomy, routine intravenous (IV) fluids and routine repeat caesareans—decreased, while new methods of inducing labour, safer drugs and safer means to pain relief became widespread. In 1994, under the leadership of Lamaze International, the Coalition for the Improvement of Maternity Services (CIMS)—representing thirty national organisations of midwives, maternity nurses, childbirth educators, lactation consultants and others—came together to begin work on a Mother-Friendly Childbirth Initiative. (See Recommended Resources and Appendix I.) The initiative promoted a cost-effective, research-based, woman-centred model of maternity care focusing on prevention and wellness.

On the other hand, attendance at childbirth classes declined in the 1990s. Childbirth educators, faced with lower class enrollments, realised that their approach was not meeting the needs of expectant couples with increasingly busy lives. Many educators shortened their classes; some offered one- or two-day 'crash' courses on weekends. In doing so, however, some important material was left out. For example, concepts of informed choice were de-emphasised, as was training in self-help and non-drug methods of pain relief. (Ironically, the 1990s also saw the development of numerous new and effective non-drug methods and aids to reduce labour pain.) Numerous expectant parents stopped participating in childbirth decision-making and left it to their caregivers. Some turned to other sources—such as the Internet, books and videotapes—for much of the information and discussion that had formerly been an important part of childbirth classes. Currently, leaders in childbirth education are making efforts to restore the relevancy and completeness of childbirth education in a form that suits the lifestyles and learning styles of today's expectant and new parents. The goal is to ensure that women and their partners will participate knowledgeably and confidently in both their childbirth experiences and maternity care.

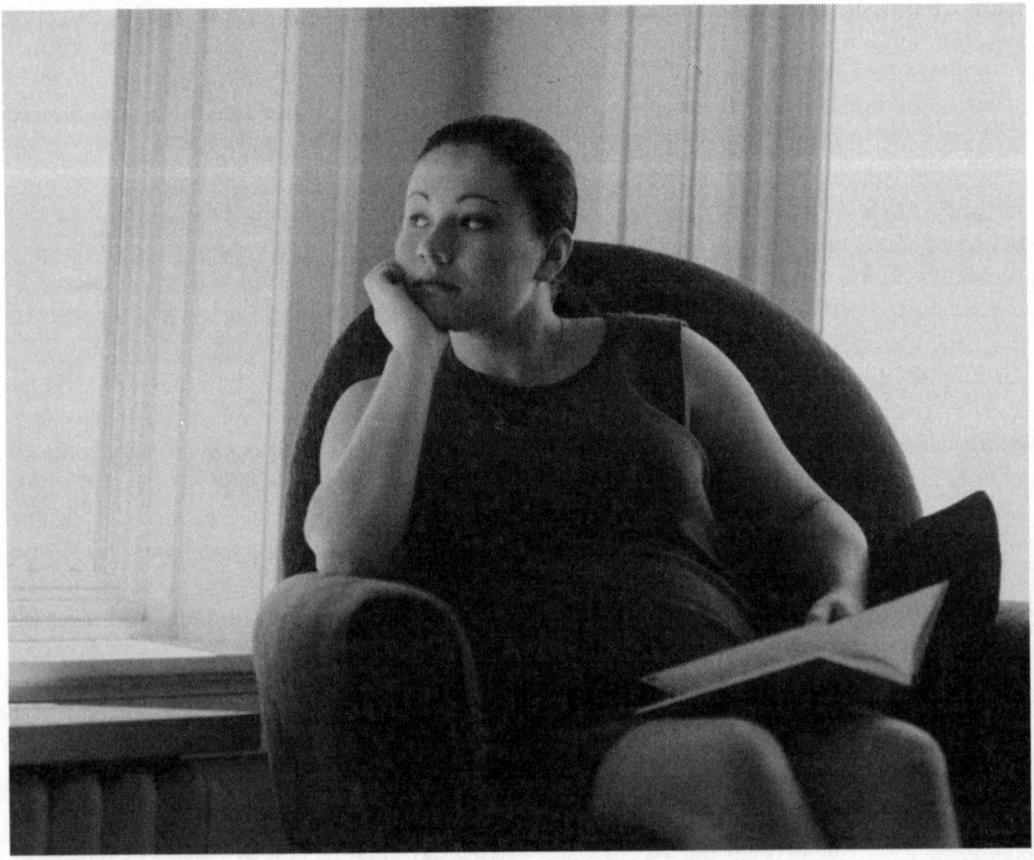

The more you learn about childbirth the better prepared you'll feel.

Pain in Childbirth

When asked to describe labour contractions and the sensations of birth, new mothers use words such as *painful, exhilarating, exhausting, uncomfortable, frightening, awesome, empowering, tedious, manageable, overwhelming* and *beautiful.* The pain of childbirth, which is in the forefront of most women's minds when they think about labour and birth, has been attributed to several factors:[1]

- Reduced oxygen supply to the uterine muscle. (Labour pain is more intense if the interval between contractions is short, preventing full replenishment of oxygen to the uterine muscle.)
- Stretching of the cervix (effacement and dilation)
- Pressure of the baby on nerves in and near the cervix and vagina
- Tension and stretching of the supporting ligaments of the uterus and pelvic joints during contractions and descent of the baby
- Pressure on the urethra, bladder and rectum
- Stretching of the pelvic floor muscles and vaginal tissues
- Fear and anxiety, which can cause the release of excessive stress hormones (epinephrine, norepinephrine and others), resulting in a longer and more painful labour[2]

The perception of pain in labour varies greatly from one woman to another. Many predisposing factors can increase or decrease the degree of labour pain a woman perceives, including her:

- Previous experiences with pain, medical care and childbirth
- Knowledge about birth (facts and myths) gained from people, books and other media
- Cultural background
- General health
- Perception of herself as one who can or cannot deal with pain

During the labour itself, further variables make each woman's perception of pain unique. Some of these are:

- Frequency of contractions
- Size and position of baby
- Length of labour
- Freedom to move about
- Degree of fatigue, anxiety and fear
- Sense of aloneness versus support
- Degree of confidence and preparedness

The comfort measures described in this chapter may decrease labour pain, reduce a woman's perception of pain or help her cope well with it. Becoming familiar with and using these measures gives many women a sense of mastery during the unpredictable and uncontrollable process of labour and childbirth.

Your perception of pain during labour can be reduced if you work towards becoming knowledgeable, feel confident, and are well supported by your partner and your caregivers. Simply knowing the reasons for the pain in labour helps many women cope better with it. It may also help to see that when childbirth is normal, the pain is not a sign of injury; rather, as Sheila Kitzinger has said, it is 'pain with a purpose'. By acknowledging your pain, working in suggested ways with your body during childbirth and remembering that the pain will soon end, you will be more able to put the pain in perspective and to prevent it from overwhelming you. The coping techniques and comfort measures that follow may be used exclusively or in combination with medication.

The Gate Control Theory of Pain

The Gate Control Theory of Pain, first described in the 1960s by R. Melzack and P. D. Wall, provides a useful explanation of how pain perception can be increased or decreased. Following is a brief description of the Gate Control Theory and how it applies to childbirth pain.

Under certain circumstances, a painful stimulus feels less painful than under other circumstances. A familiar example is the head-ache that seems to go away during an exciting movie but returns when the movie ends. Or the bruise, acquired while playing a sport, that goes unnoticed until the game is over. Or the pain from dental work that is eased when music transmitted through ear-phones distracts the patient from the discomfort. In all these examples, the pain is still there, but awareness of it decreases when the brain receives other non-painful or pleasant stimuli.

The Gate Control Theory states that the balance of painful and non-painful stimuli reaching your consciousness determines the perception of pain and its severity. In childbirth, you can increase the non-painful stimuli and decrease the painful stimuli in numerous ways. The techniques described in this chapter are powerful enough to reduce (but not eliminate) your perception of pain. They may be all you need to keep your pain manageable. If not, you may choose to use pain medications along with them. Some of the techniques—such as relaxation, breathing, massage and some movements—are more effective if you practise and adapt them to suit yourself before you go into labour. Others—such as hot packs, cold packs, baths and showers—require no prior practice.

An Individualised Approach to Childbirth Preparation

Despite the insights and wisdom of all the childbirth experts and all the advice available on how to have your baby, it is really you, with the help of your partner, caregiver and others, who will develop your own personal approach to labour. You have your own learning style, your own belief system and values, and your own way of dealing with change, stress and pain. Your way may be quite different from another woman's.

For example, some people have a highly academic approach to learning about birth. They find the information fascinating and essential to their ability to cope. Others learn better through experience, discussion, observation and practice. Some women find distraction from pain to be the most effective way to cope; others focus directly on the pain; and still others mentally reframe the pain, perceiving it as something different and more acceptable than pain. Some women love to be touched, massaged, held and talked to when they are in pain. Others must be left undisturbed to explore and draw on their inner resources. You will find that the comfort techniques described in this chapter are presented within a broad framework that includes guidelines for modifying and adapting them to suit your personality, your preferences and your particular labour.

The Three Rs: Relaxation, Rhythm and Ritual

Despite the variety of ways in which individual women cope with the demands of labour, there are some basic similarities among women who cope well. By coping well, we mean that they get through their contractions without being overwhelmed. Their behaviour has these three things in common: relaxation, rhythm and ritual. We call these the Three Rs, which is really a description of the essential, universal and instinctual behaviours of women in labour. The relaxation techniques, comfort measures and breathing exercises described in this chapter will enhance your ability to utilise the Three Rs.

Relaxation

Women who cope well in labour always use relaxation, either during or between contractions, or constantly. It is quite common for these women in early labour to allow their muscles to go limp during contractions, and to move about between contractions. Later in labour, some women may become more active during contractions (swaying, rocking, being stroked) and relax and rest only between contractions. Others may remain very relaxed, still and unresponsive to what is going on around them, both during and between contractions. (For more on relaxation, see pages 177–186.)

Rhythm

Women who cope well rely on rhythm in any number of forms. For example, they may rhythmically breathe, moan or chant. They may rhythmically tap or stroke something or someone. They may rock, sway or even dance in rhythm. They may even curl and uncurl their toes in rhythm! Or, they may want someone else to talk with them, stroke them or moan with them. Rhythmic activity calms the mind with its lulling effect.

Ritual

Although the word *ritual* is usually applied to religious or cultural activities or to behavioural habits (such as a morning ritual), in the context of labour ritual refers to the repetition of a meaningful rhythmic activity. For handling contractions, childbirth educators teach rituals that include relaxation, breathing and attention-focusing. Such rituals help women in early labour establish an effective

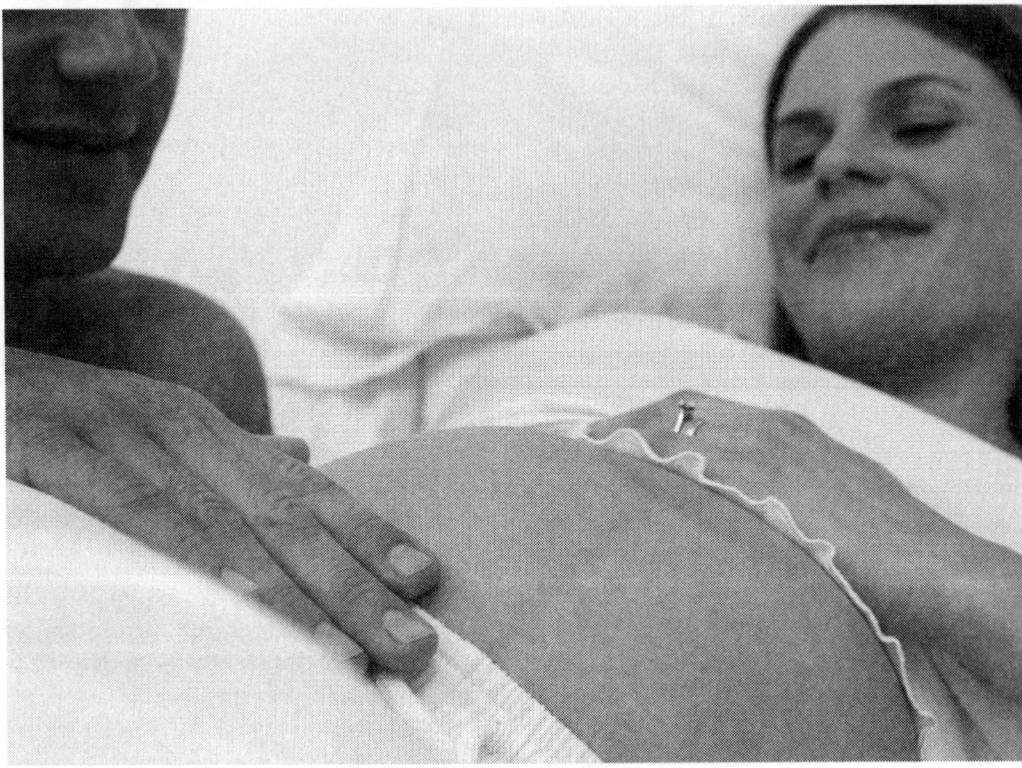

A supportive partner or friend will help you cope better with the pain.

style of coping. But as labour progresses and becomes more intense, most women adapt or add to these learned rituals in ways that reflect their own personal coping styles and that help them deal with the specific challenges of their particular labours.

If you are free to move (change positions, walk, sway, rock) and feel uninhibited in your behaviour, you will almost surely find a spontaneous ritual (usually adapted from what you have learned in childbirth classes) that you will repeat during each contraction. If your partner or someone else is a part of your ritual, that person must also consistently repeat his or her behaviour without changing it. Your partner's role may include eye contact; holding, touching or stroking you; swaying with you; saying exactly the same words over and over; or counting your breaths through each contraction.

You will change your ritual from time to time in labour. If you begin to feel overwhelmed and unable to carry on a ritual, your partner or caregiver may help you re-establish it or create a new one. The effective use of rituals shows that women can adapt to the demands of labour and get through it.

Following are examples of unplanned rituals discovered by women in labour to help them during contractions:

- Rocking in a rocking chair in rhythm with her breathing
- Silently repeating, 'Be still like the mountain; flow like the river' in rhythm with her breathing
- Partner stroking her lower leg up and down in the rhythm of her breathing
- Partner softly and rhythmically counting her breaths and pointing out when she probably passed beyond the halfway point in the contraction (For example, if she were taking about twenty breaths per contraction, when she reached the twelfth or thirteenth breath, her partner would say, 'You're on the downside'.)

Relaxation

Relaxation—the art of releasing muscle tension—is the cornerstone of comfort during labour. It is especially important to remain relaxed during the contractions of early labour, as this is the time when it is usually quite easy to do. If you consciously work to remain relaxed during these early contractions, you will be establishing a good habit that can be continued far into labour. Unfortunately, women often begin tensing with contractions right away, and then it becomes difficult to relax later when contractions become more intense. Your partner should help you recognise and release tension during these early contractions.

The ability to relax comes more easily to some than to others. With concentration and practice, however, most everyone can learn to relax. Many approaches to relaxation are presented in this chapter. Try them all, but concentrate on those that appeal to you and seem to work best for you.

Benefits of Relaxation

During labour, relaxation will help you do the following:

- **Conserve energy and reduce fatigue.** If you are not consciously relaxing your muscles, you will most likely tense them during contractions. This tensing increases your pain, wastes energy, decreases the oxygen available for the uterus and baby and tires you.
- **Calm your mind and reduce stress.** A relaxed body leads to a relaxed state of mind, which in turn helps reduce your stress response. There is evidence that distress in the labouring woman caused by anxiety, anger, fear or illness produces an excessive amount of catecholamines (stress hormones) such as epinephrine (also called adrenalin) and norepinephrine (also called noradrenalin). High blood levels of catecholamines can prolong labour by decreasing the efficiency of uterine contractions and can adversely affect the foetus by decreasing the blood flow to the uterus and placenta.[4]
- **Reduce pain.** Relaxation decreases the tension and fatigue that intensifies the pain you feel during labour and birth. It also allows maximum availability of oxygen for your uterus, which also may decrease pain,

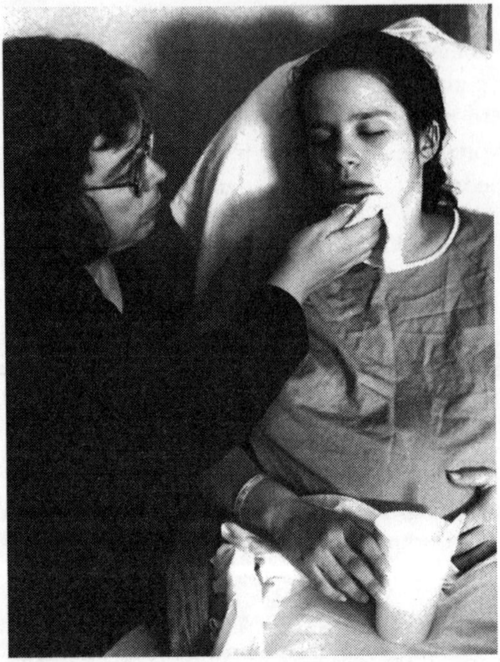

Photograph by Marilyn Nolt

Relaxation decreases tension and fatigue.

since a working muscle (the contracting uterus) becomes painful if it is deprived of oxygen. In addition, the mental concentration involved in consciously relaxing your muscles helps focus your attention away from the pain of contractions and thereby reduces your awareness of pain.

Learning to Relax

The first step in learning to relax is to become aware of how your mind and body feel when you are resting or falling asleep. Since your mind and body influence each other, you probably will notice a simultaneous release of muscular and mental tension when you relax. Your breathing pattern will be slow and even, with a slight pause between each inhalation and exhalation. This type of breathing will aid you in the relaxation exercises and during labour.

When you practise relaxation, lie down on your side with plenty of pillows to make yourself comfortable or sit in a comfortable chair with your head and arms supported. After you have learned to relax in these positions, practise relaxing while sitting up, standing and walking, since you will need to relax in a variety of positions during labour.

When you are learning relaxation skills, begin in a quiet, calm atmosphere and progress to noisier, more active surroundings. Remember that hospitals are busy places, so you will need to be able to relax in the midst of activity. At the end of a practice session, lazily stretch all your muscles and get up slowly to avoid becoming light-headed or dizzy.

The next step is to learn to recognise muscle tension. The following techniques will help you detect and reduce the unnecessary tension that may develop during labour.

Body Awareness Techniques

Tensing and Releasing Muscles

Starting position: Sit in a chair or on the floor.

Exercise: Make a tight fist with your right hand. Pay attention to how the muscles in your forearm feel. They are hard when they are tense. Touch those muscles with the fingers of your left hand. Now open your right hand and relax it. Notice how soft the muscles feel when you release the tension.

Next, raise your shoulders towards your ears. Notice how you feel when your shoulders are tense. Relax and lower your shoulders. Now release even more. Really relax. Did you notice a change? Often you can release residual muscle tension when you become aware of it.

Tensing and Releasing the Whole Body

Starting position: Lie down in a comfortable position.

Exercise: Tighten the muscles of your entire body—stiffen your abdomen, hips and legs, then your back, neck and arms. Keep the muscles contracted for about five seconds. Pay attention to how you feel—for example, tense, tight, cramped or uncomfortable.

Then let your body go limp, releasing the tension all over. You may start by relaxing your abdomen and releasing outwards towards your arms, legs and head. Think of the tension flowing out of your limbs. Breathe slowly. Sigh, relaxing even more. Feel yourself relaxing as you breathe out.

Discovering the Effect of Mind on Body

Your state of mind has a great influence on how relaxed or tense your body is. If you are anxious or frightened, your body will reflect these feelings by tensing. If you are confident and positive, your body will remain relaxed. When in pain, you can focus on these confident, positive feelings to help you release tension that might otherwise worsen your pain.

Exercise: Use the following two visualisations to help you imagine contrasting reactions to labour contractions. Notice how the visualisations can affect the tension in your body. One can make you feel tense and afraid; the other can help you relax.

1. As your contraction begins, you feel tension, first in your back. You think, 'Uh-oh. Here it comes'. This tight grip comes around to your front . . . . It's building. 'Oh no!' It's getting stronger and stronger. It hurts! You want to say, 'Owww. Make it stop. I can't do it! I can't!' You clench your fists. You stiffen your back. You grit your teeth and squint hard in an anguished expression of pain. 'Please! Make it stop!' The grip tightens around your middle. You feel weak. You feel helpless. You hold your breath. 'Won't it ever stop?' The grip begins to fade. It's leaving, but you're afraid to let go. 'Is it really gone? Is it coming back? Ohhhhh'.

How do you feel after reading the above visualisation or hearing it read to you? Are you tense, upset? For contrast, try the following visualisation of a labour contraction.

2. Your contraction comes like a wave, starting deep within you as a small swell. Vague at first, it grows . . . larger and larger, stronger and stronger. You wonder, 'What shall I do?' It's building to a peak of strength, power and pain. *Your* strength, *your* power, *your* pain. You ride the crest of this wave, letting it carry you along. As the power sweeps through you, your uterus works to open your cervix and to bring your baby closer. You do not fight the wave, you go limp, and in doing so you feel safe, supported and strong. Your face is still and peaceful. Your arms and legs are floating—limp and relaxed. You are not afraid. You are open to this power. You are *opening* to this power. And now the wave eases; it

ebbs; it flows back deep within you. You are at rest.

How do you feel as you visualise a contraction in this way? Do you find it less threatening? More empowering? Does it help you interpret the contraction more positively than the first visualisation? If so, you may wish to use such visualisations as you prepare for birth.

As you can see, your way of interpreting the pain of contractions can influence your physical response to them. It helps if you can visualise the pain as healthy pain with a positive purpose. Through knowledge and practice, you will be able to do this, and your labour will be far more fulfilling for you.

Practising with Your Partner

While you are developing an awareness of tension and relaxation, your birth partner should also learn to recognise when you are tense or relaxed. He or she can detect signs of tension in several ways:

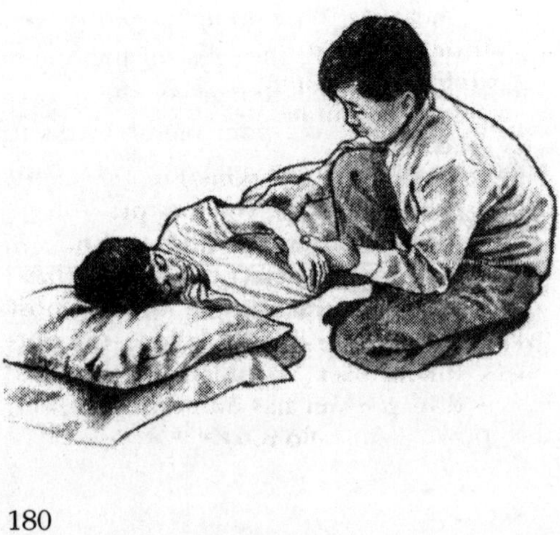

- By observing you when you are tense and when you are relaxed. How do you look when you are anxious, uncomfortable, calm, content or asleep?
- By touching or feeling various parts of your body (arms, legs, neck and face). How do your muscles feel? Hard or soft?
- By lifting one of your arms or legs, supporting it well, and moving the joints and feeling for the looseness and heaviness that accompanies relaxation. How does the limb feel to your partner when it is being moved? A relaxed arm or leg should neither help nor resist movement.

The way your partner checks you for relaxation has a lot to do with your ability to relax. If he or she touches or moves you in a gentle manner—not dropping, shaking or pinching your limbs—you will develop a sense of confidence and security. This trusting relationship carries over beautifully into labour. As you practise together, you will learn which parts of your body are most difficult to relax (called 'tension spots'). Many people under stress tighten their shoulders. Some reflect tension with a frown or anxious brow. Others clench their jaws or fists. Your tension spots should receive special attention while you are learning relaxation and during labour. Find out what eases the tension in these areas. Is it touch, massage, verbal reminders or warmth? After exploring the possibilities together, you will both know what works best in helping you relax and stay relaxed.

Once you and your partner are skilled in spotting tension and relaxing, practise by deliberately tightening a limb and having your partner try to detect the part you have tensed. Try contracting the muscles most likely to be tense during labour (buttocks, thighs, back, shoulders, face or fists). Once your partner has found the tension, have him or her help you relax.

Relaxation Techniques

Passive Relaxation

Once you can recognise tension in your muscles, the next step is to master the art of releasing tension. By focusing on different parts of your body and by releasing tension in each part, you can achieve a state of deep relaxation of both body and mind. This takes some concentration and conscious effort. When you start passive relaxation, have your partner read the following exercise in a calm, relaxed voice. He or she should read slowly, allowing you time to focus on and release each part of your body. If your partner is unavailable, there are many relaxation audiotapes available for pregnant women. (See the Recommended Resources.) Pleasant, relaxing music may also help. Once you have selected some appealing music, use the same music each time you practise, and then use it during labour to create a familiar and relaxing environment.

Practising Passive Relaxation

Find a comfortable position lying on your side or semi-sitting, with your head and all your limbs supported by the floor or bed and pillows. Take plenty of time getting as comfortable as you can, so that you do not need to use any muscle effort to hold yourself in position. Depending on the position you choose, you may want to put pillows under one or both knees, beneath your head, or under your abdomen to make you more comfortable and relaxed.

1. Take a long sigh, or yawn.

2. Now focus way down to your *toes* and *feet*. Just let go. Think how warm and relaxed they feel.

3. Think about your *ankles*—floppy and loose. Your ankles are very relaxed and comfortable.

4. And now your *calves*. Let those muscles go—loose and soft. Good.

5. Now focus on your *knees*. They are supported and relaxed—not holding your legs in any position. Your knees are very comfortable and loose.

6. Think of your *thighs*. The large, strong muscles of your thighs have let go. They are soft and heavy, and your thighs are totally supported. Good.

7. And now your *buttocks* and *perineum*. This area needs to be especially relaxed during labour and birth. Just let go. Think soft and yielding. When the time is right, your baby will make the journey down the birth canal, and the tissues of your perineum will open and let the baby slide out. You will release, allowing the perineum to give and open for the baby.

8. And now your *lower back*. Imagine that someone with strong, warm hands is giving

you a lovely rub. It feels so good. Your muscles relax to the imagined touch, and your lower back is comfortable. Feel the warmth. Feel the tension leaving.

9. And now let your thoughts flow to your *abdomen*. Let those muscles go. Let your abdomen rise and fall as you breathe in and out. Your abdomen is free. Focus on how it moves as you breathe. Good. Focus on your baby within your abdomen. Your baby is floating or wiggling in the water in your womb—a safe and interesting place where you are meeting all your baby's needs for nourishment, oxygen, warmth, movement and stimulation. Your baby hears your heartbeat, your voice, your partner's voice and all the interesting sounds from outside. What excellent care you are giving your baby! You are a wonderful mother!

10. And now your *chest*. Your chest is free. As you breathe in, bringing air into your lungs, your chest swells easily, making room for the air. As you breathe out, your chest relaxes to help the air flow out. Breathe easily and slowly, letting the air flow in and flow out, almost like sleep breathing. This easy breathing helps you relax more. The relaxation helps you breathe even more easily and slowly. Good.

Now try breathing in through your nose and out through your mouth—slowly and easily, letting the air flow in and out. At the top of the in-breath, you notice just a little tension in your chest, which is released with your out-breath. Listen as you breathe out. It sounds relaxed and calm, almost as if you were asleep. Every out-breath is a relaxing breath. Use your out-breaths to breathe away any tension. This is very much like the slow breathing you will be using during labour. Good.

11. And now your *shoulders*. Imagine you have just had a lovely massage over your shoulders and upper back. Let go. Release. Feel the warmth. Feel the tension slip away.

12. Focus on your *arms*. With your out-breath, let your arms go limp—from your shoulders all the way down your arms, to your wrists, hands, and fingers. Heavy, loose and relaxed.

13. And now your *neck*. All the muscles in your neck are soft because they do not have to hold your head in any position. Your head is heavy and completely supported, so your neck can just let go and relax. Good.

14. Focus on your *lips* and *jaw*. They are slack and relaxed. You do not have to hold your mouth closed or open. It is comfortable. No tension there.

15. And now your *eyes* and *eyelids*. You are not holding your eyes open or closed. They are the way they want to be. Your eyes are unfocused and still beneath your eyelids. Your eyelids are relaxed and heavy.

16. Focus on your *brow* and *scalp*. Think how warm and relaxed they are. Just let go. You have a calm, peaceful expression on your face, reflecting a calm, peaceful feeling inside.

17. Take a few moments to note and enjoy this feeling of calm and wellbeing. You can relax this way anytime—before sleep, during an afternoon rest or during a quiet break. This is the feeling to have in labour. During

labour, you will not lie down all the time. You will be walking, sitting up, showering and changing positions. But whenever a contraction comes, you will allow yourself to relax all the muscles you do not need to hold your position, and you will let your mind relax, giving you a feeling of peace and confidence. It is this feeling that will help you focus on the positive accomplishment of each contraction, yielding to these contractions and letting them guide you in breathing and comfort.

18. Now it is time to end this relaxation session. No need to rush. Gradually open your eyes, stretch, tune in to your surroundings and get up slowly.

Relaxation Countdown

After you have become aware of body tension and have mastered passive relaxation, learn the following technique to quickly release muscle tension. This is particularly helpful when you want to get back to sleep at night, when you are feeling stressed and when you are trying to relax after contractions during labour. In addition, your organising breath at the beginning of each contraction (see page 194) can be used as a rapid relaxation countdown.

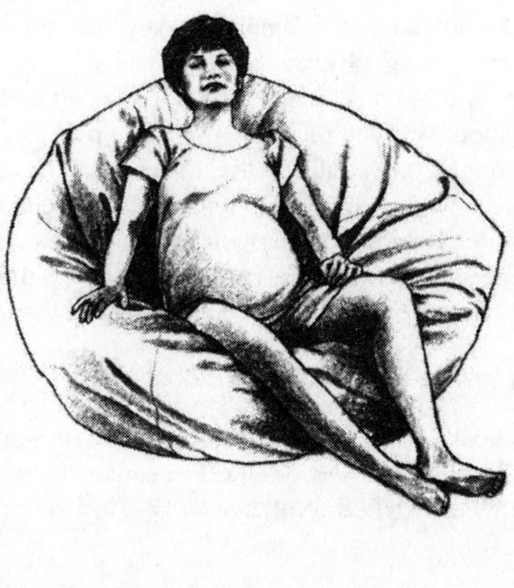

Practising the Relaxation Countdown

Breathe in through your nose. As you breathe out through your mouth, release the muscle tension throughout your body. At first, use five slow breaths to accomplish this, relaxing a different area with each breath. Then try to relax all areas on the slow exhalation of one breath. Think of this countdown as a wave of relaxation that passes down through your body from head to toe:

5. Head, neck and shoulders

4. Arms, hands and fingers

3. Chest and abdomen

2. Back, buttocks and perineum

1. Legs, feet and toes

As you practise, use as many breaths as you need to count down to total body relaxation.

Touch Relaxation

With touch relaxation, you respond to your partner's touch by relaxing or releasing tense muscles. During pregnancy, touch relaxation is a pleasurable way to practise relaxation. During labour, you use your companion's touching, stroking or massaging as a non-verbal cue to relax.

Starting position: Lie down on your side or sit in a comfortable position.

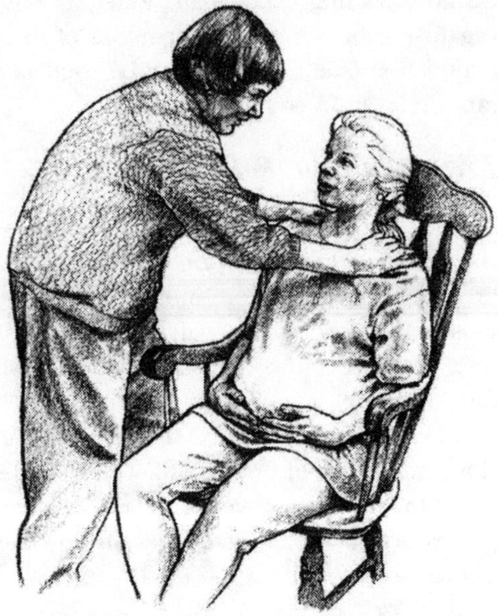

Exercise: Contract a set of muscles and have your partner touch those muscles with a firm, relaxed hand, molding his or her hand to the shape of the part of your body being tensed. Release the muscle tension and relax towards your partner's hand. Imagine the tension flowing out of your body.

Your partner can use several types of touch listed below. Find out which types you prefer, but practise all methods, since your preference could change during labour.

Still touch. Your partner holds his or her hand(s) firmly in place until he or she feels you release your tension.

Firm pressure. Your partner applies pressure with fingertips or the whole hand on the tense area. Your partner gradually releases the pressure. You respond by releasing tension as you feel your partner's gradual release.

Stroking. Your partner lightly or firmly strokes the tense area. When stroking your arms or legs, he or she strokes away from the centre of your body.

Massage. Your partner firmly rubs or kneads tense muscles. This is commonly used for neck and back rubs, but any muscle group can be massaged.

Practising Touch Relaxation

Practise tensing the following muscle groups, then releasing to your partner's touch. Learn to release to still touch, firm pressure, stroking and massage:

- Scalp
- Face
- Neck
- Shoulders
- Arms and hands
- Abdomen
- Buttocks
- Legs and feet

Active Relaxation

If you practise relaxing in many positions and during physical activity, you can prepare more realistically for labour, because in labour you will probably use many positions and be physically active. Your goal is to achieve the same relaxed feeling and mental state while active that you had with passive relaxation, when pillows, the bed or the floor were supporting your entire body.

Practising Active Relaxation

Practise relaxing in many positions—standing (upright or leaning against a wall or your partner), sitting, semi-sitting, on your hands and knees, kneeling with head and shoulders resting on the seat of a chair, squatting and lying on your side. Different positions require that some muscle groups work, while allowing release of tension in others. Only by practising in various positions will you be able to relax most effectively during labour. Imagine you are having labour contractions while you are practising relaxation and breathing patterns. By visualising the intense sensations of labour contractions, you can make each practice session a labour rehearsal.

The Roving Body Check

Sometimes, you may think you are entirely relaxed, but when you focus on a particular body part—such as your arm, leg or abdomen—you become aware that there is some tension there. The following exercise helps you release tension throughout your body, part by part. It combines the built-in tension-releasing properties of the out-breath with your own conscious release.

Practising the Roving Body Check

Find a comfortable position. While breathing slowly, rhythmically and easily in through your nose and out through your mouth, focus on one part of your body with each breath. As you breathe in, detect any tension in that part. As you breathe out, deliberately release any tension from that area. Take two breaths or more, if necessary. Then, with the next breath or two, focus on another part. Find any tension as you breathe in and release it as you breathe out. Repeat this exercise, roving from one area to another, checking for tension on the in-breath, and releasing it on the out-breath, as follows:

1. Brow
2. Jaw and lips
3. Neck
4. Shoulders
5. Right arm and hand
6. Left arm and hand
7. Upper back
8. Lower back
9. Chest and abdomen
10. Buttocks and perineum
11. Right leg and foot
12. Left leg and foot

By systematically releasing tension in each part as you release your breath, your entire body will be more relaxed at the end of the exercise than it was at the beginning.

You can use this technique during or between labour contractions. Your partner can help by telling you which part to relax with each breath, or by touching or stroking a different part for each breath. Rather than roving through your entire body with each contraction, you may prefer to have your partner focus only on your tension spots (areas where you tend to become tense when you are under stress). For example, some women tend to carry tension in their shoulders. If they can relax their shoulders, the rest of their bodies remain relaxed.

Control in Labour

For many women, the prospect of 'losing control' in labour is the most upsetting part of the whole thing. They worry that the pain will be so intense that they will panic or do or say things they will regret later. To prevent this, some plan to use anaesthesia to reduce the pain. Others work on mastering self-help techniques like those described in this chapter to lessen the pain or to keep themselves from reacting negatively to it. They also try to choose a place for birth where they will feel comfortable expressing their spontaneous sounds and engaging in necessary activities.

One of the undeniable facts about labour is that you cannot consciously control your labour or your contractions. Labour cannot be controlled any more than digestion can be controlled. However, you can usually control how you respond to it. Exceptions include a very fast painful labour that gives you almost no break between contractions and a long or complicated labour that exhausts you. In a sense, then, control in labour is a matter of coping with your labour, not controlling the labour itself. This book emphasises understanding and working in harmony with the powerful forces of labour rather than resisting or fighting them.

Women also feel loss of control when everything is done for them or to them. Many women want to participate in decisions about their care during labour and to be treated respectfully as individuals. Feeling left out makes them feel out of control. In family-centred care, the mother is consulted and her wishes are respected.

Comfort Measures for Labour

Women respond differently to labour, depending on the nature of their labours, their sense of readiness, their coping styles, and their goals and expectations. As you prepare and rehearse for labour, learn the various comfort measures and then adapt them to suit your needs. Analyse yourself and use this knowledge to develop your own style for labour. Think about what helps you relax now—music, massage, soothing voices, a bath or shower, meditation, prayer, chanting or humming, thinking about or visualising pleasant places and activities and so on. Think about the people and things that help you feel safe and comfortable—your partner, mother, sister, friend, pillow, nightgown or pyjamas; or music, flowers, a favourite object or photo and so on. Plan to use these familiar comfort measures to help you relax during labour.

Unlike most pain, which is associated with injury, illness or stress, the pain of labour is associated with a normal, healthy body function. By recognising your labour pain as productive and positive—a part of the process that brings the baby—you can help reduce the pain to a more manageable level. To cope with your pain, you may find it most helpful to 'tune into it'—focus on it, accept it and tailor your response to it. Or, you may prefer using distraction techniques, concentrating on outside stimuli, or performing mental activities to keep yourself from focusing on your pain.

Many women successfully use both tuning in and distraction. For example, in early labour they relax, breathe slowly and easily throughout their contractions, close their eyes, and visualise either something soothing and pleasant or the uterine contractions' opening the cervix and pressing the baby downwards. As labour intensifies, some maintain this ritual, while others lighten and speed up their breathing. Then, during late labour (transition), when contractions are very intense and close together, many women find that they cannot continue as before. Often, they need to open their eyes, focus on something external like their partner's face, and follow outside directions (their partner guiding their breathing rhythms with verbal directions, hand signals or by breathing with them). Sometimes, more complex breathing patterns are helpful.

The following comfort measures are based on relaxation—the key to pain control in labour. Learn and adapt them to suit your needs. You will notice that most of these measures are based on the Three Rs (relaxation, rhythm and ritual repetition of rhythmic activities).

Attention-Focusing

During labour contractions, your attention should be focused on something. Many women prefer an *internal focus*. For example, some women close their eyes and visualise the effect of contractions—the uterine muscle pulling the cervix open and the baby pressing down and further opening the cervix. Other women prefer images that are calming and pleasant (the beach, a mountaintop or a happy memory). Some women visualise themselves as being 'above' their contractions (like a gull soaring over a stormy sea), while remaining in touch with the contractions. Still others visualise each contraction as a hurdle to be overcome (a steep hill to be climbed, a footrace, a wave to ride and so on).

You may also find it helpful to look at something. This *visual focus* is often called an *external focal point*. You may wish to look at your partner's face, a picture on the wall, a reminder of the baby (perhaps a toy), an object in the room, a flower or the view from the window. Some women focus on the same thing for many contractions; others change focal points often. Some focus on a line, such as the edge of a window, and follow that line visually during the contraction.

Many women find it helpful to focus on touch. Examples of *tactile focus* include a partner's rhythmic massage, stroking of one area of the body or tight embrace.

Other women focus on sounds. Examples of an *auditory focus* include listening to a favourite musical recording, the soothing voice of a birth partner, repeated rhythms or a recording of environmental sounds such as surf, rain or a babbling brook. Many women find it helpful to vocalise in a rhythmic pattern by moaning, sighing, counting their breaths, singing, reciting poems or verses, or chanting. In the past, vocalising by labouring women was considered unacceptable, but many childbirth educators now encourage it and many hospital staffs recognise its usefulness to labouring women. Rhythmic vocalisation or vocal breathing is not the same as screaming out in fear or panic. Instead, it is an effective technique for maintaining a sense of control while releasing tension.

Some women focus quietly on a particular *mental activity* such as thinking the words of a song, poem or verse made up on the spot. For example, one second-time mother said to herself over and over as each of her contractions built to a peak, 'I think I can, I think I can'. As each contraction subsided, she repeated, 'I thought I could, I thought I could'. Another woman, on the day before she went into labour, had allowed some fudge to boil over while talking on the phone. In labour the next day, she found herself stroking her belly and rhythmically chanting to herself, 'Keep stirring and you won't boil over'.

Another focusing technique women use to get through contractions involves performing a particular *physical activity*. Examples include breathing in a complex pattern (see page 196), relaxing with the roving body check (page 185), and moving by rocking, swaying, walking, dancing, massage or stroking.

As you and your partner rehearse breathing and relaxation together during pretend contractions, try the attention-focusing techniques described above. You will probably prefer some over others. Be ready to try more than one if a particular favourite loses its appeal in labour. Also, realise that in labour you may discover an unexpected but helpful focusing technique.

Massage and Touch

Massage techniques—such as firm stroking, rubbing or kneading (squeezing and releasing)—are soothing and relaxing during both pregnancy and labour. This type of massage of the neck, shoulders, back, thighs, feet and hands can be very comforting. Another helpful form of touch for labour is firm pressure on one spot such as your hips, thighs, shoulders or hand. (Exercises using touch and massage are described on pages 183–185.)

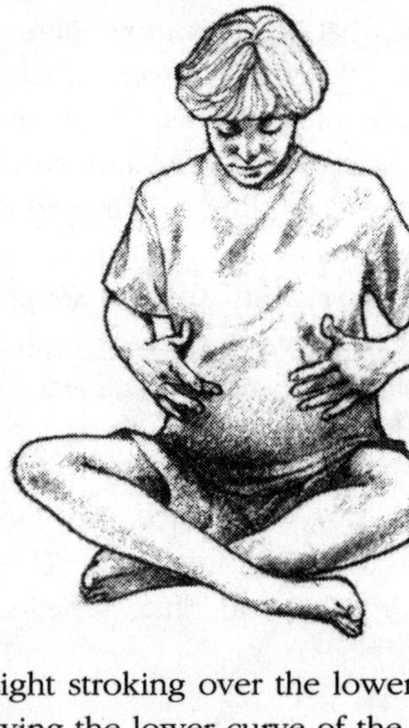

Light stroking over the lower abdomen, following the lower curve of the uterus, is a popular massage during labour. Lamaze teachers call this *effleurage*. Some people think of this massage as stroking the baby's head. Others like to stroke the abdomen in circles with both hands. Use baby powder to make your hands slide more easily. Keep the massage rhythmic, pacing it with the slow breathing. In addition to stroking your abdomen, a light, rhythmic stroking massage of your back or thighs can help with relaxation and pain relief when done on your bare skin by your partner.

Work together in pregnancy and find out how and where massage is most helpful and plan to use it in labour.

Baths and Showers

Warm water in the form of a lingering bath, whirlpool bath or shower is a marvellous comfort measure for most labouring women. Contractions are usually less painful if you are in water. You are able to relax better because of the warmth and buoyancy of the bath water or the gentle massage provided by the shower or whirlpool jets. Find out if you will have access to a bath or shower during labour. In the shower, lean against the wall or sit on a towel-covered stool so you can rest. Direct the spray where it helps most. In the tub, lean back against a bath pillow or folded towels and relax. If the bathtub is large enough, you may kneel and lean over the side or lie on your side with your head elevated on a bath pillow. In the past, it was believed that bathing after the membranes had ruptured would lead to infection (due to water entering the vagina). However, several studies show no greater incidence of infection in women who bathed during labour with ruptured membranes than in those who did so with intact membranes.[5]

Sometimes, a partner accompanies the labouring woman into the shower, or even in the tub, if it is large enough. (Your partner may wish to bring a swimsuit.) Besides relieving pain, baths and showers sometimes lower elevated blood pressure and, if you do not get into the tub too early (before 4 centimetres dilation), they often speed up slow labours.[6] Sometimes, the baby is born in the water, either because the mother is reluctant to get out of the tub or because mother and caregiver have planned a water birth. Water births are rarely allowed in Australian hospitals, although the option of using the bath for pain relief and relaxation during labour has become widely available. Many caregivers who attend births in homes or in birth centres not associated with hospitals are comfortable having births take place in water. (For more information on water birth, see Recommended Resources.)

Heat and Cold

Heat applied to the lower abdomen, back, groin or perineum can be very soothing. Electric heating pads, hot water bottles and warm compresses are good sources of heat. However, many hospitals restrict the use of heating devices brought from home, so check with your hospital. Warm compresses are simply washcloths or small towels soaked in hot water, wrung out, and quickly applied wherever you need them. As they cool, they are replaced. Covering them with plastic retains their heat longer. A warm blanket helps a woman who is chilled or trembling.

A cold pack can provide a great deal of relief. Examples include an ice bag, frozen wet washcloths, a rubber glove filled with crushed ice, a bag of frozen peas, a hollow plastic rolling pin filled with ice, 'instant' cold packs, or frozen gel packs like camper's 'ice' or the cold packs used for athletic injuries. Placed on the lower back for back pain during labour, a cold pack feels wonderful. Also, try one on your perineum immediately after birth to help reduce pain and swelling. For cold packs to bring comfort, however, you must be comfortably warm. If you are feeling chilled, the cold pack may make you more uncomfortable. In that case, it would be a good idea to use a warm blanket, robe, bath or shower to first warm you up all over, and then the local application of cold may be welcomed.

How hot or cold should the compresses be? During labour, you might easily tolerate compresses so hot or cold they could damage your skin, so your partner should use common sense. A good rule is that the person applying the hot or cold pack should be able to hold it in his or her hand for several seconds without pain. The pack should be covered with a layer or two of towelling to protect your skin. If you have anaesthesia that causes loss of sensation, avoid the use of heat or cold wherever sensation is not normal.

Movement

Moving around during labour is another extremely useful comfort measure. Changing position frequently (every thirty minutes or so, especially if progress is slow) helps relieve pain and may speed up labour by adding the benefits of gravity and by allowing changes in the shape of the pelvis. You may choose to sit, kneel, stand, lie down, get on your hands and knees, and walk. Swaying from side to side, rocking, or other rhythmic movements may also be comforting. An upright position may give you a greater sense of control and active involvement than lying down. (See pages 227–229 in Chapter 9 for a further description of positions for labour.)

The Birth Ball

A birth ball is a large inflated ball like ones normally used in physical therapy and gymnastics. Such a ball is now also used as a comfort aid and a prop to help the mother with positioning and movement during labour. You can sit on it and sway during and between contractions, especially during early labour. A birth ball is very comfortable and helps you relax your trunk and perineum. You can also place the ball on the bed and, while kneeling on the bed or standing beside it, lean over the ball for support. You may then sway rhythmically from side to side or front to back. Such movement is almost effortless and often very comforting.

Most women, unless they are very tall or very short, do best with a ball having a 65-centimetre diameter. If you are over 178

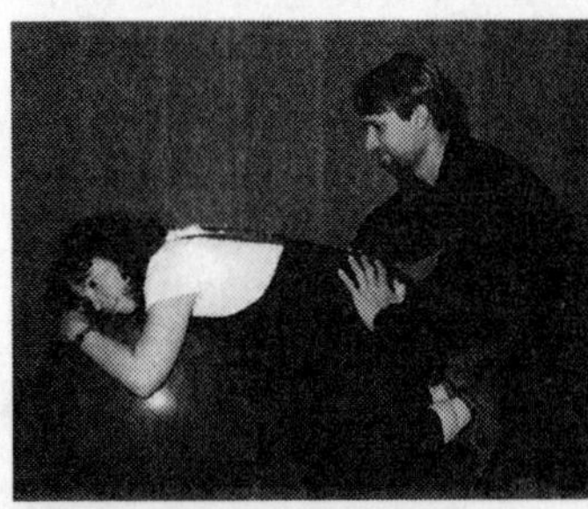

The birth ball provides a relaxing substitute for the hands-and-knees position.

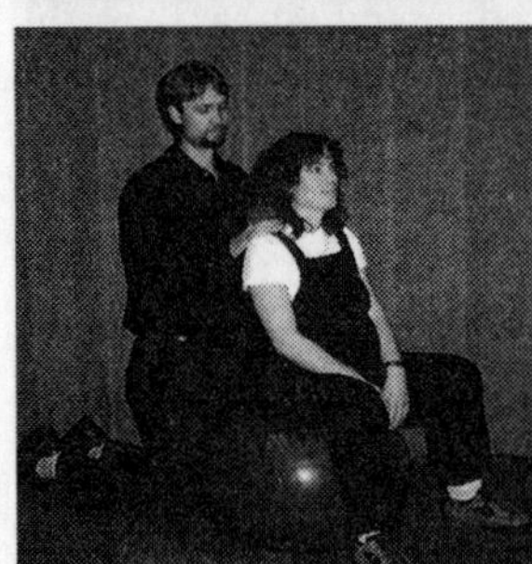

Swaying from side to side is comforting.

Photographs by David Swain

centimetres in height, the 75-centimetre size is preferable. If you are less than 158 centimetres tall, the 55-centimetre size is preferable.

It is a good idea to practise sitting on the ball before labour. While getting used to it, hold on to someone or something stable. Also, be sure to keep one hand on the ball as you lower yourself onto it. (Balls roll!) Cover the ball with a towel or pad when sitting or leaning on it, as it may have become dirty on the floor.

Many hospitals and birth centres have birth balls available. You may even wish to own one. You can inflate it to your desired firmness and sit on it at home for comfort, or use it for prenatal or post-partum exercises. Also, one of the greatest benefits comes at home after the birth, when you may soothe your fussing baby by holding the baby up to your shoulder and bouncing gently on the ball together. Be sure to use caution as you lower yourself onto the ball.

Birth balls are available for purchase from hospital physical therapy departments, some well-stocked toy stores and sporting goods stores, and by mail order from birth supply companies. Be sure to request a ball that is strong enough to hold at least 136 kilograms.

Fluid Intake

Most labouring women lose their appetites when they begin active labour, but their need and desire for liquids continues throughout labour. You should take in liquids either by drinking or, if that is not allowed (as might be the case if a caesarean or general anaesthetic is anticipated), by an intravenous (IV) drip. During a normal labour, you can drink water, tea or juice, or suck on iceblocks between contractions. By quenching your thirst, you are also meeting your body's requirements for fluids. If your caregiver does not allow liquids by mouth (which in the past was common), if your labour is prolonged or if you are vomiting, you probably will receive fluids intravenously to prevent dehydration. You can still move around, walk and shower or bathe when receiving IV fluids, if the IV unit is placed on a rolling stand. Remember to empty your bladder regularly, as a full bladder may slow labour and increase pain. If oral fluids are restricted, you may have a very dry mouth, so suck on ice, a frozen juice bar or a sour lollipop. You may also refresh your mouth and teeth with cold water, a toothbrush or mouthwash.

Comfort Measures for Back Pain

Some women experience added discomfort in labour because of severe back pain during contractions. Measures to decrease this back pain are described in Chapter 10, pages 285–290.

Breathing for Labour

All activities involving physical coordination and mental discipline (swimming, running, singing, playing a musical instrument, public speaking, yoga, meditation and so on) require that you regulate your breathing for effective and efficient performance. Labour is no different. Along with relaxation and other comfort measures, breathing rhythmically in a pattern is used during labour and birth to enhance relaxation and relieve pain. The pattern you use depends on the nature and intensity of your contractions, your preferences and your need for oxygen. By practising a variety of breathing patterns before labour, you can use them and adapt them as necessary to help calm and relax yourself during labour. Each method of childbirth preparation—Lamaze, Bradley, Kitzinger, Dick-Read and others—relies on some form of patterned breathing.

In keeping with our individualised approach, no single method is promoted here. Broad guidelines are offered, which will help you master breathing techniques that will fit your preferences and needs. Some women find abdominal breathing more comfortable than chest breathing; other women find just the opposite. The important thing is not where you breathe, but that the breathing calms and relaxes you. Through practice, experimentation and adaptation, you and your partner will find your own best way to use and adapt rhythmic breathing in labour.

Avoiding Hyperventilation

Hyperventilation occurs when the balance of oxygen and carbon dioxide in your blood is altered, causing a light-headed or dizzy feeling, or a tingling sensation in your fingers, feet or around your mouth. When breathing too deeply, too fast or both, you may exhale too much carbon dioxide, which causes hyperventilation. Tension also contributes to hyperventilation. While rarely serious, hyperventilation is uncomfortable and unnecessary because it can be prevented or easily corrected. If you have practised and mastered relaxation and breathing techniques before labour begins, it is unlikely that you will hyperventilate during labour. Rather, you will be able to adapt the pace and depth of your breathing to your changing respiratory requirements.

If hyperventilation does occur, it can be corrected by these measures:

- Re-breathing your own air (to restore your carbon dioxide to a normal level) by breathing into cupped hands, a paper bag or a surgical mask (available in the hospital).
- Holding your breath after a contraction until you feel the need to take a breath. This allows carbon dioxide levels in the blood to normalise. Do not hold your breath during a contraction (unless it is time to push your baby out).
- Relaxing and reducing tension. A shower, bath, massage, touch relaxation or music may help here.
- Setting a slower breathing rate or making breathing shallower. Your partner can help by 'conducting' (setting a rhythm with hand movements) or breathing along with you. (*Note:* If your partner hyperventilates when breathing along with you, he or she should use the above measures, too. Or, he or she may help you by talking to you in the rhythm of your breathing, or by pacing your breathing with head nodding or with rhythmic stroking of some part of your body.)

Breathing Patterns (First Stage)

There are two basic patterns of breathing for labour: *slow breathing* and *light breathing*. Plan to use them or their adaptations during labour to assist relaxation, to ensure adequate oxygenation and to enable you to change your breathing in response to the intensity of the contractions. It is most restful to begin using slow breathing when needed in early labour and to use it for as long into labour as it is helpful. Then you may want to switch to light breathing or one of the variations or adaptations that is most comfortable for you. Some women use only slow breathing throughout labour. Others use only slow and light, while still others use slow and one or more adaptations. What you do will depend on your preferences at the time and the intensity of your labour. The illustrations that accompany the descriptions of the breathing patterns in the following pages show the length and intensity of contractions (bottom line) along with visual images of the specific pattern of inhalations and exhalations (top line).

We advise learning both slow and light breathing. Then practise them along with some or all of the adaptations that are described on pages 196–198. You may use these adaptations that combine slow and light breathing, or you may find that you discover your own adaptations during labour (for example, adding sounds or words, or modifying the rhythms). The most important thing is to master the two basic patterns so that they can help you with relaxation and distraction during labour. You will be able to adapt them as needed.

Practise the breathing patterns in all the body positions shown in the chart on pages 227–229.

How to Use Breathing Patterns and Comfort Measures during Labour

When a contraction begins:

1. Signal your partner that the contraction is beginning by using a big in- and out-breath (similar to a sigh), by beginning your breathing pattern, or by telling or gesturing to your partner. Remember to release all tension as you breathe out.

2. Focus your attention (usually with a visual, tactile, auditory or mental focus, as described on pages 187–188).

3. Continue patterned breathing (slow, light or an adaptation) throughout the contraction. Use the intensity of the contraction to guide the pace of your breathing.

4. Combine breathing with other comfort measures (moaning, movement, massage, tension release, hot or cold packs, bath, shower and so on).

When the contraction ends:

1. Indicate to your partner that it is over (with a sigh of relief, words, gestures or by merely ending your patterned breathing).

2. Move around, give your partner feedback, ask for comfort items, sip liquids and get ready for the next contraction.

Slow Breathing

Use slow breathing (the first level of patterned breathing) when you reach a point in your labour when the contractions are intense enough that you can no longer walk or talk through them without having to pause. Use slow breathing for as long as you find it helpful, usually until you are well along in the first stage of labour. Shift to light breathing or a variation if you become tense and can no longer relax during contractions. Some women use only slow breathing throughout the entire first stage of labour; others use all the patterns and variations described here.

Slow breathing may be either chest breathing or abdominal breathing. More important than whether you breathe with your chest or abdomen is that the breathing helps you relax.

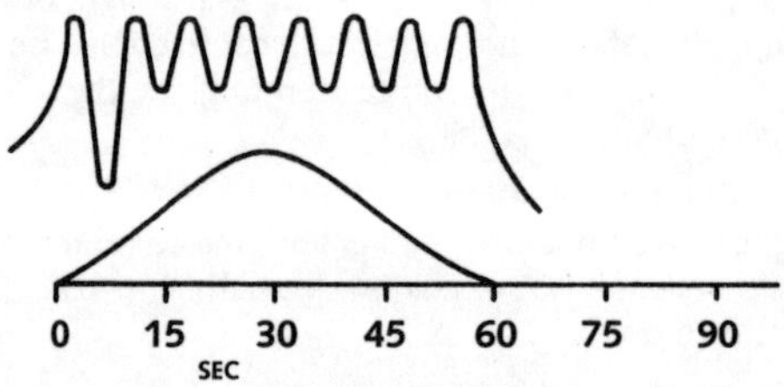

Slow breathing

How to Use Slow Breathing in Labour

1. As soon as the contraction begins, take a big breath, sighing on the exhale. This could be used as your 'organising' breath or as a signal to your partner. Release all tension as you breathe out, going limp all over—head to foot.

2. Focus your attention. (See pages 187–188.)

3. Slowly inhale through your nose (or mouth if your nose is congested) and exhale through your mouth, allowing all the air to flow out. Pause until the air seems to 'want' to come in again. Breathe about six to ten times per minute (about half your normal breathing rate).

4. Inhale quietly, but make your exhalation audible to those who are nearby, keeping your mouth slightly open and relaxed. The audible out-breath sounds like a relaxing sigh. In labour, you may vocalise or moan as you breathe out.

5. Keep your shoulders down and relaxed. Relax your chest and abdomen so they can swell as you inhale and return to normal as you exhale.

6. As the contraction ends, signal to your partner that it is over or take a final deep relaxing breath, ending with another sigh. Sometimes a yawn is a good finishing breath.

7. Relax all over, change positions, take sips of liquids and so on.

Note: While learning and practising this pattern, a few women find it uncomfortable to breathe in through the nose and out through the mouth. If that is true for you, modify the pattern to all-nose or all-mouth breathing. The most important thing is that slow breathing is comfortable and relaxing for you.

How to Rehearse Slow Breathing for Labour

Rehearse the technique described above until you become completely comfortable and consistent with it. Then you will be confident in your ability to use slow breathing to relax deeply. During labour contractions, you will

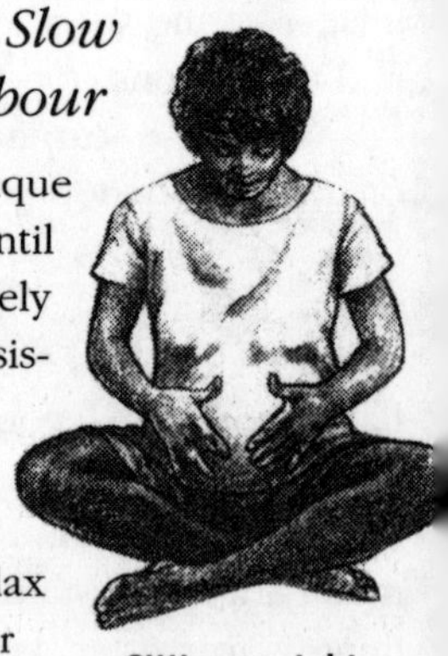

Sitting upright

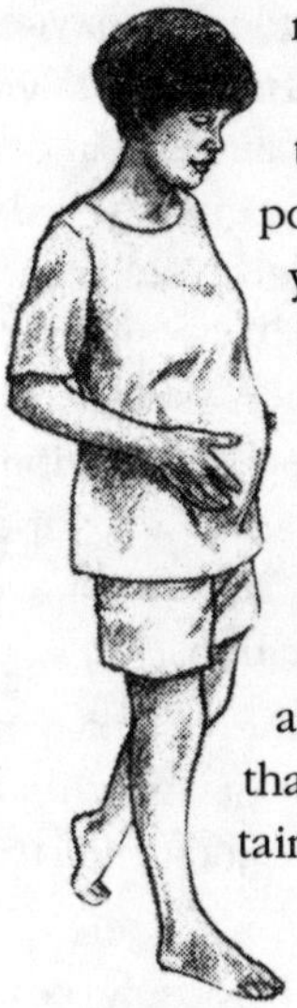

Walking

need to use this pattern for sixty to ninety seconds at a time. Practise in different positions (sitting up, lying on your side, standing, on hands and knees, and even in the car). With each out-breath, focus on relaxing a different part of your body (the roving body check, page 185) so that you relax all the parts of your body that are not necessary to maintain your position.

Light Breathing

Light breathing is very useful if and when you find that you can no longer relax during contractions, the contractions are too painful with slow breathing, or you are instinctively speeding up your breathing rate. If your partner notices that you are tensing, grimacing, clenching your fists or crying out at the peak of the contraction (even with reminders to relax), he or she might suggest that you switch to light breathing. Most women, though not all, feel the need to switch to light breathing (or one of the adaptations described on pages 196–198) at some time during the active phase of labour—especially if their contractions are very close together and very intense. Let the intensity of your contractions guide you in deciding if and when to use light breathing.

To do light breathing, breathe in and out rapidly and lightly through your mouth—about one breath every one or two seconds. Keep your breathing shallow and light. Your inhalations should be quiet, your exhalations clearly audible either as a short breath or light vocal sound. Quiet inhalations help ensure that you will not over-breathe, or hyperventilate.

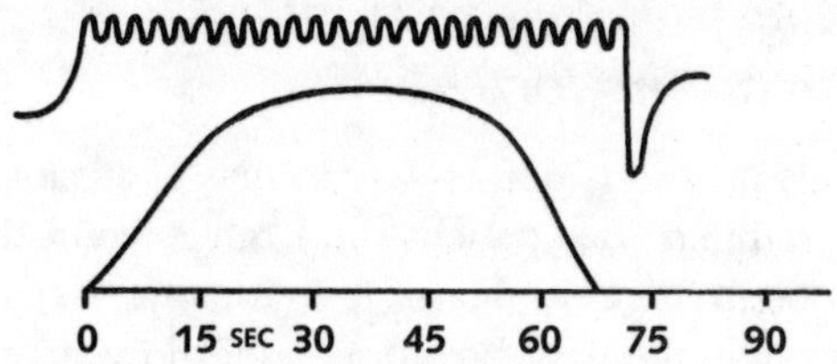

Light breathing

How to Use Light Breathing in Labour

1. Take a quick organising breath as soon as the contraction begins or signal your partner that the contraction has begun. Release all tension—go limp all over.

2. Focus your attention.

3. Begin light breathing. Allow your contraction to guide you in the rate and depth of your breathing, using a range of one breath every one or two seconds. Keep your mouth and shoulders relaxed. Continue breathing in this way until the contraction ends.

4. When the contraction ends, think of your last breath as a finishing breath (as if you are sighing the contraction away), or tell your partner that it is over.

5. Completely relax, change position, take sips of liquids and so on.

How to Rehearse Light Breathing for Labour

This pattern is not as easy to master as slow breathing. Be patient and give yourself enough time to learn it gradually. Begin learning the light breathing pattern by practicing at a rate between one breath per second and one breath every two seconds. Try breathing at different rates within that range until you are comfortable. The best way to calculate your rate is to count your breaths for ten seconds. If you count between five and ten breaths, you are in this range. Stay at that rate for thirty seconds to two minutes. When you are able to do light breathing effortlessly, comfortably and consistently for one to two minutes, you will be ready to try the adaptations described below.

At first, you may feel tense or as if you cannot get enough air. With practice, light breathing becomes easier and more comfortable. Mastering this breathing technique is like learning to breathe properly while doing the crawl stroke in swimming. Rhythmic breathing while swimming is challenging to learn, but once you learn it, it becomes almost second nature and you swim much more easily and efficiently. Mastering light breathing is not nearly as challenging as breathing with swimming, but it does take some practice. Once you master it, you will be able to use it effortlessly during contractions. You will also be able to vary the rate as necessary without getting dizzy from hyperventilation or feeling short of breath.

During labour, light breathing seems even more natural because the uterus is working so hard that you need more oxygen. Just as running makes you breathe rapidly to meet your oxygen needs, the increase in contraction intensity and frequency also increases your need for oxygen. Your breathing rate during labour will be naturally guided by your need for oxygen as well as by the pain and frequency of your contractions.

Breathing lightly through an open mouth may cause dryness, so use one or more of the following suggestions:

- As you breathe, touch the tip of your tongue to the roof of your mouth just behind your teeth. This slightly moistens the air that you breathe.
- With your fingers spread, loosely cover your nose and mouth so that your palm reflects the moisture from your breath.
- Between contractions, sip water or other fluids, or suck on ice or a frozen fruit juice bar.
- Brush your teeth or rinse your mouth occasionally.

Adaptations (Combining Slow and Light Patterns in a Variety of Ways)

Following are some ways you might adapt rhythmic breathing for your own comfort. These adaptations of slow and light breathing may be used in the first stage of labour, if you want to try something different. If at some point in labour you are feeling overwhelmed, unable to relax, in despair or exhausted, switching to one of these variations may help.

How to Use Adaptations of Slow and Light Breathing in Labour

Contraction-Tailored Breathing

In contraction-tailored breathing, you use the intensity of your contraction to guide you in the rate and depth of your breathing. If your contractions peak slowly, begin breathing slowly when the contraction begins. As the contraction intensifies, accelerate and lighten your breathing. Keep it light and rapid (one breath every one or two seconds) over the peak. As the contraction subsides, gradually slow and deepen your breathing. As with slow breathing, it helps to think of each out-breath as a relaxing breath. If your contractions peak quickly, you may skip slow breathing entirely, begin each contraction with light breathing, and modify the rate as needed.

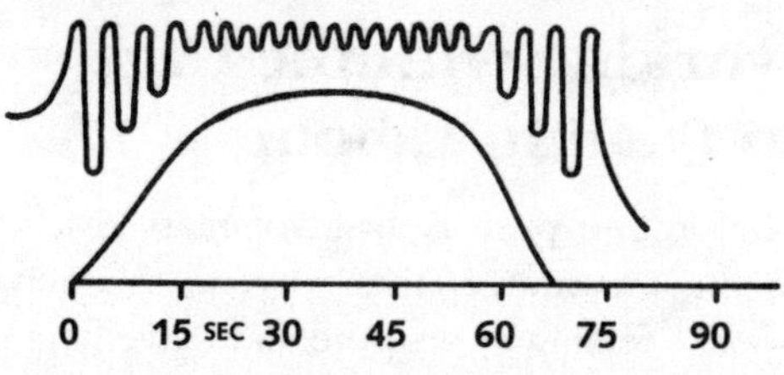

Contraction-tailored breathing

Vocal Breathing

Some women find that vocalising or verbalising during labour contractions helps them manage better. With vocal breathing, you breathe in a rhythm as described for slow and light breathing, but as you breathe out you make sounds or words (moaning, sighing, counting, singing, reciting poems, saying words, making varied sounds, chanting and so on). One mother found that counting and saying her baby's name was a way for her to maintain rhythm and a sense of control. She repeated, 'One, two, three, Max' over and over throughout each contraction. Another mother chanted, 'Epidural, epidural' over and over. She felt that as long as she could say it, she did not need it!

Most women who use vocal breathing effectively during labour use low tones. High-pitched tones often indicate suffering or fear. Your partner can check with you during contractions by asking, 'Are the sounds you are making helping?' If you indicate that they are not helping or that you are afraid, then your partner should help you lower the pitch of your sounds while maintaining the rhythm of your breathing. If high-pitched sounds are helping, then you should be encouraged to use them. Any worries about disturbing other people can usually be eased by making sure doors are closed.

Slide Breathing

Some women, especially those with asthma, find the more rapid pace of light breathing uncomfortable and tension producing. If you cannot master light breathing after trying it and focusing on using the exhalations to release tension, try slide breathing instead: Take a full slow breath in and breathe it out

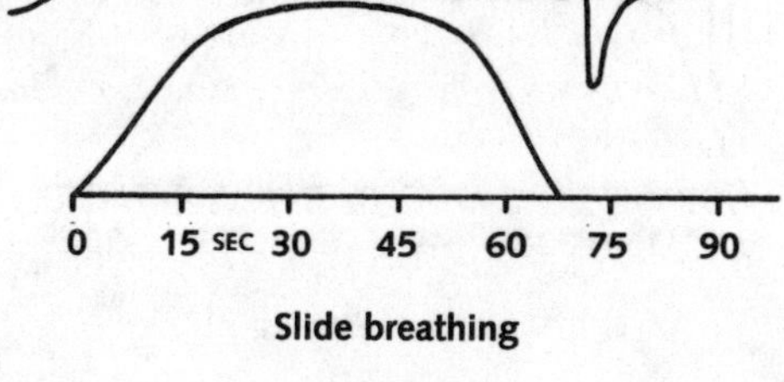

Slide breathing

by puffing lightly three or four times. Pause, breathe in, and repeat. You might say to yourself, 'IN… out-out-out-out…, IN… out-out-out-out….' Slide breathing was given its name by a pregnant woman who had asthma and could not do light breathing. She found this variation a good alternative. Though not very different physiologically from slow breathing, the change in rhythm provides a different focus and a psychological benefit.

Variable Breathing

Variable breathing is sometimes referred to as 'pant-pant-BLOW' or 'hee-hee-WHO' breathing, because it combines light, shallow breathing with a periodic longer or more pronounced exhalation. Variable breathing is helpful for those who feel short of breath with the light pattern or those who like having a structured pattern.

The pattern may consist of breathing lightly for two to five breaths (as in light breathing) followed by a longer, slower or more accented relaxed breath (the 'blow'). This last breath (the blow) helps you steady your rhythm and release tension. You do not need to take in a bigger breath before this blow, but you may appreciate a longer inhalation after the blow. Some women emphasise this blowing breath by making a long 'WHO' or 'PUH' sound as they exhale. Find the pattern you are comfortable with, and then repeat it throughout the contraction. Your partner might count for you, 'One, two, three, BLOW', or you might count to yourself for added concentration.

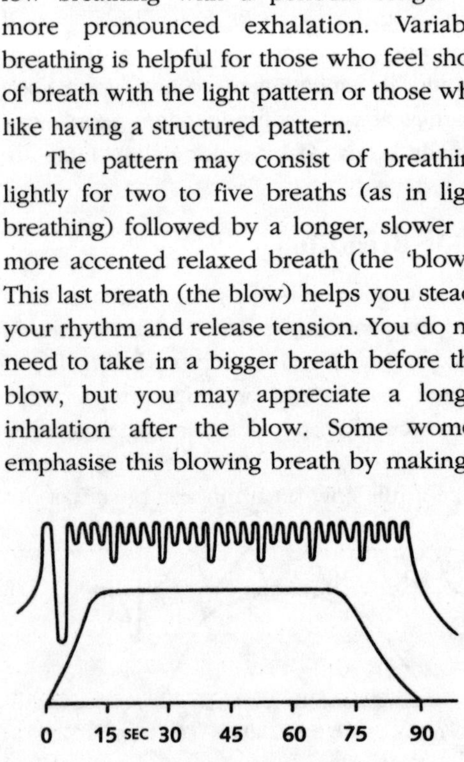

Variable breathing

How to Rehearse Breathing Adaptations for Labour

Add your favourite adaptations to your practice sessions. Late first-stage contractions might last two minutes, or they might 'piggyback' (come in pairs), so you need to be able to use light breathing or its adaptations for up to three minutes without becoming short of breath. Practise in various positions. Relax for only thirty seconds or so between practice contractions to prepare for the brief rest period between contractions in late first stage.

Working with the Urge to Push in Labour

The urge to push is an involuntary reaction to the pressure of the baby on the pelvic floor. A feeling of pressure and movement of the baby deep in the pelvis, which causes an irresistible need to bear down or strain, characterises the urge. Some women think they need to have a bowel movement when they first feel this urge. When you get an urge to push in labour, you will either hold your breath, make grunting sounds as you breathe or have a catch in every breath. You or your partner should ask your midwife to check for dilation at this time. If your cervix is fully dilated, you generally can begin bearing down and pushing when you feel the urge.

If your cervix is not fully dilated but is very thin, soft and stretchy, you should bear down only enough to satisfy the urge. If your cervix still has a thickened area (sometimes called a 'lip' or an 'anterior lip'), you may need to avoid bearing down altogether until the cervix dilates completely. Otherwise, the cervix may swell and slow labour progress. Your caregiver will guide you in what to do at this time. Although it is sometimes very difficult and uncomfortable to keep from pushing when you have a strong urge, it is not harmful to postpone pushing until the cervix has completely dilated.

How to Avoid Pushing, When Necessary

If you get a premature urge to push, lift your chin or arch your back to avoid curling your trunk and pressing your chest down onto your uterus. Either breathe deeply in and out, or blow lightly until the urge subsides. It may be helpful for you to vocalise at this time, actually saying or singing 'puh, puh', or 'hooo, hooo, hooo'. Then use your chosen breathing pattern for the rest of the contraction. This technique does not take away the strong urge to push, nor does it prevent your uterus from pushing. All it can do is keep you from adding your voluntary strength to the pushing effort. Certain positions—such as side-lying, hands and knees, and knee-chest

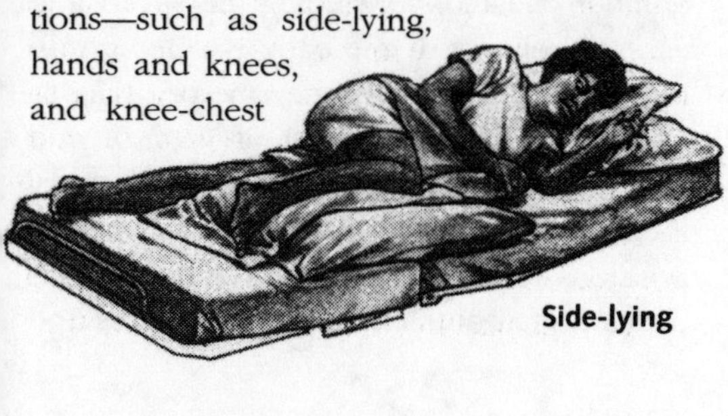

Side-lying

Hands and knees

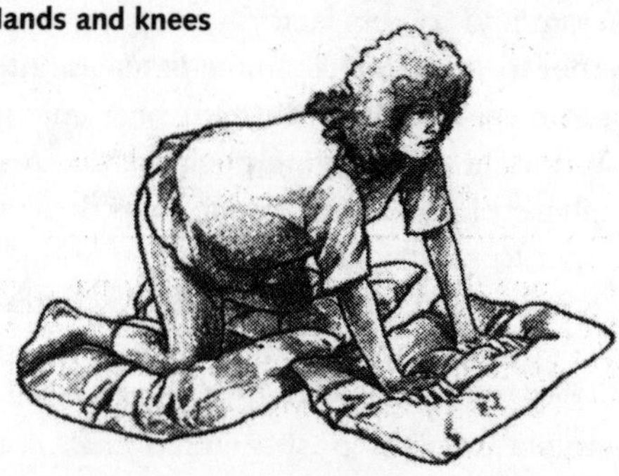

(see page 294)—often reduce the premature urge to push or make it easier to cope.

How to Rehearse Avoiding Pushing in Labour

When you are rehearsing breathing patterns, occasionally incorporate an imagined urge to push. Hold your breath or grunt as you breathe, so that your partner can also learn his or her part. When your partner recognises the urge to push, he or she can remind you to lift your chin and blow-blow-blow (or pant-pant-pant) until the imagined urge passes.

Expulsion Breathing (Second Stage)

Once the cervix is fully dilated, the second stage of labour has begun. You may or may not feel an immediate urge to bear down (or push) with your contractions. The amount and speed of your baby's descent, his station and position within your pelvis, your body position and other factors will determine whether the urge comes immediately or after a brief rest. Usually, with time or a change to an upright or squatting position, this resting phase of the second stage subsides and the urge to push increases.

Your responses to second-stage contractions depend on the sensations you feel. You will probably feel several surges—strong, irresistible urges to push—within each contraction. Each lasts a few seconds. You simply breathe, using whatever pattern suits you, until you have an urge to push and your body begins bearing down. Respond to this urge to push, bearing down for as long as you feel the urge. Then breathe lightly until either another urge comes or the contraction is over. You will probably bear down three to five times per contraction, with each effort lasting about five to seven seconds. Take advantage of the opportunity to rest and relax between contractions.

This type of pushing is called 'spontaneous bearing down' (meaning that you react spontaneously to your urge to push). This type is recommended when labour is progressing normally and the woman has had no anaesthesia. Spontaneous bearing down may be impossible when anaesthesia is used, because anaesthesia diminishes the pushing sensations and your ability to bear down effectively. When you have had anaesthesia, your birth attendant will tell you when and how to push. This is called 'directed pushing'.

When practising bearing-down techniques for the second stage, you do not need to bear down forcefully, only enough to feel the bulging of your pelvic floor. (See the exercise on page 130.) To practise more effectively, imagine what will be happening when you are pushing in actual labour. Visualise the baby descending and rotating to remind yourself of the importance of relaxing and bulging your pelvic floor.

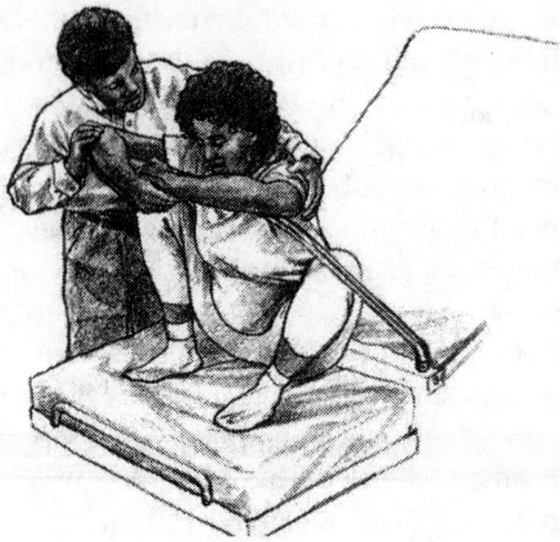

Squatting

Positions for the Second Stage

Just as movement and changing positions can be helpful for both comfort and progress in the first stage, they may be equally beneficial in the second stage. Rehearse bearing down (expulsion breathing) in the positions shown on pages 227–229.

The positions you use will depend on a number of factors, including the speed and ease of delivery. If the baby is coming rapidly, you may not have the time or desire to change positions; however, if your second stage is slow, you will have a chance to try them all. Other factors will influence the positions you try, including your birth attendant's preferences and your willingness and

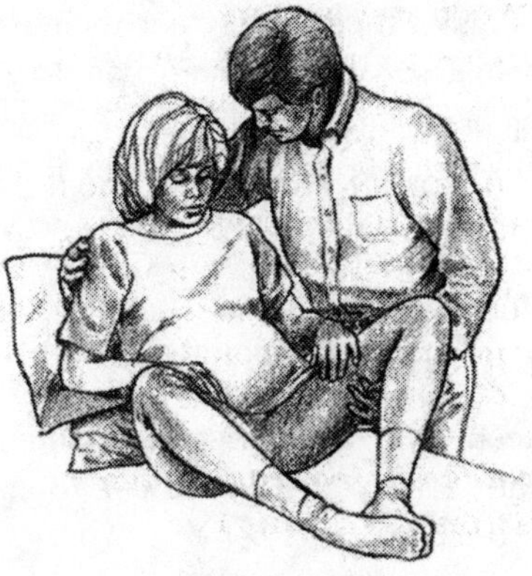

Semi-sitting

freedom to move about. Electronic foetal monitors, catheters, anaesthetics, IV equipment and narrow beds discourage mobility, but with help and encouragement you can safely move into favourable positions. Discuss delivery positions when preparing your birth plan. Although most doctors and midwives are accustomed to the semi-sitting position, they may be willing to let you try other positions, if you ask. They may be less flexible as you get close to delivery, at which point your attendant may ask you to move to the position most familiar to him or her.

Spontaneous Bearing Down (Expulsion Breathing)

How to Use Spontaneous Bearing Down in Labour

1. As the contraction begins, start a breathing pattern and try to release all unnecessary tension as you breathe out.

2. Focus on the baby moving down and out, or on another positive image.

3. Let the contraction guide you in the rate and depth of your breathing pattern. When you cannot resist the urge to push (when it 'demands' that you join in), bear down or strain while holding your breath or slowly releasing air by grunting or vocalising, whichever feels best. As you do this, you automatically tighten your abdominal muscles. Most important of all, relax the pelvic floor. (See the 'bulging' exercise on page 130.) Help your baby come down by releasing any tension in the perineum. You may need reminders to try to relax your perineum.

4. Release all your breath when you need to (usually after five to seven seconds of pushing) and breathe in and out until the urge to push comes again. Then, once again join in by bearing down. How hard you push is dictated by your sensations. (In practice, never push hard. Push just enough to feel the bulging in your perineum.) You will continue in this way until the contraction subsides. The urge to push comes and goes in waves during the contraction, giving you time in between to 'breathe for your baby' (to oxygenate your blood to provide sufficient oxygen for your baby).

5. When the contraction ends, slowly lie or sit back or stand up from a squat and take one or two relaxing breaths.

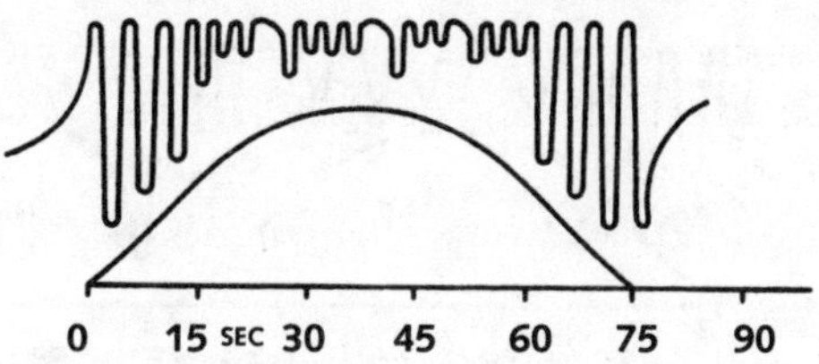

Spontaneous bearing down

Avoiding Pushing As the Head Is Born

The breathing and bearing down just described continues for each contraction until much of the baby's head can be seen (crowning), at which time you will feel the tissue of your lower vagina stretch and burn. At this point, you may need to stop bearing down to allow the vagina and perineum to stretch gradually around the baby's head as it emerges, to reduce the likelihood of tearing or a too-rapid delivery. While the stretching, burning sensation is a clear signal to stop your bearing-down effort, your doctor or midwife will also give you directions at this point, telling you when to push and when to blow to stop pushing. To avoid pushing, blow as you do when avoiding the urge to push (page 199), until the urge subsides or until you are told to bear down again.

Directed Pushing

The previous description of the second-stage bearing-down technique is based on the assumption that you will feel a spontaneous urge to push, which will guide your response to your contractions. However, if you do not feel your contractions because of anaesthesia, or if you have no urge to push (even after twenty or thirty minutes have passed and you have tried gravity-enhancing positions such as squatting, sitting, 'dangling', lap squatting or standing upright [see pages 227–229]), then you may need to follow a routine of directed pushing.

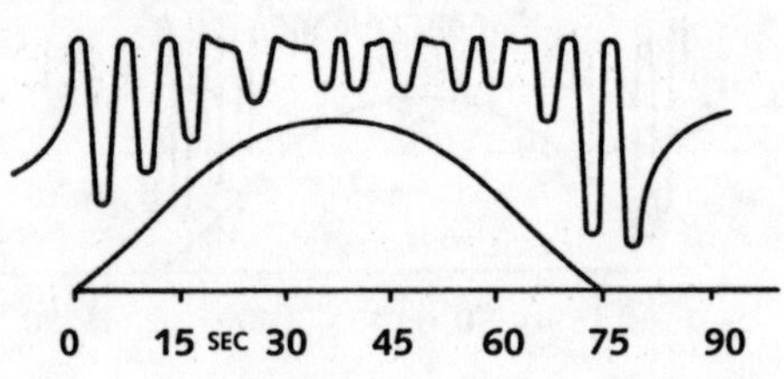

Directed pushing

How to Use Directed Pushing in Labour

In this technique, your birth attendant, nurse or partner tells you when, how long and how hard to push.

1. When the contraction begins, take two or three breaths, and when you are told to push, take a breath in and hold it. Curl forward, tucking your chin on your chest and bear down, tightening your abdominal muscles.

2. Relax your pelvic floor muscles. Bear down for five to seven seconds. Quickly release your breath, take another few breaths, and repeat the routine until the contraction subsides.

3. When the contraction ends, slowly lie or sit back, rest and breathe normally.

Note: This routine continues for each contraction until the baby's head is almost out. At this point, the doctor or midwife may tell you to stop pushing to allow the baby to pass slowly through the vaginal opening. At the attendant's direction, relax and let all the air out of your lungs. Pant or blow quickly, if necessary, to keep from bearing down.

How to Rehearse Spontaneous Bearing Down and Directed Pushing for Labour

Use the practice sessions as rehearsals, going through the contractions as described for spontaneous bearing down. Remember the importance of relaxing the perineum while bearing down. In practice, bear down only enough to allow yourself to feel bulging of the pelvic floor. In actual labour, your body guides you in how hard to bear down. Some women find it helpful to rehearse these bearing-down techniques during perineal massage.

In addition, occasionally rehearse directed pushing, with your partner counting to five or seven while you hold your breath. In labour, your caregiver may direct you in how hard to push.

Prolonged Pushing

Prolonged breath-holding and pushing were once taught for all births, whether the mother could feel her urge to push or not. It is still more familiar to many birth attendants than spontaneous pushing, and it is more widely advocated by them. Prolonged pushing differs from directed pushing in the length of time the woman is expected to hold her breath and bear down (ten seconds or more instead of five to seven seconds). This kind of pushing, especially in the supine (back-lying) position, is associated with a decrease in the oxygen available to the foetus and a drop in the mother's blood pressure, both of which can increase the need for an episiotomy. Also, prolonged pushing may cause too-rapid stretching of the vaginal tissues, increasing the possibility of a tear. Spontaneous bearing down and directed pushing efforts with breathing in between result in better oxygenation of the foetus[7] and more gradual distention of the vagina. Unless the woman uses upright positions that promote foetal descent, the second stage may last slightly longer with spontaneous or directed pushing than with prolonged pushing, but the foetus usually remains in good condition throughout.[8]

Under some circumstances (discussed in Chapter 10), the advantages of prolonged pushing may outweigh the disadvantages. These situations include a very long second stage, the inability of the woman to use a gravity-assisted position, and a large or malpositioned foetus. You may be trying to avoid the use of forceps or a vacuum extractor. Your caregiver is the best judge of this. Since you will be using prolonged pushing only under the guidance of your caregiver, and because there is little benefit in practising it, there is no need to practise it before labour.

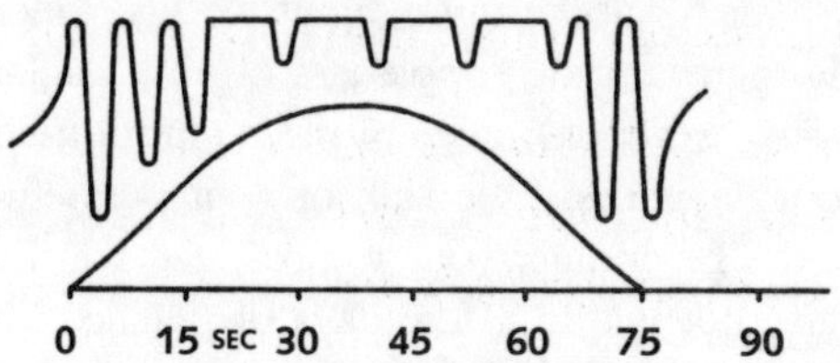

Prolonged pushing

Preparation of the Perineum (Perineal Massage)

Perineal massage (stretching the inner tissue of the lower vagina) teaches you to respond to pressure in your vagina by relaxing your pelvic floor (a useful rehearsal for birth). It is also thought to enhance the hormonal changes that soften connective tissue in late pregnancy. You are more likely to avoid an episiotomy or serious tear if you practice perineal massage.[9] (Episiotomy is discussed further in Chapters 9 and 10.)

If you are interested in avoiding an episiotomy or a tear, you may find it very helpful to massage your perineum five to seven times a week during the last five or six weeks of your pregnancy. Be sure your caregiver knows what you are doing and why. Because there are only a few studies done on perineal massage, and because it is somewhat unconventional, some caregivers are not familiar with it. Some women or couples find it distasteful and do not want to do it. Others feel it is worthwhile if it can reduce the chances of having an episiotomy or a serious tear. Some find it enjoyable, especially after doing it for a while and learning to relax.

If you have vaginitis, a genital herpes sore or other vaginal problems, you should wait until you are healed before beginning perineal massage, as it could worsen the condition.

What to Do

Either you or your partner can do the massage. Until you are familiar with the technique, use a mirror to help you see your perineum. Be sure your hands are clean and your fingernails are short. If you or your partner has rough skin, it may be more comfortable for you if disposable, protective vinyl or latex gloves are worn. You can purchase these at a pharmacy.

Make yourself comfortable in a semi-sitting position (if your partner is doing it) or standing with one foot up on the side of the tub or a chair (if you are doing it yourself).

1. Generously lubricate your thumb (if you are doing it yourself) or your partner's index fingers with oil or water-soluble jelly by squirting it from a squeeze bottle or tube. This method is preferable to dipping your fingers into the oil, since repeated dipping will contaminate the oil. Some people recommend wheat germ oil, available at health food stores, because of its high vitamin E content, but other vegetable oils or water-based lubricants, such as K-Y Jelly, can also be used. Do not use baby oil, mineral oil, petroleum jelly or hand lotion, as these are believed to be less well tolerated than vegetable or water-based products.

2. If you are doing the massage yourself, use your thumb. Your partner can use the index fingers (one at first, then both when you are more used to it). Place the fingers or thumb well inside the vagina (up to the second knuckle). Then do a Kegel (pelvic floor contraction) so that you can feel the muscle tense on your thumb or your partner's fingers. Relax your pelvic floor muscles and move either thumb or fingers within the vagina in a rhythmic U movement while gently pulling outward and downward towards the anus. Do this for about three minutes. This stretching increases the suppleness of your vaginal tissue (mucosa), the muscles surrounding your vagina and the skin of your perineum. In the beginning, your vaginal wall will feel tight, but within a few days of practice, the tissue will relax and stretch more easily.

3. Concentrate on relaxing your muscles as you feel the pressure and stretching. As you become comfortable with the massage, increase the pressure just enough to make the tissue begin to sting or burn slightly from the stretching. (This same stinging sensation occurs as the baby's head is being born.)

4. If you have any questions after trying the massage, ask your caregiver or someone who teaches or has used this technique.

Practice Time: Rehearsals for Labour

Try to use practice time for more than simply going through a number of techniques. Use this time as a rehearsal for labour. Think about and discuss when you might use the techniques and why. Review what you have learned about the emotional and physical events of labour. (Use the 'Labour and Birth Guide' on pages 248–255 to help you review.) Most of all, use this time together to explore the basic techniques you have learned, to adapt them to fit your needs and to learn how to work together.

Practising with Your Partner

Here are some suggestions for how your partner may work with you during practice. Many of these tips will be useful in labour as well.

- To signal the beginning of a contraction, tell your partner or begin a breathing pattern. You can also have your partner say, 'Contraction begins', 'Here we go' or something similar. It is a good idea for you to take turns 'starting' the contractions during practice. You both will get used to responding whether you are ready or not. (This is more like a true labour situation.) When the practice or real contraction ends, you may say, 'It's over', and your partner may acknowledge it by saying, 'Contraction ends', 'Blow it away', 'It's gone' or something similar. Explore these options and select a ritual that works best for you.
- Having your partner count your breaths during the contraction and interject encouraging words at the same time can be very helpful. For example, your partner can say, 'One, let's get started. Two, that's the way. Three, let go of your shoulders. Four, just like that', and so on. The number of breaths you need to take to get through each contraction will not vary significantly from one contraction to the next. Therefore, you can figure out roughly how many breaths it takes to get through each contraction. Your partner can then point out to you when you have passed the halfway point. One woman said of her partner, 'He cut my contractions in half, because I knew when I had passed the peak I could make it the rest of the way'.
- To simulate the intensity of labour contractions, you might try holding an ice cube in one hand for sixty seconds while using rhythmic breathing. Then switch the ice cube to the other hand and hold it for

sixty seconds without doing the breathing. Many women are surprised to discover how much better they tolerate the cold if they are concentrating on doing rhythmic breathing. It will be reassuring to both of you to discover how these skills reduce your awareness of pain.

- While practising the techniques, your partner should be able to detect any tension and help you regain a relaxed state. Touching, massaging, talking, breathing with you, steadying your rhythm by conducting (using his or her hand to set a pace for breathing) and reminding you to move around are all ways your partner can help you during practice and during actual labour.
- Your partner's facial expression, tone of voice and way of touching you can affect how you respond. Loud or worried tones of voice, a troubled expression or tense or nervous rubbing all convey anxiety. On the other hand, a soothing voice, a confident facial expression and a relaxed calming touch communicate reassuring messages. Help your partner become aware of the non-verbal messages he or she is sending.

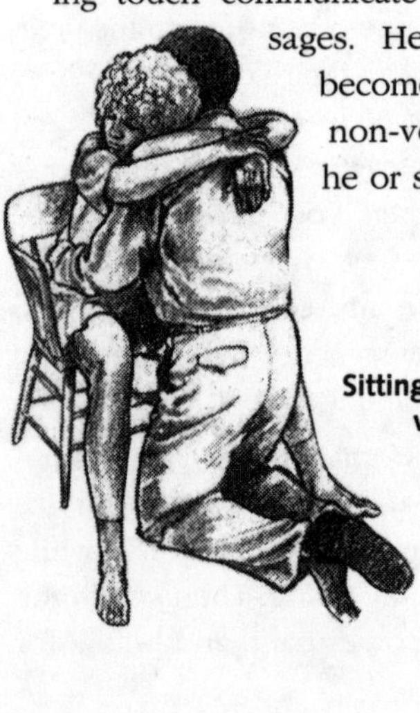

Sitting, leaning forward with support

How Much Should You Practise?

You probably do not have to practise every day to master these techniques, especially if you are attending childbirth classes together. Spend enough time practising to become completely comfortable with each breathing pattern and relaxation technique and to figure out any adaptations you want to use. Then review them periodically so they become familiar and easy for you. Some people need or want to practise more than others. The techniques will be more helpful if you have mastered them well ahead of time.

Suggested Practice Sequence

The following learning sequence will help you master the techniques discussed in this chapter and in Chapter 10. You may take a few months to complete the sequence or you may begin closer to your due date and condense it into several weeks. Either way, practising these exercises, breathing patterns and relaxation techniques will prepare you for the birth of your baby.

1. Conditioning exercises (pages 129–134). Add the variations and continue practising these exercises until the birth.

2. Comfort measures for pregnancy (pages 134–138). Use the ones that decrease any discomforts of pregnancy and those that seem appropriate for you.

3. Body awareness exercises (pages 178–180)

4. Passive relaxation (pages 181–183). Practise alone or with your partner.

5. Relaxation countdown (page 183). Start by practising this using several breaths and work towards relaxing with one breath.

6. Perineal massage (pages 203–205)

7. Slow breathing (pages 193–195)

8. Touch relaxation (pages 183–184)

9. Roving body check (page 185). Practise both by yourself and with your partner's direction (saying the area or touching the area).

10. Slow breathing and roving body check (pages 185 and 193–195)

11. Attention-focusing (pages 187–188)

12. Possible positions for first stage of labour (pages 227–228). Practise slow breathing in a contraction pattern using each position (side-lying, sitting, standing, slow dancing, on hands and knees, and sitting on or leaning over a birth ball).

13. Light breathing (pages 195–196). Experiment with depth and rate to find what works for you.

14. Adaptations of slow and light breathing—contraction-tailored, vocal, slide and variable breathing—(pages 196–199)

15. Variety of positions for first stage of labour (pages 227–228) while practising the adaptations of slow and light breathing

16. Ways to decrease back pain in labour (pages 285–289). Practise the double hip squeeze, counterpressure and lunge. Combine these with practise of all breathing patterns.

17. Panting to avoid pushing (with a premature urge to push) during the peak of a contraction in late first stage of labour (pages 198–199)

18. Expulsion breathing—spontaneous bearing down and directed pushing—(pages 199–203). Learn and rehearse both breathing patterns. Practise gently bearing down and incorporate the pelvic floor bulging exercise (page 130). Occasionally, practise panting to avoid pushing in the middle of a practice contraction.

19. Positions for second stage of labour (pages 227–229). Try the positions and then use them while practising expulsion breathing.

20. Labour rehearsal. Practise all the coping techniques during a series of contractions (pages 174–207, 227–229 and 285–289). Your partner can assist by observing you and helping you relax fully in all positions.

Chapter 9

Labour and Birth

During labour, your uterus contracts, your cervix thins (effaces) and opens (dilates), your baby rotates and moves down the birth canal, and you give birth to your baby, placenta, umbilical cord and amniotic sac. The entire process, which usually takes from a few hours to a day or more, is the transition to parenthood for you and the transition to an independent existence for your baby. Labour is the climax of pregnancy, when many seemingly separate systems work in harmony to bring about birth.

The onset of labour seems to be under the joint control of the hormonal (endocrine) systems of mother and baby. These systems function in synchrony so that most of the time the baby is ready to be born at about the same time the mother is physically and emotionally ready to give birth and to nourish and nurture her baby. Corticotropin-releasing hormone (CRH) regulates the timing of the birth by triggering the changes in the mother's uterus and in the foetus that must precede labour. Both the foetal brain and the placenta produce CRH. The rate at which the hormone is released is sometimes called 'the foeto-placental clock'. The clock is faster in some women than in others, which helps explain why healthy term babies are born at any time between thirty-seven and forty-two weeks gestation.

The sequence of events set off by CRH includes a late pregnancy increase in oestrogen production. Before then, the balance between the hormones oestrogen and progesterone keeps the cervix tightly closed and prevents the uterus from contracting in a coordinated fashion. In late pregnancy, increases in oestrogen produce the following changes in the uterus:

- Increased sensitivity of the uterine muscle to oxytocin (the hormone that causes the uterus to contract)
- Increased maternal production of prostaglandins (substances that ripen or soften the cervix)
- Increased uterine activity and more noticeable contractions

Also in late pregnancy, CRH causes the foetal adrenal glands to mature and begin producing cortisol. Cortisol stimulates the foetal lungs to mature and ensures that they will remain inflated after birth when the newborn begins breathing.

Although this physiological interaction between mother, placenta and foetus is complex and not yet fully understood, recent research indicates that the foeto-placental clock plays a crucial role in the timing of foetal maturity and in triggering the mechanisms that begin labour.[1] The foeto-placental clock may be altered by such events as illness or infection in the mother, heavy smoking or use of other drugs,

Events of Late Pregnancy: A Collaboration of Foetus, Mother and Placenta

During the last 6–8 weeks of pregnancy, numerous complex interrelated events take place, as shown below. Birth is the climax. Each component of the foetal-maternal-placental unit contributes by triggering changes in other components, thereby continuing the process that results in the birth of a mature and capable baby to a mother who is ready to nourish and nurture her baby. Cortico-releasing hormone (CRH), produced by the placenta and the foetal brain, initiates these changes that lead to birth. The timing is usually perfect, although in 10–12 percent of births the timing falters and a premature baby is born.

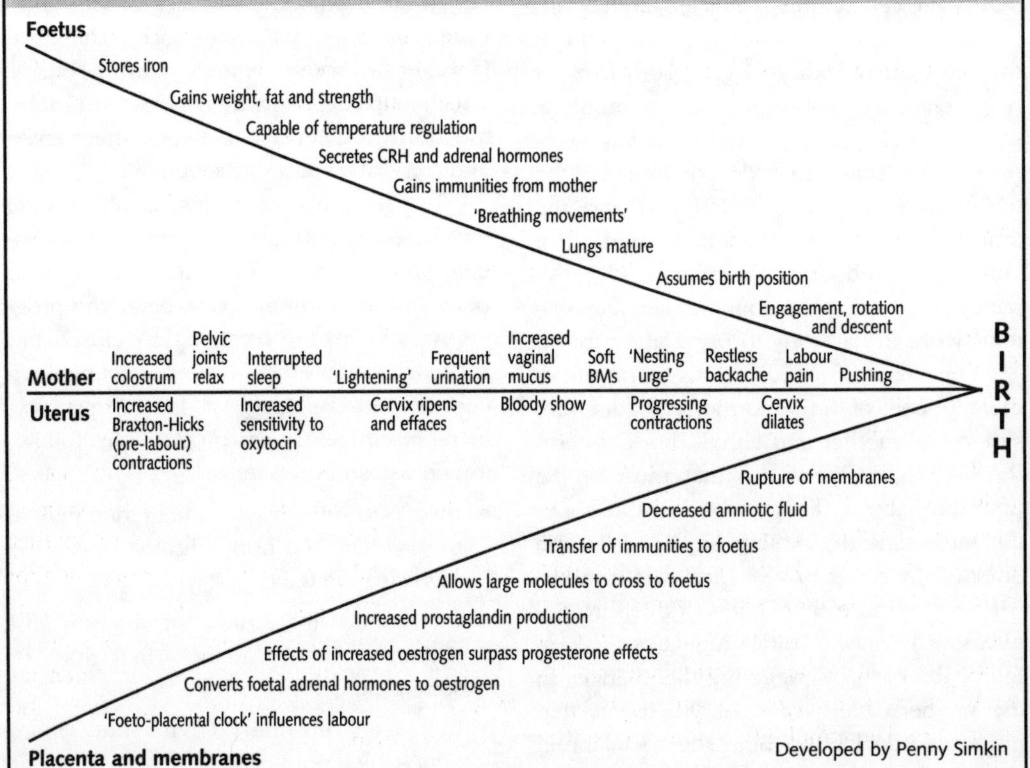

Developed by Penny Simkin

extremely stressful life circumstances or other factors. The intricate timing of the onset of labour is also altered by induction of labour for both medical and non-medical reasons. Non-medical inductions are somewhat controversial. (See Chapter 10 for more discussion of labour induction.) As you approach the end of your pregnancy, you may wish you could have the baby sooner. You may feel awkward, tired, fat, hot and uncomfortable. But try to remember that even if you pass your due date, labour has probably not begun because the baby is not yet ready to be born.

The Last Weeks of Pregnancy

During the last weeks of pregnancy, your body goes through changes that prepare you to give birth and to nourish your baby. Your breasts produce more colostrum (the baby's first food after birth). Your uterus becomes more irritable and contracts more frequently, both spontaneously and in response to activity and minor disturbances such as walking, sneezing and bumping your abdomen. These mild contractions, influenced by the changing hormonal balance, contribute to cervical changes such as ripening (softening) and effacement (thinning). Before labour begins, your cervix may have dilated 1 or 2 centimetres (or even more if you have given birth before). The ligaments and cartilage in your pelvis relax, allowing greater mobility in the joints. This makes it possible for your pelvic bones to spread during labour and birth to give your baby a bit more room in the birth canal. At the same time, vaginal secretions increase and the tissues of the vaginal wall become more elastic. All these changes are essential to the baby's passage.

Foetal development late in pregnancy not only sets in motion some of the mechanisms that initiate labour, it also prepares the baby for life outside the uterus. He stores iron at a rapid rate in the last weeks of pregnancy, taking in enough to supplement the small amounts in breast milk and to meet his needs for the next four to six months. The baby adds fat and develops the mechanism needed to maintain his own body temperature. He gains weight and strength. His foetal lungs mature, ensuring that he will be able to breathe without difficulty.

As the placenta ages, the membrane that separates the foetal blood from the maternal blood becomes more permeable to large molecules. This permits antibodies and immunoglobulins to cross from your bloodstream to your baby's, providing months of protection for the baby against diseases to which you are immune. If you breastfeed, you will continue to provide such protection for as long as you nurse your baby.

Your baby's readiness for survival outside your body coincides with his production of various substances that feed back to your circulation and play a key role in triggering the changes involved in starting labour. Your own physical and psychological readiness for labour is the other key. Usually, when the time is right for both you and your baby, labour begins.

Things to Do before the Birth

The following lists will help you get ready for a hospital or birth-centre birth. If you are planning a home birth, much from these lists will still be relevant; in addition, ask your midwife or doctor what preparations to make in your home and what supplies to have on hand.

Early Preparation

1. Prepare a birth plan and go over it with your doctor or midwife. (Use Chapter 7 as a guide.) Your childbirth educator can help you write it or answer questions, but make sure your birth plan reflects what is important to you.

2. Tour your hospital or backup hospital if you are planning a birth-centre or home birth.

3. Pre-register at the hospital. (This may be unnecessary if you are planning an out-of-hospital birth.) You or your partner will sign admission forms, including possibly a general consent form. Most general consent forms used in hospitals are intimidating and make it seem as if you are giving the hospital permission to do whatever they want to do to you or your baby. Try to read this form before labour and ask for clarification of any items that make you uncomfortable. Some patients simply cross out or reword the items that concern them and initial those changes before signing the form. Some add a statement that they want to be informed of reasons, risks, benefits and alternatives before any treatment or procedure is done. It might be helpful to know that the general consent form is not the only one you sign. If you or your baby develops a problem requiring major procedures—such as caesarean section, other surgery, a septic work-up or (in some hospitals) epidural anaesthesia—you will probably be asked to sign another consent form specific to the procedure.

Pack Your Bags for the Hospital or Birth Centre

For easy access, pack the following items in a bag separate from your suitcase:

For Use during Labour:

- Lip gloss or balm
- Toothbrushes (for you and your partner) and toothpaste
- Warm socks in case your feet get cold
- Baby powder or massage oil
- This book
- Nightgown or long T-shirt to wear in labour (if you prefer not to wear a hospital gown)
- Hot water bottle
- Rolling pin or other item for pressure on back (A blue icepack could provide pressure and cold.)
- Birth ball (if hospital or birth centre does not have one)
- Favourite juice, tea or iceblocks (if not provided)
- Partner's snack

- Partner's swimsuit (so partner can accompany you in the shower or bath)
- Phone numbers of people to call after the birth
- Optional: camera and film, tape recorder and audiotapes, video recorder and blank videotapes to record the birth (Check with the hospital staff and your caregiver regarding any policies on these items.)
- Personal comfort items (pillow from home, pictures, flowers and so on)
- Tapes or compact discs of relaxing music (Check with the hospital staff about available equipment and policies.)

For Post-partum Stay:

- Nightgowns or pyjamas for nursing (You may prefer hospital gowns.)
- Robe and slippers (You may prefer the hospital's.)
- Cosmetic and grooming aids
- Nursing bra
- Going-home clothes (a comfortable size, as you will probably not be back to your pre-pregnant size yet)
- Other personal items

For Baby:

- Nappies and waterproof nappy cover, or disposable nappies
- Undershirt or one-piece body suit
- Nightgown or stretch suit
- Receiving blanket
- Outside blanket and cap
- Car seat for ride home (properly installed in the car before labour)

Key Concepts for Understanding Labour

At some time during late pregnancy or early labour, the baby moves down within your uterus and assumes his birth position, and your cervix changes in preparation for labour. In this section we cover the terminology used by care providers in describing and assessing these events and changes.

Presentation and Position

Your caregiver uses the following terms to describe how your baby is lying within your uterus:

- *Presentation* describes the part of the baby that is lying over the cervix and that will be delivered first. For example, the most favourable and most common presentation (occurring 95 percent of the time) is the *vertex* presentation, in which the crown (or top) of the baby's head is down over the cervix. Other presentations are the *frank breech* (buttocks), *footling breech* (one or two feet), *complete breech* (buttocks and feet), *shoulder, face* and *brow* presentations. (These rarer presentations, which may cause difficulties in labour, are discussed in Chapter 10.)
- *Position* refers to the direction towards which the back of the baby's head (or

other presenting part) lies within your body. The possible positions are *anterior*, referring to your front; *posterior*, referring to your back; and *transverse*, referring to your side.

If your doctor or midwife tells you the baby is *occiput anterior*, it means that the back of the baby's head (the occiput) is pointing directly towards your anterior (front). Here are some other common descriptions of the baby's presentation and position:

Left (or right) occiput anterior (LOA or ROA). The back of the baby's head is towards your left (or right) front.

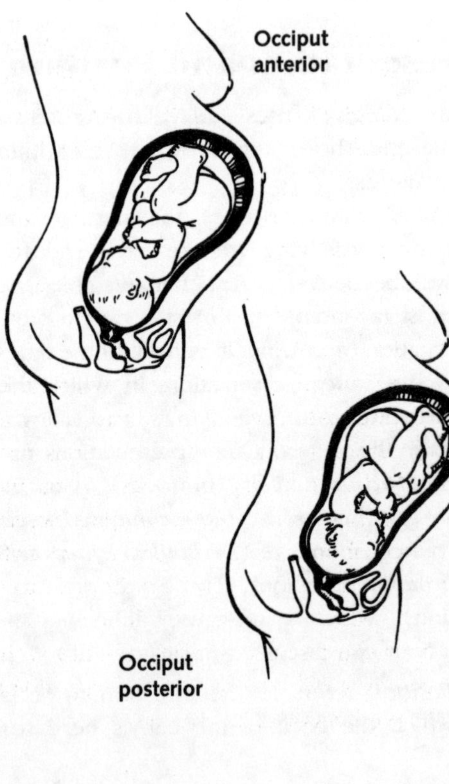

Occiput posterior (OP). The back of the baby's head is directly towards your back.

Right (or left) occiput posterior (ROP or LOP). The back of the baby's head is towards your right (or left) back.

Right (or left) occiput transverse (ROT or LOT). The back of the baby's head is towards your right (or left) side.

Right (or left) sacrum anterior (RSA or LSA). The baby's tail bone or buttocks (sacrum) is towards your right (or left) front. A breech presentation is described in this way.

During labour, the presentation of the baby rarely changes; however, the position of the baby usually does change. The head usually rotates to an OA position (or more rarely to an OP position).

Station and Descent

Station refers to the location of the foetal presenting part (usually the baby's head) in relation to the ischial spines, which are bones marking the middle of the true pelvis. (See illustration.) For example, if the top of the head is at 0 station, it means that it has descended to the middle of the pelvis. If the head is still very high ('floating' above the level of the pubic bone), it might be as high as a –4 (minus four) station (4 centimetres above the mid-pelvis). If it is at a –1 or –2 station, the top of the head is 1 or 2 centimetres above the mid-pelvis. If the head is at a +1 (plus one) or +2 (plus two) station, it is 1 or 2 centimetres below the mid-pelvis. When the head is at the vaginal opening and on its way out, it is at a +4 station. This downward movement of the baby is called *descent*. Complete descent means that the baby moves from the highest station (–4) down to the lowest station (+4) and is then born. For *primigravidas* (women pregnant for the first time), some descent—either gradual or sudden—usually takes place several weeks before the onset of labour (though this is not always the case). For *multigravidas* (women who have been pregnant more than once), it is not unusual for labour to begin with the baby still floating or rather high in the pelvis. For both primigravidas and multigravidas, most descent takes place during late labour after the cervix has opened and as the mother pushes.

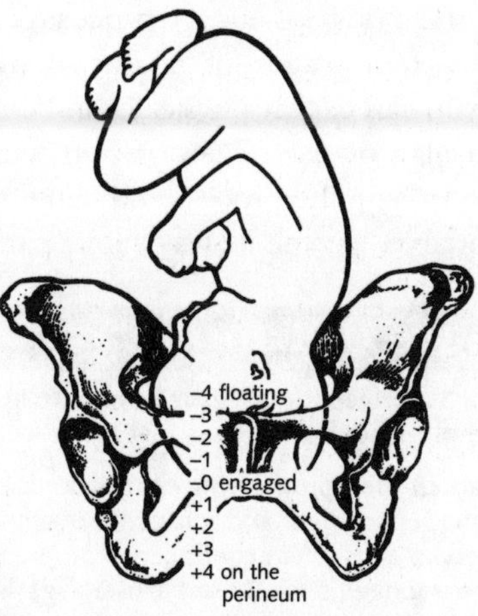

Pelvic station

Many women begin labour at a –1 or 0 station, meaning that some descent has already taken place. Other terms used to describe the descent that takes place in late pregnancy include *lightening* and *dropping*, which refer to the relief of pressure in the woman's chest and upper abdomen, and to a noticeable change in her contour (carrying the baby lower). *Engagement*, which can be determined only with a vaginal exam, means that the presenting part is 'engaged', or at 0 station, and fixed in the pelvis.

Cervical Changes

The following changes in the cervix take place gradually, beginning before labour and ending when the baby is about to be born. Your caregiver assesses these changes during a vaginal exam to evaluate your readiness for labour or your progress in labour. Because the assessments are subjective, they may vary from one caregiver to another. It may be confusing or discouraging to be examined within a short period of time by two people whose assessments differ. If the same caregiver checks your cervix each time, the assessment of progress is more reliable.

- *The cervix moves forward.* Usually weeks before labour, the cervix is high and posterior (pointing towards your back); it gradually moves down and forward to an anterior position.
- *The cervix ripens, or softens,* beginning in late pregnancy. Before ripening takes place, the cervix is firm. During pregnancy and pre-labour, when your cervix is still firm, it contracts right along with the uterus during uterine contractions (Braxton-Hicks contractions).[2] Once ripening has occurred, the cervical changes begin (the cervix passively thins and stretches open). For some women, cervical ripening begins weeks before labour, while for others it starts only a few days before. This may help explain why some women have strong and frequent contractions in late pregnancy without any dilation (opening) of the cervix, while others do have dilation.

- *The cervix effaces, thins or shortens.* For a primigravida, a substantial degree of effacement usually occurs before significant dilation (opening) takes place. This is less likely with a multigravida, whose cervix usually effaces and dilates at the same time. Effacement is determined during a vaginal exam and is measured in one of two ways: percentage of effacement or length of cervix in centimetres. 'Zero percent effacement' means the cervix is 3–4 centimetres long and has not begun to thin or shorten; '50 percent effacement', or 2 centimetres long, means the cervix has thinned about halfway; '100 percent effacement', or 'paper-thin', means the cervix has thinned completely. Be sure you do not confuse centimetres of length of the cervix with centimetres of dilation.
- *The cervix dilates, or opens.* Although the cervix usually dilates before labour begins (1 or 2 centimetres in the primigravida or as much as 4 centimetres in the multigravida), most dilation takes place during labour. Dilation is estimated during a vaginal exam and is measured in centimetres. When the cervix is opened only a fingertip, it is 1 centimetre dilated; at the halfway point, it is 5 centimetres; when fully dilated, it is about 10 centimetres.

The Six Steps to Birth

The following six steps must take place before a vaginal birth. The first three usually begin weeks or days before labour, the last three during labour. (See pages 213–216 for further explanation of these key concepts.)

1. The cervix moves forward.
2. The cervix ripens, or softens.
3. The cervix effaces, thins or shortens.
4. The cervix dilates, or opens.
5. The foetal head rotates.
6. The foetus descends through the pelvis.

Childbirth: The Physiological Process

The rest of this chapter contains a description of a normal and healthy childbirth. It presents the physiological process, which includes four stages of labour along with what you can expect physically and emotionally. It also offers suggestions on what you can do to help the process and make it more comfortable, as well as ways your partner or

Stages of Labour

Labour is divided into distinct stages according to the physiological changes that take place.

Pre-labour (non-progressing contractions) causes ripening, effacement and forward movement of the cervix; ends when contractions progress (become longer, stronger and closer together).

First stage (dilation) begins with progressing contractions and ends when the cervix is completely open.

Second stage (descent and birth) begins when the cervix is fully dilated and ends when the baby is born.

Third stage (delivery of the placenta) begins with the birth of the baby and ends with the delivery of the placenta.

Fourth stage (recovery) begins after the placenta is born and ends one to several hours later when the mother's condition stabilises.

other support people may help you. Chapter 10 deals with labour variations that are more challenging or complicated, along with interventions your doctor or midwife might want to use to correct difficulties. Chapters 8 and 12 discuss the use of comfort measures and pain medications for labour.

First Stage of Labour: Dilation

At some point during your pregnancy (usually within two weeks before or after your due date), you will recognise that you are in labour. You will probably miss the exact moment labour begins, but it is not necessary to pinpoint that moment, as the process starts gradually and most of the early signs are subtle. Usually, it takes a period of time (a few hours to a few days) for labour signs to become clear enough for you to recognise. If you experience any signs of labour (see chart on page 218) before thirty-seven weeks gestation, call your caregiver immediately. (See Chapter 3 for more discussion of preterm labour.)

The first stage of labour is subdivided into three phases: latent, active and transition. The phases become shorter and more intense as labour progresses. Each phase is distinguished by its own physiological and emotional characteristics. If you and your partner understand the process, you will be better prepared to recognise each phase and cope with your labour. Once the labour process begins, you move through the first stage into the second stage, and the baby and placenta are born. Then you can rest and rejoice in your baby.

Signs of Labour

By familiarising yourself with the signs of labour listed in the chart on page 218, you will probably recognise labour and not be caught by surprise. You will also be more able to recognise when you are not yet in labour. The signs of labour are listed in three categories: possible signs, preliminary signs and positive signs. You may or may not experience all of these signs of labour. The possible signs may come and go and are not reliable predictors of labour. They may, however, serve to warn you that labour may begin soon. Some of the preliminary signs indicate that you are in pre-labour and that important cervical changes are taking place, such as the cervix moving forward, ripening or effacing. The positive signs indicate that your cervix is actually dilating, which is what *labour* actually means.

Possible Signs

- *Backache that comes and goes.* This backache is often accompanied by a feeling of uneasiness or restlessness—an inability to feel comfortable in any position for very long. It differs from the postural backache that most pregnant women experience after standing or sitting for a while. It may resemble the backache often experienced before a menstrual period. A restless backache may occur off and on for days before or along with other signs of labour. If restless backache is the only symptom you have, do not get too excited, as it alone is not enough to constitute labour or even pre-labour.

Signs of Labour

The signs of labour are categorised as possible signs, preliminary signs and positive signs. These categories will help you decide when you are truly in labour. Please note that you may not experience all these signs and that they do not necessarily occur in a particular order. If you are unsure, call your caregiver or the hospital.

Category	Signs	Comments (also see pages 217–221)
Possible signs of labour (These may or may not be early signs of labour; time will tell.)	**Backache.** Vague, low, nagging; may come and go	May be caused by early contractions
	Cramps in lower abdomen. Like menstrual cramps; may be accompanied by discomfort in thighs	May be intermittent or continuous
	Soft bowel movements. Several in several hours; may be accompanied by intestinal cramps or digestive upset	May be related to increase in circulating prostaglandins, which ripen your cervix while causing these other symptoms
	Nesting urge. An unusual burst of energy resulting in great activity and a desire to complete preparations for baby	Think of this extra energy as a sign that you will have strength and stamina to handle labour; try to avoid exhausting activity
Preliminary signs of labour (These are signs of progress, but are still associated with very early labour or pre-labour.)	**Non-progressing contractions.** Tend to remain about the same length, strength and frequency. These pre-labour contractions may last for a short time or continue for hours before they go away or begin to progress (see below).	Accomplish softening and thinning (effacement) of cervix, although most dilation does not occur until you have positive signs
	Bloody show. Passage of slippery blood-tinged mucus from vagina	Associated with thinning (effacement) and early opening (dilation) of cervix; may occur days before other signs or not until progressing labour contractions have begun; continues throughout labour
	Leaking of amniotic fluid from vagina. Caused by a small rupture of membranes (ROM)	Sometimes stops when membranes seal, or continues on and off for hours or days (See precautions on pages 220–221.)
Positive signs of labour (These are the clearest signs that your cervix is dilating.)	**Progressing contractions.** Become longer, stronger, and/or closer together with time; are usually described as 'painful' or 'very strong' and are felt in the abdomen, back or both	These dilate the cervix, are not reduced by mother's activity and do not subside because of a change in activity. Use the Early Labour Record (page 221) to determine the contraction pattern.
	Gush of amniotic fluid from vagina. Caused by a large rupture of membranes (ROM)	Often accompanied or soon followed by progressing contractions (See precautions on pages 220–221.)
	Dilation of cervix. Opening of the cervix in response to the progressing contractions	This sign is not felt by the mother, but is confirmed by vaginal exam.

- *Abdominal cramping that is mild to moderate in discomfort.* Some women find it similar to menstrual cramps. These cramps may or may not progress into distinct contractions of the uterus.
- *Frequent, soft bowel movements.* Sometimes mistaken for an intestinal upset, this is probably a prostaglandin-induced change, which clears the lower digestive tract and makes more room for the baby to move down. Diarrhoea-like symptoms on or near your due date are a possible sign of labour.
- *A nesting urge.* A sudden burst of energy focused on getting the 'nest' ready. Whether it is scrubbing every floor in the house, marathon shopping, paying all the bills or sprucing up the baby's room, there is a sense of urgency: 'If it doesn't get done now, I'll never ever do it'. Women often do not recognise their nesting urge until after the birth, when they look back and recall having had so much energy and such a need to complete a certain task.

Preliminary Signs

- *Non-progressing contractions of the uterus.* These are regular contractions that may continue for hours without changing in intensity, frequency or duration. They are often referred to as pre-labour contractions. Sometimes they are quite strong, long (up to two minutes) or frequent (as close as five minutes apart). They are more likely to be mild and eight to twenty minutes apart. Such non-progressing contractions do not dilate the cervix, but they are probably preparing the cervix for dilation (bringing it forward, causing ripening and effacement). (See page 216 on 'The Six Steps to Birth'.) It is important to remain patient and try to maintain normal activity—eat, drink and alternate between rest and distracting activities.
- *Passage of slippery mucus mixed with some blood ('bloody show').* Throughout pregnancy, the cervix contains thick mucus, which may be loosened and released in late pregnancy when the cervix begins thinning and opening. Sometimes this appears as a sticky mucous plug. However, most women never notice such a plug. More often the mucus becomes thin and more liquid. The medical term for this thin watery discharge is *leukorrhea.* It may be tinged with blood because small blood vessels in the cervix break as it thins and opens. This bloody show can appear before any other signs of labour or may not appear until hours after contractions have begun. Bloody show continues as labour progresses. You may wonder how much blood is typical. Here is a good rule of thumb: If it is more mucus than blood, it is 'show'. If it is more blood than mucus, or if blood is dripping out, it may be due to a somewhat larger blood vessel breaking. If so, you should call your caregiver. In late pregnancy, women often pass some brownish, bloody discharge within twenty-four hours after a vaginal exam, because the exam often causes some cervical bleeding. Sexual intercourse sometimes causes the same thing. It is easy to mistake this discharge for the show. If you are unsure whether the discharge is show or not, note the appearance of the blood. If it is show, it is

pink or bright red and mixed with mucus; after an exam or intercourse, it is usually brownish, like old blood.

- *Leaking of amniotic fluid from your vagina.* The bag of waters (membranes or amniotic sac) sometimes begins to leak before labour. Sometimes the bag breaks with a sudden gush. (See below.) Leaking or a gush of amniotic fluid before labour occurs in approximately 10 percent of women. If you notice leaking as opposed to gushing, it may mean a small hole in the bag has developed high in your uterus, and amniotic fluid (the water) is seeping out. Your underwear seems damp and you notice a little leaking when walking or changing position. Let your caregiver know. He or she may want to see you and make sure it is amniotic fluid (as opposed to urine or mucus). If your caregiver knows or suspects you are at risk for Group B strep (GBS), he or she will want to give you antibiotics. (See pages 63 and 67 for more on GBS.)

Positive Signs

- *Progressing contractions of the uterus.* These are contractions that become longer, stronger and/or closer together as time passes. Progressing contractions dilate the cervix and push the foetus down and out of the uterus. In early labour, contractions are usually felt as abdominal tightening with some backache. As labour advances, contractions usually become painful. Some multigravidas have 'on again, off again' contractions for several hours per day or night before they finally get into a continuing progressive pattern. This can be very confusing. To determine if your contractions are progressing or not, time them and keep a written record. (See the sample 'Early Labour Record' on page 221.) It can show you if your contractions are becoming longer, stronger, and/or closer together.
- *Rupture of the membranes (ROM) with a gush.* (This is also called 'breaking of the bag of waters'.) In most pregnancies, the membranes do not rupture until the active phase of labour or later. The bag of waters breaking with a gush is more dramatic than when the bag begins to leak. At times preceded by a sudden 'pop', ½–1 cup of amniotic fluid gushes from the vagina. Sometimes, women think they have lost control of their bladders. When ROM occurs with a gush, labour contractions usually start within hours. If your membranes rupture before labour, follow these guidelines:

  1. Note the time, colour and odour, and describe the general amount of fluid (a trickle or a gush). Amniotic fluid is clear and practically odourless. A strong foul odour could mean infection. Brownish or greenish fluid may be a sign that the baby has been stressed. (See page 259 for more explanation.)

  2. Notify your caregiver or call the maternity nurses immediately. Some caregivers induce labour soon after ROM, if it occurs at term. Others wait to see if you will go into labour spontaneously or if you can get labour started by yourself. (For suggestions, see 'What You Can Do to Start or Speed Up a Slow Labour' on

pages 263–265.) If ROM occurs before term, your caregiver may try to prevent labour. If you are at risk or have tested positive for Group B strep, you will be given antibiotics to prevent an infection in the baby. (See page 67.)

3. Do not put anything into your vagina (no tampon to control the flow, no fingers and no intercourse) because doing so increases the possibility of infection. Because the risk of infection is higher if ROM has occurred, most caregivers limit the number of vaginal exams during labour in order to reduce the chance of infection. After ROM, baths have not been found to increase infection.[3]

Caution: On rare occasions, the cord prolapses (slips through the cervix into the vagina) when the membranes rupture with a gush. This is a true emergency because the baby may press against the cord and cut off his oxygen supply. (See page 294 for further information on prolapsed cord.)

- *Changes in the cervix confirmed by vaginal exam.* Your caregiver performs this exam to determine what changes have taken place in the position, ripening, effacement or dilation of your cervix. If your membranes have ruptured, your caregiver may postpone this exam until there are very clear signs of active labour.

Early Labour Record

To help you decide if you are truly in labour, keep track of what is happening by using an Early Labour Record form like the one below. You may find this form helpful in deciding when to call your caregiver or when to go to the hospital or birth centre. Many women begin timing contractions when they cannot walk or talk throughout a contraction or when they need to use patterned breathing.

To time contractions, you need a watch or clock with a second hand. When the contraction begins, write down the time in the Time column. When the contraction ends, figure out how many seconds it lasted *(dura-*

Early Labour Record (sample)

Contractions on April 29

Time	Duration	Interval or Frequency	Comments
Starting time	How many seconds long?	How many minutes since the beginning of the last one?	Intensity of contractions, food eaten, breathing level, bloody show, status of membranes, other events
1:54 A.M.	40 seconds	–	Bloody show started at 6 P.M.
2:03 A.M.	45 seconds	9 minutes	Can't sleep
2:10 A.M.	45 seconds	7 minutes	Loose BM, backache
2:17 A.M.	50 seconds	7 minutes	Stronger!

tion). *Interval* refers to the length of time between the beginning of one contraction and the beginning of the next. That same length of time describes the *frequency*, which refers to how often the contractions are coming (for example, every five minutes).

Time six or eight contractions in a row. If there is no progression in your contractions (if they do not become longer, stronger and/or closer together), stop timing for a while. Resume timing later when there seems to be a change. If the contractions have not clearly progressed, then you are probably still in pre-labour.

In Labour

When labour is established, your contractions are progressing and your cervix is dilating. You are now in the first stage of labour, which normally lasts from two to twenty-four hours. The average length of the first stage for a primigravida is twelve and one-half hours; for a multigravida, seven and one-third hours. Your first labour is likely to be longer than subsequent labours. Prepare yourself for a short, average and long first stage, since it is impossible to predict how long it will take. Think about how different a short, intense labour would be from a long, drawn out labour, including how your concerns and needs for support would differ.

Labour Contractions

By the end of pregnancy, your uterus has become the largest and strongest muscle in your body. When it contracts, your uterus hardens and bulges like any other muscle, shortening the muscle fibres in the body of the uterus and pulling the cervix open. Under the control of various hormonal and other physiological factors, labour contractions are involuntary and continue intermittently throughout labour. Each contraction follows a wave-like pattern: it builds to a peak, then gradually goes away, allowing the uterus to rest for a time.

Early in labour, contractions may feel like a dull lower backache or menstrual cramps. These early contractions are usually (though not always) short and mild, lasting thirty to forty seconds, and the interval between them may be as long as fifteen or twenty minutes. However, some labours begin with contractions closer together and rather intense. As labour advances, you will feel the contractions more in your abdomen or in your lower back, or both. Sometimes backache persists even between contractions.

These powerful contractions become stronger and longer as labour progresses. By the end of the first stage, contractions are usually very intense and last as long as 90 to 120 seconds, and the interval between them may be as short as two to three minutes.

The Latent Phase

The latent phase is usually the longest phase of the first stage, in which the contractions are further apart, shorter and less intense than during the later phases. During this phase, your cervix will efface and dilate to approximately 4 centimetres. You will probably spend most of this phase at or near home, doing whatever activity is appropriate for the time of day—resting if it is nighttime, keeping busy if it is daytime. You and your partner will also probably spend a good portion of this phase wondering whether or not you are in labour. Keeping an Early Labour Record (page 221) will help you decide.

Getting through the Latent Phase

During this phase, it is best for you not to be alone. Try to remain active or, if you are tired, to rest. You will probably feel excited and a bit nervous. In fact, the greatest problem for most first-time parents (and even multigravidas) is overreacting to early labour by focusing too much on each contraction, tensing unnecessarily, and assuming the labour is progressing much faster than it really is. Try to keep busy doing things that are fun, calming or distracting, but not exhausting. Pack your bag with any last-minute items (see suggestions on pages 212–213) or prepare your home if you are planning a home birth. Focus on relaxing your muscles and your mind during contractions. Have a massage. Take a long shower. (Do not underestimate the soothing, pain-relieving properties of a shower.) It is best to postpone using the bath until your cervix is 4–5 centimetres dilated, unless progress is very slow and you are exhausted; then the bath may stop contractions for a while. Immersion in water in very early labour tends to slow early labour progress and is associated with increased need for Syntocinon to augment labour and for anaesthesia for pain relief.[4] Later in labour, however, immersion in water is recommended because it can relieve pain and increase labour progress.

Eat and drink easy-to-digest, appealing foods such as soup or broth, fruit, yoghurt, pasta, toast and herbal tea, unless you know you are going to have a caesarean. (See Chapter 11 for information on a planned caesarean.) Pass the time with pleasant, distracting activities: Go for a walk, visit with friends, listen to music, watch a movie, dance, or play cards or other games. Plan for an early labour project—for example, working on a hobby, preparing some one-dish meals to freeze and enjoy after the birth, or baking bread or a birthday cake. Such activities can help keep you from becoming preoccupied with your contractions too soon.

After a period of time (hours or even a day or more), you will reach a point where you can no longer be distracted from the contractions—you cannot continue walking or talking through them without

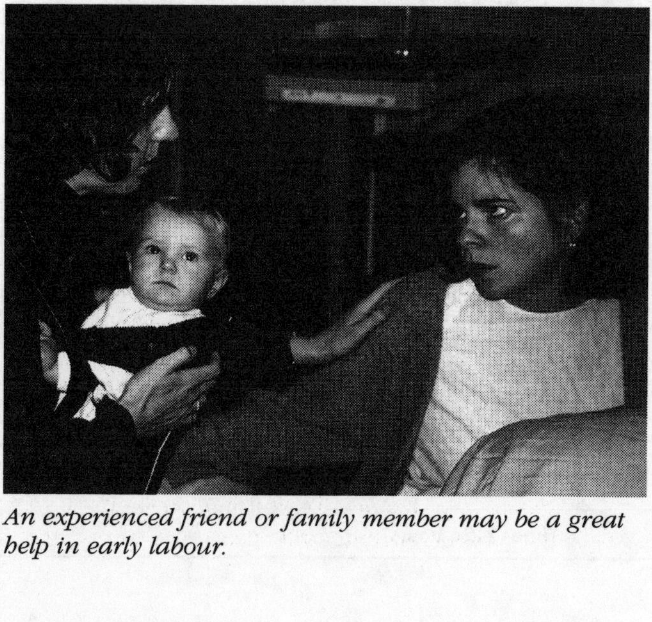

Photograph by Penny Simkin

An experienced friend or family member may be a great help in early labour.

having to pause over the peak. Then it is time to begin using the three Rs—relaxation, rhythm and ritual. During each contraction, begin using relaxed breathing that includes an exhalation with a sigh; release tension from a different part of your body with each out-breath, and focus your attention on something positive. (See Chapter 8 for a description of slow breathing and self-comforting techniques.)

Between contractions, resume whatever you were doing. Your partner may be busy with last-minute arrangements and phone calls, but should be prepared to focus on you during contractions. He or she can provide feedback if you show signs of tension. Touch relaxation, the roving body check, or simply a soothing tone of voice or calm presence may help you remain calm and confident during contractions. The importance of work-

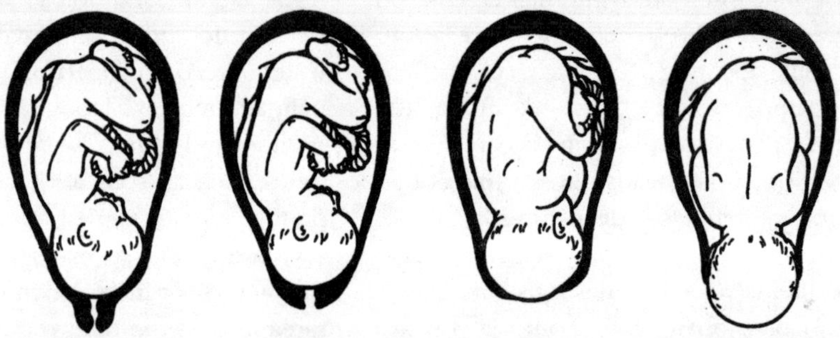

Effacement:	**none**	**50%**	**90%**	**100%**
Dilation:	**none**	**2–3 cm**	**5 cm**	**9 cm**

First Stage of Labour

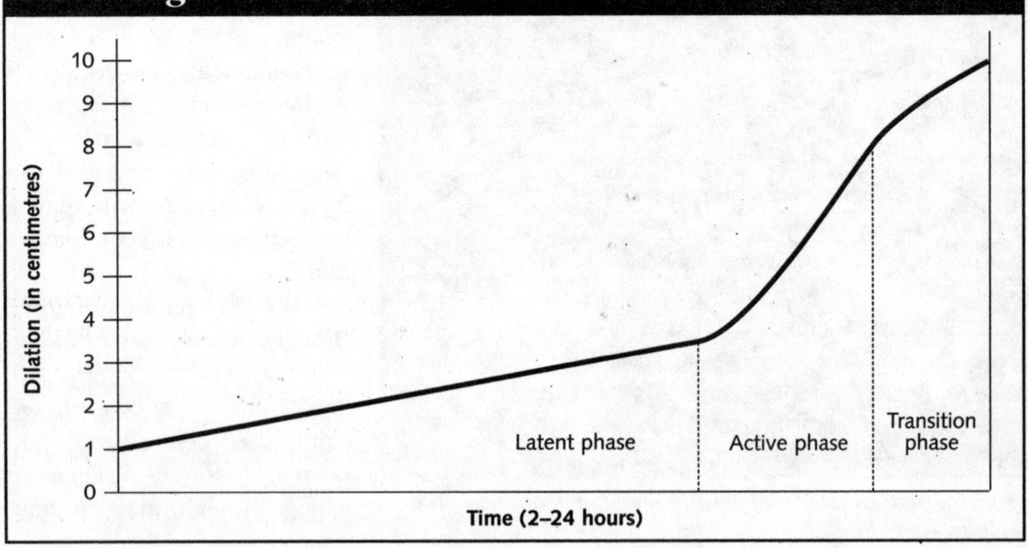

ing well as a team in early labour cannot be overemphasised. Remain physically relaxed, even limp, during contractions; focus your mind on calming thoughts or visualisations, pleasant music, photos, pictures or videos. If you start off well in labour, you are likely to continue well. If you start off by tensing, worrying or feeling at odds with your body or partner, it is more difficult to cope later.

The Active Phase

As the latent phase draws to a close, your labour pattern changes. Your contractions will probably be painful, though manageable, each lasting a minute or more and coming close together—three to five minutes apart. When you enter the active phase, dilation usually speeds up and you accomplish more with each of these intense, painful contractions. This is the time when most people go to the hospital or birth centre, or when the midwife or doctor would like to arrive for a home birth. Of course, you cannot know how far dilated your cervix is, so rely on your contraction pattern and intensity to guide you.

Getting through the Active Phase

Getting into active labour is emotionally challenging for many women, because the labour is so much more intense than it was earlier, and progress has been relatively slow to this point. As you look back on how long it took to get to 4 or 5 centimetres, you will feel discouraged, thinking it will take that much more time to get to 10 centimetres! You may wish you could call it quits for the day. You may feel trapped in the labour as you realise there is no way out but to go on and com-

When to Call Your Caregiver

During the last month of your pregnancy, ask your caregiver when and whom to call. You may be asked to call the hospital maternity unit (especially at night) or your midwife or doctor directly.

- If this is your first baby, you should call when your membranes rupture or when the contractions are intense—lasting a full minute and requiring total concentration and patterned breathing. By this time, contractions may be about five minutes apart or less.
- If you have had one or more children before, you should call when your membranes rupture or when you are experiencing regular contractions and several of the possible or preliminary signs of labour (for example, contractions with soft bowel movements, bloody show and so on).
- If you have a condition that requires more early labour observation in the hospital, call whenever you suspect labour. Your caregiver should have told you if you have such a condition (for example, positive Group B strep status, a herpes sore, high blood pressure or others).
- Even without evidence of true labour, you may always call if you are anxious, have questions, live far away or have received specific instructions from your caregiver.

When you do call, be ready to report the information you recorded in your Early Labour Record.

- How many seconds long your contractions are (duration)
- How many minutes apart they are, from the start of one to the start of the next one (interval or frequency)
- How strong the contractions seem (intensity)
- How long your contractions have been like this
- Status of membranes (Have they ruptured?)
- Presence of bloody show
- Other information or conditions that would help your caregiver (or another on-call caregiver) know about you and your pregnancy

plete the process. The contractions will continue and escalate until your cervix is fully dilated. This realisation, sometimes called the 'moment of truth', represents a crisis of sorts. You realise, as you have not up to this point, that you cannot control the process of labour. At first, you may struggle emotionally: 'It's so hard. I don't think I can do this'. You may weep; you may feel overwhelmed. These are typical reactions to this more demanding and, fortunately, more productive phase of labour. In the latent phase, your spirits were high; in the active phase, you become serious, quiet and preoccupied with the contractions. Earlier, your partner's jokes were funny and the conversation entertaining; now you cannot listen. You may even feel resentful of any small talk around you.

As you become more centred on your labour, your partner should move in closer, focus more on your labour and share your serious, quiet mood. He or she should help you relax, find comfortable positions, and maintain your focus, breathing and rhythmic activity. Most importantly, your partner can help you interpret what is going on. You may be discouraged because it seems as if labour is progressing as slowly as before, yet the contractions are demanding so much more of you. It is the knowledge that you are finally getting somewhere that renews your confidence and optimism and puts a more positive perspective on the pain.

Arrival at the Hospital or Birth Centre

Once you decide to go to the hospital or birth centre, call ahead to tell them you are coming. Gather your bag, your birth plan and any last-minute items (a pillow and blanket, plus a towel if your bag of waters is leaking) and go. Do not drive yourself. If your partner is not available, have a backup plan for someone else to take you. Be sure you know which hospital entrance to use. In the middle of the night, the emergency room may be the only open entrance. Find out ahead of time.

Once in the hospital, you can take a wheelchair or walk to the maternity floor. Try to think of this trip to the hospital or birth centre as a trip to find out more about what is going on and whether it is time for you to be at the birthplace. The staff does not want to admit you before you need clinical supervision. A nurse usually greets you, takes you to a small room (often called the 'triage' or observation room) where she or he assesses your condition, your labour, and your baby's wellbeing and decides whether you should be admitted. If it appears that you are still in very early labour (or prelabour), the nurse may suggest that you leave the hospital or birth centre for a while, until the labour pattern changes. This is usually a good idea. If you get to the hospital or birth centre too early and stay, labour is likely to dominate your thoughts and can seem extremely long and discouraging; at home, you can keep busy in a familiar place until you need to be in the birthplace.

It is sometimes very discouraging to learn that your contractions have not resulted in significant dilation and to be sent home, especially if you have missed sleep and have found the contractions uncomfortable and difficult to cope with. You may think that no one

Positions and Movements for Labour and Birth

Position or Movement		What This Position or Movement Does
Standing	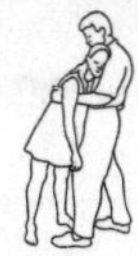	• Takes advantage of gravity during and between contractions • Can help contractions be less painful and more productive • Helps foetus be well aligned with angle of pelvis • May speed labour if woman has been lying down • May increase urge to push in second stage
Walking	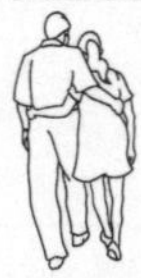	*Same as standing, plus:* • Causes changes in pelvic joints, encouraging rotation and descent • Can be tiring if done for long periods
Standing and leaning forward on partner, bed or birth ball	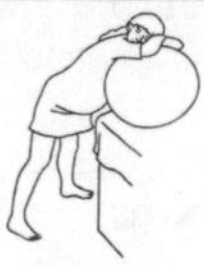	*Same as standing, plus:* • Relieves backache • Is good position for back rub • May be more restful than standing • Encourages rotation of occiput posterior (OP) foetus
Slow dancing (See page 287.)	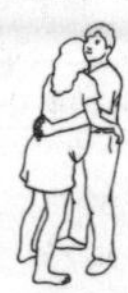	*Same as standing, plus:* • Causes changes in pelvic joints, encouraging rotation and descent • Increases mother's sense of wellbeing as she is embraced by loved one • Adds comfort through rhythm and music • Is good position for partner to give back pressure to relieve back pain
Lunge (See page 287.)	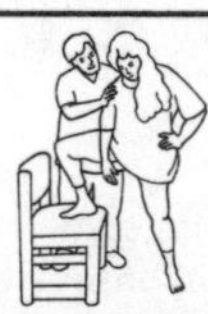	• Widens one side of pelvis (side towards which lunge is made) • Encourages rotation of occiput posterior (OP) foetus • Can be done in standing or kneeling position
Sitting upright	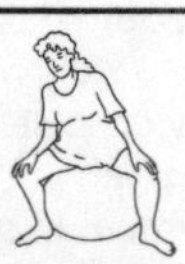	• Is good resting position • Uses gravity somewhat
Sitting on toilet or commode	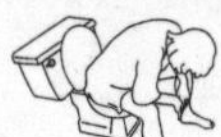	*Same as sitting upright, plus:* • Helps with pushing because of association with bearing down for bowel movements • May help relax perineum for effective bearing down
Semi-sitting	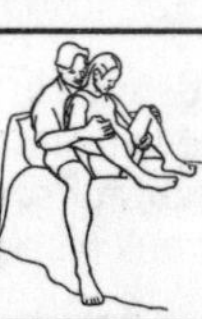	*Same as sitting upright, plus:* • Is possible position for vaginal exams • May increase back pain • Is easy position to get into (on bed or delivery table) • Is a common delivery position

Positions and Movements for Labour and Birth

Position or Movement	What This Position or Movement Does
Sitting, rocking in chair 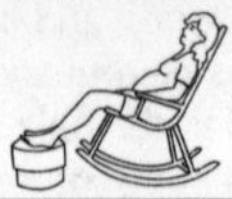	*Same as sitting upright, plus:* • May speed labour because of rocking movement
Sitting, leaning forward with support 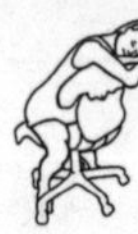	*Same as sitting upright, plus:* • Relieves backache • Is good position for back rub
Hands and knees 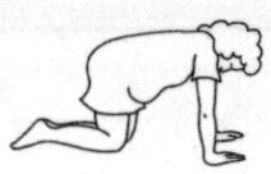	• Helps relieve backache • May protect foetus in case of cord problems • Assists rotation of baby in occiput posterior (OP) position • Allows for pelvic rocking • Is possible position for vaginal exams • Takes pressure off haemorrhoids • May reduce premature urge to push • May slow a rapid second stage; is gravity neutral
Open knee-chest position (See page 285.) 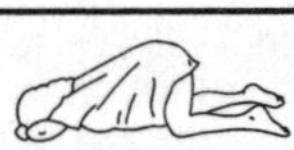	• Encourages baby's head out of the pelvis during contractions, which may be desirable with prolapsed cord • Sometimes recommended in early labour if contractions are frequent and accompanied by back pain and no progress in dilation (encourages OP baby's head out of the pelvis) • Reduces pressure on swollen cervix • Not to be used in post partum
Side-lying 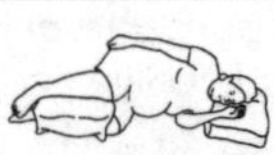	• Is very good resting position • May reduce back pain • Helps lower elevated blood pressure • Is safe position if pain medications have been used • May promote progress of labour when alternated with walking • Is gravity neutral • Useful to slow a very rapid second stage • Takes pressure off haemorrhoids • Allows posterior sacral movement in second stage
The Following Are Primarily Second-Stage Positions:	
Squatting 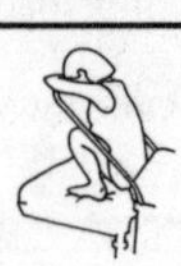	• May relieve backache • Takes advantage of gravity • Widens pelvic outlet (may diminish pelvic inlet, therefore not good in first stage) • May enhance rotation and descent in a difficult birth • Is helpful if mother does not feel an urge to push • Allows freedom to shift weight for comfort • Takes advantage of upper trunk pressing on fundus

Positions and Movements for Labour and Birth

Position or Movement		What This Position or Movement Does
The Following Are Primarily Second-Stage Positions:		
Lap squatting **(See page 291.)**	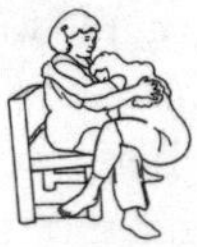	*Same as squatting, plus:* • Reduces strain on knees and ankles, compared to squatting • Allows more support, less effort for exhausted mother • Enhances feelings of wellbeing, as mother is held close by a loved one
Supported squat **(See page 291.)**	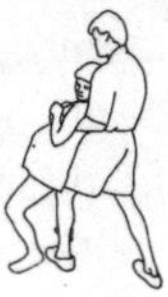	• Eliminates restriction of pelvic joint mobility that can be caused by external pressure (from bed, chair and so on) or by stretching of the hip joints (from squatting, pulling legs back and so on) • Takes advantage of gravity • Lengthens mother's trunk, allowing more room for foetus to manoeuvre into position • Allows foetus to move the joints of the pelvis to enhance rotation and descent • Requires great strength in partner
Dangle **(See page 291.)**	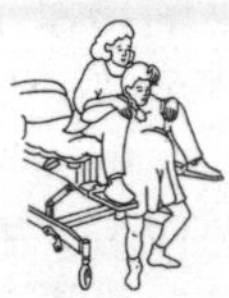	• Is same as supported squat, except much easier on the partner • Requires woman to stand during second stage

listened to you, and you may feel concerned, angry or frustrated. You may worry that you will not get back to the hospital in time.

Do express your feelings to the admitting nurse. She or he may be able to reassure you, help you with coping strategies, give you a sleeping pill to take when you get home, or suggest other options besides returning home (for example, walking near the hospital, going to the cafeteria or watching television in the lobby) to wait until labour signs increase. Try to constructively use the information that your labour has not progressed enough to be admitted. Focus on coping strategies. Can you relax better during contractions? Can you find some better distractions? Can you get some rest? (Check Chapter 8 for more on coping strategies.)

Once you are admitted, the midwife will ask questions about what is happening and about your medical history; she or he will check your weight, pulse, blood pressure, temperature, the baby's heart rate and position, your contractions and possibly (with a vaginal exam) the dilation of your cervix. If it is unclear whether your bag of waters has broken, you may have a special exam called a 'sterile speculum exam'. If your bag of waters has broken, the vaginal exams may be postponed. (See page 221.) The midwife will also get urine and possibly blood samples. If you are making progress in labour, you will go to your room and change into a hospital gown or your own gown or T-shirt.

Initial Procedures for a Home Birth

Once you call your midwife or doctor for a home birth, she or he will arrive and make similar assessments to those described for hospital admission. If you are progressing in labour, the caregiver will bring in the essential implements, medications, an oxygen tank and other equipment. She or he may remain with you from then on or, if labour is still quite early and you are comfortable on your own, may leave for a while. Your caregiver may work with an assistant who may remain with you.

Working with Your Labour

After these initial procedures, make yourself comfortable. Continue your ritual (rhythmic movement and breathing patterns, tension release, and attention-focusing) and use comfort measures as appropriate. Try pressure and cold packs on your back or hot compresses on your lower abdomen, groin and back. Go to the bathroom at least once an hour; a full bladder is uncomfortable and can slow labour. Change position frequently. Unless you are very tired and need to rest or unless the contractions are coming so fast you cannot move, try to walk and sit rather than lie in bed. Some labouring women make the mistake of staying immobile in bed throughout labour. Lying down may increase the pain of contractions and slow the progress of labour.[5] Take advantage of gravity by standing and walking for at least part of the time. (See the chart on pages 227–229 for pictures and a discussion of positions.) You may want to alternate activity with rest. It is important to get fluids, so drink something after each contraction or suck on an iceblock or ice. To gauge your progress, at each vaginal exam ask about effacement and dilation of your cervix as well as the station and position of your baby.

The breathing and relaxation taught in this book and in childbirth classes can be very helpful as you get into labour. Most women adapt and personalise these techniques and add other unique ones as they go through labour. Many women discover their own rituals once they have passed beyond the hurdle of getting into active labour. (See page 175 for a description of some of these spontaneous rituals.)

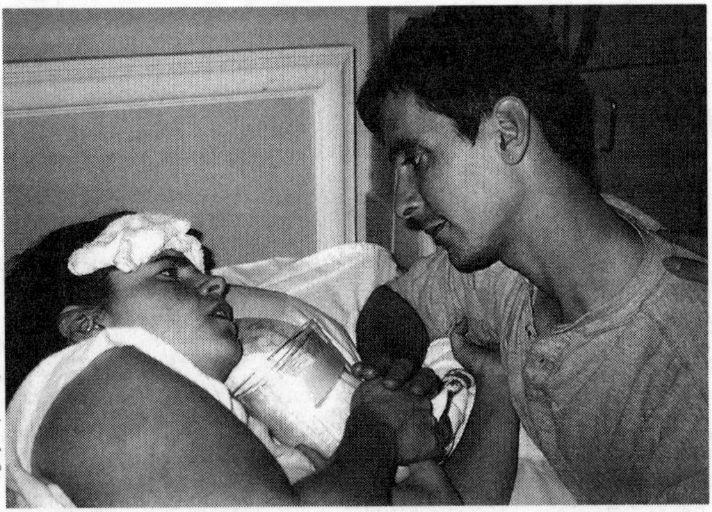

Photograph by Penny Simkin

In active labour, your partner moves closer and becomes more involved.

Labouring without Pain Medications

If you prefer to avoid or minimise your use of pain medications, the following suggestions will help:

- Before labour, line up a supportive birth partner or birth team and rehearse the relaxation and self-help comfort techniques with them. (See Chapter 8.)
- Be sure the staff knows your wishes. Ask them to help you have an unmedicated childbirth. Ask them not to offer you medication, even if you appear to be in pain. Ask them instead to help you and your partner with encouragement, advice about your labour progress and ideas for comfort measures. You will, of course, receive medication if you ask for it.
- When your cervix reaches 6 or 7 centimetres, assess how you are coping. If you are able to relax between (if not during) contractions and are able to use patterned breathing, movement or some other ritual or rhythmic coping activity consistently during contractions, you are doing very well. Do not expect to feel peaceful and relaxed during contractions. Remember that as labour intensifies, progress almost always speeds up. (See the graph on page 224.) Labour's intensity is an encouraging sign of progress.
- By about 7–8 centimetres, your contractions are about as painful as they will become (though they may come closer together). Even though you may need a lot of help from your partner, nurse or midwife, you will probably be able to manage the rest of your labour without pain medications—especially if you are able to handle the contractions at 7 or 8 centimetres—if labour continues to follow a normal course and it is your desire to do so.
- If difficulties arise or if you become exhausted and discouraged during labour and start to think about pain medication, ask these questions: How far dilated am I? How is labour progressing? Is it likely to last much longer? Can I continue for a while? Would other coping techniques and comfort measures help? Should I change breathing patterns? Can I postpone medication for three to five more contractions and then reassess? Can my partner help me more? The answers will help you make the best decision.
- If you want to minimise the use of pain medications, use the labour coping skills (described in Chapter 8) for as long as possible in labour. In addition, ask for the lowest dose possible and use more only if needed.

As you enter the active phase, you may become physically active or vocal during contractions. Your partner may become more involved—holding you, stroking you, talking rhythmically or gazing into your eyes. Your partner can also help by offering you something to drink, reminding you to move around and go to the bathroom, and reminding you to relax between contractions. On the other hand, you may become very still and quiet, relying on internal mental activities such as visualisations or silent prayers/statements. You may only want your partner to remain close and hold your hand, or you may need absolute silence and no touch from your partner or others. There is no right or wrong ritual. What is most important is that you feel secure and have the freedom to find your best way to cope at this challenging time.

You will want to continue slow breathing (see page 193) for as long as it helps you relax. When you switch to light breathing or one of the adaptations (see pages 195–198), you may get just the boost you need. Use a new breathing pattern if your breathing begins to sound tense or laboured, if you are unable to keep the rate slow, or if you find you cannot maintain your ritual, even after renewed efforts and more active encouragement from your partner. You may find light

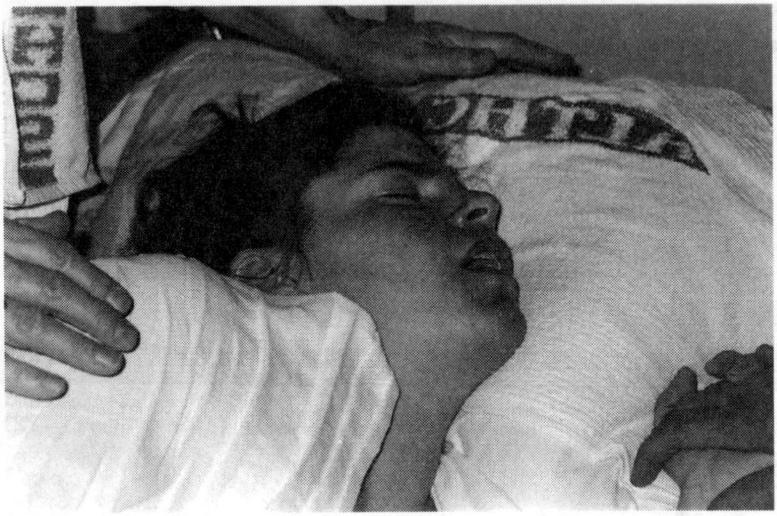

Photograph by Penny Simkin

During transition, you are totally consumed by your efforts to cope.

which may include temporary fear, nausea, agitation and trembling.[6] Contractions may last 90 to 120 seconds with only 30-second rests in between. The transition phase is relatively short, usually lasting between five and twenty contractions. These contractions—the longest of your labour—usually give you the shortest rest in between.

breathing or one of its variations better suited to the more intense contractions, in much the same way short quick breaths are better suited to demanding physical exercise such as running. By tuning in to your contractions, you can adapt the breathing patterns as needed; in this way, you can continue getting enough oxygen while calming yourself with the rhythm of your breathing.

The Transition Phase

The transition phase will probably represent the peak of difficulty in your labour, not necessarily because the pain is greater, but because at this time your contractions are longer and closer together, there is more pressure in your pelvis, and the accompanying physical and emotional signs are intense. In fact, at this time a surge of adrenalin (epinephrine) and other stress hormones occurs, often causing a 'fight or flight' response, The assistance and concentrated support of others will help you get through the intensity of transition.

During this phase, you are truly in a transition from first to second stage. Not only is your cervix dilating the last couple of centimetres, but the baby is beginning to descend. The baby's head slips through your cervix and into your vagina. Your body shows some of the signs of the second stage, although labour is still technically in the first stage. You will probably have some very intense new emotions and physical sensations in this phase. You will probably be tired, restless, irritable and totally consumed by your efforts to cope. You may lose your rhythmic ritual at this time. Your diaphragm may be stimulated by the involuntary spasms that are the precursors of bearing down. As a result, you may begin hiccuping, grunting or belching. Nausea and vomiting are common. You may find yourself holding your breath and straining at times during each contraction. This is what is known as 'the urge to push'. The baby's head, pressing against your rectum, may feel like you need to have a bowel movement. You may feel confused about whether you should push or not. You may feel aching in your back or thighs. Trembling in your legs, which may spread throughout your body, and a heavy discharge of bloody mucus from your vagina reflect the increased downward pressure. Despite the intensity and pain of the contractions of transition, you may doze off during the short rests between contractions, as if your body is conserving every bit of energy for the work of contractions. Dozing is helpful, but the moment the next contraction begins, your partner should immediately help you focus and begin breathing so the contraction does not get ahead of you.

During transition, you become very focused on your labour; nothing else matters. You may feel frightened by the intensity of labour and very dependent on those around you. You may feel transition will last forever, that you cannot take any more. But as one woman said, 'When you can't take any more, there's no more to take'. Transition pushes you to your limits, but with good support and the knowledge of where you are and what you need to do, you will meet the challenge.

Getting through Transition

Recognition is one of the keys to coping with transition. If you are experiencing the extreme sensations of transition and believe you are only 5 or 6 centimetres dilated, you will probably become discouraged. Remember that labour is a progressive process. 'You are not where you were at the last vaginal exam—you are beyond that', is a guideline to remember after you have passed the latent phase, especially if your sensations and emotional responses change during contractions. Know the signs of transition described above and be ready for them any time after you enter the active phase of labour. When a woman and her partner know where she is in labour, they are heartened by her progress and see the pain and difficulties of transition in a more positive light. Transition is bringing the baby closer.

Understanding the normal feelings, reactions and events of transition is another key. Pain, fear, nausea, trembling, despair, dependence, crying, an urge to push and difficulty maintaining your ritual are normal responses, probably associated with the adrenalin surge of transition. They do not mean anything is abnormal. It is when you think that your labour is worse than it is supposed to be that you begin to worry and seek relief with pain medications or anaesthesia. Pain medications, of course, are an option, but do not take them because you fear your transition is abnormal. Your partner may also be troubled by your expression of pain and discouragement; both of you will need reassurance and encouragement from your nurse and caregiver. You need to know that you and your baby are all right, that your sensations are normal, that you are coping well, and that this difficult time will be short.

Finally, more active support and direction from your partner, nurse and caregiver will help you through transition. Your partner might 'take charge' by getting you to look at him or her, pacing or conducting your breathing with hand movements or by breathing with you. He or she gets very close to you, helps you focus and encourages your every breath. This helps you regain your rhythm and continue a ritual. If you begin to feel like pushing, try not to hold your breath and strain until your nurse or midwife can assess you. While it is usually okay to bear down or push, sometimes your cervix is not dilated enough to make it worthwhile to do so, and pushing may cause swelling of your cervix. If you are asked not to push, try blowing or panting to keep from holding your breath. Changing positions to hands and knees, side-lying or more upright positions may relieve this premature urge to push. Many women like being held close at this time; others do not want to be touched at all but find visual and verbal contact very helpful. Hot, moist towels on your lower abdomen can be soothing. If you are sweating, your partner can fan you or wipe your face, neck and chest with a cool or cold moist cloth.

You can get through transition without pain medications, especially if you have a desire to do so, have prepared in advance, and have good support, knowledge of comfort measures and information about what is happening. Your goal is not necessarily to remain calm, still and relaxed during these contractions, but to maintain a coping ritual, which may include rhythmic movements, breathing and sounds. Between contractions, your goal is to relax and rest, if only for a few seconds. Be assured that you will not change character or lose the ability to respond to clear, simple directions. Your birth partner should not mistake rhythmic moans, groans or other sounds during transition for cries of agony. If, however, you lose the rhythm in your sounds, your partner should 'take charge', as described above, to help you regain the rhythm. Many women find transition easier to manage if they vocalise or make noise during contractions. If so, they should be encouraged to make these sounds. Some women sway, tap, stroke or rock rhythmically, or want their partner to stroke them or murmur in a rhythm. Others go into a state of deep relaxation and remain very still and quiet during their contractions. There is no single correct way to handle transition; responses to childbirth pain are very individual. The important thing is to continue a ritual, and the role of your partner is to help you do that. Getting through this brief, intense period leads into the second stage, which brings very positive changes in your mental state and physical sensations.

Women sometimes find that transition is too much for them; the pain is too great, they are exhausted, or they lose control or panic. If this happens to you, pain medication is usually an option.

Second Stage of Labour: Birth of the Baby

After dilation is complete, transition ends and the second stage of labour begins. A new sequence of events begins: The baby gradually leaves the uterus, rotates within the pelvis, descends through the vagina, and is born.

The second stage lasts from fifteen minutes to over three hours. For the primigravida, the average time is one and one half to two hours. The multigravida's second stage is usually faster than it was with her first birth. As with the first stage, the second stage can be divided into three phases: the latent or resting phase, the active or descent phase and the transition (or crowning and birth) phase. These three phases share some characteristics with the three phases of the first stage. High spirits, little pain and slow progress characterise the latent phases of both stages. The active phases are characterised by intense contractions, total mental absorption and good progress. Both transition phases are characterised by intense sensations and confusion over what to do.

Signs of Second Stage

The urge to push. This urge—the most significant sign of second stage—coincides roughly with full dilation. Although some women experience the urge to push before full dilation, others experience it sometime later, and a few not at all. (See pages 198–199 on how to handle a premature urge to push.) The urge to push is a combination of powerful sensations and reflex actions caused by the pressure of the baby in the vagina during contractions. The urge to push is a strongly felt need to grunt or hold your breath and bear down. It occurs several times within a contraction and is responsible for your pressing the baby downwards. It is involuntary, compelling, and difficult to control the same way that a sneeze or vomiting is difficult to control. In all these instances, you feel a build-up, you give in to it, and it happens. Resisting it may postpone it, but only temporarily. For many women, joining in with the urge to push is one of the most satisfying aspects of the entire birth experience. For others, it is disturbing and painful.

Relief from sensations of first-stage transition. This is another sign of second stage. The pain lessens. You calm down, think clearly again, get a second wind, cheer up and become more aware of those around you. Now you can collect yourself for pushing your baby out of your body. During the first stage, you cooperate with your labour contractions by relaxing as much as possible and using positions and movement to enhance the process. During the second stage, you cooperate with your labour by voluntarily bearing down and moving into helpful positions.

Key Concepts

Two key concepts should guide you and the staff during the second stage:

The importance of not rushing. Although both you and the staff are anxious to get the baby out, it is best not to rush. Follow your body's signals; bear down or push spontaneously as the urge demands, and allow time for your vagina to open. Pushing hard and long without an urge only tires you out and does not speed the birth.[7] By not rushing, your vagina can stretch open more gradually, decreasing the likelihood of damage.[8] You will also use your energy more efficiently. By joining in, holding your breath and bearing down only when you cannot resist the urge to push, you will be working in harmony with your uterus and not wasting your effort. Your caregiver can help you focus your bearing-down efforts in this way.

If you follow your urge to push, you will bear down for five to six seconds at a time and take several breaths between bearing-down efforts. This allows you to take in more oxygen and make more oxygen available to your baby than if you hold your breath and strain as long as possible. Although there is very little exchange of oxygen across the placenta during contractions, when the uterus relaxes, exchange resumes and the foetus benefits.[9]

It often seems as though the staff is in a rush to get your baby out, imploring you to push as long and hard as you can without regard for your urge to push. Prolonged, maximal bearing down in a normal labour, with or without anaesthesia, is usually not necessary and sometimes causes problems (maternal exhaustion, foetal distress, failure of the baby to rotate, arrest of descent, overstretching of pelvic ligaments and muscles, and possible perineal tears) that would not have occurred with spontaneous bearing down.[10] Prolonged maximal pushing is best reserved for times when progress is inadequate or the baby is already in distress and other interventions (forceps, vacuum extractor or caesarean) are being considered. Discuss this with your caregiver in advance and with the nurses when you arrive at the hospital. Include your wishes in your birth plan. (See pages 199–203 for more discussion of the various bearing-down techniques.)

The importance of different positions. Progress and comfort should guide your choice of position. Feel free during the second stage to use positions that are comfortable, that alter progress (either by enhancing slow progress or slowing too-rapid progress) or that provide other advantages.

Positions for Second Stage

When the second stage is progressing at a reasonable pace—not too fast or slow—use whatever positions seem most comfortable. Sometimes, you have to get into another position, even if it is uncomfortable, especially if the position you are using adversely affects the baby's heart rate or impairs descent. This new position may make medical intervention, such as a vacuum extractor or forceps, unnecessary. If the second stage is going very fast, try a gravity-neutral position, such as side-lying, to help slow it down. If you make no progress in one position, try another. Positions that take advantage of gravity are an asset and may aid progress and descent.

You may be asked to get into the position favoured by your doctor or midwife. Some caregivers are very flexible and can conduct deliveries with women on their backs, sides,

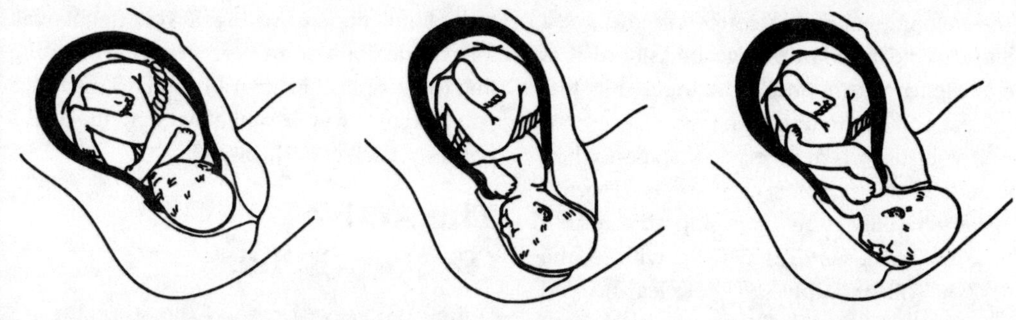

Latent (resting) Active (descent) Transition (crowning)

Second Stage of Labour

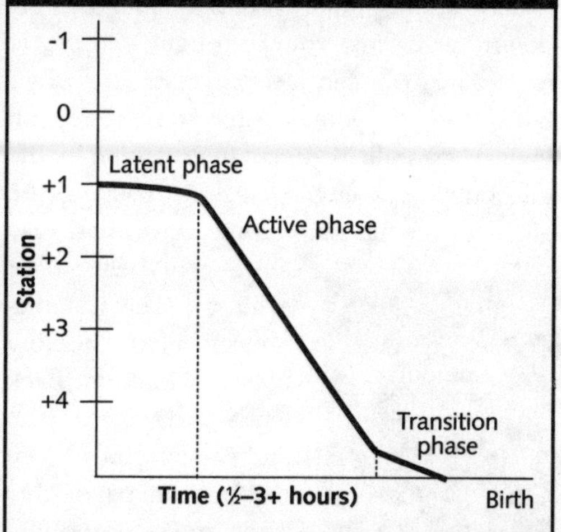

hands and knees, or squatting. Others prefer only one position for delivery, usually semi-sitting or lying on the back. When women are asked to lie on their backs with their heads raised and their legs flexed and drawn up, it may be more convenient for the birth attendant, but it is not always the best position for the mother's comfort or labour progress.

It is a good idea to know all the positions and their advantages and disadvantages; be prepared and willing to change positions every twenty to thirty minutes. (See the chart on pages 227–229 for descriptions of the variety of positions for second stage.)

The Latent (Resting) Phase

The latent or resting phase of the second stage is characterised by a lull in uterine activity, a brief rest for you, a pause after the intensity and confusion of first-stage transition, and excitement over your baby's imminent arrival. You will become clear-headed and energetic. Contractions may be weak and further apart for ten or twenty minutes, descent may slow or stop temporarily, and your urge to push may be non-existent or easily satisfied with slight bearing-down efforts. This resting phase may take place because your baby's head has slipped through your cervix into your birth canal, which causes your uterus, which had previously fit tightly around your baby, to become a bit slack. It often takes a few minutes for your uterus to adjust and to tighten down around your baby's body. (See the illustration above.) Then, strong contractions resume and your urge to push becomes powerful. This temporary lull is normal and very welcome as a chance to rest and get a second wind after first-stage transition; it is no cause for alarm. Sheila Kitzinger calls this the 'rest-and-be-thankful phase'.

If your baby is at a very low station when the second stage begins, or if she is descending very rapidly, you may skip this resting phase or find it very brief. Even without the rest, you will probably still feel clear-headed and renewed emotionally as you move into the active phase of the second stage. If the latent phase lasts for more than fifteen or twenty minutes, your caregiver may ask you to try a gravity-enhancing position—such as sitting, squatting or standing—to encourage an urge to push. You may also be asked to push (hold your breath and strain) even though you feel no urge to do so. This may be frustrating for both you and the staff, as progress rarely occurs in the absence of effective contractions.[11] Asking if you might wait for contractions or an urge to push (or listing that as an option in your birth plan) may give you a chance to rest while awaiting the active phase of the second stage.

The Active (Descent) Phase

During the active phase of the second stage, you become alert, your baby descends, and you feel powerful contractions and an irresistible urge to push. Women's feelings vary widely at this time. You may find bearing down with all your strength extremely rewarding. You can feel progress. The baby's head distends your vagina and presses on your rectal wall. You may feel alarmed by the full, bulging, stretching feeling. You may be afraid to let the baby come down and may tense your pelvic floor against it. This is sometimes called 'holding back'. Holding back tends to increase pain and slow progress. (See the box on page 239.) The most important thing for you to do during pushing efforts is to relax your pelvic floor and bulge your perineum (as in the pelvic floor bulging exercise on page 130). Prenatal perineal massage (page 203), in which you relax your perineum while it is being stretched, is

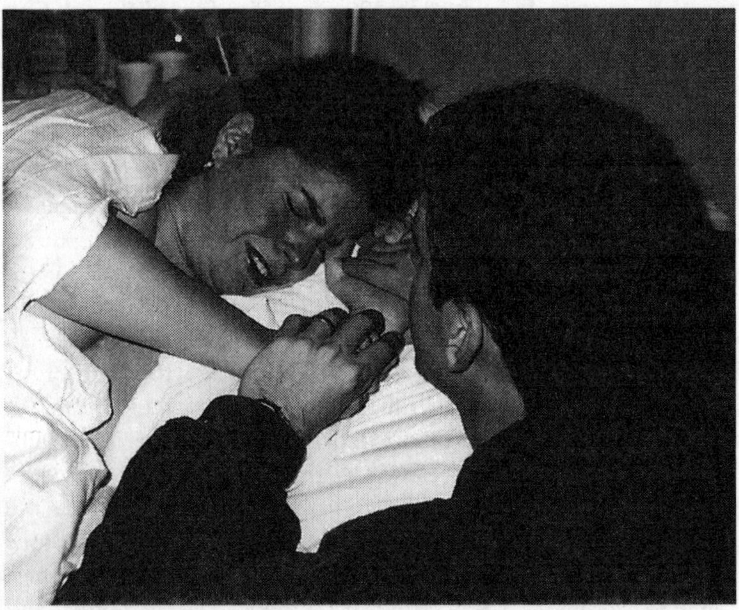

Photograph by Penny Simkin

During delivery, you bear down with all your strength.

About 'Holding Back'

Almost every woman goes through a brief period during the second stage of labour when she tenses her pelvic floor as a reaction to the stretching sensations of the baby's head in the birth canal. This 'holding back' is normal and usually passes quickly once the woman feels the baby moving down. Sometimes, she must tell herself to let go; once she does let go, the pain decreases and she has no further desire to hold back.

Sometimes, however, holding back is more prolonged and based on one or more of the following:

- Fear that the stretching will get worse, will hurt more and will lead to damage to her vaginal outlet
- Modesty issues, especially when people seem to be staring at her perineum
- Fear of passing a bowel movement onto the bed, and making a 'mess' while pushing. This does happen fairly often, but usually only a small amount is passed. It is less likely to occur if she has emptied her bowels spontaneously early in labour.
- Fear that the baby may fly out so fast that the caregiver cannot catch her. If the lower end of the bed has been removed and the woman's legs are in foot rests or leg rests, she may worry that her baby will land on the floor.

Helping the woman who is holding back:

Warm compresses (washcloths soaked in warm water and wrung out) placed directly on the perineum by the nurse or caregiver help to ease these fears. The moist heat promotes relaxation of the perineum and relieves the stretching sensation. The compresses can also be used to wipe away and dispose of any faeces. A clean compress then replaces the old one. The sensation of the caregiver pressing the cloth on the perineum reassures the woman that the caregiver is right there to gradually guide the baby out.

excellent preparation for second stage. Your partner's reminders to 'relax', 'let the baby out', 'open up', 'bulge your bottom' or 'ease the baby out' are very important at this time, certainly more important than directions to 'push, push, push'.

Sometimes, it takes several contractions before you feel that you have learned how to push effectively. Your nurse or midwife may press warm, moist towels against your perineum to help you relax and appropriately direct your bearing-down efforts. You may request warm compresses in your birth plan. Clenching your jaw and clamping your lips together is a sign that you are probably also tensing the muscles in your vagina. By relaxing your face, particularly your mouth, you may be more able to let go below. Some-times, even though it hurts, you have to push anyway. If you allow yourself to let go and push despite the pain, you will find it feels better than holding back.

As the active phase progresses, your perineum begins to bulge, your labia part and your vagina opens as your baby's head descends with each bearing-down effort. Between efforts, your vagina partially closes and your baby's head retreats. Your baby moves further down and her head becomes clearly visible. The joy and anticipation you now feel will give you renewed strength. You may be able to see your baby's head in a mirror. You may want to reach down and touch it. These concrete reminders will help you bear down more efficiently. During this phase, your baby descends and usually completes rotation to the occiput anterior position. Sometimes for a few contractions during this phase, your baby's head looks and feels strange—soft, slippery, wrinkled and gray-blue. This may be alarming to both you and your partner. The wrinkles are caused by the normal squeezing of the head by the vagina; the loose skin of the baby's scalp forms wrinkles until the baby's head moves down a little further. The gray-blue colour of the skin is normal at this time; it will become pink or tan within seconds after birth.

The Transition (Crowning) Phase

The third phase of the second stage is the transition or *crowning* phase, when your baby passes from inside to outside your body. It begins when your baby's head begins to crown (it no longer retreats between bearing-down efforts). This phase, which includes the maximum stretching of your vaginal opening, is characterised by a stinging, burning sensation sometimes called the 'rim of fire.' Forceful bearing down at this time increases the pain and the likelihood of a serious tear of your vagina or perineum. Think of the 'rim of fire' as your body's signal to ease your bearing-down efforts.

Depending on the speed of your delivery, you may be directed by your caregiver to give small pushes, to push between contractions or to avoid any pushing at this time. To help avoid pushing, try to breathe through the contractions with long deep breaths or with light panting or blowing (do not hold your breath), and relax your vagina as the baby's head crowns and emerges. Some birth attendants support the perineum with warm compresses or massage it with oil or another lubricant to assist gradual stretching, or they maintain pressure on the baby's head to keep it from coming too rapidly. Though the practice of episiotomy is declining, some caregivers frequently perform an episiotomy at this point. This surgical incision of the perineum enlarges the vaginal outlet as the perineum is stretching. (See pages 291–293 for discussion of episiotomy.)

Ways You Can Protect Your Perineum from a Serious Tear or an Episiotomy

Many women worry about damage to their vaginal tissues from a tear or an episiotomy during birth. Here are some things you can do in advance and during labour to protect your perineum:

- Choose a caregiver who prefers to avoid episiotomies.
- Eat nutritious foods during pregnancy, as good nutrition promotes healthy tissues.
- Perform perineal massage regularly for a few weeks before the birth. (See page 203.)
- During pushing, use spontaneous bearing down or short (five to seven seconds) bearing-down efforts.
- During delivery, use positions that make birth more efficient. (See pages 227–229.)
- During delivery, work with your caregiver and use light panting to avoid pushing while the baby's head and shoulders are born.

Birth

Your baby's head emerges bluish-gray and soaking wet, first the top of her head to her ears, then her brow and face. After her head is out, it rotates to the side. This allows her

Birth

The head shows (1), gradually emerges (2), crowns (3), and is born (4). The baby then rotates to one side, allowing the shoulders to fit through the pelvis (5 and 6).

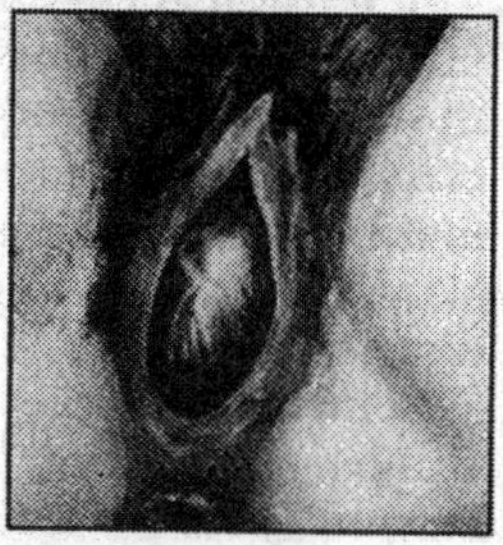

1

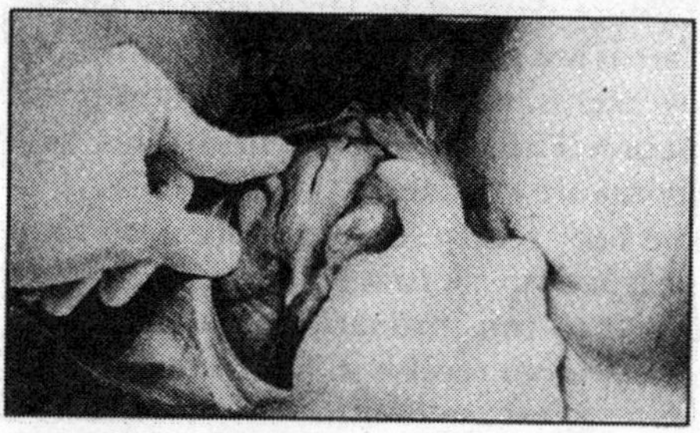

2

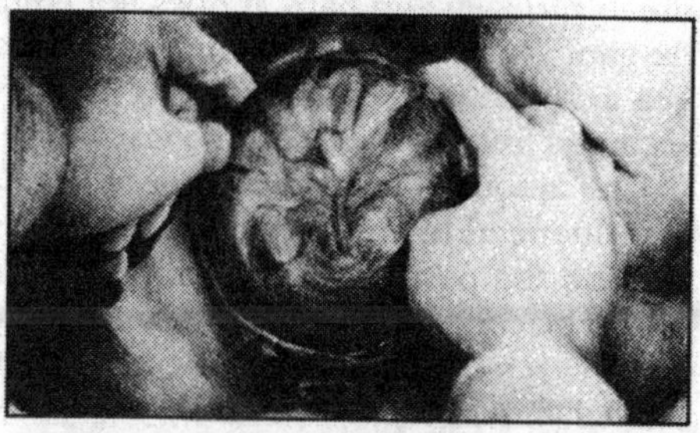

3

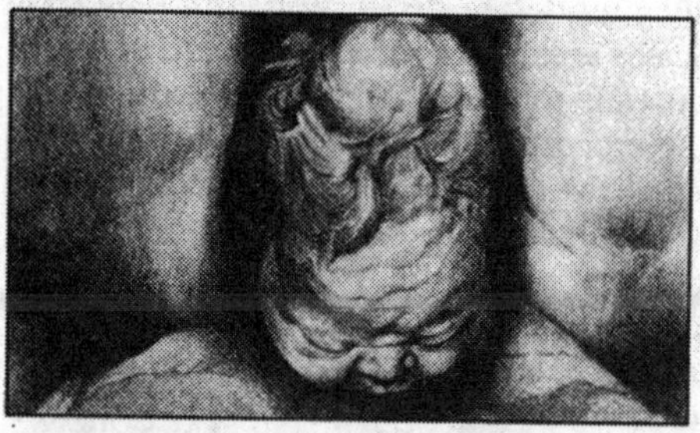

4

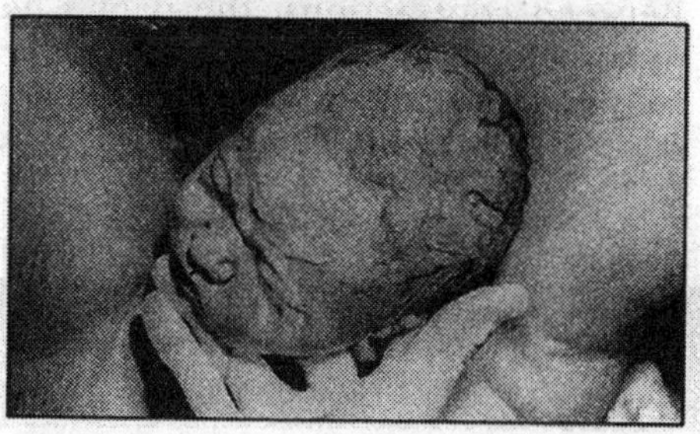

5

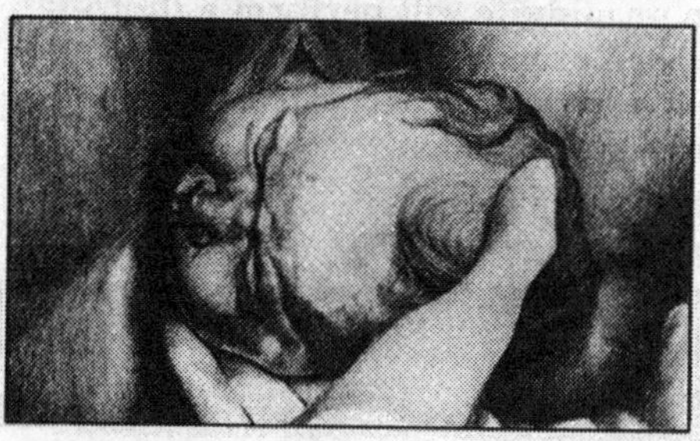

6

Then—suddenly—the baby slips out, wet, warm, blinking and crying. The caregiver clamps the cord and may suction the baby's nose and mouth (7).

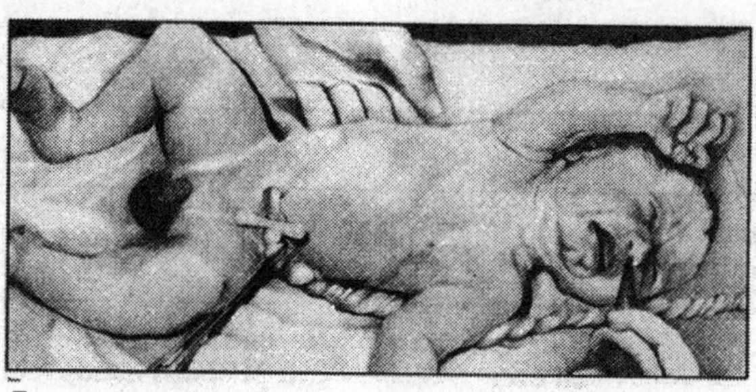

7

shoulders to slip more easily through the pelvis. One shoulder emerges, and then the rest of the baby comes rather quickly. You or your partner may want to help lift the baby out. The entire baby may appear bluish at first and may be streaked with blood and mucus. She may also be partially covered with white, lotion-like vernix. Her first breath comes within seconds, and her skin begins to turn to more normal flesh tones. All babies, whether dark- or light-skinned, go through these colour changes in the first minutes of life, as their respiration and circulation become stable. To assist respiration by clearing your baby's airways of mucus, blood, meconium or amniotic fluid, your doctor or midwife may suction your baby's nose and mouth as soon as her head is out and again later. Some babies do not need this suction, but it is often done as a precautionary measure. (See Chapter 14 for more information about the external appearance of a newborn.) Your baby may be dried and immediately placed on your abdomen or in your arms to await the delivery of your placenta.

How do you feel, now that the baby is born? Women's reactions vary. You may feel disbelieving at first, then grateful and relieved that the baby is out and that the painful contractions are over. These feelings may initially predominate over your interest in the baby, especially if it has been a long, tiring labour. Or, you may focus immediately on your baby. Many women are surprised, awed or full of wonder at their baby's appearance. The first moments—waiting for the baby to begin breathing and crying—are suspenseful. Smiles of relief and joy greet the baby's first cry. Then you await the birth of the placenta. You may find yourself unable to focus entirely on your baby because your caregiver is inspecting your perineum and checking for separation of your placenta, which may be painful and distracting. The full impact—the feelings of fulfilment and love for your baby and your partner—may not come until after your placenta is born and your caregiver has finished the afterbirth tasks. Then you can devote yourself completely to your baby.

Your partner may be overwhelmed with emotion at this time—happiness, exhaustion, relief, and deep joy and love for you and the baby. Tears may flow. And now the baby will become the focus of attention.

Third Stage of Labour: Delivery of the Placenta

The third stage, the shortest and least painful of all, begins with the birth of your baby and ends when your placenta is born. It lasts ten to thirty minutes. After your baby is born, the midwife will give you an injection into your thigh or intravenously. This is to help the uterus to contract and expel the placenta. You may need to continue relaxation and patterned breathing because the uterus sometimes cramps vigorously. You may, on the other hand, be so engrossed in your baby that you hardly notice the third stage. Often, your caregiver will direct you to give a few small pushes to deliver the placenta. Some parents appreciate seeing the placenta after it is delivered; they enjoy being shown the foetal and maternal surfaces, the membranes, and the umbilical cord.

Newborn Assessment with Apgar Score

Immediately after the birth, your baby will receive close medical attention. As soon as the baby's breathing is established and he is dried off, your caregiver performs a routine newborn assessment. Your baby's overall condition is evaluated twice (at one minute after birth and again five minutes later) using the Apgar score, a grading system devised by Dr Virginia Apgar to identify those babies who need immediate medical attention. Five areas are graded, each with a maximum of two points, making ten the highest possible score. The chart below illustrates how newborns are evaluated using the Apgar scoring.

The baby receives a total score each time the test is done. A first (one-minute) score of seven to ten indicates that the baby is in good condition. Babies seldom receive a ten on the first score; most babies' hands and feet are bluish for a while, lowering their Apgar score. A score of six may mean the baby needs extra medical attention and more observation. The second (five-minute) score is usually higher than the first, indicating improvement with time and/or medical assistance. Further Apgar scores are sometimes done, if a previous score was low, to assess whether medical treatment is succeeding. While Apgar scores are helpful, especially in detecting babies who need extra immediate medical attention, they are not perfect indicators of the baby's overall health or long-term wellbeing. A paediatrician or midwife and your nurse will perform a thorough newborn exam (within twenty-four hours) to provide a more accurate assessment of your baby's condition.

Clamping and Cutting the Cord

The umbilical cord is cut soon after the birth. It is first clamped in two places and then cut with scissors between the two clamps. Sometimes the father or partner makes the cut. The exact timing of cord clamping and cutting is a subject of some disagreement.

Apgar Scoring

Sign	0 points	1 point	2 points
Heart rate	Absent	Below 100/minute	Above 100/minute
Respiratory effort	Absent	Slow, irregular	Good, crying
Muscle tone	Limp	Arms and legs flexed	Active movement
Reflex irritability (baby's reaction to nose being suctioned)	No response	Grimace	Sneezing, coughing, pulling away
Skin colour	Blue-gray, pale all over	Normal skin colour, except bluish hands and feet	Normal skin colour all over

Some people believe that by delaying the clamping of the cord, the baby receives more oxygen. This is not true, because even though blood continues to flow back and forth between placenta and baby, it does not contain oxygen. The placenta ceases transferring oxygen long before it is delivered, since it often separates from the wall of the uterus within minutes of the baby's birth.

The amount of blood passing to the baby is influenced by the timing of cord clamping and the position of the baby in relation to the placenta. When the uterus contracts, it squeezes blood out of the placenta through the cord into the baby's body. If the cord is clamped at that time, the baby will have a higher blood volume. Between contractions, the baby's heart pumps blood back to the placenta (it is the baby's heartbeat that causes the cord to pulsate). If the cord is clamped between contractions, the baby's blood volume is lower. The shift of blood between the placenta and baby can also be affected by gravity. If the baby is held high above the placenta, more blood flows from baby to placenta. If the baby is held below the placenta, blood flows from placenta to baby. If the baby is placed on the mother's abdomen, it is at approximately the same level as the placenta and gravity is not a factor. Within a few minutes, exposure of the cord to the air causes expansion of Wharton's jelly (a substance present within the cord), which in turn compresses the blood vessels in the cord. From then on, there is no movement of blood in either direction. If the baby is born into warm water, the expansion of Wharton's jelly may be delayed and transfer of blood between placenta and baby may continue longer.

Timing of cord clamping and cutting, then, probably does not affect the baby's oxygen levels very much but does influence the blood volume. Whether clamping takes place between contractions, during a contraction or after the cord stops pulsating will influence the volume of blood within the baby's circulatory system. To achieve the optimal blood volume, the caregiver places the baby at the level of the placenta (on the mother's abdomen) until the cord stops pulsating.

Discuss the timing of cord clamping with your doctor or midwife and be sure to include your preferences in your birth plan. There are some circumstances when the cord must be cut before the baby is fully born (such as a short cord or a cord wrapped tightly around the baby's neck). Other times, the cord must be cut immediately after the birth to allow for treatment of other problems the baby may have.

Umbilical Cord Blood Collection and Storage

Umbilical cord blood, obtained from the cord just after birth, is a rich source of 'stem cells', which generate and continually renew supplies of red cells, platelets and white cells. These cells are components of blood that make it possible for us to use the oxygen we breathe, to clot blood and to fight infection. Bone marrow is another source of stem cells. Stem cells are useful as a source of healthy cells in the treatment of such disorders as childhood leukemias and severe inherited anaemias. Stem cells can also be used to replace the blood cells of cancer victims whose bone marrow has been destroyed by chemotherapy treatments. Cord blood stem cells have other potential uses as well.

Cord blood can be extracted from the umbilical cord immediately after birth. The stem cells are then separated from the blood and stored either in a blood bank for later use by the public or in a private storage facility for later use, if needed, by the child or the child's family. The stem cells from umbilical cord blood, because they are immature (or 'naive', as they are called), are easier to match than the more mature stem cells from bone marrow. Therefore, cord blood transplants may make stem cells more accessible to those who are difficult to match.

Although there is still much to learn and many problems to be overcome, cord blood transplant is a promising procedure that is rapidly gaining the interest of both scientists and the public. In Australia, private companies can arrange for the storage of cord blood. There are fees for this service. If you are interested in learning more about cord blood collection, donation or storage, several months before your due date ask your caregiver or contact your local blood bank.

Fourth Stage of Labour: Recovery

The fourth stage begins just after the placenta is born and lasts until your condition is stable, as indicated by your blood pressure, pulse, *lochia* (the normal vaginal discharge of blood from the uterus) and uterine tone. Your pelvic floor will be checked for swelling and bleeding. The fourth stage usually takes about one or two hours. It may last longer if you had anaesthesia, if labour was difficult or prolonged, or if delivery was by caesarean.

Your emotions at this time probably include profound relief that labour is over, joy or even euphoria with your baby and appreciation for those who have helped you through this meaningful experience. On the other hand, you may need a bit of time to get used to the fact that you are no longer in labour, and you may not be quite ready to hold your baby. It usually does not take long, however, before your baby monopolises your attention.

Your caregiver is concerned with your physical wellbeing at this time and has several things to do before it is time for you to settle in quietly with your partner and baby. Your caregiver will check your perineum and vaginal canal soon after the delivery of your placenta. You will be asked to lie on your back with your legs spread; your caregiver will then shine a light on your perineum and check inside and out for bleeding. If necessary, your caregiver will place stitches to hasten healing. This takes a few minutes to a half hour. Unless you have already received anaesthesia, your caregiver will inject your perineum with local anaesthetic. The injections, which may sting briefly when given, are often unexpected. While the anaesthesia is injected, you may need the help of your partner or nurse for a minute or two to resume the same breathing you were using in labour. The stitching itself should be painless.

If you have an intact perineum or a very shallow tear, there is no need for stitches, but you may have some swelling or bruising in the area. Whether you have stitches or not, you will appreciate an ice pack placed on your perineum to reduce any swelling and relieve discomfort from bruising or stitching. Then, at last, you may bask in the excitement and joy of holding and feeding your baby.

After the birth, the uterus immediately begins the process of *involution,* or returning to its non-pregnant state. By continuing to contract, the uterus shuts off the open blood vessels at the placental site. This closing prevents excessive blood loss and promotes the sloughing off of the extra uterine lining that built up during the pregnancy. You will quickly begin passing lochia and will need to wear a sanitary pad.

Your nurse or midwife will check your uterus frequently to make sure that your fundus (the top of the uterus) remains firm after the birth. If it is relaxed, you may lose too much blood, so she or he will massage your uterus firmly to cause it to contract. Because such massage can be quite painful, you may want to check your fundus and, if it seems soft or you cannot feel it, massage the area yourself. Ask your nurse to show you how to feel your fundus. This way you can keep your uterus firm with less discomfort. Do not ignore fundal massage on the first day after birth, because the uterus can bleed excessively if it is not firm. After that, you may periodically check to see if your uterus needs massage to keep it contracted.

To Massage Your Uterus

Empty your bladder. Lie flat on your back and check your uterus by pressing on your abdomen about the level of your navel (belly button). If your uterus is as firm as a grapefruit, you do not need to massage it. If you cannot feel your uterus, massage as follows:

With one hand slightly cupped, massage your lower abdomen firmly with small circular movements until you feel your uterus contract and become firm. It may be painful. If you cannot make your uterus contract, tell your nurse or midwife.

During the first minutes after birth, you may experience trembling in your legs, pain as your uterus contracts (called *afterpains*—a common occurrence, especially in multiparas), and swelling and discomfort in your perineum from the stretching or stitches. A warm blanket helps relieve trembling, and an ice pack on your perineum reduces discomfort and may control swelling. Use slow breathing if necessary for the afterpains. You may feel hungry and thirsty—not at all surprising, since you have been working hard and have probably missed some meals.

You will probably hold your baby and let her nuzzle at your breast. Many babies are ready to suckle within thirty to sixty minutes. (See page 431 for advice on the first feeding.)

Your New Family

While your body is settling down after the birth, your family is settling down also. You, your partner, and any other family members or close friends will savour these first moments with the baby. The labour stimulates a state of wakefulness and alertness in the baby that may last for several hours. During this time, your baby is likely to be calm and alert, and she will begin observing and sensing the new sounds, smells, sights, touches and tastes around her. If the light is not too bright, she stares, particularly at

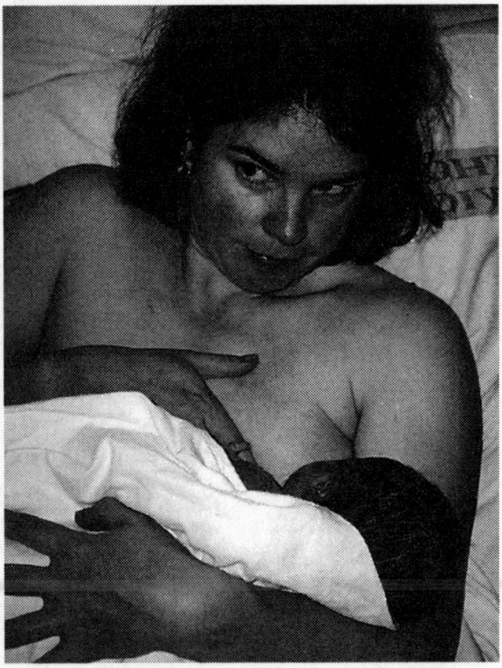

Photograph by Penny Simkin

The strength of your baby's first suckling comes as a surprise.

faces. You can ask to dim the lights or use your hand to create a shadow over your baby's eyes to shield them from the bright light. As your baby cuddles with you, gazes into your face or suckles at your breast, you will probably find her fascinating and irresistible. These moments are a time of falling in love and are a significant step in bonding, or attachment. Your partner will also want to hold her close, perhaps skin-to-skin, and enjoy these first moments together.

Most family-centred hospitals do not send healthy babies to the nursery. Instead, the babies stay with their mothers and go to the nursery only if they develop problems. Routine observations or procedures can be performed on the normal newborn in the presence and even in the arms of the mother or partner. Check your hospital's policies. If healthy newborns are routinely sent to the nursery, ask your doctor or midwife for an order to delay your baby's admission to the nursery so that you may have time together.

After one to several hours, the baby usually falls deeply asleep. You and your partner may do the same. The initial exhilaration that you feel after the birth usually gives way to fatigue. At this time, someone who is awake and alert should periodically observe the vital signs—such as colour, pulse, respiration, blood pressure and temperature—of both you and your baby. In the hospital, a nurse will do the job. After a home birth, the observations are made initially by the midwife or a birth assistant and later by an informed and rested friend or relative. Your partner may be as tired as you and may be unable to take on these responsibilities until he or she gets some sleep.

Your adjustments to your non-pregnant state and to the new state of parenthood now begin. Your real baby has replaced your imagined baby, and you will experience many physical and emotional changes. In addition, you and your partner begin the important work of talking with each other, the staff, and your other support help to review, understand and gain perspective on your labour and birth experiences.

Labour and Birth Guide

Stage 1: Effacement and Dilation of Cervix, Rotation of Baby

	Pre-labour	Latent Phase	Active Phase	Transition
Cervical changes	• Some forward movement, ripening, partial effacement, possible dilation to 1–2 cm	• Further ripening and effacement, dilation to approximately 4 cm	• Dilation to approximately 7 cm	• Dilation to 10 cm; may be uneven, temporarily causing a 'lip' of cervix
Baby's position	• Usually head comes first and is low in pelvis: occipt transverse (OT), occiput anterior (OA) or occiput posterior (OP)	• Same as pre-labour	• Baby begins to rotate to occiput anterior (OA).	• Baby begins to descend further in pelvis; head begins to 'mold' to fit through pelvis.
Contraction pattern	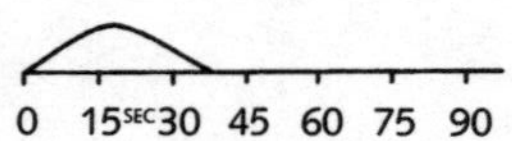	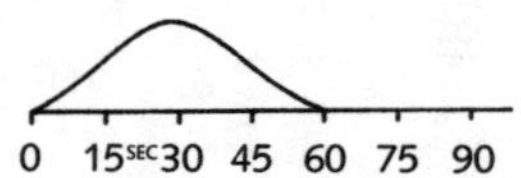	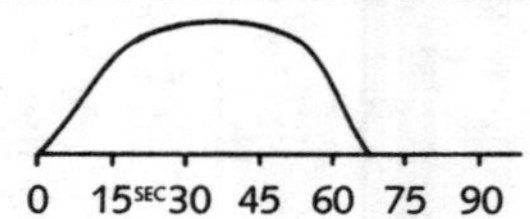	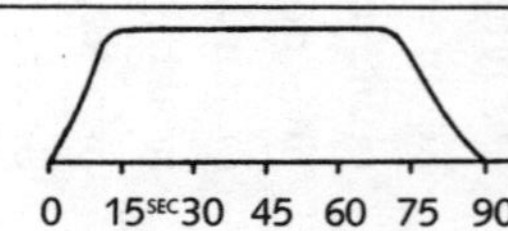
Frequency	• Variable, range from 3–30 minutes apart	• About 10–12 minutes (or less) apart	• About 5 minutes (or less) apart	• About 2–3 minutes apart
Duration	• Variable	• About 30–40 seconds long	• About 60 seconds long	• Range from 60–120 seconds long

Labour and Birth Guide

Stage 1: Effacement and Dilation of Cervix, Rotation of Baby

	Pre-labour	Latent Phase	Active Phase	Transition
Possible physical signs	• Pre-labour may last a short time or persist for days. *Possible signs of labour:* • Low abdominal cramps • 'Restless' backache • Increased energy (nesting urge) • Soft, loose bowel movements *Preliminary signs of labour:* • Non-progressing contractions (may go away with change in activity, sometimes very painful) • Blood-tinged mucus from vagina • Small chance of leaking (or gush) of fluid from vagina (rupture of membranes)	*Positive signs of labour:* • Progressing contractions (becoming longer, stronger and more frequent) • Continuing passage of blood-tinged mucus (show) • Possible rupture of membranes	• Contractions continue progressing, becoming longer (more than 1 minute), stronger and more frequent (less than 5 minutes apart) • Peak of pain intensity reached by 7 cm • More blood-tinged mucus • Membranes may rupture	• Very intense, long contractions • Very little rest between contractions (30 seconds to 2 minutes) • Pressure on vagina and rectum • Possible urge to push • Nausea, vomiting • Leg cramps • Trembling • Sensitivity to touch • Drowsiness • Cold feet • Flushed face, hot flashes • Rupture of membranes (usually occurs by this time)
Possible emotional responses	• Confusion about whether this is labour or not • Mixed feelings (exhilaration, excitement, self-doubt, anxiety) • Distractible during contractions • May overestimate labour progress and start rituals or go to the hospital too early	• Uncertain whether in labour • Excited, talkative • Confident, optimistic (or) • Apprehensive, distressed • Possibly distractible during contractions • May focus on contractions, 'overreact' to early labour	• Serious, focused, uninterested in anything but labour • Cannot tolerate small talk or distracting conversation • Feels trapped, discouraged and tired; may weep • Recognises that labour is not within her control	• Restless, irritable • Weepy, easily upset, angry • Panicky, afraid of pain and intensity of labour • Difficulty with relaxation, rhythm and ritual • Overwhelmed, ready to give up, at her limit

Labour and Birth Guide

Stage 1: Effacement and Dilation of Cervix, Rotation of Baby

	Pre-labour	Latent Phase	Active Phase	Transition
What to do: mother	• Prepare and pack your bag. • Alternate pleasant, mild, distracting activity with rest or nap. • Work on a project (prepare meals, arrange baby clothes, paint or sew). • Take a walk. • Take a shower. • Eat and drink normally. • Visit friends, listen to music. • At night, sleep (or rest), if possible. • Usually no breathing pattern needed; if needed, use slow breathing. • If prolonged, painful and exhausting, try strategies to ease pain and promote comfort. (See page 186.)	• Alternate rest and activity (appropriate to time of day). • Use the Three Rs (relaxation, rhythm and ritual) when unable to walk or talk through contractions. • Begin with a ritual of slow breathing, tension release and attention-focusing during contractions. • Try to remain relaxed between contractions. • Eat and drink (sensibly) as desired. • Empty your bladder every hour. • Bathe or shower for cleanliness. (A long bath may slow contractions.) • Call doctor or midwife (if membranes rupture, with progressing contractions, or other concerns).	• Go to hospital or birth centre (or caregiver arrives at home); settle in and discuss birth plan. • Use positions of comfort. • Use ritual, rhythmic movement and breathing patterns, attention-focusing, or visualisation during contractions. • Begin light breathing or an adaptation of slow and light breathing (if or when slow breathing no longer helps). • Repeat anything (ritual) that helps in each contraction. • Relax between contractions. • Drink liquids; suck ice or ice-blocks. • Empty bladder every hour. • Use measures to relieve backache (see page 287) or to promote labour progress (see page 283), if necessary.	• Change position as needed for comfort. • Continue light breathing or use an adaptation. • Maintain a rhythm with breathing patterns, movement and moaning. • Try to stick with your ritual; if you cannot, adapt it. • Maintain an internal or external focus. • Pant, if necessary, to control premature urge to push. • Take contractions one at a time. • Remember: transition is intense, but short.

Labour and Birth Guide

Stage 1: Effacement and Dilation of Cervix, Rotation of Baby

	Pre-labour	Latent Phase	Active Phase	Transition
What to do: partner	• Help her pack. • Give her moral support. • Rest or sleep (at night). • Encourage mild activity and naps during the day. • Distract her, if necessary. (Go to a movie or walk with her.) • Carry a pager or cell phone to be sure you can be reached while away. • Periodically time a series of 5–6 contractions. • Use massage; help her relax. • Take care of last-minute details (phone calls, gasoline in car, comfort items and snacks for yourself).	• Help pass the time with walking, talking, music, TV, games, meal preparation for after birth and so on. • Time and record a series of 5–6 contractions. • Help her relax as necessary. • Suggest comfort measures as indicated (massage, back rub, food, fluids). • Help her prepare to go to hospital or get ready for home birth. • Give her your undivided attention during contractions, if needed. • Offer encouragement and give feedback on her use of coping skills.	• Remain calm; show your love; help her feel safe and secure. • Identify her ritual and help her maintain it. • Give her your undivided attention with every contraction. (Do not ask her questions during contractions.) • Use soothing touch and voice, stroking, massage, cold or hot pack. • Use verbal encouragement. • Offer ice, liquids. • Remind her to urinate. • Use measures to alleviate back pain, if needed. • Tune in and work with her rhythm.	• Know the signs of transition. • Encourage and reassure her; give her simple directions. • Remind her that transition is short. • Compliment her; avoid criticising her. • Stay with her. • If she cannot maintain ritual, take charge by establishing eye contact, conducting her rhythmic breathing, and speaking calmly and rhythmically. • Comfort her if she weeps or protests about the intensity of contractions. • Hold her tight or do not touch her, depending on her response.

Labour and Birth Guide

Stage 2: Birth of Baby

	Resting (Latent) Phase	Descent (Active) Phase	Crowning and Birth
What is happening?	• Baby's head leaves uterus and descends into birth canal. • Uterus slackens around baby's trunk and needs time to catch up or tighten around baby. • This phase is sometimes short and goes unnoticed. • Mother does not feel contractions or pain for 5–30 minutes.	• Contraction strength returns. • Baby rotates and descends. • Baby's head moves down during bearing-down efforts and retreats between efforts. • Caregiver supports perineum and may direct bearing-down efforts.	• Baby's head no longer retreats between bearing-down efforts. • Head steadily emerges, crown first, then brow and face; head rotates; shoulders are born; then baby quickly slides out. • Caregiver may support perineum and direct mother when and when not to push. • Baby is dried, suctioned and placed with mother or in own bed.
Possible physical signs	• No urge to push • Relief from pain: decreased or absent	• Increasingly powerful urge to push • Great pressure in vagina that remains between contractions	• Stretching • Burning sensation at vaginal outlet (may subside before birth, as stretching causes diminished sensation)
Possible emotional responses	• Renewed energy, enthusiasm, hope and 'second wind' (or) • Relaxation and drowsiness • Readiness to 'get on with it'. • More awareness of surroundings • Sense of humour (may return temporarily)	• Exhilaration to be doing something to hasten the birth • Alarm at the pressure in the vagina, possible involuntary 'holding back' • Appreciation of encouragement, calm reminders of what to do • Discouragement, impatience if progress is slow • Involuntary breath-holding, straining or grunting	• Confusion, alarm with burning sensations • Desire for someone to 'do something' to help • Wave of fear, anxiety to get the baby out, often followed by awe and concentration as baby emerges • Desire to know if baby is whole and healthy • Relief that labour is over • Curiosity to get to know baby, desire to hold baby

Labour and Birth Guide

Stage 2: Birth of Baby

	Resting (Latent) Phase	Descent (Active) Phase	Crowning and Birth
What to do: mother	• Rest and enjoy the break. • Wait for the urge to push. • Change to an upright position or hands and knees if resting phase lasts more than 15 minutes.	• Bear down for 5–7 seconds when urge to push is irresistible; breathe lightly between pushing efforts. • Rest between contractions. • Follow directions of nurse or caregiver. • Focus on relaxing the perineum (not holding back). • Try a variety of positions if progress is slow.	• Follow caregiver's directions for pushing (may include asking to ease your bearing-down efforts as the baby's head emerges). • Touch baby's head or watch birth in mirror, if desired. • Enjoy touching the baby skin-to-skin. • Rejoice in the birth of the baby!
What to do: partner	• Enjoy the break; stay close by her. • Wait patiently. • Review bearing-down techniques and the importance of releasing pelvic floor tension. • Help her into another position, if desired or if resting phase goes on too long. • Provide comfort (sips of water or juice, mouthwash).	• Don't rush her or raise your voice. • Remind her to bulge or relax perineum while pushing. • Help her with appropriate positions while pushing and with relaxing positions between contractions. • Continue using comfort measures. (Offer ice, wipe brow with cool cloth, provide lip moisturiser.) • Ask for warm compresses for her perineum and mirror if she wants to see baby's head. • If she needs help pushing effectively, suggest she keep her eyes open and look down where the baby will come out.	• Let the caregiver guide her pushing efforts. • Don't rush her. • Support her position. • Share in the joy of the birth!

Labour and Birth Guide

	Stage 3: Delivery of Placenta	Stage 4: Recovery (First Hours after Birth)
What is happening?	• Placenta separates from uterine wall. • Placenta is expelled. • Baby's condition is assessed (Apgar scores); baby either placed with parents or given any needed care.	• Mother, partner and baby enjoy first contact. • Mother's perineum is checked, stitched if necessary; ice pack is placed on perineum. • Baby feeds. • Baby is given vitamin K. • Baby is weighed, measured, assessed, nappied and wrapped in a blanket. • Mother's and baby's vital signs are checked; wellbeing evaluated. • Mother's uterus is checked for firmness; vaginal flow (lochia) evaluated. • Family has private time together.
Physical signs	• Mild to moderate contractions • Uncontrollable shaking	• Possible shaking • Pain with inspection of vagina or administration of local anaesthetic and possible stitches • Hunger • Afterpains (painful uterine contractions, especially with multigravidas who are breastfeeding) • Heavy lochia • Perineal discomfort, swelling • Possible difficulty with urination
Possibe emotional responses	• Excitement • Engrossment with baby • Fatigue • Relief • Surprise or dismay if contractions are painful	• Excitement, elation • Fatigue, exhaustion • Relief • 'Empty' feeling • Surprise or fascination with appearance of baby • Desire to see and hold baby • Disappointment if there is pain with vaginal inspection and repair • Desire to talk and review labour and birth

Labour and Birth Guide

	Stage 3: Delivery of Placenta	Stage 4: Recovery (First Hours after Birth)
What to do: mother	• Use breathing patterns as necessary. • Push placenta out as directed. • Hold baby skin-to-skin. • Relax and enjoy baby. • Watch initial examination and care of baby. • Ask to see placenta, if desired.	• Rest, relax. • Interact with baby (cuddle, stroke, kiss, talk to and feed). • Drink or eat. • Massage top of uterus (fundus).
What to do: partner	• Help with breathing pattern, if needed. • Cut cord, if desired and possible. • Hold baby or help mother hold baby. • Watch initial examination and care of baby.	• Hold, touch, talk to baby; enjoy family time. • Provide comfort to new mother as needed. (Give back rubs, help her change position, offer fluids.) • Talk about the birth experience with mother and praise her efforts. • Possibly go to the nursery with baby, if baby is taken there. • Call family and friends.

Chapter 10

Labour Variations, Complications and Interventions

Each birth experience is unique. Some labours and births are very short, some are long and discouraging, and some pose problems for mother or baby. You can expect that your experience will be different from your mother's, your sister's or even your own prior experiences. Because no one can predict what kind of labour and birth you will have, you will want to prepare yourself as much as possible and include your ideas and wishes in your birth plan. This chapter discusses variations and complications in labour and birth and how they can be handled by your own special efforts and by your caregiver's assistance.

A labour *variation* presents challenges beyond the typical labour that are still within the wide range of normal. A variation in itself does not pose dangers to either mother or baby, but it does pose problems that require the mother and her partner to draw more deeply on their resources.

A labour *complication* presents problems that cannot be solved by the extra efforts of the mother and her partner. Such labours require medical assistance and intervention to ensure an optimal outcome. Sometimes, a variation becomes a complication when, despite all the mother's efforts, the problem remains unsolved. Other complications are emergencies that pose immediate problems for mother or baby and require prompt medical attention.

A labour *intervention* is an action taken by your caregiver to identify, prevent or treat a medical problem. Medical interventions include tests, procedures and medications that are selected by your caregiver according to the problem. This chapter explains factors or problems that may cause labour variations and complications. It also shows how you can adjust, cope with and even correct some of the problems. In addition, it describes common medical or surgical interventions that your caregiver may recommend for dealing with a problem. This knowledge, along with sensitive and experienced emotional support, can take many of the surprises out of an atypical labour and help make it satisfying.

Monitoring Techniques

By monitoring your condition and that of your baby during labour, your doctor or midwife becomes aware of labour variations and can detect most complications. The monitoring techniques described below help identify variations and complications, and they help your caregiver decide how to manage your labour, especially if it is a difficult one.

Monitoring the Mother

Periodic vaginal exams by the nurse or caregiver determine the effacement and dilation of your cervix and the station, presentation and position of your foetus. The results are recorded on a time chart or labour graph that shows how your labour is progressing. The frequency and intensity of your contractions will be observed by the nurse or midwife, who will assess them either by feeling your contractions with her hand or by using an electronic monitor (see pages 310–311).

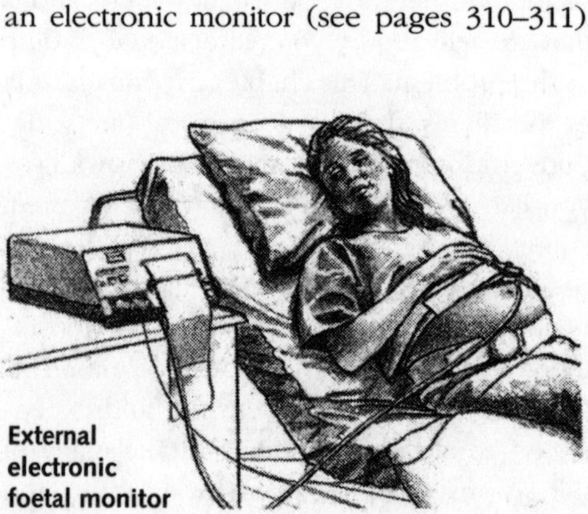

External electronic foetal monitor

Throughout labour, your nurse or midwife will assess and record your blood pressure, temperature, pulse, urine output and fluid intake. All assessments are recorded either by hand on a paper record or by keyboard into a computer.

Monitoring the Foetus

Foetal Heart Rate Monitoring

In labour, the foetal heart rate (FHR) is influenced by uterine contractions, foetal movements, the administration of medications, your body temperature, your position and other factors. The normal FHR range is generally considered to be between 120 and 160 beats per minute. The foetus has the ability to speed or slow his heart rate in response to changes in the availability of oxygen. Depending on the maturity and health of the foetus, his reserves and thus his ability to compensate vary. If a lack of oxygen continues over time, the foetus's reserves may be exhausted. He may no longer be able to compensate and may experience what is known as 'foetal distress'. The term *foetal distress* refers to the foetus whose heart rate patterns indicate a lack of oxygen and a need for further testing or intervention. The FHR is monitored to identify the foetus who may be in distress. When indicated, further testing assists the caregiver in identifying those few babies who are not compensating adequately and who need immediate medical intervention.

The foetal heart rate can be monitored either by *auscultation* or by *electronic foetal monitoring* (EFM). With auscultation, the caregiver or nurse listens to the foetal heartbeats during and between contractions with a special foetal stethoscope or with a hand-held ultrasound stethoscope called a 'Doppler'. He or she counts the heartbeats, notes any speeding up or slowing down, and records the findings each time the FHR is checked.

With EFM, the mother has two sensing devices placed either on her abdomen (external EFM) or within her uterus (internal EFM). One of these devices picks up the baby's heartbeat; the other picks up changes in uterine tone (which indicate contractions). These sensors may be connected to video screens in the mother's room and/or at the nurses' station. They are also connected to a machine that detects and prints out a sheet that displays two graphs that indicate the foetal heart rate and the intensity of the contractions. The caregiver checks the video screen (which shows second-by-second numbers) or the printout to assess the baby's wellbeing and the mother's contraction pattern.

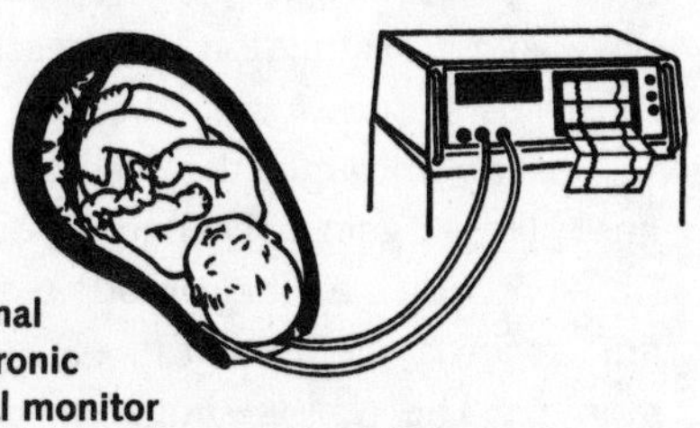

Internal electronic foetal monitor

Auscultation and electronic foetal monitoring are about equal in their ability to assess foetal wellbeing, although most caregivers prefer to use continuous EFM with high-risk labouring women. Each type of monitoring requires a specific set of skills. With auscultation, hearing and touch are the senses used to gain information. With electronic foetal monitoring, sight and to a lesser extent hearing are the operative senses. Auscultation requires more direct contact between the nurse/caregiver and the mother, while EFM allows one nurse at the nurses' station to keep track of several labouring women at the same time. EFM using telemetry (in which a wireless transmitter sends data to a monitor) allows the mother to be out of bed and out of her room while being continuously monitored. If the hospital is short-staffed, EFM is advantageous as long as the recordings are checked frequently. From the mother's point of view, auscultation may seem more personal because the nurse is looking at and touching her instead of watching a monitor. (See pages 309–311 for more information on the different types of monitoring.)

Amniotic Fluid Evaluation

When the mother's membranes rupture (bag of waters breaks), the appearance of the amniotic fluid gives useful information about the baby's condition. A strong odour may indicate an infection. A green or dark colour means the baby has expelled meconium from his bowels, which may be a warning sign that the foetus has been stressed. If meconium is present, your caregiver will assess the foetal heart tones frequently to check for foetal wellbeing. As soon as your baby's head is born and before he takes his first breath, your caregiver will probably suction your baby's nose, mouth and trachea (windpipe). The suctioning is done to help prevent your baby from breathing in the meconium, which could cause breathing problems or (rarely) pneumonia. As soon as the baby is completely born, your caregiver will cut the cord and move the baby to the newborn care area in the room. Here, a specialist may view the baby's trachea and vocal cords for meconium and suction them again as necessary. If you do not hear your baby cry right away, try not to worry. If your amniotic fluid contains meconium, your caregiver may not want your baby to breathe or cry immediately. Meconium in the amniotic fluid occurs in approximately 20 percent of labours.

Foetal Stimulation Test

If foetal heart rate monitoring raises concerns about the wellbeing of the foetus, your caregiver may seek to confirm foetal distress with a foetal stimulation test, which is reliable, simple and inexpensive. By pressing or scratching your foetus's scalp during a vaginal exam (foetal scalp stimulation test) or by creating a loud noise outside your abdomen (fetal acoustic stimulation test), your caregiver can check the baby's condition. If the foetal heart rate speeds up, it is a good sign that your baby is all right. If not, it may indicate foetal distress. The foetal scalp stimulation test is more commonly used than the one using sound.

Foetal Scalp Blood Sample

Taking a foetal scalp blood sample is another way to assess foetal wellbeing if your caregiver suspects foetal complications because of FHR changes. A sample of scalp blood from a small cut in the foetus's head is taken and analysed for changes in the blood due to a lack of oxygen. This test, though helpful, is invasive to the baby and uncomfortable for the mother (it feels like a lengthy vaginal exam). The result of the test is available soon after the sample is collected. It allows for a more accurate assessment of the baby's wellbeing and is sometimes repeated in labour.

Foetal Oxygen Saturation Monitoring

The newest technology for assessing foetal wellbeing when monitor tracing is not reassuring is foetal oxygen saturation monitoring. Oxygen saturation refers to the amount of oxygen in the blood in relation to the maximum amount possible. It is measured as a percentage of the maximum. In a newborn or adult, an oxygen saturation of 96 percent or higher is considered normal, whereas in a foetus, a level of 30 percent or higher is normal.

Foetal oxygen saturation is measured continuously by a sensor that the nurse or caregiver inserts through the vagina and cervix and places against the baby's cheek. The skin sensor measures blood oxygen levels and records them on the electronic foetal monitor. The test is similar to pulse oximetry, which has been used for years to measure oxygen saturation in newborns and adults. (See the chart on page 308 for further description of both foetal oxygen saturation monitoring and pulse oximetry.) Few units in Australia use this routinely.

The Need or Wish to Start Labour

Labour is sometimes started (induced) before it begins spontaneously. Sometimes there are medical reasons to do so (for example, if problems arise in late pregnancy for either the mother or the foetus). The doctor or midwife and parents usually make the decision to induce labour after the mother is examined, lab tests are run, and testing for foetal wellbeing and maturity has been performed. (See Chapter 3.)

Some of the most common *medical reasons* for starting labour include:

- Prolonged pregnancy
- Prolonged ruptured membranes
- Foetus who is no longer growing or thriving in the uterus
- Particular illnesses in the mother, such as pregnancy-induced hypertension (PIH) or diabetes

When any of these conditions is suspected or known, the mother and foetus are watched closely. If it appears that one or the other might be harmed if the pregnancy continues, labour is started.

Inductions are also done for *non-medical reasons* (also called 'elective' or 'planned' inductions). These reasons include the following:

- Convenience for the caregiver or mother is the most common reason for elective induction. For example, choosing a day when the woman's primary doctor or midwife is on call may appeal to some women who do not want an unknown caregiver for their birth. Planned inductions appeal to some caregivers because they like to attend their clients' births but cannot do so when they are not on call.
- The predictability of inductions appeals to many women, especially those with other children, those who have had a previous rapid birth, those who live far from the hospital, or those who depend on working friends or relatives to help out during a fixed vacation time.
- For women having frequent outbreaks of genital herpes, a plan to induce labour between outbreaks may avoid a caesarean birth. (See page 69 for more on herpes.)
- Sometimes, women find the last weeks of pregnancy very uncomfortable and want to end it.
- Both women and caregivers sometimes fear that if they wait for labour to begin, the baby may grow too big to fit through the pelvis. They may hope that induction will allow an easier birth or will prevent a caesarean. However, this hope has not been borne out in scientific investigations. Studies have found a large margin of error (as much as 10 percent) in ultrasound estimates of foetal weight and size. In addition, an arrest of labour and a caesarean delivery are actually more likely when labour is induced (because of a suspected large baby) than when labour begins spontaneously.[1]
- Frequently, women and their caregivers go ahead with an induction because there is no clear reason not to. The pregnancy

may be at thirty-seven to forty-two weeks (term), the cervix ripe, and the baby apparently large enough. The question becomes, 'Why not?' rather than 'Why?'.

The methods of induction used today are more reliable than in the past, when elective inductions were considered unsafe. Although the temptation may be great to schedule an induction, consider the following before deciding:

- Your body has its own 'foeto-placental clock', which greatly influences the baby's readiness for birth. Babies continue to mature and develop during the last weeks of pregnancy and may benefit from a few more days in the uterus. (See pages 209–211 for further explanation.)
- Induction is not a risk-free procedure, and there is no guarantee that it will be successful. The chances of a caesarean are higher for those who are induced than for those with spontaneous onset of labour, especially in first-time mothers[3] and for those women with an unripe cervix.
- You will probably be asked to call in before going to the hospital for the planned induction. If the maternity unit is especially busy when your induction is scheduled, they may tell you to wait and call back in a few hours to see if they have room for you. The hospital staff cannot, of course, predict the number of women who will be in labour at any time. Still, it may be frustrating and demoralising to have prepared yourself to have your baby on a specific day, only to have the plans changed at the last minute.
- An induction can take as little as six to eight hours or as long as a day or more. A long or unsuccessful induction is more likely if the induction begins when the cervix is unripe. It may require several trips to the hospital to have prostaglandins or dilators inserted in or around your cervix before you are admitted for induction. Syntocinon, the drug most commonly used to stimulate contractions, sometimes acts slowly; many hours may pass before contractions begin. You may take magazines, needlework or other projects to pass the time.
- Continuous electronic foetal monitoring is required once you are admitted, which may restrict your options for self-help comfort measures and pain relief. For example, walking and other movements, bathing, and massage of your back and abdomen are cumbersome and sometimes impossible with EFM.
- You may not be allowed to eat while Syntocinon is running, though you can probably have clear liquids to drink. If it is a long wait before contractions begin, hunger is a problem.
- Induced labours, even in early labour, may be more painful than spontaneous labours. Sometimes the intensity of the contractions can be eased by reducing the induction medication, but not always.

If induction is suggested to you, be sure to ask the key questions about the procedure (page 52) so that you will know if the induction is medically indicated or elective. Weigh all the factors so that you will be able to make an informed decision. When offered an induction for convenience and when fully informed of the risks and benefits of the procedure, some women decide to postpone it or wait for the onset of spontaneous labour. Others schedule the induction after deciding that the reasons for going ahead outweigh the potential drawbacks.

If either a medical or elective induction is decided upon and scheduled, there may be time for you to start your labour on your own, if desired, by trying the self-help techniques described below and in greater detail in the charts on pages 268–274. Discuss the idea with your caregiver before trying them. If you are successful, you will avoid the disadvantages of a medical induction, or you may at least cause enough cervical changes to make a medical induction easier and more likely to succeed. If you do not have time to use these techniques, if you do not wish to try them or if they are unsuccessful, then your caregiver has a variety of methods of inducing labour. (These are described on pages 265–267 and in the charts on pages 268–274.)

What You Can Do to Start or Speed Up a Slow Labour

When it is important that labour start or when labour is progressing too slowly, you may try these measures. *Consult your caregiver before trying any of these techniques.* They have the advantage of being simpler and easier than a medical induction; however, they are less likely to succeed than the medical methods and may carry some risks or unpleasant side effects. In addition to the brief descriptions of the techniques below, the charts on pages 268–274 give more details on how to do them, how effective and safe they are, and how much we know (or do not know) about them. *Please note:* If you really want to try some of the following techniques but are concerned that your caregiver may not support you when you ask, choose the wording of your question carefully. Instead of asking, 'Do you think I should try some self-help induction methods such as…?' try asking, 'Is there any medical reason why I shouldn't try some self-help induction methods…?'.

Walking

Long walks (thirty minutes or several hours) may help start labour; however, they are more effective in keeping labour going than in starting it. If it is important for you to go into labour soon, try the other more effective and less tiring methods listed below.

Acupressure

Firm finger or thumb pressure over particular acupressure points sometimes starts or accelerates contractions. The two points most commonly suggested are the Spleen 6 and Hoku points. (Locations, precautions and techniques are described on page 269.) *Caution:* Because pressure on these points can cause contractions, avoid using it on

Acupressure points

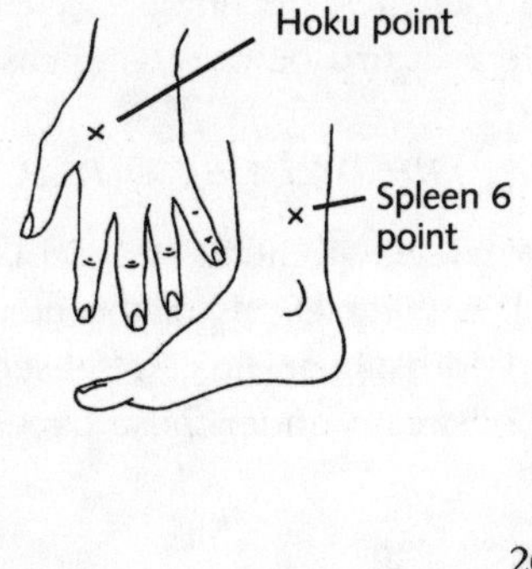

yourself until it is appropriate for you to go into labour. To practise finding the acupressure points, try them on a non-pregnant friend or your partner.

Bowel Stimulation (Enemas and Castor Oil)

You can sometimes start labour by stimulating your bowels to empty. Doing so is thought to increase the production of prostaglandins, causing your cervix to ripen.

One of the old methods for starting labour was the use of an *enema*, though it has never been shown in scientific studies to induce labour. If you want to try it, you can buy a compact, self-administered enema at the drugstore. Some caregivers suggest an enema before a planned induction to empty the bowels (which usually empty by themselves before spontaneous labour).

Castor oil is a strong laxative that causes powerful contractions of the bowel. Castor oil induction has been used with some success for years.[4] The contractions may begin soon after you take it or not until hours later. Castor oil may cause painful intestinal cramping and diarrhoea and could aggravate haemorrhoids; some women have only cramping and diarrhoea with few or no contractions. See the table for directions but, as with all these techniques, check with your caregiver first before trying castor oil.

Orgasm or Intercourse

Sexual excitement, particularly orgasm, causes contractions of the uterus. Oxytocin and prostaglandins, released into your bloodstream under these circumstances, act on the uterus and cervix. Prostaglandins are also present in semen, and after intercourse they act directly on the cervix. Manual or oral stimulation of the clitoris, even without orgasm, may also be effective in starting labour. Intercourse, manual stimulation and oral-genital stimulation can be done as long as the membranes are intact and it is comfortable for you and your partner. If your membranes have broken, only clitoral stimulation should be done, as nothing should enter the vagina. If you choose these techniques, make them as pleasant as possible. Try to forget your aim of starting labour and enjoy the sexual experience.

Nipple Stimulation

Stimulating your nipples causes the release of oxytocin, which contracts your uterus and often succeeds in either ripening the cervix or starting labour. You may have to repeat this measure off and on over a few hours or longer.

Caution: Occasionally, nipple stimulation causes contractions that last too long (more than sixty seconds), come too frequently (more than two in ten minutes) or are too intense and painful. The baby may not tolerate them. Some caregivers discourage nipple stimulation for women having vaginal birth after caesarean (VBAC).

To protect against these potential problems, you and your caregiver may decide to have you do nipple stimulation first in the hospital or clinic while your contractions and the baby's heart rate are measured by an electronic foetal monitor. This is how one test of foetal wellbeing (the contraction stress test) is carried out. If all is well, you can go home and continue nipple stimulation. Some caregivers are more comfortable with nipple stimulation if such a test is done first. Another way to protect against contractions that are too long, too strong or too frequent is to time the length and interval of the contractions caused by nipple stimulation. If they are painful or last longer than one minute, or if they occur more frequently than every five minutes, decrease the nipple stimulation (from both breasts to only one, or from continuous to intermittent).

- *Use self-stimulation.* Lightly stroke or brush one nipple with your fingertips or a washcloth, or roll the nipple between your fingers. Begin with one nipple. Within a few minutes, you will probably feel contractions. If not, stimulate both nipples. Because contractions may stop when you stop nipple stimulation, you may have to continue stroking or nipple rolling on and off for hours, especially if you are trying to start labour soon. If your aim is to ripen your cervix and you are not under pressure to go right into labour (for example, if an induction is scheduled within a few days), you might stroke your nipples or gently massage your breasts with warm, moist towels for an hour, three times a day, for several days.[5] Do not stimulate your nipples so vigorously that your breasts become sore. Stroking, nipple rolling and caressing should be gentle and light.
- *Use an electric or manual breast pump* for ten to twenty minutes per breast. Electric pumps are often available in the hospital.[6]
- *Caressing and oral stimulation by your partner* may cause contractions. Try this for as long as you find it effective and pleasant, or until contractions become strong.

Herbal Tea and Tinctures

Some caregivers recommend teas or various tinctures to induce labour. These should be used only with the knowledge and guidance of your caregiver, since they contain active ingredients that enter the bloodstream and have potential undesired side effects. Therefore, they represent a medical approach to inducing labour. For example, one of the most common herbal induction agents, blue cohosh tea, causes your uterus to contract, but it can also cause your blood pressure to rise to unsafe levels.[7] (See the chart on page 272.)

Medical Induction of Labour

There are several methods used by physicians and midwives to start labour: stripping the membranes, cervical dilators, artificial rupture of membranes (AROM), various forms of prostaglandins and intravenous Syntocinon. (For a description of these methods, see the charts on pages 268 and 272.)

The choice of method depends on the condition of your cervix. It is *favourable for induction* if it is soft (ripe), anterior, and partially effaced and dilated. It is *unfavourable* if it is firm (unripe), thick and posterior. The philosophy and preferences of your caregiver and hospital also influence the choice of method. If you are scheduled for an induction, find out which method will be used so you will know what to expect.

- *Stripping (or sweeping) the membranes* is a quick and relatively non-invasive procedure. It is painful (like a very vigorous vaginal exam) but has been found to reduce the time until labour begins.[8] Your caregiver might want to try this if you are at or beyond your due date and your cervix is very ripe and dilated enough to allow insertion of your caregiver's finger. (See page 270.)
- *Cervical dilators* are popular in some areas as a way to ripen the cervix and cause some dilation. They may hasten the onset of labour. A Foley balloon catheter or water-absorbent materials, such as Laminaria, are placed within the cervix. (See page 270.)
- *Prostaglandins* come in a variety of forms (gel, a tampon-like device or a tablet). They are relatively non-invasive and are used especially when the cervix is unripe, firm and/or posterior ('unfavourable for induction'). Misoprostol, a recent addition to the prostaglandin agents used to ripen the cervix, is a different type of prostaglandin and is more likely than other prostaglandins to cause contractions along with cervical ripening. Sometimes, misoprostol (brand name Cytotec) is all that is needed to start labour and complete the birth. It can be given orally by pill or inserted into or next to the cervix in a gelatin capsule. The effects of misoprostol can be unpredictable, however. Sometimes it seems to work very smoothly, but sometimes it causes sudden onset of long, painful contractions that do not ease until the birth. Once administered, removal of misoprostol is difficult (a vaginal douche may have to be used), and side effects of uterine hyper-stimulation and foetal distress are not unusual. Women are often shocked and distressed by these effects. Dosage and timing are factors in the safety of misoprostol, and many concerned practitioners are reluctant to use it until optimal doses are scientifically established.[9] (See page 274.)
- *Artificial rupture of the membranes (AROM),* also called *amniotomy,* is a form of induction sometimes done alone or along with Syntocinon, if your cervix is found to be favourable for the procedure. AROM is rarely successful if your cervix is unfavourable. When combined with Syntocinon, AROM increases the success rate of induction when compared to using Syntocinon alone. Therefore, if the induction is medically indicated, it may be desirable to use AROM. On the other hand, AROM represents a 'commitment to delivery'. In other words, once the membranes are ruptured, the labour must proceed, and an unsuccessful induction (for example, no labour progress) means that a caesarean will be performed. As long as your membranes remain intact, if the induction is being done for a non-medical reason and is unsuccessful, the induction might be discontinued for a few days and a caesarean possibly averted. (See page 271.)

Even if AROM was not performed to start labour, it is frequently done once labour has begun in hopes of speeding

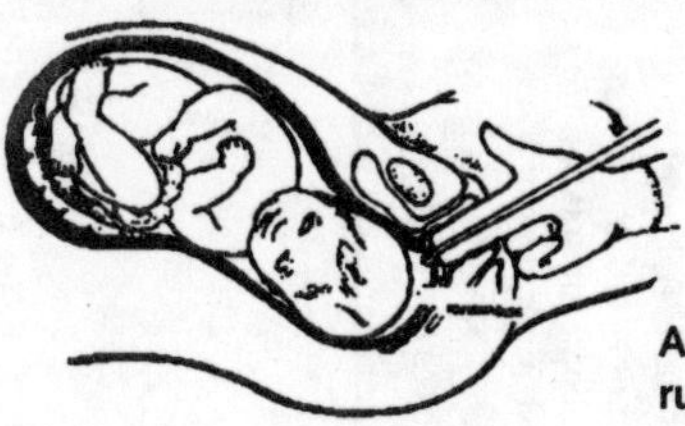

Artificial rupture of membranes

the process. Sometimes, the bag of waters is bulging through the cervix during contractions, and breaking it causes the baby's head to press firmly on the cervix. Contractions often become suddenly more painful, and labour progress does indeed speed up. Without AROM, the membranes often remain intact until the second stage of labour. If the baby's head is mal-positioned, intact membranes may provide some cushioning and a little room for the baby's head to wiggle into a more favourable position. Removing the cushion by rupturing the membranes sometimes fixes the baby's head and impairs these subtle movements, possibly causing a longer or more painful labour.[10] (See page 309.)

- *Intravenous (IV) Syntocinon infusion* is almost always used for medical induction. Syntocinon causes the uterus to contract, but it does not ripen the cervix. Therefore, when the cervix is thick, posterior and unripe, use of prostaglandin precedes the Syntocinon infusion. With this method, the prostaglandin is inserted in or next to the cervix once or twice or more within a period of a day or two. Then intravenous Syntocinon is given. The dosage is usually low at the beginning and increased periodically until the desired contraction pattern (three contractions in ten minutes) is reached. If the induction is going very slowly and the woman's membranes are intact, the Syntocinon is often discontinued at night to allow the mother to eat and sleep. This gradual approach, even though it may avoid a caesarean, can be emotionally and physically draining for the mother and her partner. Extra support and patience are essential with this type of induction. (See page 274 for more on Syntocinon.)

Non-Drug Methods of Cervical Ripening and/or Labour Induction

Most of the following methods have been used for many decades. However, they are slower in ripening the cervix and less effective in inducing labour than combinations of prostaglandins, Syntocinon and amniotomy. If the need for induction is urgent for the wellbeing of mother and baby, the methods below are not the best choice. However, if the need is less urgent, these inexpensive, less invasive, low-risk methods might be considered. (Also, see the chart on page 272, 'Herbs and Drugs for Cervical Ripening and/or Labour Induction'.)

Method/How It Is Done	How It Is Thought to Work	Benefits and/or Purposes	Possible Risks and/or Disadvantages	Comments
Sexual intercourse, clitoral stimulation, orgasm We assume you know how to do these…	• Orgasm with or without intercourse is associated with the release of oxytocin, which causes contractions. • Semen contains prostaglandins, which ripen the cervix.	• Even if it does not start labour, sex may ripen the cervix. • May be more pleasurable for most people than other methods	• Orgasm is sometimes difficult to achieve when trying to start labour. • Contractions may subside shortly after lovemaking stops.	• Intercourse should not occur once membranes are ruptured, because the chance of infection in mother or foetus increases. • See page 264 for more information.
Nipple stimulation Mother or partner lightly strokes one or both nipples, pauses during contractions, and resumes after the contractions. May continue nipple stimulation for hours. Other options for nipple stimulation include using a breast pumpor oral stimulation.	• Increases oxytocin production and causes contractions • May not ripen cervix (which is caused by prostaglandin), but sometimes starts labour if cervix is ripe	• May be able to avoid other forms of induction	• Difficult to regulate 'dose' of oxytocin • Some cases of foetal distress have been reported with foetuses already known to be at high risk. • Mother may tire of nipple stimulation. • Contractions may stop when nipple stimulation is discontinued, which may be discouraging.	• Should not be done by a woman at high risk • Should be discontinued if contractions come more frequently than every four minutes or last longer than one minute • Some caregivers prefer that the foetal heart rate be monitored closely during nipple stimulation for a few contractions at the beginning. • See pages 264–265.

Non-Drug Methods of Cervical Ripening and/or Labour Induction

Method/How It Is Done	How It Is Thought to Work	Benefits and/or Purposes	Possible Risks and/or Disadvantages	Comments
Enema Small volume of pre-mixed solution is squirted into rectum by mother or nurse.	• Stimulates prostaglandin production from contractions of bowel	• If successful, avoids need for other induction methods • Does not require close monitoring • May ripen cervix even if it does not start labour	• Discomfort to mother • Rarely successful in starting labour • Some women find enemas objectionable.	• Rarely used today • Sometimes used before Syntocinon induction to empty bowels (which usually happens as part of spontaneous onset of labour) • See page 264.
Acupuncture (manual or electrical stimulation) Needles are applied at specific acupuncture points. Needles are then spun and/or heated; electrical current may also be added.	• Unblocks energy flow lines along critical meridians. Blocked energy is thought to impair the onset of labour. • Western medicine has no clear explanation for how acupuncture works.	• If successful, avoids need for other induction methods • May appeal especially to those interested in Chinese medicine or complementary (alternative) medicine	• Requires additional training for caregiver or referral to an acupuncturist (additional cost) • Uncertainty regarding success rate and possible risks	• Acupuncture is not understood or used by most North American medical practitioners. • Scientific evaluation for this purpose is lacking; effectiveness is unknown.
Acupressure Finger pressure on two specific points: • *Spleen 6:* on lower leg, 4 finger breadths above one or both inner ankle bones • *Hoku:* on bony point at the V of the fleshy notch on the back of the hand between base of thumb and forefinger Apply pressure in on-off cycles of 10–60 seconds each for up to 6 cycles.	• Thought to be similar to though less effective than acupuncture (described above)	• If successful, starts contractions or increases their frequency.	• Should not be practised by women before term, as may increase risk of preterm labour	• No scientific evaluation of its effectiveness • See page 263 for illustrations of acupressure points.

Non-Drug Methods of Cervical Ripening and/or Labour Induction

Method/How It Is Done	How It Is Thought to Work	Benefits and/or Purposes	Possible Risks and/or Disadvantages	Comments
Laminaria Thin, highly absorbent material (dried seaweed is in Laminaria) is inserted into cervix where it remains for hours. Water absorbed from surrounding tissue causes the material to swell and expand the cervical opening.	• Mechanically dilates cervix gradually • May stimulate prostaglandin production	• Less invasive than some other forms of induction • Does not require close monitoring • Can be used more than once • Can be used outside the hospital	• Low rate of success • Once Laminaria is removed, cervix often closes again. • Mother may have to remain in bed (to keep material from falling out). • Infection and unintentional ROM more likely than with some other methods.	• Use is declining because newer induction methods are more successful. • See page 266.
Balloon catheter A Foley balloon catheter (same as that used to empty the bladder) is inserted through the cervix, filled with 30 ml saline, and pulled back so the balloon presses against the internal cervical opening.	• Mechanically dilates the cervix • May stimulate prostaglandin production	• Can be removed easily and quickly • Does not require hospitalisation or close monitoring	• Unintentional ROM more likely than with less invasive methods • Few studies of effectiveness have been done.	• Although used infrequently today, has a growing group of enthusiastic proponents • Requires further study • The balloon slips out when the cervix has opened. • Can be left in for hours or days • See page 266.
Stripping (sweeping) the membranes Caregiver inserts a finger into the internal cervical opening and separates membranes from the lower uterine segment. If cervix is too closed, it is massaged vigorously.	• Increases prostaglandin production after 37 weeks	• Particularly useful if cervix is unfavourable for induction • Reduces the need for other methods of induction when mother is past due date • Can be repeated • Can be done outside the hospital	• Increased risk of infection and unintentional ROM • Bleeding if placenta is previa or low-lying • Painful for mother	• Women often pass brownish discharge hours later and confuse it with 'bloody show'. • See page 266.

Non-Drug Methods of Cervical Ripening and/or Labour Induction

Method/How It Is Done	How It Is Thought to Work	Benefits and/or Purposes	Possible Risks and/or Disadvantages	Comments
Amniotomy (Artificial Rupture of Membranes—AROM) *(also used to speed labour; see page 309)* Caregiver inserts an amniotomy hook through the cervix and makes a hole in the membranes, releasing amniotic fluid. Procedure is often done in conjunction with Syntocinon for induction.	• Increases prostaglandin production • If foetal head moves down with AROM, there may be some mechanical pressure-induced dilation.	• When used with Syntocinon, reduces length of labour, compared to Syntocinon alone • The procedure is no more painful than a vaginal exam. • Allows caregiver to check amniotic fluid for meconium, to assess foetal well-being	• Increased risk of maternal or foetal infection • Increased risk of prolapsed cord (if foetus is at a high station) • Once AROM has been done, there is a commitment to delivery (the baby must be born, even by caesarean, if labour goes on too long). • Requires some dilation of the cervix before it can be done • Increased risk of foetal distress due to cord compression • If done to speed labour, may increase discomfort of contractions • If baby's head is subtly mal-positioned, AROM may prevent it from correcting itself, thus prolonging labour.	• If induction with AROM is unsuccessful, a caesarean is necessary because of the risk of infection. If induction without AROM is unsuccessful, the Syntocinon can be turned off and the woman can rest and possibly avoid a caesarean. • AROM is sometimes done in spontaneous labour to speed progress; it is sometimes successful. • AROM is necessary for internal electronic foetal monitoring. (See page 311.) • Intravenous antibiotics may be used if membranes are ruptured for several hours. • See page 266 for more information.

Herbs and Drugs for Cervical Ripening and/or Labour Induction

If induction of labour becomes necessary, the first step is to be sure the cervix is ripe, effaced and ready to dilate. If it is not ripe, prostaglandins or other substances may be used to prepare the cervix for induction with Syntocinon (discussed below). Sometimes, the ripening agents not only ripen the cervix, they start the labour without the need for Syntocinon. Some self-induction and manual and mechanical techniques that are not included in this chart are described in another chart, 'Non-Drug Methods of Cervical Ripening and/or Labour Induction'. Please consult a knowledgeable practitioner when using these agents and methods.

Types and Names of Specific Agents	How Given	Benefits and/or Purposes	Possible Risks and/or Disadvantages	Comments
Cervical Ripening Agents				
Herbal preparations • Blue and/or black cohosh • Evening primrose oil • Other herbs	*Cohosh:* • Tea • Tincture (drops) under the tongue hourly until cervix is ripe *Evening primrose:* • Capsules by mouth • Oil applied directly to cervix	• Hastens ripening of cervix • Teas, tinctures and capsules can be self-administered by mother.	• Scientific evidence is lacking; success rates are unknown. • Side effects may include stomach upsets, increased blood pressure, nausea and others.	• These preparations are not used in conventional obstetrics but are popular with some midwives and alternative practitioners. An herbalist may be consulted for guidance. • Do not use these agents if you have high blood pressure.
Homeopathic solutions • Caulophyllum (tincture from blue cohosh) • Cimicituga • Pulsatilla • Other preparations	• Tablets taken orally or tinctures placed under the tongue, beginning as early as 36 weeks, increasing the dose until 40 weeks	• Hastens ripening of the cervix • Can be self-administered by mother	• Scientific evidence is lacking; success rates are unknown. • In the small doses administered, no side effects are thought to exist.	• These preparations are not used in conventional obstetrics, but are popular with some midwives and alternative practitioners. • Homeopathy uses very small doses of medication, based on the theory that homeopathic doses stimulate the body to take over the desired function. Choice of agent and dosage is based on many characteristics of the woman. • A trained, experienced homeopathic physician should supervise treatment.

Herbs and Drugs for Cervical Ripening and/or Labour Induction

Types and Names of Specific Agents	How Given	Benefits and/or Purposes	Possible Risks and/or Disadvantages	Comments
Castor oil	• The woman swallows 56 g castor oil mixed with 56 g orange juice and 1 tsp baking soda, then repeats using half the amount 1 and 2 hours later. • In eggs scrambled in 56 g castor oil; then, 1 and 2 hours later, in eggs scrambled in 28 g castor oil	• Hastens ripening of cervix; may start labour within 2–8 hours; empties bowel	• Causes intestinal cramps, diarrhoea for several hours • Little scientific evaluation of effectiveness • Frequently does not succeed • Has a bad taste	• May work by stimulating prostaglandin production • Best if started very early in the morning • Check with health care provider before using this intervention • See page 264.
Prostaglandin E2 (PGE2) • Prostaglandin gel • Prostin	• PGE2 gel may be mixed in a hospital pharmacy in varying doses and inserted into the vagina in or around the cervix with a syringe. Dose may be repeated after 4 and 8 hours. • Prostin, a commercially produced gel, is placed within or around the cervix with a syringe. Dose may be repeated after 6 and 12 hours.	• Hastens ripening of cervix; may trigger onset of labour • Women may be able to go home between doses of gel, after being observed and monitored for 1–2 hours. • Improves success of induction with Syntocinon	• Uterine hyper-stimulation and foetal distress, requiring quick removal and administration of a uterine inhibitor • Possible nausea, vomiting or diarrhoea • Pain at site of PGE2 • Requires caution if used in women with asthma, glaucoma, liver or kidney disease	• Hospital pharmacy preparations were all that were available until 1993, when commercial preparations became available. • Removal of gel by douching is awkward, slow and uncomfortable. • Syntocinon is usually begun about 1–2 hours after discontinuation of prostaglandin.

Herbs and Drugs for Cervical Ripening and/or Labour Induction

Types and Names of Specific Agents	How Given	Benefits and/or Purposes	Possible Risks and/or Disadvantages	Comments
Synthetic PGE (misoprostol) • Cytotec	• Tablet is placed in the vagina behind the cervix, or given orally.	• Low cost • Easy to administer • Can be repeated every 3 hours • Has lower rate of failed induction than other induction methods • More likely to start labour than Prostin	• Excessive, frequent uterine contractions • Requires repeated vaginal entry for repeated doses	• Misoprostol is the most recently introduced agent for cervical ripening and labour induction. • Few scientific trials have been done to establish optimal dosage, effectiveness and safety for mother or baby. • Not to be used for women who have had a prior caesarean
Labour Induction/Augmentation Agents				
Synthetic oxytocin • Syntocinon	• By IV, with an infusion pump to control dosage	• Causes uterine contractions and dilation of the cervix	• Uterine hyper-stimulation • Foetal distress • Longer labour in hospital and possibly greater pain than with spontaneous labour • Excessive fluid retention • Requires continuous electronic foetal monitoring, close nursing care	• Induction of labour is different from augmentation (speeding a slow labour). • Does not succeed if the cervix is unripe ('failed induction'), which leads to a caesarean • When done for convenience, benefits may not outweigh risks. • Early induction without clear due date may cause premature birth.

Drugs to Contract the Uterus after Birth

Types and Names of Specific Agents	How Given	Benefits and/or Purposes	Possible Risks and/or Disadvantages	Comments
Synthetic oxytocin • Syntocinon • Syntometrine **Ergot alkaloids** • Ergometrine **Prostaglandin F2x**	• By IV, intramuscular injection or by mouth (method varies according to drug) • Most caregivers routinely give a drug to contract the uterus as the baby is being born.	• Causes uterine contractions, to reduce the possibility of excessive bleeding after birth	• Nausea and vomiting • Headache • Possible increased chance of retained placenta or elevated blood pressure • Rare side effects include cardiac arrest, eclampsia (post partum) and pulmonary oedema.	• Nipple stimulation (by breastfeeding or with manual stimulation) and fundal massage are other ways to encourage the uterus to contract post partum.

Short, Fast Labour

Occasionally, labour lasts less than three hours. This *precipitate labour* is rare, especially in first-time mothers. Though a short labour may sound appealing, a precipitate labour presents its own special problems and challenges. The latent phase of a precipitate labour passes unnoticed or so quietly and uneventfully that you often miss the early signs of labour. Suddenly, you find yourself in active, hard labour without time to prepare psychologically. The first noticeable contractions can be long and very painful. You may feel confused, unprepared and even panicky. You may quickly lose faith in your ability to handle labour.

If you had been planning a hospital birth, you hurry off to the hospital while trying to cope with these strong, almost continuous labour contractions, all the time thinking that if this is early labour, the so-called easy part, how will you ever cope with the demands of active labour! You may feel overwhelmed by the thought of what is yet to come. At the hospital, you will probably be met with a flurry of activity and an unfamiliar doctor or midwife. You may feel anxious if your partner was unable to accompany you. Even if he or she is with you, you may feel alone and afraid. In fact, you may feel like giving up and taking all the medication available to you to make the pain go away. Your partner will be caught off guard, too, and may be shocked by the sudden intensity of your labour and surprised by your reaction to what he or she believes is early labour.

What You Can Do

Do not give up on yourself. Trust your ability to get through this. Try not to tense with your contractions. Try slow breathing; if that does not help, go to the light breathing. Have a vaginal exam before you make any decision about pain medication. You may have dilated to 8 or 10 centimetres. If labour has progressed this rapidly, birth will soon follow and anaesthesia may be unnecessary or may take effect too late to help you. You will need to focus on your self-help comfort measures. What you need most are reassurances that this labour is normal and frequent updates on your labour progress. You also need help from your partner or nurse in handling the painful contractions. In a rapid labour, your contractions will be intense and very effective, and you may have the urge to push before the hospital staff is ready. If this happens, lie on your side (rather than using an upright position) and pant or gently bear down.[11] Doing this will give your birth canal and perineum more time to stretch, will decrease the likelihood of tearing, and will help protect your baby's head from being pressed through the vagina too rapidly.

After the birth, you will probably feel relieved that you and the baby are safe, but stunned that everything is over so quickly. You may need to discuss what happened. Talk with the staff and your partner to put the pieces together. You may also experience disappointment because your labour passed so quickly and you were not able to appreciate it, use all the breathing and relaxation techniques, or share it with your partner as you had planned.

Rapid Birth without Medical Help

Sometimes, labour progresses too rapidly for you to get to the hospital in time or for your midwife to arrive for a home birth. Babies are occasionally born without professional care under these circumstances. What if you are alone or with only your partner when the baby starts to come? Initially, you may panic and temporarily forget all you know about labour, birth and coping techniques.

If the baby is truly about to be born, it is far better for you to stay at home, unattended, where it is warm and where you have some essential supplies, than to attempt to rush to the hospital. If the baby starts to come during your ride to the hospital, the driver will have to pull over to the side of the road, help you deliver your baby, and then continue to the hospital. Usually, babies born under these circumstances are in excellent condition, but the following guidelines will help you and your partner during such an emergency, to ensure the best possible outcome. The first question is: How will you know that the baby is really coming?

Signs That the Baby Is Really Coming

- You feel your body pushing (involuntary breath-holding and straining) and you cannot stop it.

- You or your partner sees the baby's head or presenting part at the vaginal opening.
- You feel the baby coming out.

Getting Help

- If you are alone when you have the above signs that birth is imminent, try to get help from someone nearby. If possible, call 000. Do not drive a car yourself.
- If you are riding in a car, the driver should pull over and do as many of the following as possible. If you are at home, the speed of your labour will dictate how much you can do before the birth.
- If you have not already done so, you or your partner should call the emergency care number (000) and request assistance. Tell them your baby is being born and give your location. Avoid sounding too calm—let them know they should come quickly. Paramedics are trained to handle emergency childbirth.
- You or your partner should call your caregiver's office or the labour-and-delivery unit of your hospital. Ask for help or emergency instructions.
- Call for someone to help you at home—your partner, a relative, a neighbour or a friend. Even children can help if they are told specifically what to do.

Before the Birth

Follow as many of these suggestions as time allows:

- Remove the clothing from the lower half of your body.
- Lie on your side or in a semi-sitting position in as warm and comfortable a place as possible (in bed or on the seat of your car) with clean towels or any clean piece of clothing under your buttocks. Be sure you are positioned so that there is a safe, clean place for the baby to land as he is born, so there will be no problem if the baby comes out too fast for an inexperienced person to 'catch' him. You or your partner may be able to gently press a hand on the baby's head as it comes out, to keep the baby from coming out too suddenly.
- Remain as relaxed as possible. Let your uterus do the work. Try not to push or bear down with the contractions; pant or blow through them.
- Your partner or attendant should quickly but calmly gather clean sheets, towels, receiving blankets, handkerchiefs and tissues. If none are available, use your own or your partner's jacket, shirt or other clothing. Keep these supplies nearby. If possible, put the towels or receiving blankets in a clothes dryer or warm (not hot) oven so they will be warm when the baby arrives. Do not use up all your warm and dry items during the birth. Save some to wrap the baby.
- Your partner should thoroughly wash his or her hands and arms up to the elbows.

During the Birth

When you and your partner first see the baby's scalp at the vagina, it will be wet and somewhat wrinkled, and it may be streaked with blood and vernix. The pressure of the baby's head bulges your perineum and opens your anus. With the contractions, you will see more and more of the baby's head. With labour progressing so rapidly, try not to bear down. Instead, raise your chin and pant or 'puh, puh' as lightly and rapidly as you can. Sometimes, as your baby's head descends, you will pass some stool (bowel movement). If this happens, your partner or attendant should wipe it away with tissues or toilet paper to keep the area clean. He or she should remind you to keep your thighs and pelvic floor muscles relaxed. As the head emerges from the vagina and as 'crowning' begins, make extra efforts to relax, pant and keep from pushing. If the head is delivered slowly, it lessens the risk of injury to the perineum.

Once the head has fully emerged, your partner or attendant should use the clean handkerchief or tissues to wipe away excess mucus from around the baby's nose and mouth. If the membranes cover the baby's face, he or she should break them with a fingernail and peel them away. Wipe the baby's face. Many babies are quite blue at first but turn pink quickly after birth once they start crying.

Your baby's head will probably be born facing your back. After the head is born, the baby will turn 90 degrees to face your thigh so the shoulders can be born. At this time, your partner or attendant can gently support the baby's head but should not pull on it. He or she should feel the baby's neck to see if the umbilical cord is around it. If so, the cord may slow the birth. Your partner or attendant should gently try to release the cord by slipping it over the baby's head.

With the next contractions, you can bear down smoothly to deliver the shoulders and the rest of the baby's body. You or your partner can support the rest of the baby's body; remember that it will be wet and slippery.

After the Birth

Care of the Baby

Usually, the baby begins breathing and crying immediately. Place the baby on her side or stomach on your bare abdomen, with her head slightly lower than her body, to drain any mucus remaining in her nose and mouth. Be sure her nose and mouth are clear so that she can breathe. Wipe away any mucus and dry the baby completely, especially her head, to help keep her warm. Cover her head with a hat or blanket to prevent further heat loss. She will stay warmest with her skin next to yours (with no blanket between you) and a warm blanket or any available cover over both of you.

Do not cut the cord. It is safer to wait until a doctor or midwife can clamp it properly and cut it with proper equipment. There is no rush because the blood vessels within the cord begin to close when the cord is exposed to air, automatically stopping the blood flow. You will know the blood flow has stopped when the cord stops pulsating.

Care of the Mother

Your contractions will resume after a slight lull, and they will cause the placenta to separate from the uterine wall and slide down into the vagina. Bear down to deliver it. You can kneel or squat if it does not come out easily. Do not pull on the cord. The placenta will normally come out within twenty minutes without difficulty. Place the placenta in a bowl or wrap it in a towel or newspapers and place it next to you. Place a sanitary pad, folded nappy or small towel on your perineum to absorb the heavy vaginal flow.

You can start breastfeeding right away. Doing so makes your uterus contract and reduces bleeding. Even if the baby does not suck, her nuzzling at your breast may cause your uterus to contract. Your uterus will be at the level of your navel, and should feel firm like a large grapefruit. If your uterus is not firm and the baby is not nursing, stroke your nipples or have your partner do it. In addition, massage your lower abdomen firmly until your uterus contracts. Do not continue the massage if your uterus is firm, but check it from time to time and massage again, if necessary.

You should get medical attention immediately. The baby's cord needs to be clamped and cut, and the baby should be checked. You should also be checked to make sure you delivered the entire placenta, your uterus remains contracted and there are no vaginal injuries. While you tend to the baby, have someone call the emergency aid number (000) if it has not already been called.

Quick Checklist for Emergency Birth

You should do these tasks if you are alone. If you have a partner or helper, then this person will assist you when appropriate.

1. Get help, if possible. Call your partner, the hospital and/or 000.
2. Gather clean sheets, towels, paper towels, tissues and extra clothing to be used during the birth and for the baby.
3. You and your partner should wash your hands, if possible.
4. Remove all clothing from your buttocks and vaginal area.
5. Lie down on your side or sit leaning back. Make sure you are in a clean place with enough room for the baby to rest as she slips out of the birth canal.
6. Put a sheet, towel or some clothing under your buttocks.
7. Try not to hold your breath if your body is pushing. Keep panting through each contraction until the baby is born.
8. After the baby comes out:
   - Wipe away any mucus from her nose and mouth.
   - Wipe her head and body to dry her.
   - Place her on your bare abdomen or chest.
   - Cover the baby using cloths, towels or clothing.
9. Do not cut the cord.
10. Breastfeed the baby, if possible.
11. If you are at home, await the birth of the placenta. If you are in a car, have your partner or another person drive you and the baby to the hospital.
12. Place the placenta nearby (still attached to the cord and the baby) in a bowl, newspaper or cloth.
13. Place towels or a pad between your legs to absorb the blood flow.
14. Get medical help as soon as possible to check both you and the baby.

Possible Problems

- *Baby does not breathe spontaneously.* Place the baby's head lower than her body and rub her back or chest briskly but gently. If she does not respond within thirty seconds, hold her ankles together and smack her soles sharply. If the baby still does not breathe, check for mucus in her mouth with your finger, then place the baby on her back and tilt her head back to straighten her airway from face to chest.

Place your mouth over her nose and mouth and your fingers on her chest. Blow gently until you feel or see her chest rise a little. *Do not blow hard.* Remove your mouth. Continue this sequence, one blow every three seconds, until the baby responds or medical help arrives. This is mouth-to-mouth resuscitation for an infant—one of the techniques used in infant CPR (cardiopulmonary resuscitation). Every parent should learn how to do infant CPR. Check with your hospital, fire department or St Johns Ambulance to find a course.

- *Excessive bleeding from the birth canal.* Some bleeding normally occurs after labour and delivery, both before and after the birth of the placenta. However, if you lose more than 2 cups of blood, you may be haemorrhaging. Haemorrhage is characterised by a steady flow of blood and symptoms of shock in the mother (rapid pulse, pale skin, trembling, faintness, cold, sweating). If you or your partner suspects haemorrhage, firmly massage the top of your uterus until it contracts, and encourage the baby to nurse (or stroke your nipples). To avoid shock, lie down. Your partner should raise the lower half of your body by placing pillows under your hips. If the bleeding appears to come from tears at the vaginal opening, press an ice pack and towels firmly against the perineum. Continue applying firm pressure. Call the hospital or 000 for assistance or go in to a hospital where the staff will assess you and give appropriate medical assistance.
- *Placenta does not come.* If the placenta does not come within twenty to thirty minutes, stand up or kneel to get the help of gravity. If it still does not come and no help has arrived, you or your partner will need to call the hospital for guidance. Do not pull on the cord.

In an emergency situation, your options are limited. Luckily, in most areas experienced paramedics are only minutes away. If an emergency home birth becomes necessary, remember what you have learned about relaxation, breathing techniques and the birth process. An emergency birth can be hectic, but if you respond calmly and wisely, the experience will always be precious to you, despite its unconventionality.

Prolonged Labour (First Stage)

A labour that lasts longer than twenty-four hours after progressing contractions begin is considered to be prolonged. (See page 220 for more on progressing contractions.) Prolonged labours are more common than fast ones and can be discouraging, tiring and worrisome. They are also a strain on your partner because of the lack of sleep, need for food, concerns for your wellbeing and a sense of helplessness in making it better for you. Your caregiver is more attentive when labour is prolonged, and is likely to suggest medication or interventions to monitor the baby more closely, to augment (strengthen) your contractions and to make you more comfortable. You can help yourself through such a labour if you understand what is going on so that you can pace yourself realistically, and if you know some self-comforting techniques and ways to correct the causes of prolonged labour. A sensitive, attentive midwife or other caring support people can advise and nourish both of you and give your partner a break.

More important to your caregiver than the length of labour is the phase of labour in which the progress slows. A long pre-labour (a long period of continuous non-progressing contractions) or a long latent phase can be very hard on you, but it is likely to correct itself and evolve into a normal labour pattern by the time you reach 4 or 5 centimetres. On the other hand, if your labour slows or stops in the active phase or later, your caregiver will be more concerned and will probably want to try medical ways to speed it up.

Prolonged Pre-labour or Latent Phase

If dilation is slow in getting started or you are experiencing a long latent phase, do not assume that your entire labour will be prolonged. In most cases, labour will progress normally once you reach the active phase. The most probable causes for a slow-to-start labour are the following:

- Your cervix has not yet undergone some of the changes that prepare it to dilate. In other words, it has not yet moved forward, ripened or effaced. (See 'The Six Steps to Birth', page 216.) Your early contractions must accomplish these things before they can effectively open the cervix. Your cervix needs time, and you need patience and stamina. Remember that a slow early labour is not a complication; labour progress often improves once the latent phase is finally complete.
- A scarred cervix (from previous surgery, cone biopsy or other procedures on the cervix) sometimes delays its dilation. A long period of frequent and intense contractions may be necessary to overcome the resistance caused by scar tissue. When dilation finally begins, the labour usually proceeds normally.
- A mal-positioned baby, most commonly an occiput posterior baby, is often associated with back pain and a prolonged pre-labour. Your contraction pattern may seem very irregular, or you may notice that your contractions come in pairs followed by a longer pause (referred to as 'coupling' of contractions). Once the baby's position improves the back pain disappears, the contraction pattern improves and progress speeds up.
- Emotional stress, anxiety or tension may also contribute to a prolonged pre-labour or latent phase of labour.

What You Can Do

Each time you have a vaginal exam, find out whether your cervix has undergone the early changes necessary for dilation to take place. Ask if your cervix has moved from posterior to anterior, whether it is ripe and how much effacement has taken place. If it has not yet changed very much, you will need to pace yourself psychologically to accept that your cervix needs time to prepare to dilate.

Try not to become discouraged or depressed. Visualise the contractions bringing your cervix forward, ripening and effacing it. Try to accept your slow progress as temporary and appropriate under the circumstances. Nurture yourself with food and drink. Alternate among distracting, restful and labour-stimulating activities. You probably cannot sleep (if you could there would be no problem!), but you may find you can get more rest in a tub (filled high with warm water) than anywhere else. Baths also sometimes temporarily slow a non-productive labour pattern, thus giving you more rest. Once you have rested, try the various methods of stimulating labour. (See pages 263–265.) Try distractions such as a movie, a walk outdoors, food preparation, a shopping trip, or a visit with friends or relatives. Think of something to do that helps keep your mind off the contractions. You do not need to time every contraction. Time four or five contractions in a row, then wait a few hours or until the labour has changed before timing another series of contractions.

If you have slow progress, back pain, and/or painful and irregular or 'coupling' contractions, assume that your baby is occiput posterior and try to relieve your pain and help your baby rotate to the more favourable occiput anterior position using the techniques described on pages 285–290. If worry, emotional stress and tension are prolonging your early labour, it is most helpful to have kind, patient support people and nurses or caregivers around you. Of course, it is always helpful if you have identified nagging fears, concerns or self-doubts ahead of time and have addressed them. A previous difficult birth experience; stress in your relationship with your partner, caregiver or family members; fears about your own or your baby's wellbeing; and many other factors create emotional stress that sometimes interferes with labour progress. If you can talk to your caregiver, counsellor or childbirth educator about such feelings and disclose them in your birth plan, you may be able to identify ways to help you feel safer and less stressed during labour. You may also use your relaxation techniques and slow breathing to calm yourself and ease the pain.

Medical Care

If your contractions become exhausting or continue without progress for more than twenty-four hours, you and your caregiver may turn to medical interventions. There are two major approaches: attempting to stop the contractions and help you rest with medications, or stimulating more effective contractions. Such drugs as tranquillisers, sedatives or pethidine may be used to try to stop contractions or help you rest. These drugs should not be used without good reason, because they reach the baby and have effects on the baby similar to those on the mother (sleepiness, unclear thinking, lowered oxygen levels and other effects). To stimulate effective contractions, your caregiver may suggest procedures such as stripping the membranes, mechanically ripening or dilating your cervix, breaking your bag of waters, ripening your cervix with prostaglandins or inducing labour with Syntocinon.

If you have had previous surgery on your cervix and your early labour is very painful with little or no progress over a period of hours, assume that scar tissue is the cause. The same measures as those described above may be used to help you rest or to ripen your cervix. In addition, once your cervix has begun to change, your caregiver may open it a few centimetres with his or her fingers. Though painful, this procedure is done rather quickly and, if successful, causes your cervix to begin dilating; labour progress may then continue normally. You may request pain medications—such as IV or intramuscular narcotics or spinal narcotics ('walking epidural')—earlier in labour than you might if your cervix were dilating more rapidly.

Prolonged Active Phase

Labour that slows or stops once the active phase (4 centimetres or more) has begun may present more serious clinical problems than a prolonged latent phase. A prolonged active phase can result from inefficient uterine contractions, an unfavourable presentation or position of the baby, a small pelvis or a combination of these factors. Immobility, restriction to bed, a full bladder, some medications, fear, anxiety and stress may also contribute to a prolonged active phase.

What You Can Do

The solution will depend on the problem. For example, a full bladder can delay the baby's rotation and descent (and increase your pain), so empty your bladder every hour. If you have received drugs that may have slowed your labour, allow time for them to wear off, if it is safe to do so. If you have been lying still in one position, try walking or standing (positions that make use of gravity), or try shifting positions in bed from lying on one side or another to sitting or to resting on your hands and knees. You can use these positions even if you are attached to an IV line and an electronic foetal monitor. To enhance contraction effectiveness, try nipple stimulation, walking and standing. To improve the position of the baby within your pelvis, try the techniques described on pages 285–287.

Factors such as how rested you are, the amount of pain you have, your state of mind and the quality of emotional support you have will influence whether and how long you can use the measures mentioned above.

If you are discouraged, tired, anxious or fearful, you will need reassurance, encouragement, help with relaxation, and other comfort measures such as a bath, massage or shower. Ask for help, not only from your partner, but also from the staff. Do not neglect these resources—they can sustain you.

Medical Care

During a prolonged active phase, you can expect your caregivers to closely evaluate the progress of your labour and the wellbeing of your baby. You will probably have more vaginal exams to check for progress in dilation, descent or rotation. Your caregiver will want to monitor your baby's heart rate more, probably with the electronic foetal monitor. IV fluids to prevent dehydration and medications for relaxation and pain relief become more likely and more welcome if your labour is unduly long. Your doctor or midwife may rupture your membranes in an attempt to speed the labour, or administer Syntocinon to increase the frequency and intensity of your contractions.

Even if you had been planning a home or birth-centre birth, you will go to the hospital if you need Syntocinon or if your baby is having trouble tolerating labour. Prolonged active labour is the most common reason for transfer to the hospital during labour.

If the baby is under stress, as indicated by the foetal heart rate in response to contractions, or if labour continues to lag, even with Syntocinon, you and your doctor may decide a caesarean birth is necessary.

The Occiput Posterior and Other Unfavourable Foetal Positions

One of the most common reasons for a prolonged active phase is the occiput posterior (OP) position, in which the back of the baby's head is towards the mother's back. Approximately one woman in four begins labour with the baby in the OP position; this is associated with longer labours because the baby must rotate further to get to the anterior position. Dilation and descent may not take place as efficiently when the baby is OP. By transition, however, most babies in the OP position have turned to an occiput anterior position (OA), though some turn even later. Other 'persistent' occiput posterior babies are born in that position with their faces towards their mother's front (sometimes called a 'sunny-side-up' delivery). If your baby is OP, you may have considerable back pain during and sometimes between contractions, because the hard round part of your baby's head (the occiput) presses on your sacrum (lower back), straining the sacroiliac joints and causing pain in the entire lower back area.

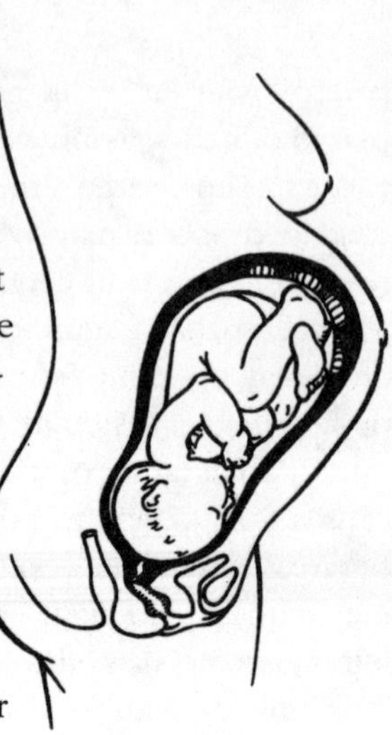

Occiput posterior

Sometimes a prolonged active labour is caused by a different, subtler mal-position than the OP position. The baby's head may be tilted slightly to one side. This is called *asynclitism*. In asynclitism, the baby's head does not press evenly against the cervix or fit through the pelvis as well as when the head is centred on the cervix. Asynclitism is difficult to diagnose. It is not as clearly associated with back pain as is the OP position. The best clues are a delay in dilation or uneven dilation—resulting in a cervical 'lip' (in which a part of the cervix does not dilate, while the rest of it dilates completely)—or the cervix may swell and seem to close. After the birth of an asynclitic baby, the shape of his head is also a good clue. If there is some off-centre elongation or swelling of the top of the head, it indicates which part of the head was coming first. When the baby's head is tilted, it is similar to the baby having a large head; the presenting part is larger than when the vertex (top centre of the baby's head) is coming first.

What You Can Do

It is not really necessary for you to know if your baby is asynclitic, OP or mal-positioned in some other way. (See page 284.) When you and your caregiver recognise that you have a backache during contractions and/or have a very slow progressing labour, you will select several of the measures described on the following pages, based on your signs and symptoms. Once the baby rotates to the occiput anterior position, the back pain usually subsides. Rotation can take place anytime during labour—sometimes quite early, sometimes very late.

The two main aims with a mal-positioned baby are to correct the baby's position and deal with any back pain, if it occurs.

To Correct the Baby's Position

- Try to find out the position of the baby (for example, right or left occiput posterior). This information is helpful but not crucial to success in turning the baby. You may be able to tell by noting where you feel most small movements (kicking and punching). Because the baby's hand and foot movements are probably opposite where his back is, feeling those movements in the front of your abdomen may indicate that he is in an OP position. If you feel movements more in your right front rather than your left front, the baby is likely to be in a left occiput posterior position. Also, your midwife or doctor can usually tell the position by palpating your abdomen to locate your baby's back, or by feeling the baby's head during a vaginal exam.
- *For pre-labour and in early labour*, use the following positions and movements to help turn the baby: open knee-chest, leaning forward, pelvic rocking and abdominal lifting. (See below for descriptive details.)
- *In active labour and during second stage*, use all the positions except the open knee-chest position.

Maternal Positions and Movements Used with an Occiput Posterior (OP) Foetal Position:

Some of the following positions are marked with an asterisk (*). With these positions and movements, knowing whether your baby is LOP or ROP is helpful. If you do not know if your baby is LOP or ROP, try them on each side for a few contractions, and use the side that feels most comfortable. With the positions and movements not marked by an asterisk, you do not need to know whether the baby is LOP or ROP.

1. Open knee-chest.
From a hands-and-knees position, move your knees backwards

and outwards and then lower your head and chest to the floor or bed. Be sure your buttocks are high in the air and your thighs are angled away from your belly so that your knees are slightly behind your buttocks. Try to remain in that position for thirty to forty-five minutes. Your partner can help you maintain the position by kneeling beside you (facing your head), placing his or her hands on your shoulders, and pulling up and back slightly. This position may help re-position an OP baby if it is used during very early labour.

2. Leaning forward.

Forward-leaning positions—such as being on hands and knees or kneeling; standing; or sitting while leaning over a birth ball, the labour bed or a counter—may help rotate the baby. They also relieve back pain caused by the pressure of the baby's head on your sacrum.

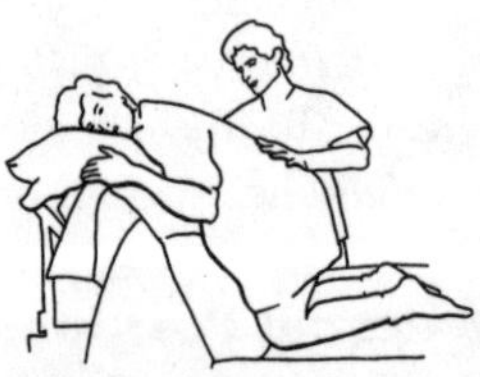

3. Pelvic rocking.

While kneeling and leaning forward, rock your pelvis forward and back (see page 133 for a description) or in a circle. The rocking helps dislodge the baby within your pelvis, and the position encourages rotation from the OP position.

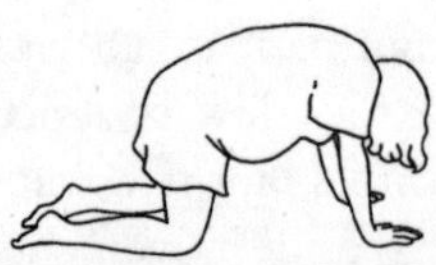

4. Abdominal lifting.

While standing, interlock your fingers and place your hands against your pubic bone. During the contractions, lift your abdomen up and slightly in while bending your knees. This often relieves back pain while improving the position of your baby in your pelvis.

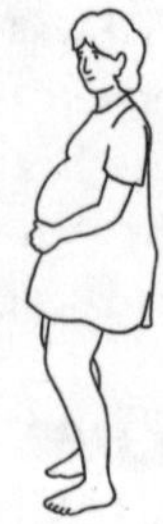

5. Abdominal stroking.*

While you are on hands and knees, your partner can reach beneath your abdomen and firmly and repeatedly stroke across your abdomen in the direction the baby should rotate (from the side of your body where the baby's back is to the other side). The stroking should feel good. It is usually better to do it between, not during, contractions. Cease the movement if you feel any discomfort, and do not try the movement if you do not know the baby's position.

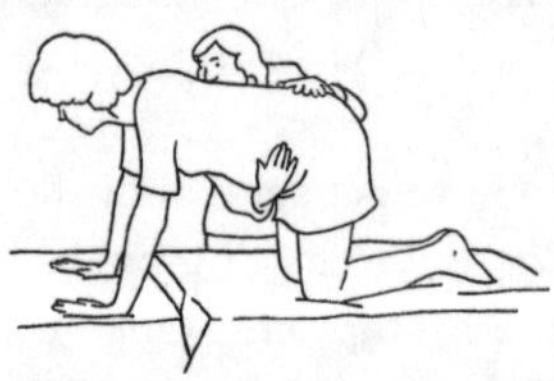

6. Standing, walking and stair climbing.

Take advantage of gravity in encouraging descent of the baby. In addition, the alignment of the baby with the pelvis is thought to be most favourable for descent when you are in an upright position. Walking or stair climbing allows some movement within the pelvic joints, which may also encourage rotation of the baby.

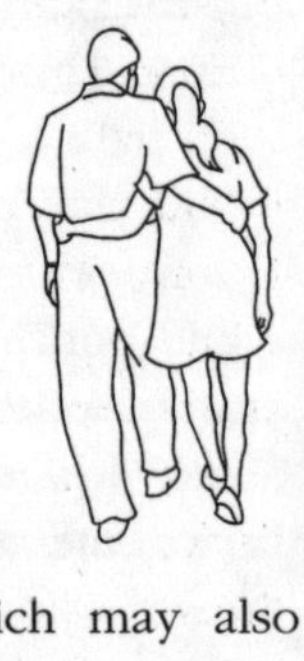

7. Slow dancing.
Standing and swaying side to side while being embraced by your partner is a pleasant alternative to walking.

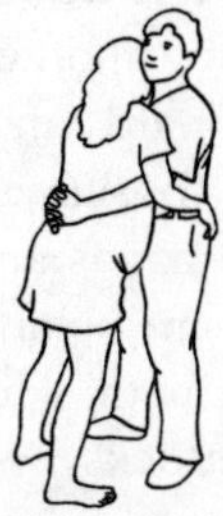

8. The lunge.*
Stand near a chair positioned next to your right or left side. Place the foot closer to the chair on the chair seat, extending your leg to that side. Make sure the chair cannot slide away. Remaining upright, slowly lunge or lean sideways towards the chair (bending the knee of the leg on the chair). You should feel the insides of both thighs stretching. Stay in the lunge for a slow count of five, and then return to upright. Repeat during contractions for five or six contractions in a row. If you know the baby's position, lunge towards the side where her back is. If you do not know the baby's position, try lunging in each direction and then continue with the direction that is most comfortable.

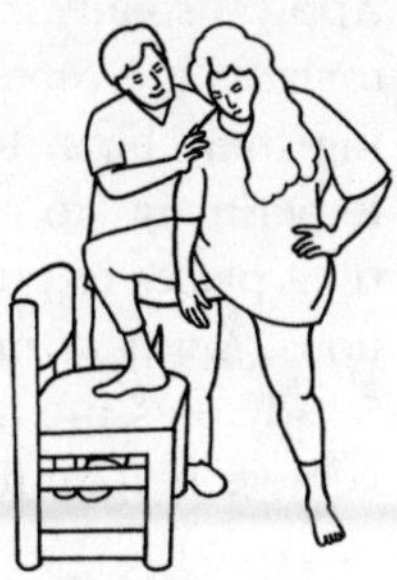

9. Side-lying.*
Lie on your side with both hips and knees flexed and with a pillow between your knees. Lie on the *same* side as the side where your baby's occiput is. If the baby is left OP, lie on your left side; if right OP, lie on your right side; if direct OP, try either side and look for some rotation of the baby's back towards that side.

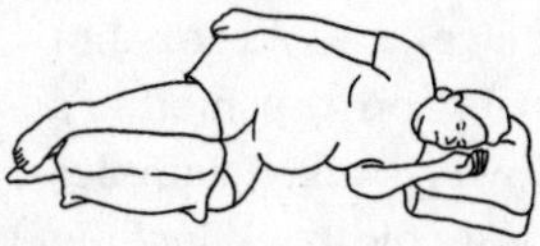

10. Semi-prone.*
Lie on your side with your lower arm behind you and your lower leg straight out. Flex your upper hip and knee, rest your knee on a doubled-up pillow, and roll towards your front. Lie on the side *opposite* the baby's occiput. If your baby is left OP, lie on your right side; if right OP, lie on your left side.

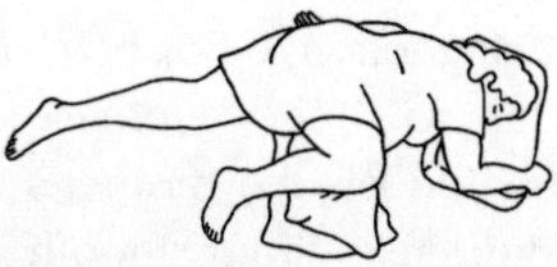

To Relieve Back Pain

- To reduce the pressure of the baby's head on your back during labour contractions, use positions that take advantage of gravity (hands-and-knees, leaning forward, side-lying and semi-prone) or use movements that decrease back pain (abdominal lifting and the lunge).
- Have your partner use the following measures to make you more comfortable and to reduce back pain. The techniques that use external pressure by the partner may work because they change the shape of the pelvis that has been affected by the internal pressure of the mal-positioned foetal head. If any measure causes more pain or does not help, the partner should discontinue it.

Techniques Used by the Partner and Comfort Measures to Relieve Back Pain

1. Massage of the lower back and buttocks.

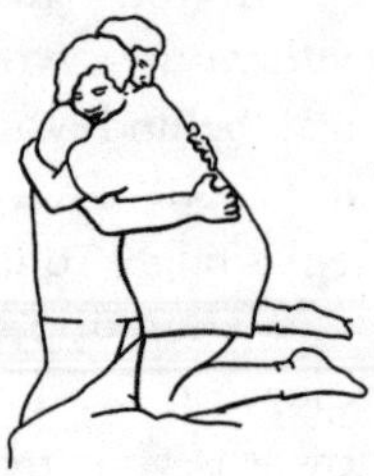

Using lotion, oil or powder to help decrease friction on the mother's skin, use firm, smooth stroking or kneading massage. She will tell you how she wants you to do it.

2. Counterpressure.

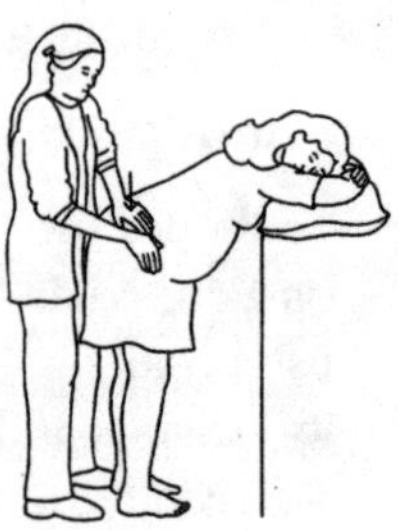

Holding the front of the mother's hip with one hand (to help her maintain balance), press steadily and firmly (with your fist or the heel of your hand) in one spot in the lower back or buttocks area. She will help you know what spot to press—it varies from woman to woman and over time within the same labour. Try pressing in several places. She will tell you when you have found a spot that brings relief.

For best results, press quite hard during every contraction. This measure is very helpful in coping with back pain. Between contractions, you may massage the area or use cold or hot compresses. (See description at right.)

3. The double hip squeeze.

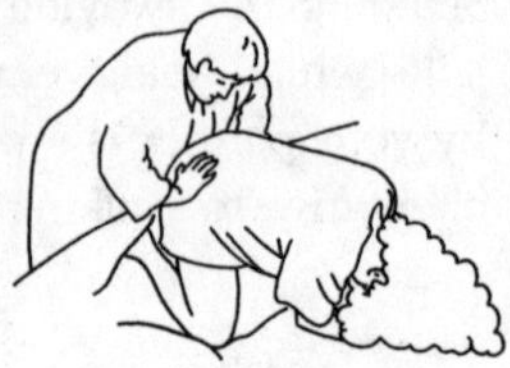

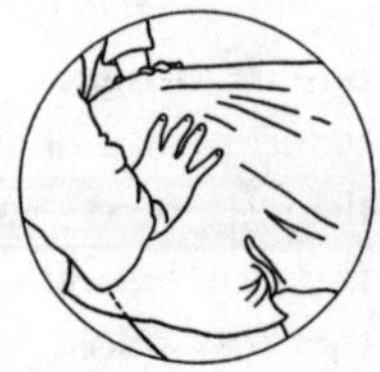

The mother leans forward and kneels or positions herself on hands and knees. From behind, press on both sides of her buttocks with the palms of your hands. Apply steady pressure towards the centre (pressing her hips together). Experiment to find the right places to press. Do this during contractions. Apply as much pressure as she needs. Steady pressure throughout each contraction is more helpful than pressing on and off.

4. The knee press.

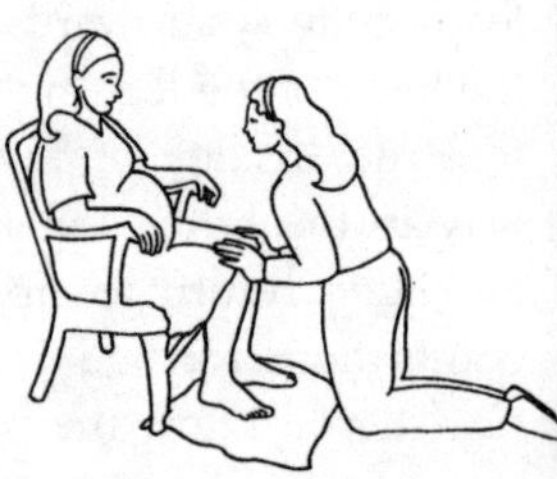

The mother sits upright in a chair that will not slide. You kneel on the floor in front of her and cup one hand over each knee and lean towards her so that you are pressing straight back towards her hip joints. This action releases tension and discomfort in her lower back.

5. Cold or hot compresses.

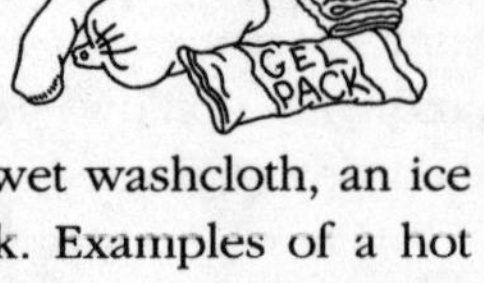

Place a cold or hot pack on the mother's lower back. Examples of a cold pack include a cold cloth, a frozen wet washcloth, an ice bag or a cold gel pack. Examples of a hot pack include a hot water bottle, a warm moist towel wrapped in plastic, a heated rice-filled pack or a warm blanket.

Cold is usually more effective because of its numbing effects. Before applying a cold pack, *be sure the mother is warm.* If her hands, feet and nose are cold, wrap her in a warm blanket and put socks on her before applying the cold pack. *Be sure there are one or more layers of cloth between her skin and the cold or hot pack,* both to protect her skin and to help ensure a gradual, rather than sudden, increase in cold or warmth.

6. Bath or shower.

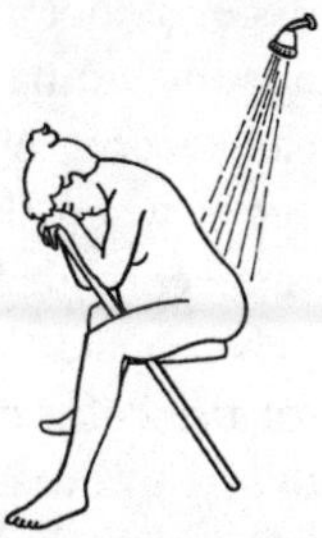

Both baths and showers are relaxing and often help a great deal with back pain. Directing the shower against the mother's lower back helps immensely.

7. Rolling pressure over the lower back.

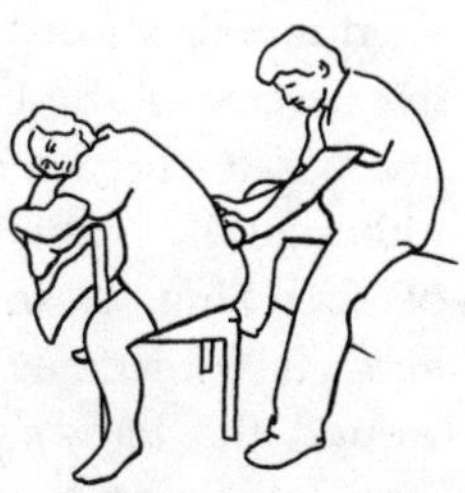

A rolling pin—or better yet, a hollow rolling pin filled with ice, a can of frozen juice or a cold can of soft drink—rolled over the mother's lower back is soothing during and between contractions. To ensure having a cold 'roller' in the hospital room, you may want to keep a few cans of soft drink on ice in a bowl or small cooler.

Medical Care

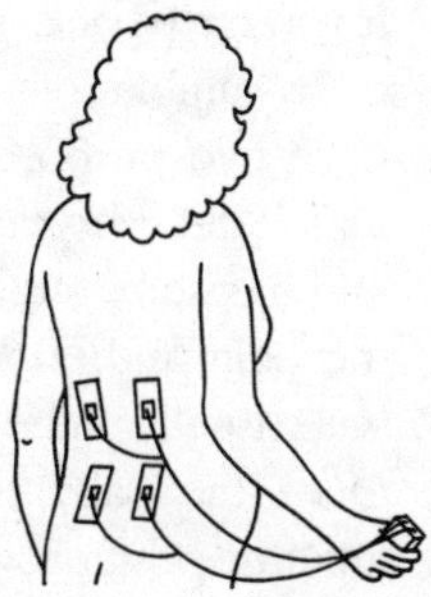

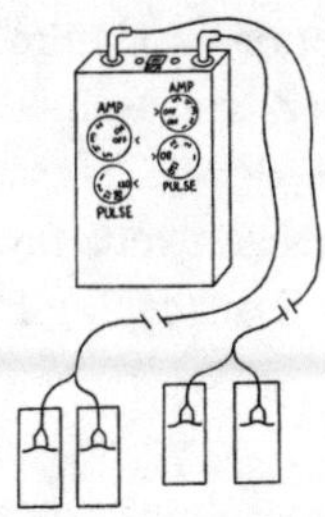

Transcutaneous electrical nerve stimulation (TENS) can be used during contractions as a method of back pain relief. Four stimulating pads placed on the mother's back are connected to a small hand-held generator that produces buzzing or prickly sensations over the back. The TENS unit has several dials that control the intensity of the sensation and change the pattern of the stimulation (quick or slow pulses, 'bursts', waves and other patterns). Either you or your partner holds and controls the unit. When the contraction begins, you turn up the intensity to the desired level. The sensations reduce your awareness of the back pain. When the contraction ends, you turn the unit down. Some women have found TENS helpful while others have not. If your caregiver is unfamiliar with TENS, a physiotherapist can advise you on its use during labour.

Medication for pain relief. You may also ask for pain medications if you have severe back pain. (See Chapter 12 for discussion of medication options.)

Conclusion

If you have back pain in labour because of an unfavourable foetal position, your efforts will have two purposes: to get the baby to turn and to relieve your back pain. The positions and measures suggested above will help ease the pain and, along with your contractions, will usually encourage the baby to rotate. Once the baby has rotated to the occiput anterior position, the back pain usually subsides. Rotation can take place anytime during labour—sometimes quite early, sometimes very late. Sometimes, with a persistent OP, the doctor assists rotation manually or with forceps. Very few babies do not rotate and are born facing forward ('sunny-side-up').

Prolonged Labour (Second Stage)

Sometimes labour progress slows or stops after the cervix is fully dilated, for many of the same reasons that cause a prolonged active phase. In these cases, the prolonged second stage may be handled with the same measures.

In addition, there are other possible problems that can arise only in the second stage. If not resolved, these problems may need to be handled by performing a caesarean section. A delay in the second stage can occur when the pelvic inlet (upper part) is large enough for the baby to enter, but the pelvic outlet (lower part) is not large enough for the baby to easily rotate and descend. If this is the case, problems do not arise until late in labour when the baby is quite low in the pelvis.

Another possible (but rare) problem is a short umbilical cord, which sometimes limits the descent of the baby or causes the foetal heart rate to slow during contractions. Although the umbilical cord is quite capable of stretching, it sometimes cannot stretch enough. Sometimes, a cord that is wrapped around the baby's neck or trunk has the same effect as a short cord. However, in most cases when the cord is wrapped around the baby, it is still long enough not to be a problem.

A third (also rare) problem occurs if the birth of the baby's shoulders is delayed *(shoulder dystocia)* after the birth of the head. This serious complication arises when the shoulders are so broad or in such a position that they do not fit through the pelvis. It is usually not possible to do a caesarean section after the head is out. Instead, skilled manoeuvres by the doctor or midwife, with the cooperation of the mother, are used to rotate the baby and deliver the shoulders. Time is of the essence, since the baby's oxygen supply from the cord may be reduced.

What You Can Do

If your baby is not descending during the second stage, you should change to gravity-enhancing positions (pages 227–229). If there is no apparent progress after twenty to thirty minutes in one position, change again. Do not continue doing something if it is not effective. Squatting, lap squatting, the supported squat or the 'dangle' are perhaps the best aids to descent, since they not only use gravity but also allow maximum enlargement of the pelvic outlet.[13] These positions may provide enough room for a baby in the occiput posterior position to rotate, or they may enlarge a relatively small pelvic outlet enough for the baby to pass through. You may also try the standing, semi-sitting and hands-and-knees positions. If you cannot use these positions because of caregiver preference or an epidural that limits your movements, or if they do not work, you might ask to try the exaggerated lithotomy position (flat on your back with your knees drawn up towards your shoulders). This position may help the baby move beneath the pubic bone.[14]

If tension in your perineum seems to interfere with effective bearing down, even with warm compresses and reminders to relax, sitting on the toilet may encourage release of the perineum.

If using various positions does not enhance progress, you may need to use prolonged pushing with more forceful bearing down to get the baby moving. At this time, the advantages of prolonged pushing may outweigh the disadvantages described in the discussion of expulsion breathing in Chapter 8. Your birth attendant directs your pushing at this time. Sometimes, an epidural prolongs the second stage. (See page 355 for discussion of pushing with an epidural.)

Medical Care

Close medical observation is necessary if the second stage is prolonged. Your caregiver will carefully monitor the foetal heart rate. If the foetus seems to be tolerating the contractions and positions, your caregiver will usually encourage you to continue your efforts. But if your attempts are unsuccessful, if you are exhausted and unable to push effectively, if you have received medications that inhibit your efforts and slow your labour, if Syntocinon augmentation is not helping, or if your baby is responding poorly, procedures such as vacuum extraction, episiotomy, forceps delivery and caesarean section may be used.

An *episiotomy* is a surgical incision of the perineum that is performed just before the baby's head comes out, as the perineum

Episiotomy

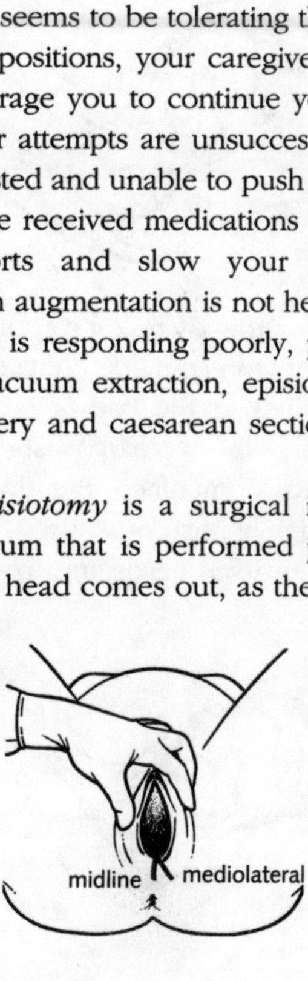

is stretching. An episiotomy enlarges your vaginal outlet and has been found to shorten the time to delivery by five to fifteen minutes, which may be important if the baby is in distress. An episiotomy may also be needed if forceps are used. In Australia, a mediolateral episiotomy is more common than the midline incision (towards the rectum). After birth, the episiotomy is repaired with sutures. You will probably have moderate to severe pain during the first post-partum days, after which it should steadily decline. (See page 367 for more on healing and comfort after an episiotomy or a spontaneous tear.)

Vacuum extractor

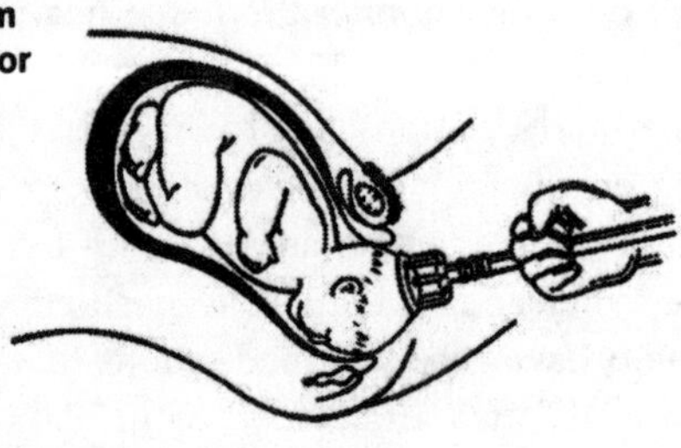

The *vacuum extractor* (a silicone suction cup) and *forceps* (steel tongs) are instruments applied to the baby's head. During contractions, the woman pushes and the doctor pulls. Sometimes, the doctor's help makes a vaginal birth possible. These instruments, when used according to established

Forceps

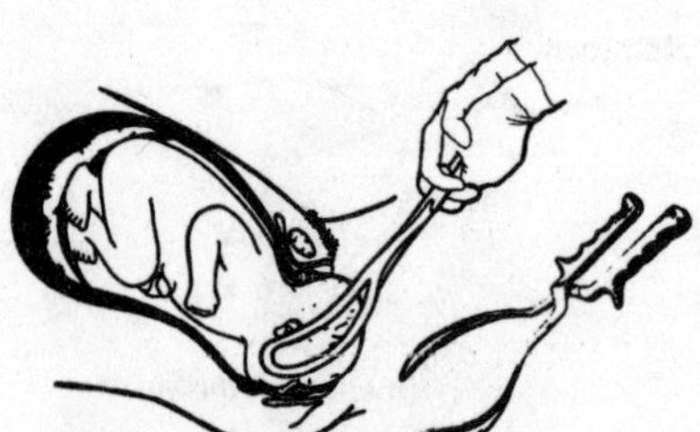

safety protocols, are generally safe for babies. Bruises, swelling and abrasions on the baby's head do sometimes occur. To protect the baby, the caregiver discontinues use of the instruments if it is obvious that the baby is not moving down. A caesarean is the next step. (See pages 314–315 for more on episiotomy, vacuum extraction and forceps; see Chapter 11 for more on caesareans.)

Routine Episiotomy

The use of episiotomy, once a standard practice, has declined in recent years. Some caregivers who still perform routine episiotomies have rates as high as 80 percent, but most caregivers have rates below 30 percent. When reserved for situations in which there are problems in delivery, the episiotomy rate ranges between 10 and 20 percent. Many midwives' episiotomy rates are below 10 percent. The reason for the decline is that scientific studies performed in the 1990s found no benefit, and some real risks, to routine episiotomy.[15] They found that many of the long-held beliefs about the advantages of routine episiotomy simply could not be confirmed by these studies.

If this matter is important to you, discuss it with your caregiver at a prenatal visit. Rather than asking if he or she does routine episiotomies, ask his or her opinion on episiotomy and how often women need one. Those caregivers with high episiotomy rates tend to believe that a tear is always worse than an episiotomy, and that an intact perineum has been over-stretched and is therefore worse than one that has had an episiotomy. Those with low rates believe an intact perineum, which can be expected about half the time, is the best result. They point out that most spontaneous tears are smaller than the average episiotomy and that serious large tears are more likely with an episiotomy than without one. If you wish to avoid an episiotomy, you should realise that you have a 50 percent chance of a spontaneous tear, but that most tears are smaller or about the same as the average episiotomy. Besides choosing the right caregiver, you can do other things to help safely avoid an episiotomy. (See the box on page 240 for suggestions on how to avoid a spontaneous tear and an episiotomy.)

Third-Stage Variations and Complications

Post-partum haemorrhage is the most common problem during the third stage of labour. It is defined as a loss of at least 500 millilitres (about 2 cups) of blood during the first twenty-four hours after birth.

The three major causes of post-partum haemorrhage are *uterine atony* (poor uterine muscle tone), *lacerations* or tears of the cervix or vagina, and *retention of the placenta* or placental fragments. Of these, uterine atony is the most frequent cause of haemorrhage. The treatment of post-partum haemorrhage depends on the cause. If the bleeding is serious, you may need intravenous fluids or a blood transfusion.

Uterine Atony

Your caregiver will massage your uterus to encourage it to contract after birth. Nursing your baby or lightly stroking your nipples stimulates the release of oxytocin, which in turn also helps your uterus contract. If these measures do not control bleeding, your doctor or midwife may give you medications, such as Syntocinon, to promote uterine contractions. (See page 275.)

Lacerations

Lacerations or tears of the cervix, vagina or perineum sometimes occur with or without an episiotomy. They will be sutured to control bleeding. Occasionally, packing the vagina with sterile gauze is also required to stop bleeding.

Retained Placenta

If the placenta or fragments of it are retained in the uterus, they interfere with post-partum uterine contractions, allowing the blood vessels at the placental site to bleed freely. Your caregiver will remove the placenta, clots or fragments, administer Syntocinon and massage your uterus. You can help by massaging your uterus yourself and by breastfeeding your baby.

Very rarely, the placenta cannot be separated from the uterine wall *(placenta accreta)*. The only safe treatment for this rare but serious complication may be a hysterectomy (removal of the uterus).

Prolapsed Cord

Though rare, a *prolapsed cord* is an extremely serious complication. If the umbilical cord slips through the cervix into the vagina ahead of the baby, it can be pinched between the baby and the partly opened cervix or the mother's bony pelvis. Especially during contractions, this compression of the cord can drastically reduce oxygen to the foetus, which is life threatening for the baby.

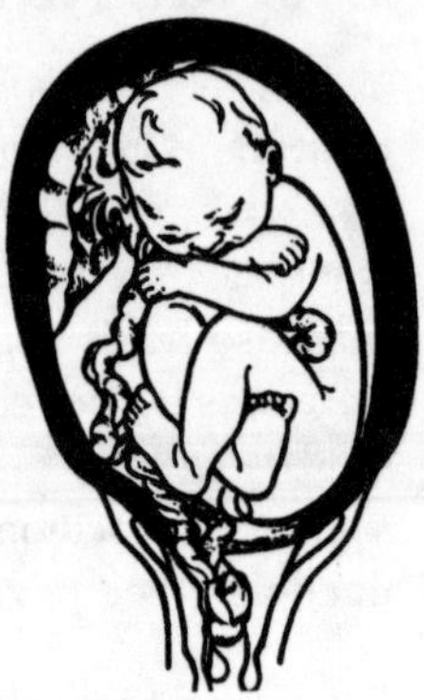

Prolapsed Cord

A prolapsed cord is most likely (though still rare) if your membranes suddenly rupture and there is a space around the baby for the cord to slip down. This can occur if your baby is premature; if you are pregnant with twins, triplets or more; if your baby is in a breech or transverse presentation; or if her head is 'floating' and not engaged in your pelvis.

At your prenatal checkups in late pregnancy, ask your caregiver if your baby is breech or transverse, or if her head is high. Your caregiver can often tell by feeling your baby through your abdominal wall. If you know that your baby's head is high or that she is breech or transverse, and your membranes break with a gush, you should take the following precautions until medical care is available:

- Get into a knee-chest position in which gravity can move the baby away from your cervix and off the cord, which may have prolapsed. You may or may not be able to feel the cord in your vagina.

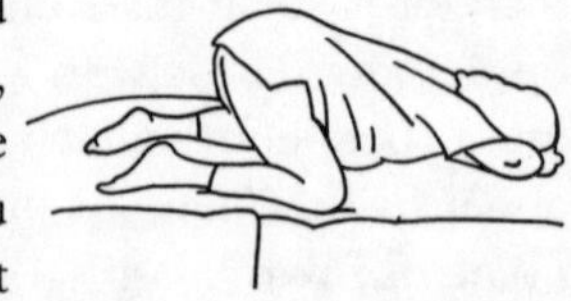

- Someone needs to arrange for immediate transportation to the hospital.
- After walking to the car, you should remain in the knee-chest position in the car or ambulance.
- When you arrive at the hospital, tell the staff that you may have a prolapsed cord.

A nurse will check for a prolapsed cord and, if necessary, put her or his hand in your vagina to hold the baby off the cord. A caesarean delivery will be performed as soon as possible. If no prolapse is found, everyone will heave a sigh of relief, your caregiver will be impressed and will reassure you that you did just the right things, and you will resume coping with your labour.

As frightening as the prospect of a prolapsed cord is, by understanding what it is and what you can do to minimise the dangers, you may be able to save your baby's life.

Difficult Foetal Presentations

About 5 percent of the time, the baby is in a presentation other than vertex. Face and brow presentations occur in less than one in two hundred pregnancies and usually prolong labour. The shoulder presentation (transverse lie) occurs rarely in about one in five hundred births. Because a baby in this position only occasionally turns to a head-down presentation, a caesarean delivery is usually necessary.

Finally, the breech presentation (with head up and buttocks, legs or feet over the cervix) occurs in three to four per one hundred pregnancies. (The incidence rises with prematurity or twins.) This is the most common type of difficult presentation.

Breech Presentation

There are three types of breech presentation: *frank* (buttocks down with legs straight up towards the face), *complete* (sitting cross-legged), and *footling* (one or both feet down). The frank breech is the most common. Although vaginal breech deliveries can turn out well, they are riskier to the baby than the vertex presentation. A breech presentation increases the chances of a prolapsed cord, because the baby's buttocks or feet do not cover the cervix and thus do not prevent the umbilical cord from being swept below the baby or even into the vagina. This situation is most likely to occur when the membranes rupture with a gush.

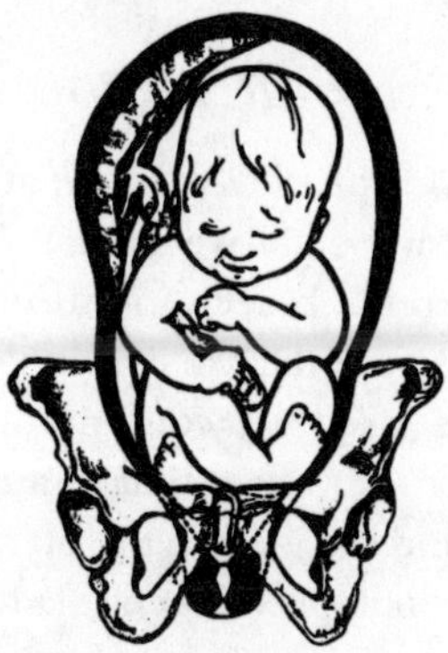

Complete breech

Because the baby's feet and body are delivered before his head in a breech birth, the baby's head can compress the cord at the cervix or within the birth canal, reducing the oxygen available from the placenta to the baby. An added risk exists because the baby's feet and buttocks are small enough that they can be born before the cervix dilates enough for the birth of the head. This may result in foetal distress and a delay in the birth of the head. Another rare foetal risk is spinal cord injury, which may occur if the head of the foetus is hyper-extended (bent back). Because of these potential increased complications, caesarean births have become the usual mode of delivery of breech babies.

What You Can Do

Try to keep informed about your baby's presentation and position, which are checked at each prenatal visit during late pregnancy. Most babies assume their birth position by thirty-four to thirty-six weeks. Others turn later, even during labour. If your baby is breech at thirty-six weeks, you may try the 'breech tilt' position or use sound to encourage your baby to turn.

Breech Tilt Position

The breech tilt position involves tilting your body so your hips are higher than your head. Before doing so, check with your caregiver for any medical reasons that might make it unwise. Usually, if you are in good health and the baby is thriving, caregivers encourage using the breech tilt position. Lie on your back with your knees bent and your feet flat on the floor. Raise your pelvis, and slide enough firm cushions beneath your buttocks to raise them 25–40 centimetres above your head. Ask your partner to help with the cushions. You may also lie head down on an ironing board or a similar flat board tilted with one end on a chair, the other on the floor. If the board is at all wobbly, have someone stay with you to steady the board and help you get on and off. Lie in this position for about ten minutes three times a day when the baby is active. To ease discomfort, make sure your stomach and bladder are empty. Try to relax your abdominal muscles and visualise your baby turning a 'somersault' so his head comes towards your cervix. Your baby will probably squirm as his head presses into the fundus. This technique does not always work; in fact, even though many women swear by it, research findings have not shown that the technique increases the chances of turning a baby.[16] However, since there is little chance of harm, you may wish to try it.

Use of Sound

This harmless technique is comfortable, unlike the breech tilt position. Using sound involves placing earphones from a tape player just above your pubic bone and playing music for the baby during his active periods. Or, your partner can talk to the baby with his or her head in your lap. The music or voice should be at a volume that is comfortable for you to listen to. You can use this technique for as long as you like. The rationale is this: We know that babies can hear well and that they respond to sound coming from outside the womb. They already know your partner's voice. We think that if the baby hears pleasing or familiar sounds coming from low in the uterus, he might move his head down to hear them better. While not always successful, numerous women who have tried this technique have reported that their babies turned. While it is possible that the babies would have turned spontaneously, this harmless and enjoyable technique may be useful.

Medical Care

If your attempts to turn the baby to a head-first presentation by trying the breech tilt position or using sound have not been successful, your caregiver may try external version and will begin discussing your delivery options.

External Version

This procedure, done at about thirty-seven to thirty-eight weeks, involves turning the baby from a breech to a head-down presentation. Before the version is performed, ultrasound is used to confirm that the baby is still breech, to estimate amniotic fluid volume, and to visualise the uterus and the site of placental attachment. External version is not recommended with certain conditions: with low fluid volume, with uterine abnormalities or when the placenta is on the anterior wall of the uterus. A non-stress test is usually done before and after the version to determine the baby's wellbeing. A *tocolytic* drug (for example, Salbutamol) is given to relax your uterus. Some doctors use epidural anaesthesia to reduce the discomfort of the procedure. Then, using ultrasound for guidance and to observe the foetal heart rate, your caregiver presses and pushes on the baby through your abdomen, turning him to a head-down position.

If the baby shows signs of foetal distress (as indicated by his heart rate), the procedure is stopped. In the unlikely event that the placenta begins to separate during the version or the baby remains in distress after the procedure is stopped, a caesarean section might have to be performed. Sometimes, the version is unsuccessful (the baby does not turn). Sometimes, after a successful version, the baby turns back later. Studies of external version indicate that it is a safe procedure that succeeds about 60 percent of the time.[17]

The pressure on your abdomen that is required for an external version is sometimes quite uncomfortable. Relaxing your abdominal muscles helps you tolerate the procedure and allows your caregiver the time that is needed to turn the baby. Bring your partner with you to help you relax and use patterned breathing. He or she should maintain eye contact with you and encourage you to maintain a rhythm with your breathing.

Vaginal or Caesarean Birth for the Breech

Vaginal births of breech babies are unusual today in Australia because of a combination of factors. Complications for the baby associated with vaginal breech birth have led to increased reliance on caesarean delivery, especially since the 1970s, when improvements in the surgery led to increased caesarean rates for all reasons. As vaginal breech births declined, fewer doctors developed the technical skills to conduct them, and this led to further decline of vaginal breech births. A recent large scientific study comparing outcomes of caesarean and vaginal deliveries found that babies born by caesarean had better outcomes.[18] The results from this study seem to have removed any lingering doubt about the safest route of delivery for breech babies.[19] And while some doctors still have skills in vaginal delivery of the breech baby, pressure from peers and medical-legal concerns may cause them to stop performing them.

Most women with breech babies are limited to having a caesarean birth. If your attempts at turning the baby are unsuccessful and he remains breech, you will have to shift your focus to planning a caesarean and making it the best caesarean birth ever. (See Chapter 7 about birth plans and discuss your preferred options with your caregiver.)

Pregnancy-Induced Hypertension

If you have pregnancy-induced hypertension (PIH), your caregiver will manage your labour to keep your blood pressure down and prevent eclampsia. Induction of labour is commonly done. Restriction to bed or recommending that you stay on your left side in bed is likely, although some caregivers believe that time in the shower or bathtub also helps to keep your blood pressure down. Drug therapy lowers blood pressure and helps prevent seizures. (See the chart on page 298 for information on drug therapy used with PIH.) Some caregivers recommend an epidural because of its side effect of lowering blood pressure. However, this practice has not been shown to be effective in treating PIH. (See page 75 in Chapter 3 for more on PIH.)

Medications Used in the Management of Preterm Labour and Pregnancy-Induced Hypertension

These are the drugs used in Australia to help prevent preterm birth, to promote foetal lung maturity in case of preterm birth, and to prevent and treat high blood pressure during pregnancy and birth. Similar drugs with different names may be used in countries outside Australia.

Category, Drug Type and Drug Names	When/How Given	Benefits and/or Purposes	Possible Risks and/or Side Effects	Comments
Medications Used to Slow or Stop Preterm Labour Contractions				
Beta-mimetic agents • Salbutamol	• Between 20 and 35 weeks gestation if preterm labour is suspected • Salbutamol is given intravenously when started; later, if contractions stop, it may be taken orally.	• Causes tocolysis (relaxation of uterus) • Stops preterm contractions and may prevent or postpone preterm labour • May be used to relax the uterus before external version of a breech baby	• If active labour is established, tocolytics are ineffective. *To mother:* • Rapid heart rate or palpitations • Hypotension (drop in blood pressure) • Pulmonary oedema (fluid in the lungs) • Shortness of breath • Nausea and vomiting • Headache • Thirst • Nervousness and tremours • Elevated insulin and glucose levels with long-term salbutamol therapy • Prolonged therapy may cause a decreased response to the drug (desensitisation) and recurrence of preterm labour. *To foetus and newborn:* • Rapid heart rate • Newborn hypoglycemia and hyper-insulinism	• Dosage adjustments can be made to reduce unwanted effects. • Contraindications include maternal cardiac rhythm disturbances, cardiac disease, poorly controlled diabetes or hypertension. • Subcutaneous pump with low doses of salbutamol minimises possibility of desensitisation. • These drugs may postpone delivery for only 2–7 days.

Medications Used in the Management of Preterm Labour and Pregnancy-Induced Hypertension

Category, Drug Type and Drug Names	When/How Given	Benefits and/or Purposes	Possible Risks and/or Side Effects	Comments
Calcium channel blockers • nifedipine (Procardia)	• Between 20 and 35 weeks gestation if preterm labour is suspected • Given orally	• Causes tocolysis (relaxation of uterus)	*To mother:* • Transient hypotension • Possible liver problems (rare) • Temporary headache	• May be comparable to salbutamol in effectiveness • Should not be used with magnesium sulphate; doing so can lead to severe muscular problems and can increase risk of toxicity
Prostaglandin inhibitors • indomethacin (Indocid)	• Given as a suppository if preterm labour is suspected	• Inhibits prostaglandin synthesis • May postpone preterm delivery for at least 2 days and reduce incidence of low birth weight	*To mother:* • Peptic ulcer and gastrointestinal bleeding • Thrombocytopenia (decreased blood platelets) • Prolonged bleeding time • Allergic reaction (rashes) • Nausea, vomiting, heartburn and diarrhoea • Headache, dizziness • Signs of infection (fever) can be masked. *To foetus:* • Drug crosses to foetus. • Reduction in amniotic fluid volume *To newborn:* • Prolonged bleeding time • Premature closure of ductus arteriosus • Persistent pulmonary hypertension • Transient impairment of kidney function	

Medications Used in the Management of Preterm Labour and Pregnancy-Induced Hypertension

Category, Drug Type and Drug Names	When/How Given	Benefits and/or Purposes	Possible Risks and/or Side Effects	Comments
Antibiotics • erythromycin • ampicillin • clindamycin • cefoxitin	• Intravenously or intramuscularly if infection is suspected	• Reduces the incidence of infection, especially with preterm rupture of the membranes (PROM) • Prevents or treats infection	*To mother:* • Allergic reactions • Yeast infection • Occasional irritation of the vein (phlebitis)	• Mother needs to report any antibiotic allergy to caregiver. • Use of antibiotics to prevent preterm labour in the absence of PROM or positive test for bacteria is controversial.

Medications Used to Promote Foetal Lung Maturity

Category, Drug Type and Drug Names	When/How Given	Benefits and/or Purposes	Possible Risks and/or Side Effects	Comments
Corticosteroids • betamethasone • dexamethasone	• Given intramuscularly when preterm birth seems inevitable and foetal lungs are immature • May be repeated if preterm labour contractions recur	• Hastens foetal lung maturity • Reduces risk of respiratory distress syndrome (RDS) in the baby and need for mechanical ventilation (breathing) • Reduces risk of haemorrhage in the brain of the baby • Reduces risk of early death in a premature baby	*To mother:* • Pulmonary oedema (may be more due to the accompanying use of labour-inhibiting drugs [see above]) • When pregnancy is complicated by pre-eclampsia, diabetes or other serious illnesses, the need for elective delivery for the mother's benefit must be balanced with the desirability of extra hours or days of corticosteroid treatment for the baby's benefit.	• Greatest benefit comes if baby is born between 1 and 7 days following the first dose. • May reduce length and cost of stay in the hospital for baby • Because drug exposure is short-term, adverse effects of drug are limited.

Medications Used in the Management of Preterm Labour and Pregnancy-Induced Hypertension

Category, Drug Type and Drug Names	When/How Given	Benefits and/or Purposes	Possible Risks and/or Side Effects	Comments
Medications Used to Manage Pregnancy-Induced Hypertension (PIH)				
Anticonvulsants (for seizure prevention) • magnesium sulphate	• Given intravenously or intramuscularly when mother has severe pre-eclampsia or PIH • Initially, mother receives a large dose to quickly raise blood levels to a therapeutic level, and then magnesium sulphate is given in an IV solution by continuous infusion.	• Prevents or controls seizures by depressing central nervous system function	*To mother:* • Same as those listed for magnesium sulphate when used to prevent preterm labour (see above) *To foetus and newborn:* • Same as those listed for magnesium sulphate when used to prevent preterm labour (see above)	• Drug crosses to foetus and levels are close to those in mother.
Antihypertensives (to lower blood pressure) • hydralazine (Apresoline) • labetalol (Normodyne, Trandate) • nifedipine (Procardia)	• Hydralazine is given intravenously, intramuscularly or by mouth. • Labetalol is given intravenously or by mouth. • Nifedipine is given by mouth.	• Lowers blood pressure by dilating blood vessels throughout the mother's body • Helps treat high blood pressure during pregnancy and childbirth	*To mother:* • Hydralazine may cause headache, flushing, rapid or irregular heart rate, nausea, vomiting, diarrhoea or difficulties with urination. • Labetalol may cause slowing of heart rate, shortness of breath and drowsiness. • Nifedipine may cause transient hypotension (low blood pressure) and possible liver problems. *To foetus and newborn:* • Use of hydralazine has been associated with foetal tachycardia (rapid heart rate). • The effects of labetalol include neonatal hypotension (low blood pressure), slow heart rate and hypoglycemia (low blood sugar).	• Labetalol is contraindicated in women with asthma or with certain cardiac problems. • Nifedipine should not be used with magnesium sulphate.

Preterm (Premature) Birth

A preterm birth, by definition occurs before the thirty-seventh week of gestation. If you experience any of the signs of preterm labour (see page 61), call your caregiver. After evaluating your condition, your baby's wellbeing, and the condition of your cervix, your caregiver may decide to try to stop labour. The methods used to prevent premature labour (described on pages 298–301) are more likely to succeed if preterm contractions are detected early, before the cervix has dilated 2 centimetres. Some women are identified early in pregnancy as being at high risk for a premature birth, because the cervix is not tightly closed and firm. They also may have had previous miscarriages or very early deliveries. In such cases, the caregiver may recommend a cervical cerclage (a 'purse-string suture') that holds the cervix tightly closed. The suture is removed a few weeks before the woman's due date.

When labour and birth before thirty-five weeks gestation appear inevitable or necessary, the focus of care shifts to assessment of foetal lung maturity and prevention of respiratory distress syndrome (RDS)—the most common complication of preterm birth. As the lungs may not yet be mature, you will be given corticosteroids to hasten the baby's lung maturity. Your caregiver will try to prevent labour for a day or more to give time for the steroids to act. This treatment has reduced the incidence of respiratory distress by 40–60 percent. (See the chart on page 301 for more on antenatal corticosteroids for lung maturity.)

Your caregiver's goal in managing preterm labour is to get the best possible outcome. If your baby is very premature, it may be necessary for you to have your baby in a hospital that has an intensive care nursery and highly trained nurses and neonatologists available all the time. This may mean transfer from a rural area to a larger tertiary hospital. You will be considered at high risk. Your baby's heart rate will be assessed very frequently or by continuous monitoring. Systemic pain medications that affect foetal heart rate and depress newborn respirations will probably be discouraged. Therefore, in early labour you should plan to use relaxation and breathing patterns for pain relief. In active labour or during birth, you may continue these techniques or you may request regional anaesthesia (epidural).

Since the health of your baby is paramount and she may need medical attention, you may not be able to hold her immediately after birth. Most premature infants are taken to a special care nursery. Special care is necessary until the baby is able to feed on her own and her lungs are mature. The problem with immature lungs is that the baby, who is small and relatively weak, has to work very hard to keep her lungs inflated. Treatment for immature lungs may involve extra oxygen, mechanical assistance with breathing and administration of surfactant. *Surfactant* is usually formed in the foetal lungs in late pregnancy. A premature infant has missed this important substance that helps the lung lining develop to the point where the lungs can remain partially inflated during exhalation, as they do when the lungs are mature. Surfactant, given into the lungs after birth, reduces the surface tension within the lungs and helps them remain open.

Depending on how small and immature the baby is, her care may involve prolonged hospitalisation and possibly long periods of separation from you. In most hospitals, parents are encouraged to visit and care for their babies. Participating in the care of your baby benefits both of you. (For more information on care of the premature infant, see page 409.)

Kangaroo Care

Kangaroo care is a philosophy of newborn care that places babies, even very small or sick babies, with their parents as much as possible. As soon as the baby's condition is stable, the parents are encouraged to hold their baby quietly several times a day. The baby is placed skin-to-skin with the parent, who may be sitting in a rocker next to the baby's bed. Even when the baby has several 'lifelines' to various monitors, IV solutions, and tubes for oxygen and food, she can be placed with her mother or father and will benefit from their smell, the sound of their heartbeats and the warmth they provide. With kangaroo care, a baby's growth improves and parents enjoy being close and showing love to their baby.

Twins, Triplets and More

The birth of twins, triplets or more babies (referred to as multiples, multiple pregnancy or multiple birth) is more complicated than the birth of a single baby. The added demands on the mother to grow more than one baby, the stretching of her uterus, and the combined weights of the babies and their placentas often cause premature labour. The probability of complications—such as pre-eclampsia, prematurity, small size for gestational age, breech presentation, prolonged labour and prolapsed cord—is higher in multiple pregnancies. Sometimes, the over-stretched uterus cannot contract efficiently, which slows labour progress and increases the risk of post-partum haemorrhage. Preterm rupture of the membranes is more common with multiples and is another cause of prematurity. These difficulties increase as the number of babies increases.

Although labour with multiples often progresses normally, caregivers are more wary because of the number of difficulties that can arise. You should expect more medical supervision and more interventions than are usual with the birth of a single baby at term. Some caregivers plan to induce labour or deliver the babies by caesarean at thirty-seven to thirty-nine weeks, in hopes of selecting an optimal time for the babies' and mother's wellbeing. Other caregivers await the spontaneous onset of labour and try not to induce until after forty weeks, in the belief that the physiological process should be encouraged. Epidural anaesthesia may be recommended in case the birth of the second twin needs assistance that may be painful for you. The caesarean rate for twins is higher than for single babies, and the rate goes up with the number of babies. In fact, it is rare for triplets or more to be born vaginally at term. (See Chapter 11 for a complete description of caesarean birth.)

Vaginal Birth of Twins

The most common and most favourable presentations for the vaginal birth of twins are with both babies' heads down (vertex). Ultrasound during labour helps identify the positions of the babies. The results help your caregiver determine the best type of birth—vaginal or caesarean. If both babies are breech, a caesarean is usually performed. If the first baby is head down and the other one is breech, the second baby might be turned after the vaginal birth of the first baby or delivered in the breech presentation. The second twin is usually born within five to thirty minutes after the first, and the delivery of the placenta(s) occurs after both twins are born. The babies are usually born in the operating room, in case a quick caesarean becomes necessary.

When a Baby Dies or Is Seriously Ill

Birth defects, congenital problems, stillbirth, and death resulting from genetic or developmental abnormalities, birth trauma and infection are uncommon but do occasionally occur. If your baby dies or has a serious long-term problem, your agony, sadness and despair will be deep and long-lasting. Being prepared by deciding during pregnancy what you would do if your baby dies or is deformed can help you in the first painful days.

Newborn Death

If your baby dies before you go into labour, you have to consider how you want the labour managed. Will labour be induced? If so, when? Do you want to write a special birth plan? Do you want to be awake and participate in the birth? Would relatives or other support people be helpful to you and your partner? If you have an unexpected stillbirth or your baby dies soon after birth, you will have the following options to consider: Would you prefer to recover in a relatively private area on the post-partum floor separate from other mothers and babies, or somewhere else in the hospital? Would you prefer to take an early discharge? Do you want an autopsy done to help find the cause of the baby's death? Ask your caregiver or childbirth educator how families are cared for after a stillbirth.

What might make your memories of your baby more meaningful? Many counsellors recommend that parents see and hold their dead or dying baby. Naming or baptising the baby, obtaining photographs, footprints or a lock of hair are ways to acknowledge the baby's life and to provide memories. A funeral or memorial service provides an opportunity for family and friends to come together to grieve, to say good-bye to the baby, and to express their concern and love for you. Later, you may want to join a support group of parents who have experienced a similar loss. The groups are there for you as long as you need them. While nothing takes away the pain of losing a baby, this support can help you emotionally at a very difficult time.

Seriously Ill Newborn

If your baby has a birth defect, is premature or is very ill, you have other decisions to make. In most cases, you or your partner can spend time with your baby, even if he is in a special care nursery. If the baby is transferred to a hospital that specialises in seriously ill babies, your partner may have to divide his or her time between visiting you and the baby. You may be able to have an early discharge from your hospital so that you may visit your baby. You may want to provide your baby with the special nourishment of your colostrum and breast milk, either by breastfeeding or by pumping your milk to be fed to your baby.

You will have many questions about your baby's condition, the treatment, and what to expect now and in the future. You may feel impatient with the staff for not telling you more or for not having the answers you so desperately crave. The intensive care atmosphere and all the people and machines involved in your baby's care may be confusing and exhausting for you. It helps to write down your questions as they come up and to keep a log of what is done and what various professionals tell you. Despite all the stress and exhaustion you feel, you can help your baby by being with him and contributing to his care when it is possible.

Caring for Yourselves

Parent support groups exist for those whose babies are premature or disabled, or whose babies have died. They are immensely helpful with emotional and practical support.

If your baby dies or has health problems, you will at some time need to review and reflect on the birth experience. Recalling the events with your partner, childbirth educator, the attending nurse or your caregiver and writing your birth story can help you put the pieces together. A counsellor, therapist, the hospital chaplain, or your priest, rabbi or minister can help you work through your emotions. Friends and family can help you with the numerous practical details that must be attended to: care of other children; transportation; food preparation; notification of business associates, friends and relatives; answering the phone; and more. (Helpful books are listed in the Recommended Resources.)

If your baby dies or has health problems, you will need time to grieve. Grieving is painful and exhausting, but it must be experienced. You and your partner will experience and re-experience many feelings—numbness, sadness, shock, disbelief, fear, anger, blame and guilt. Eventually, after months or years, you will reach a level of acceptance, although the sorrow will linger. Be gentle with yourselves. Give yourselves time to heal emotionally and physically. Lean on the people and the community resources that are most supportive. Try to discuss your feelings with each other frequently because, understandably, your pace and reactions to grief may be different.

Good memories will exist as well as painful ones. Allow yourselves to acknowledge your baby's life and savour the good memories from pregnancy, the birth or the time you had with your baby. Your baby is a special part of you and will always exist in your memories as an important person in your lives.

Medical Interventions in Labour and Birth

Medical interventions in labour are procedures carried out by your caregiver or nurse to alter the course of labour, provide diagnostic information, or prevent or treat complications. All interventions and medications carry some degree of risk along with their benefits, and should be used only when necessary. There is disagreement within the obstetrical community over the routine use of some interventions. During pregnancy, check with your caregiver to learn which interventions are routine (and why). You will also want to find out what interventions and medications are most likely if a problem arises and you need medical assistance. Your birth plan should include your preferences regarding the use of interventions, while reflecting your flexibility if the unforeseen occurs. The chart at the end of this chapter describes the purposes, benefits and risks of various common interventions, medications and procedures. The information will help you write your birth plan and make informed choices during labour.

After reading a chapter like this, you may have the impression that labour and birth are never normal! You need to remember that in healthy pregnant women, 60–70 percent of labours are perfectly normal; another 10–20 percent require interventions but result in normal births. Only about one in ten women (10 percent) will require major interventions, and most of these situations still result in healthy mothers and babies. Women who are at high risk during pregnancy may require more obstetrical interventions during labour. Being informed about possible variations and complications, available medical interventions and various self-help techniques can help you work with the medical staff towards the safest and most satisfying childbirth possible.

Obstetrical Interventions during Childbirth

These interventions are used during labour and birth to diagnose, prevent or treat a problem for mother or baby. Some interventions are more routinely used than others. Use the information below to aid your discussion with your caregiver when planning your birth and to learn what to expect if a problem arises and one or more interventions are suggested during childbirth.

Intervention/How It Is Done	Benefits and/or Purposes	Risks and/or Disadvantages	Comments
Intravenous (IV) fluids A needle is inserted into a vein in the forearm or back of the hand. A thin plastic tube is inserted through the needle, and the needle is removed. Fluids are then dripped continuously from the IV bag into the vein.	• Maintains hydration (adequate fluid intake) when you are not allowed to drink liquids or are unable to keep them down • Helps maintain blood pressure if regional anaesthesia is used or if you bleed too much • Allows immediate access to a vein if medication or a blood transfusion is necessary • Needed for administration of Syntocinon (to augment or induce labour) • Provides some calories for energy, if fluid contains dextrose (sugar)	• Restricts easy movement during labour; walking is more difficult (unless a heparin lock is used). • May result in infiltration (fluids leaking into tissues surrounding vein near puncture site), causing tenderness and swelling • If excessive amounts of fluid are given, fluid overload (blood chemistry disturbances) and excessive swelling in early post partum (especially in legs and breasts) • If mother receives large amounts of fluid containing dextrose (sugar), baby may become hypoglycemic at birth and require special care.	• Unnecessary if you are drinking sufficient fluids, receiving no medication or anaesthesia, and labour is progressing normally • Drinking liquids is sometimes limited or prohibited, especially after an epidural. Feelings of thirst and dry mouth occur, but ice can help alleviate the discomfort. • Some caregivers and institutions routinely allow only IV fluids (nothing by mouth) from admission until after delivery. Such policies are not supported by scientific evidence. • With a high volume of IV fluids to the mother, the baby may be born with excessive tissue fluid. These babies are heavier at birth and then may lose a higher percentage of their birth weight than babies whose mothers did not get high volumes of IV fluids. If infant weight loss in the first few days exceeds 10 percent, the mother's IV fluid intake in labour should be considered (as well as evaluating breast milk intake).[20]

Obstetrical Interventions during Childbirth

Intervention/How It Is Done	Benefits and/or Purposes	Risks and/or Disadvantages	Comments
Artificial rupture of membranes (AROM) During a vaginal exam, the caregiver makes a small tear in the membranes using a specially designed instrument called an 'amnihook'.	• May start labour (See page 266.) • May speed labour progress by allowing presenting part to fit snugly against cervix, stimulating contractions and enhancing dilation • Enables caregiver or nurse to see consistency and colour of amniotic fluid to help assess foetal wellbeing • Necessary for use of internal electronic foetal monitoring (foetal scalp electrode and intrauterine pressure catheter) and foetal oxygen sensor in foetal oxygen saturation monitoring	• Increases risk of infection • Increases use of other interventions (Syntocinon) if labour does not start or speed up with AROM • May increase discomfort of uterine contractions • Associated with greater umbilical cord compression, moulding of foetal head and drops in foetal heart rate during contractions • If presenting part is high, AROM may cause cord prolapse. (See page 294.)	• There is no pain during this procedure other than the discomfort of a vaginal exam. • AROM in early labour is associated with shorter labours (40 minutes on average), but when the foetus is mal-positioned (OP), it may not speed labour. • After the membranes rupture, vaginal exams should be kept to a minimum to reduce the likelihood of infection. • Labouring in the bathtub after the membranes are ruptured has been found not to increase infection.[21] • Caregivers usually want a woman to be in active labour or to give birth within 24 hours after AROM.
Foetal heart rate monitoring ***A. Listening (auscultation) with foetal stethoscope*** Caregiver (usually a nurse) listens to the baby's heartbeat through your abdominal wall using a special stethoscope before, during and after a contraction. The foetal heart rate (FHR) is usually counted every 15–30 minutes during the first stage of labour and more frequently during the second stage.	• Enables assessment of FHR • Non-invasive • Allows you to be mobile and active • Encourages frequent attention from your caregiver or nurse • Is an excellent way to determine foetal positions when determining location of heart tones	• Heart tones may be difficult to hear. • May require you to lie supine (flat) in bed in order to hear heart tones • Does not provide continuous printed record of FHR and contraction pattern, and requires staff to record FHR on your chart • Pressure of stethoscope against your abdomen may be uncomfortable. • Assessing relationship between FHR and contraction is more difficult than with EFM. (See below.)	• Because FHR is more difficult to hear with this device than with ultrasonic devices, the caregiver must place stethoscope very close to the baby's heart. This has the added advantage of assisting the caregiver in determining the baby's position (OP or OA). • Most caregivers today rarely use the foetal stethoscope, if at all. They prefer the following methods.

Obstetrical Interventions during Childbirth

Intervention/How It Is Done	Benefits and/or Purposes	Risks and/or Disadvantages	Comments
Foetal heart rate monitoring ***B. Listening (auscultation) with a hand-held ultrasonic foetal stethoscope*** Often called a Doppler, this device is placed on your abdomen and audibly and/or visually transmits the foetal heart tone. The caregiver counts as described above.	• Enables assessment of FHR • Is most comfortable method of FHR monitoring • Encourages frequent attention from your caregiver or nurse • Allows you to be mobile and active • Is more sensitive in picking up foetal heart tones than foetal stethoscope • Volume can be increased so others in room may hear.	• Does not provide a continuous record of FHR and contraction pattern, and requires staff to record FHR manually • Assessing relationship between FHR and contraction is more difficult than with EFM. (See below.)	• Waterproof Doppler devices are available for monitoring women who are labouring in the water.
Foetal heart rate monitoring ***C. External electronic foetal monitor (EFM)*** An ultrasound device, held in place by a belt around your abdomen, sends and receives soundwaves to detect foetal heart rate. Another belt holds a pressure-sensitive device (a tocodynamometer) in place over your fundus to detect uterine contractions. These devices are attached by wires to a monitor that displays and permanently records the FHR and uterine contractions. They are also often connected to screens in the nurses' station where more than one woman's recordings can be watched at the same time. Monitoring can be intermittent (10–20 minutes every hour) or continuous.	• Enables assessment of how contractions affect FHR • Enables assessment of foetal well-being when complications arise or when Syntocinon or other medical interventions are used • Provides information needed to determine whether more sophisticated monitoring is warranted • Provides information on frequency of uterine contractions • Provides a continuous printed record of FHR and contraction pattern • Helps labour partner know when contractions begin so he or she can help you start a breathing pattern • Does not require artificial rupture of membranes	• Requires further assessments before changing medical management, because certain conditions affect its accuracy • Needs frequent readjustment when you or baby moves • May be uncomfortable and restrict your movement (the immobility may slow labour) • Decreases your ability to use abdominal or back massage • Does not provide accurate measurement of strength of contractions • May tempt your labour partner to watch monitor instead of you • May lead to less personal contact between nurse and labouring woman	• Scientific trials comparing periodic auscultation with continuous EFM have found them comparable as a surveillance method in terms of neonatal outcomes.[22] • Though auscultation is a safe method of foetal monitoring, most nurses and caregivers have not been trained in auscultation skills and prefer to read EFM tracings. • EFM cannot distinguish mother's heart rate from foetal heart tones; a sudden drop in FHR may actually be due to the foetus moving and the mother's heart rate being picked up.

Obstetrical Interventions during Childbirth

Intervention/How It Is Done	Benefits and/or Purposes	Risks and/or Disadvantages	Comments
Foetal heart rate monitoring ***D. Telemetry unit for external monitoring*** The recording devices are the same as described above, but they are connected to a tiny wireless transmitter (a telemetry unit), which you carry or wear on a belt. The transmitter sends data to a monitor located in your labour room or in the nurses' station.	• Same as with external electronic monitoring described above • In addition, allows you more movement, including walking around maternity area	• Same as with external electronic foetal monitoring, except that it allows mobility	• Most hospitals have few telemetry units. If your hospital usually uses continuous EFM and you want to be able to walk, request a telemetry unit in your birth plan, on the phone when you call before going to the hospital, or as soon as you arrive. • Waterproof monitor parts are available in some hospitals, so telemetry can be used in the tub or shower.
Foetal heart rate monitoring ***E. Internal electronic foetal monitor (EFM)*** The foetal heart rate (FHR) is measured by a scalp electrode inserted into the skin of the foetal head (or other presenting part). Wires from the electrode transmit the baby's heart rate to the monitor, which displays and records it. Uterine contractions are measured by placing an intrauterine pressure catheter (IUPC) into the uterus. During contractions, the increase in intrauterine pressure is measured, displayed visually and recorded on the printout. Telemetry can also be used with internal EFM.	• Enables accurate assessment of how contractions affect FHR • Enables assessment of foetal well-being when complications arise during induction or augmentation with Syntocinon, or when other interventions are used • Provides information on intensity and frequency of uterine contractions • Provides information needed to determine if further medical assistance or testing is warranted • Helps labour partner know when contractions begin so he or she can help you start a breathing pattern • Is more accurate than external monitor • Is less restrictive of your movements in bed than external monitor	• Requires rupture of membranes • Restricts free movement, especially walking during labour • May cause infection of uterus and/or infection of baby's scalp • Interpretation of FHR patterns varies among practitioners; foetal distress is sometimes diagnosed when not actually present. • Pressure catheter may need frequent adjustment with the mother's change of position.	• Sometimes, a combination of internal and external electronic monitoring is used (for example, the internal foetal scalp electrode and the external tocodynamometer). • As external EFM ultrasound sensors have improved, the use of internal scalp electrodes has diminished. • As with external EFM, studies comparing periodic auscultation and internal EFM found no differences in newborn outcome, except for labours in which oxytocin (Syntocinon) was used.[23] • The sounds of the internal FHR are more distinct (sounding like 'clop, clop, clop') than those with the external EFM (which has a shushing sound). • Because of the additional risks, internal EFM is only used when external EFM is not giving adequate information.

Obstetrical Interventions during Childbirth

Intervention/How It Is Done	Benefits and/or Purposes	Risks and/or Disadvantages	Comments
Foetal scalp blood sampling A small cut is made in the baby's scalp and a sample of the baby's blood is removed and tested for its oxygen and carbon dioxide levels, acid-base balance (pH) and other factors.	• Allows further assessment of foetal wellbeing if EFM indicates problems • Prevents an unnecessary caesarean birth if foetal blood values are shown to be normal	• Time-consuming procedure • Uncomfortable for mother and possibly for baby • Invasive • May cause scalp infection in baby • Results take from 2 to 30 minutes to obtain. • Not all hospitals have necessary facilities to perform tests 24 hours a day.	• Foetal oxygen saturation monitoring is being promoted for the same purposes. (See FOSM section below.)
Foetal scalp stimulation test This test is done when EFM indicates possible foetal distress. During a vaginal exam, the caregiver presses on or scratches the foetal scalp. The foetal heart rate response to such stimulation is observed. A reactive heart rate (rises 15 beats per minute for 15 seconds) is a reliable sign that the foetus is compensating well. If the heart rate is not reactive, the foetus probably has very few reserves.	• Allows accurate assessment of foetal wellbeing if EFM indicates problems • Sometimes prevents an unnecessary caesarean birth if test indicates foetal wellbeing • Non-invasive to the foetus • Rapid and reliable test that can be repeated whenever desired • No cost	• Requires a vaginal exam	• This simple test helps to distinguish foetal 'stress' (in which the foetus is able to handle the temporary shortage of oxygen caused by contractions) from foetal distress (in which the foetus no longer has the ability to compensate). • Compared to foetal scalp blood sampling and foetal oxygen saturation monitoring, this test is much simpler, quicker, less expensive and as reliable.

Obstetrical Interventions during Childbirth

Intervention/How It Is Done	Benefits and/or Purposes	Risks and/or Disadvantages	Comments
Foetal oxygen saturation monitoring (FOSM) Once membranes are ruptured and foetal distress is suspected, the caregiver inserts a sensor through the cervix alongside the foetus's cheek. The sensor continually measures the oxygen in the foetal blood and is connected to a recording device on the EFM printer so that oxygen levels may be monitored continuously.[24]	• Provides another way (along with scalp blood sampling and foetal stimulation) to determine if FHR decelerations are causing actual distress in the foetus or not • Offers continual assessment of foetal oxygen status (as opposed to the 'spot checks' offered by scalp blood sampling and foetal stimulation) • Non-invasive to the foetus and less uncomfortable for the mother than foetal scalp blood sampling • May prevent unnecessary caesarean for foetal distress	• Extremely expensive compared to quick, no-cost foetal stimulation test (which can be easily repeated whenever desirable) • Requires purchase of specially equipped new electronic foetal monitors • Accurate placement of the sensor is difficult. • Requires use of internal EFM	• The sensor must be placed against the baby's cheek. If not placed properly or if it gets vernix on it, no data is transmitted and the sensor must be adjusted or replaced. • One randomised controlled trial showed that caesareans for foetal distress were reduced by half when EFM plus foetal oxygen saturation monitoring were used as opposed to EFM alone.[25] • FOSM was introduced in 2000; assessing its rightful place in obstetrics will take a number of years. • As of 2000, researchers recommend that FOSM be used only in the presence of non-reassuring EFM tracings. • Works just like the pulse oximeter used on the mother's finger. (See below.)
Pulse oximetry A sensor is clipped to the mother's finger to detect oxygen level in the blood. The sensor is attached to a monitor that visually exhibits the blood oxygen level. If too low, the woman is asked to breathe more deeply or is given oxygen by mask.	• Enables caregiver to continually assess whether mother has adequate oxygen • Useful during epidural analgesia/anaesthesia and during a caesarean to ensure that the woman's oxygen levels allow adequate oxygen transfer to the foetus • Is non-invasive and easily applied	• None, except for minor inconvenience of the device squeezing a finger	• Pulse oximetry is also used with newborn babies whose APGAR scores are low or who have breathing problems. The sensor is attached to the baby's skin, usually on the foot.

Obstetrical Interventions during Childbirth

Intervention/How It Is Done	Benefits and/or Purposes	Risks and/or Disadvantages	Comments
Amnio-infusion When amniotic fluid volume is low from ruptured membranes or from diminished production of fluid, sterile saline solution may be injected into the uterus via an intrauterine pressure catheter (like the one used to measure contraction strength with internal EFM).	• Reduces foetal distress • Allows labour to continue when a caesarean might otherwise be the only solution • Dilutes meconium in the fluid and helps avoid problems from the newborn inhaling meconium • If umbilical cord is being compressed during contractions and causing foetal distress, the added fluid cushions the cord and protects against foetal distress.	• Requires that mother remain in bed • Invasive • Requires artificial rupture of membranes • Possible risk of foetal hypothermia (low temperature), over-distention of uterus or intrauterine infection	• When cord compression occurs or meconium is present, amnio-infusion reduces incidence of FHR decelerations, caesareans for foetal distress and low Apgar scores. • Fluid may be injected repeatedly or continuously.
Episiotomy A surgical incision is made into the perineum from the vagina towards the rectum (midline or mediolateral) just before the birth of the baby's head.	• Enlarges birth canal • May speed delivery of baby by a few minutes, an advantage with foetal distress • Provides a straight incision, which is easier to repair than some large tears • Provides more space for application of forceps or vacuum extractor • Reduces compression from vaginal tissues on head of a premature baby • Decreases the likelihood of a spontaneous tear in front of the vagina	• Causes discomfort in early post-partum period • Sometimes performed routinely when not necessary • May delay mother-infant interaction (holding or nursing) as episiotomy is repaired (same delay may occur in repair of a spontaneous tear) • Site of incision may become infected or bleed (also true of spontaneous tear). • May cause pain with intercourse for several months after birth • More likely to extend and seriously tear perineum than if an episiotomy is not performed. Very large tears almost always happen when an episiotomy extends after it has been done.	• Episiotomy rates declined rapidly in the 1990s after publication of scientific trials comparing routine episiotomy to selective episiotomy. Rates less than 15 percent are reported in some groups of midwives, family doctors and obstetricians. • The trials found that pelvic floor strength 3 years after birth was not improved with episiotomy. • When an episiotomy is not done, the likelihood of an intact perineum (no tear) ranges from 25 to 60 percent, depending on the skill of the caregiver. And, even when a spontaneous tear occurs, it is usually smaller or no larger than the average episiotomy.[26] • Healing from a tear is more rapid and post-partum pain is less than with most episiotomies.[27]

Obstetrical Interventions during Childbirth

Intervention/How It Is Done	Benefits and/or Purposes	Risks and/or Disadvantages	Comments
Vacuum extractor Used in second stage, a plastic cap-like device is applied to the baby's head. A tube connects the cap to a vacuum pump that creates suction. During contractions, the caregiver pulls on a handle attached to the cap to assist the baby's descent. The amount of suction is controlled so that the cap releases from the baby's head if the caregiver pulls too hard. This feature protects the head from serious injury.	• Helps descent of baby's head • Under some circumstances, can be applied when foetus is at a higher station than is safe for use of forceps • Requires less space in vagina than forceps • Less need for episiotomy and anaesthesia than with forceps	• May cause bruising or swelling of baby's soft scalp tissues or of the mother's perineum • Not as helpful with rotation as forceps	• If several attempts with the vacuum extractor fail, a caesarean is done. • The woman may be asked to push as hard as she can while the vacuum (and forceps) are being used to enhance the chances of a vaginal delivery.
Forceps Two spoon-like instruments are inserted, one at a time, into the vagina and applied to each side of the baby's head. The doctor turns and/or pulls on the handles to aid rotation and descent. Used only in second stage when the baby is at a low station.	• Helps rotate baby's head to an anterior position • Helps bring baby down when anaesthesia is used or bearing-down efforts are insufficient • May be used to facilitate birth of head with a breech vaginal birth • Speeds delivery if foetus is in trouble	• Usually requires an episiotomy • May bruise soft tissues of baby's head or face • Usually requires regional or local anaesthesia • May bruise or tear vaginal tissues	• Some skilled caregivers use forceps without episiotomy or anaesthesia. • The decision between forceps and vacuum extraction is usually made by the doctor and is based on his or her skill and experience. • If forceps attempts fail, a caesarean is done. • Forceps injuries to the baby are less likely today because, rather than running the risk of a difficult forceps delivery, the doctor performs a caesarean.

Chapter 11

Caesarean Birth and Vaginal Birth after a Previous Caesarean

A caesarean section (also called a C-section or caesarean birth) is a surgical procedure used to deliver your baby through incisions in the abdomen and uterus. A caesarean, although major abdominal surgery, is preferable to a vaginal birth if labour or a vaginal birth is considered too difficult or dangerous for either you or your baby. Under most circumstances, however, a vaginal birth is safer for both mother and baby, even if the mother has already had one or more caesareans. This chapter describes reasons for a caesarean birth, the surgical procedure, and the physical and emotional recovery. A discussion of vaginal births after caesareans (VBACs)—including benefits, concerns and preparation—is also provided.

Caesarean Birth

The caesarean rate rose steadily in Australia from 1970, when approximately one woman in twenty (5.5 percent) had a caesarean birth, until the 1980s, when one woman in five (20 percent) had the surgery. These increased levels concerned many experts because the higher caesarean rates did not result in the expected improvements in infant and maternal outcomes. In the 1990s, the rate fluctuated between 21 percent and 24 percent. Although some prominent obstetricians defend high caesarean rates,[1] most leading public and professional organisations call for efforts to reduce the caesarean rate. Based on a review of international literature, the U.S. Department of Health and Human Services and the World Health Organisation set a goal of reducing the caesarean rate to 15 percent by the year 2000. Despite the fact that this goal was not reached, experts continue to suggest ways to reduce the caesarean rate without jeopardising the health of mother and baby. The chart on page 319 is based on these suggestions and describes ways to increase a woman's chances of having a vaginal birth. If these key recommendations are utilised by expectant mothers and encouraged by maternity care providers, the caesarean rate will likely be reduced.

Weighing the Benefits and Risks of Caesareans

Why the concern over a high caesarean rate? At first glance, it appears that the caesarean section is a quick, safe and easy way to deliver a baby. A caesarean is more convenient, faster and more predictable than a vaginal birth. The procedure itself is usually not painful because the mother is under anaesthesia. These facts make the caesarean attractive to both parents and caregivers. A closer look, however, reveals major disadvantages and risks that make it appropriate to limit caesareans to cases when a vaginal birth is either unsafe or impossible.

Risks or Side Effects of Caesarean Birth Include:

- Possible problems with anaesthesia used for surgery and with medications for pain relief after the caesarean
- Increased incidence of infection and need for antibiotics
- More blood loss and increased risk of haemorrhage, which may cause anaemia or require a blood transfusion
- Longer hospitalisation, which increases the cost of childbirth
- Post-operative pain that lasts weeks or months and makes caring for yourself, your baby and any other children more difficult.
- Risk of problems from scar tissue or adhesions inside the abdomen
- Possible injury to other organs (bowel or bladder) and risk of blood clots in the leg and pelvic area
- Increased risk of breathing and temperature problems for the new baby
- Higher rate of subsequent infertility than that for women who have had a vaginal birth
- Increased risk of placenta praevia or retained placenta in future pregnancies
- Increased likelihood of another caesarean for the next birth

When making a decision about a caesarean, you and your doctor should weigh these risks against the potential benefits. The risks of a caesarean birth are of course worth taking in situations in which a vaginal birth would present even greater risks to the mother or baby.

Reasons for a Caesarean Birth

A caesarean may be performed for any of the following reasons:

Failure to progress (or 'prolonged labour'). Contractions are of poor quality, dilation is not progressing and/or the baby is not descending, even after attempts have been made to rest the uterus or to stimulate stronger contractions. The diagnosis of failure to progress cannot be made reliably until the active phase of labour (after 5 centimetres dilation), since a normal latent phase (0 to 4 or 5 centimetres) is often very slow.

To Improve Your Chances for a Vaginal Birth

1. Take good care of yourself (good nutrition, moderate exercise, avoidance of drugs and tobacco, and so on) so that you enter labour in the best possible health. Both your pre-pregnant weight and your pregnancy weight gain affect your risk for a caesarean. Therefore, lose extra pounds before becoming pregnant and work with your caregiver to maintain an optimal weight gain during pregnancy.
2. Prepare a birth plan with your caregiver to help ensure that you both are working together to decrease your chances of having a caesarean. (See Chapter 7.)
3. Avoid labour induction for non-medical reasons such as being 'tired of being pregnant', convenience for yourself or the medical staff, fearing that the baby is growing too big or being a few days past your due date. (See page 261.)
4. Find a caregiver whom you trust, who has low caesarean rates, and who encourages you to use self-help techniques in labour. (See Chapter 8.)
5. If your baby remains in a breech presentation, talk with your caregiver about an external version to turn your baby to a head-down position. (See page 295.)
6. Take childbirth preparation classes that emphasise the normalcy of birth and encourage your participation in decision-making and in the use of self-help methods to relieve pain and promote labour progress.
7. Wait to be admitted into the hospital until you are in active labour. Learn to differentiate between pre-labour and true labour so you feel confident in staying home until active labour. (See page 218.)
8. Plan to rely on medical interventions only when clearly necessary, since these tend to alter the course of normal labour. Such interventions include artificial rupture of membranes, IV fluids, continuous electronic foetal monitoring and Syntocinon. (See page 308.)
9. Use labour coping skills instead of medications to manage pain. (See Chapter 8.) If medications for pain relief are used, try to delay or minimise their use. A light and late epidural has less slowing effect on labour progress than one given in early labour. (See page 347.)
10. Plan to be up and about during labour. Change your position and activity about every thirty minutes if labour progress slows. Instead of lying on the labour bed for long periods of time, try walking, sitting and taking a shower or bath.
11. If you have had a caesarean previously, plan and prepare for a vaginal birth the next time rather than a repeat caesarean. Take a childbirth review class that promotes vaginal births after caesareans (VBACs) and assists you with psychological preparation and practical information.

There are times when the above measures are employed, but a caesarean delivery is still necessary for a safe outcome. You and your partner should know what to expect with a caesarean and what choices are available.

Mal-presentation or mal-position. The baby's placement in the uterus is unfavourable for a vaginal birth. Examples of mal-presentations include the transverse lie (baby lying horizontally), breech presentations and face or brow presentation. Mal-positions include the persistent occiput posterior position (see page 284) or asynclitism (baby's head tilted so that it does not fit through the pelvis).

Cephalo-pelvic disproportion (CPD). The baby's head is too large, the mother's pelvic structure too small or a combination of the two. CPD can rarely be diagnosed before labour, because even if the baby is large or the mother's pelvis is somewhat small, the baby's head moulds and the pelvic joints spread during labour, both of which create more room. If plenty of time has been allowed and contractions have been of good quality, but there is still no progress, then a diagnosis of CPD can be made. Sometimes, it is difficult to distinguish CPD from a mal-position.

Foetal distress. Particular changes in the foetal heart rate may indicate problems for the baby. These heart rate changes may occur with cord compression or with decreased flow of oxygenated blood to the placenta. Observing the foetal heart rate response to scalp stimulation (see page 260) or using foetal oxygen saturation monitoring (see page 260) can help the caregiver tell whether the baby is compensating well or is beginning to suffer from lack of oxygen. If the baby is no longer able to compensate, a caesarean is necessary.

The major concern with lack of oxygen to the baby is that it may cause damage to the brain (cerebral palsy) or to other vital organs. While it is possible for brain damage to occur during birth, numerous studies have found that, in most cases, brain damage actually takes place during pregnancy before labour begins.[2] These conditions are not detectable in the protected environment of the uterus. Everything appears fine until the stress of labour, when abnormal foetal heart rate patterns appear, or after birth, when abnormal neurological signs develop. Caesareans cannot prevent or cure these pre-existing problems.

Fetal problems. A caesarean birth may reduce problems for a baby with congenital defects. For example, a baby with a spinal cord defect (spina bifida) has a reduced risk of paralysis if born by caesarean. Screening tests in pregnancy (see page 80) help detect this problem.

Prolapsed cord. When the umbilical cord descends through the cervix before the baby, the baby's head or body may pinch the cord and drastically reduce his oxygen supply, necessitating immediate caesarean delivery. (See page 294 for more on prolapsed cord.)

Placenta praevia. The placenta covers or partially covers the cervix. As the cervix dilates, the placenta separates from the uterus, causing painless bleeding in the mother. This could result in decreased oxygen to the foetus. A safe vaginal birth is not possible with a placenta praevia, because the placenta would come out before the baby.

Placental abruption. The placenta prematurely separates from the uterine wall. This may cause vaginal bleeding or hidden bleeding with constant abdominal pain. The separation decreases the foetus's oxygen supply and, depending on how much of the placenta has detached, a caesarean may be necessary.

Maternal disease. If you have heart disease or certain other serious medical conditions, you may not be able to withstand the stress of labour and vaginal birth. Occasionally, the location or size of uterine fibroids is the reason for a caesarean birth. The presence of a herpes sore in or near the vagina at the time of labour is also an indication for a caesarean birth, since the baby may acquire the infection when passing through the birth canal. A mother who is HIV positive decreases her risk of passing the virus to her baby when she has a planned caesarean birth.

Repeat caesarean. Another caesarean may be performed if the reason for a previous caesarean still exists or if the doctor or patient prefers a caesarean birth. Since the 1980s, elective (chosen without a medical reason) repeat caesareans have been the primary reason for the rise in the caesarean rate. Now, pregnant women may be encouraged to have a vaginal birth, unless there is a medical indication for a repeat caesarean. A discussion of vaginal birth after caesarean (VBAC) appears at the end of this chapter.

The Planned (Elective) Caesarean Birth

Sometimes, a caesarean birth is planned in advance for an existing medical reason. Your doctor may wait until you go into labour and then perform the surgery. If labour is allowed to begin spontaneously, your baby is more likely to avoid breathing problems and be closer to full-term. A baby with a breech presentation is an example of a problem that is managed this way. On the other hand, after considering your due date, the foetal size and maturity, and the urgency of need, your doctor may schedule the surgery before your due date. If there are doubts about the maturity of your baby's lungs, foetal maturity tests may be done. (See page 81.) Placenta praevia is an example of a problem that is usually managed this way.

With a scheduled caesarean, routine blood and urine tests are done. The anaesthesiologist discusses the type of anaesthesia and pre-operative and post-operative medications he or she will use and asks about your allergies or sensitivities to drugs. The thought of surgery may make you feel nervous and afraid. It helps to have your partner with you at this time. Calm yourself by using slow breathing and relaxation techniques. Envision yourself holding your baby after the birth. Feel free to ask questions and make requests. Review the section in this book that describes the caesarean procedure. (See pages 323–327.) Discuss your birth plan for caesarean birth and your partner's role with your physician, the nurses and the anaesthesiologist. All this can make your caesarean birth experience more positive and less frightening.

The Unplanned or Emergency Caesarean Birth

Most caesareans are unplanned. In other words, they occur after difficulties arise during labour. Hospitals should be equipped and staffed to perform caesareans within thirty minutes—day or night—so the fact that a caesarean is unplanned does not mean the hospital is unprepared. Most unplanned caesareans are done for failure to progress in labour or for foetal distress. These problems do not usually arise suddenly. They develop gradually, and there is time to try other measures to speed labour or get more oxygen to the baby. Only when these measures fail is a caesarean done. A quick response time is not critical under these circumstances. On rare occasions, an emergency arises (for example, a prolapsed cord or serious haemorrhage), and the mother's or baby's survival depends on a caesarean delivery within minutes. Under such rare circumstances, the hospital's ability to respond very quickly is crucial. Ask your caregiver about your hospital's response time.

Before the Caesarean Birth

Whether the caesarean is planned or unplanned, you will usually be asked to sign a consent form stating that you understand the reasons for and the risks and benefits of the caesarean and that you give the staff your permission to do it. A nurse then shaves your abdomen and the upper portion of your pubic hair. She or he may give you an antacid medication to drink. This is a precaution for the unlikely possibility that you will vomit and inhale the vomited material. (The more acidic the vomitus, the greater the damage to your lungs.) The nurse starts an intravenous (IV) drip in a vein in your hand or arm. The IV remains in place for a few to

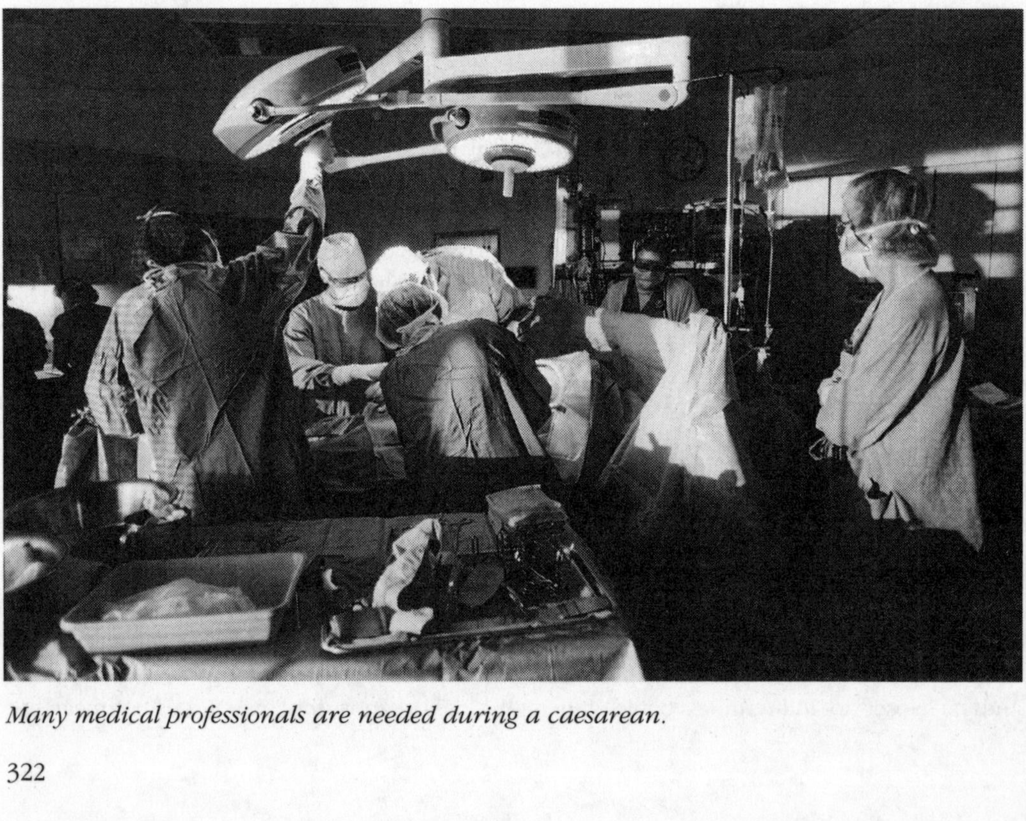

Many medical professionals are needed during a caesarean.

twenty-four hours after the delivery. The nurse also inserts a thin, flexible tube (a catheter) through your urethra into your bladder to keep it empty. The catheter is removed within twenty-four hours after the surgery. Because insertion of the catheter may be uncomfortable, the nurse usually waits to insert it until the anaesthetic has taken effect.

You may be surprised by the large number of people in the delivery room. Besides you and your partner, there are the surgeon, an assistant doctor, a midwife, an anaesthesiologist or nurse anaesthetist, a scrub technician, a circulating nurse and possibly a doctor for the baby. They all have specific jobs to do and you may be impressed by the rapid and precise teamwork of this group of professionals.

Your partner stands or is seated at the head of the delivery table. In this position, he or she can hold your hand, talk to you and remind you to use relaxation and slow breathing to calm yourself.

Most doctors use regional anaesthesia (spinal, epidural or combined spinal-epidural), which allows you to be awake without feeling pain. A *spinal* or a *combined spinal-epidural* numbs you from your lower chest to your toes, and you cannot move your legs. An *epidural* numbs you in the same area, but you may be aware of pressure or pulling during the surgery. Nausea, burning sensations, shoulder pain, trembling, a drop in blood pressure and shortness of breath are all common reactions to regional anaesthetics. To decrease these side effects, the anaesthesiologist can alter the anaesthetic drugs or give you other medications to relieve the discomforts, although some may make you drowsy and unable to enjoy your baby for the first few hours. Occasionally, the regional anaesthesia is either inadequate in providing pain relief, or the level of anaesthesia is too high. (See Chapter 12 for a discussion of these complications.)

In those extremely rare cases of life-threatening emergencies in which immediate intervention is required, *general anaesthesia* is used because it acts quickly. General anaesthesia may also be used if a regional block is unsuccessful or if you are allergic to the medication used for regional blocks. Small or rural hospitals sometimes use general anaesthesia because they do not have round-the-clock regional anaesthesia personnel. (See pages 344–357 for more information on anaesthesia.)

The Surgery

During the surgery, you lie on your back, usually with a wedge under one hip to move the uterus off the large blood vessels and to reduce the likelihood of supine hypotension. (See page 126.) The nurse washes your abdomen with an antiseptic, drapes a sterile sheet over your body, and places a surgical drape or screen between your head and abdomen to prevent you from viewing the surgery or reaching down and touching the surgical area. Some hospitals have drapes with plastic windows in them. You cannot watch the surgery through this window, but you can see as the baby is lifted up and out of your abdomen. Otherwise, you can ask the nurse to lower the drape for the moment of birth. A caesarean takes about one hour, but the baby is usually born ten to fifteen minutes after surgery begins.

During a caesarean, the doctor makes two incisions: one through the abdominal wall (skin, fat and connective tissue) and the other through the uterus. Your abdominal muscles are usually not cut; they are spread apart. The incisions may be both vertical, both transverse (horizontal), or one may be vertical and one transverse. It is important for future births that you know which type of uterine incision you had previously, so ask the doctor to write it down for you.

Skin Incisions

There are two types of skin incisions for a caesarean. The *transverse skin incision* (or bikini cut) is the more common of the two; it is made horizontally just above the pubic bone. The *midline incision* is made vertically between your navel and pubic bone. It allows for a quick delivery in an emergency, or may be preferable under circumstances such as some cases of maternal obesity.

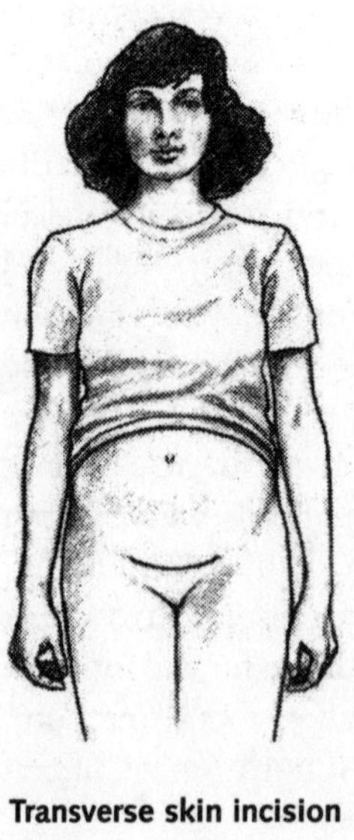

Transverse skin incision

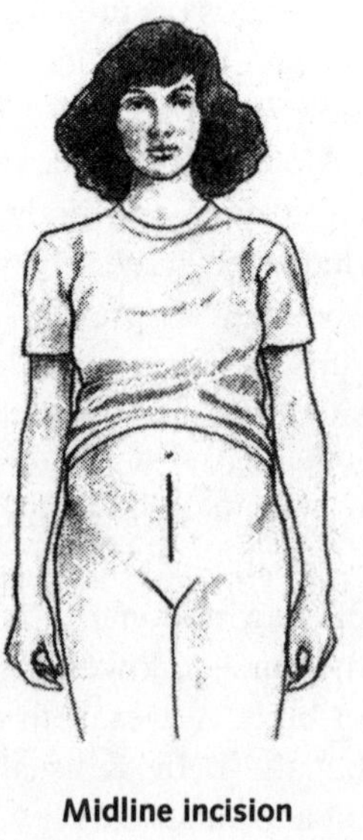

Midline incision

Uterine Incisions

There are three types of uterine incisions. The *classical incision* is made vertically in the upper part of the uterus. It is rarely done today except for placenta praevia or when the foetus is in a transverse presentation or has specific birth defects. Vaginal delivery for future births is not recommended if you have had a classical incision.

The most common uterine incision is the *low transverse incision*. Associated with less blood loss and reduced risk for post-partum infection, this incision requires a little more time to perform than the classical. After a low transverse incision, future vaginal births are encouraged, because the risk of this incision opening during a future labour is low (less than one in a hundred).

The *lower segment vertical incision* is not commonly performed except when the lower part of the uterus has not developed or thinned enough to allow a transverse incision (as in some premature births). Most lower segment vertical incisions go up into the muscle of the lower part of the uterus and therefore lose the advantages of a lower segment incision.

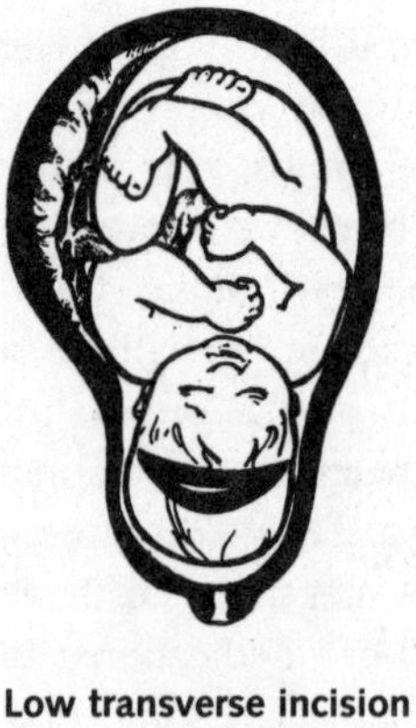

Low transverse incision

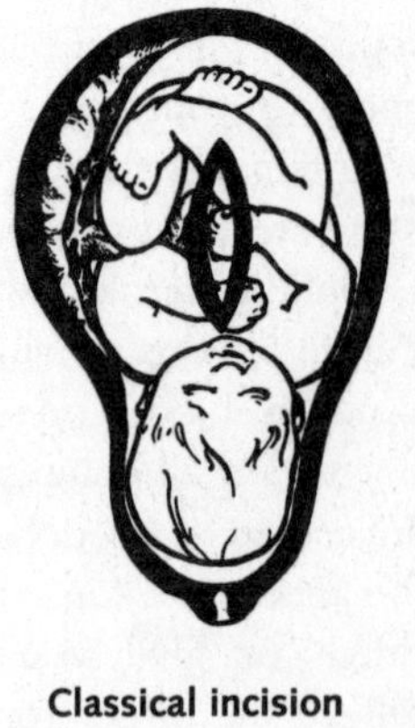

Classical incision

To control bleeding from the incisions, the doctor cauterises (seals by burning) the ends of the cut blood vessels. This causes an odour that you may smell. Your doctor then suctions out the amniotic fluid from your uterus. You may hear this. The doctor usually removes the baby headfirst and suctions the nose and mouth to remove fluid and mucus, just as after a vaginal birth. Then the doctor cuts the cord, shows your baby to you briefly and hands him to the baby's nurse. The baby is placed in a warmed bassinet, dried off, evaluated with the Apgar score (page 243), examined and given any necessary medical care. Syntocinon is added to your IV to cause your uterus to contract, which prevents excessive bleeding. As your placenta is removed, you may feel some pressure or tugging, but often your attention is focused on your new baby.

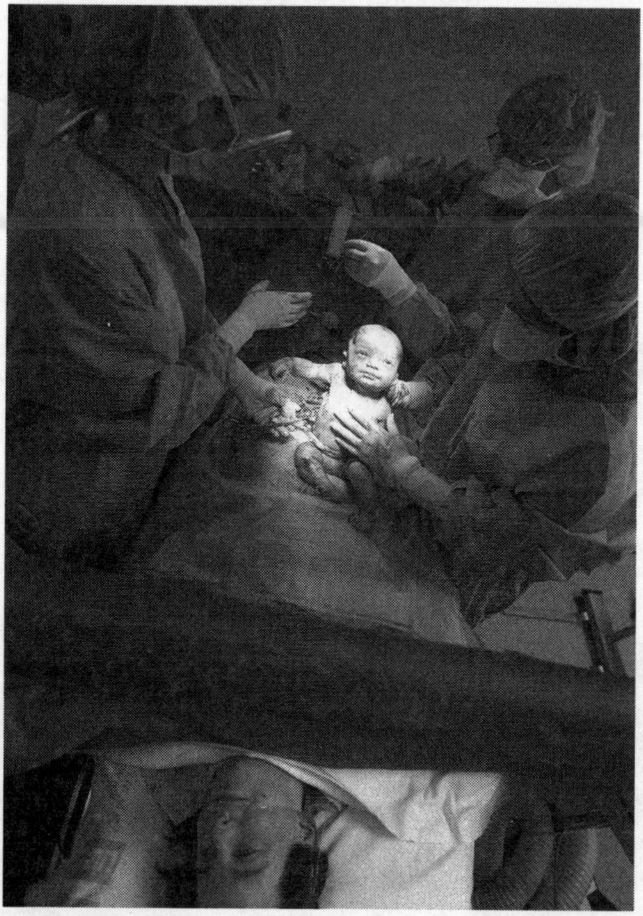

Photograph by Paul Joseph Brown

The baby is placed on the mother's abdomen in the first moments after birth.

After the Caesarean Birth

After the baby and placenta are removed, the doctor inspects your uterus and begins the repair—a procedure that usually takes about thirty to forty-five minutes. The incisions in your uterus and abdomen are sutured with absorbable thread. The skin is closed with absorbable or non-absorbable thread, or with staples or clips that are removed before you go home. A bandage is placed over the incision. The Syntocinon in your IV will be continued to keep your uterus contracted.

If you had regional anaesthesia, you will probably feel queasy or nauseated during the repair. You may tremble all over. It is not clear why these reactions occur, but they usually pass within a few minutes to an hour. You may be given medication for nausea and trembling. This medication may make you drowsy or put you to sleep. If so, you may be unaware of your baby's initial calm, alert period and may be unable to nurse until you awaken. Ask in advance about these post-operative medications. You may state in your birth plan that you want to be consulted before drugs for nausea or trembling are administered. Warm blankets also help reduce trembling. If you had general anaesthesia, you will remain unconscious throughout the repair and for an hour or so afterward.

If the baby's condition is good, your partner can hold the baby, and both of you can see and touch her. Sometimes, the baby can be placed on your chest while your partner helps you hold her. As long as your baby is breathing well and is generally healthy, she may remain with you during the few hours of your recovery, so you can hold, admire and breastfeed her. (See pages 431–434 for help with the initial breastfeeding.) The nurses will observe the baby quite closely for the next hours, watching for breathing problems, a drop in body temperature or any other suspected problems.

During your recovery (either in your hospital room or in a special recovery room), the nurse will check your blood pressure, your incision, the firmness of your uterus and the amount of lochia on your pad. You will be observed closely until the anaesthesia wears off (two to four hours). You will then be monitored periodically until you go home.

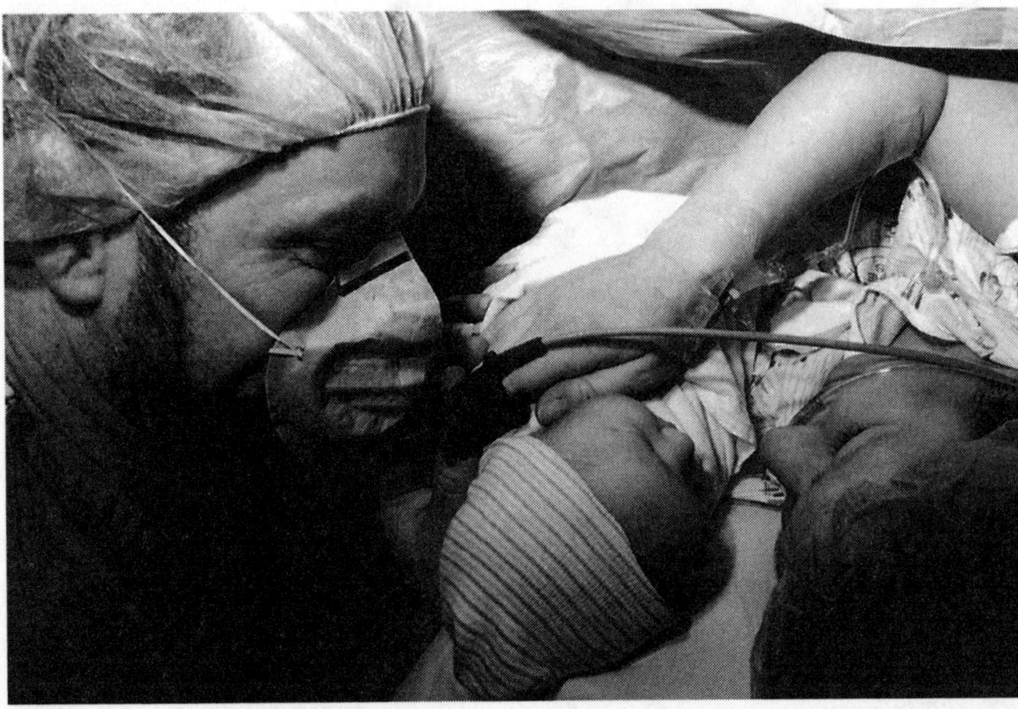

After the caesarean, the family gathers for the first time.

If you had a spinal or epidural anaesthetic, there is a very small risk of a spinal headache. In that case, you will probably be told to lie flat for eight to twelve hours, or you may be given a blood patch. (See page 356.) If you had general anaesthesia, your throat and neck may be sore for a few days from the insertion of the airway tube used to administer the anaesthetic.

Pain Medication after a Caesarean Birth

Pain in your incision will probably bother you quite a lot at first, but it will gradually go away. You will probably need pain medications for several days to a week. You might feel you should use as little medication as possible, but if pain keeps you from moving around and caring for your baby, it might be wise to use enough medication to allow you to do these things. Only low concentrations of the medication will get to your baby via your breast milk, so the effects on your baby will be very slight.

Pain medications come in a variety of forms: pills, injections, self-administered intravenous doses, and spinal or epidural narcotics (given in the delivery room). (See pages 356–358 for a complete discussion of post-caesarean pain medications.)

Recovery from a Caesarean Birth

The first few days after a caesarean are the most difficult. Even little things like rolling over, laughing, coughing, breathing deeply and reaching for the bedside phone are difficult at first. Following are a few hints to make you more comfortable during the early days of your recovery:

Rolling over. Here is a trick that makes rolling from your back to your side easier and less painful: Bend your knees and hips (one leg at a time) so that your feet are flat on the bed. Press your feet into the bed and lift your hips so that your body is straight from shoulders to knees. Twist your hips to one side while rolling the upper part of your body to the same side. Now you are lying on your side. This way of rolling over puts less strain on your incision.

Deep breathing. Breathing deeply with a forceful exhalation is painful, but it should be done (especially if you had general anaesthesia) to clear the mucus that accumulates in your chest and sometimes causes infection. This clearing can be done by breathing out forcefully or using a special device provided by the hospital. Use the following technique to help you breathe deeply with the least pain: Support your incision gently and firmly with your hands, a small pillow or a folded towel. Take in a deep breath. Breathe out quickly, pulling your abdomen in rather than pushing it out. Exhale quickly into the tube on the device, if you have one. When your chest is clear, you no longer need to perform this technique or use the device.

Standing and walking. Your first venture out of bed will take place a few to twenty-four hours after the birth. Your nurse or an aide will help you sit up, then stand. You will probably feel weak, dizzy and light-headed the first few times you get up. You can reduce the dizziness by doing some ankle circling and leg bends to improve your circulation before getting up. Take your time. Give yourself a few moments to get used to each new position as you go from lying down to standing.

Try the following to move from lying in bed to standing up: After rolling to your side near the edge of your bed, let your legs dangle over the edge of the bed and push yourself up to a sitting position. Stay there a while and do some more ankle circling. When you are ready, place your feet on the floor and stand (with someone helping you). Stand as tall and straight as you can. It will not harm your incision even though it feels as if it is pulling and it hurts. Once you are used to the standing position, take a short walk. Each time you get out of bed, you will find it a little easier. Try to increase the distance you walk each time.

Abdominal gas. Abdominal gas is sometimes a problem after a caesarean or any abdominal surgery. If you have it, you become bloated and may have sharp abdominal pains until you pass the gas. The accumulation of gas is caused by a slowdown of intestinal activity that may occur as a result of the surgery. You may not be given food until the nurse notes intestinal activity, which is usually within hours after surgery. Physical movement in and out of bed, deep breathing and rocking in a chair may help prevent or alleviate gas build-up. You may also wish to avoid foods and beverages that cause you gas.

Urination. You may have difficulty urinating after having had a bladder catheter, anaesthesia and abdominal surgery. Your nurse will suggest ways to help you urinate. (See page 368.) If you are unable to urinate within a reasonable amount of time, you will need to be re-catheterised with the 'in-out' method: The nurse inserts a thinner catheter, drains the urine and then removes the catheter. As time passes, you will once again pass urine on your own.

Breastfeeding. It is possible and desirable to breastfeed after a caesarean, but finding a comfortable position can be a problem. To protect your incision from the weight and wiggling of your baby, experiment with the following positions: use the football or clutch hold, lie on your side, or place a pillow over your incision before holding your baby on your lap for feeding. (See Chapter 15.)

If your hospital has a family-centred philosophy, your partner may be allowed to stay in your room with you. If your partner cannot stay, the nurse will help you with baby care as you recover from surgery.

You will probably stay in the hospital two or three days. Your recovery will not be complete by then, however. You will still be sore, weak and tired. If possible, arrange to have help at home for the first few weeks. You will recover much more quickly if you have help with meals, baby care and household tasks. You should not drive a car until you can drive safely, are not in pain and have stopped using narcotic pain relievers. Your caregiver can give you specific guidelines. When your physical condition permits and you have the time and energy, you may begin the post-partum exercises described on pages 138–143. Check with your caregiver about when to begin.

Emotional Reactions to Caesareans

If the caesarean is planned in advance, you have days or weeks beforehand to get used to the idea. If you had desired and planned a vaginal birth, you have to adjust emotionally to the change in plans. If a problem develops gradually in labour, you may have hours during which you realise that the vaginal birth may not be possible. If an emergency requires an immediate caesarean, you may be shocked and completely unprepared emotionally. Everything happens so fast that you and your partner are simply swept along without enough explanation or time for questions.

After it is all over, you will think and wonder about your caesarean. There may be gaps in what you recall, especially if labour was exhausting or if the caesarean was done suddenly. If the outcome was not good—if your baby died or is ill or if your recovery is impaired by infection or poor healing—you will have little time at first to reflect on the caesarean. Shock, grief, illness and the numerous decisions to be made will occupy your attention completely. If everything turned out well, your gratefulness to be alive with a healthy baby will probably be your predominant feeling for a while. Later, although you may feel relieved and thankful for your baby, you may also find yourself depressed, disappointed in yourself or your partner, or angry with your doctor or the nursing staff. You may feel an emptiness when you recall the birth, where you had hoped and expected to feel a sense of fulfilment and joy.

This lonely, let-down feeling may be shared by your partner, but your partner may come to terms with it more quickly than you and may worry about your continued concerns. If possible, talk honestly and openly about the birth and your feelings—it can help.

It takes time to let go of a vision, more time for some than for others. The following factors help many women adjust more easily: having known in advance that a caesarean was likely or planned, having had confidence in the doctor who made the decision, having had time to try measures to solve whatever problem existed and realising that they were not succeeding, having been treated kindly and respectfully by the staff, and having had the opportunity afterwards to review the labour and the caesarean with the caregiver or nurse.

Besides reviewing the reasons for the caesarean and filling in any gaps in your understanding or memory of the events, you should ask your caregiver two questions that will be important for future births:

1. What type of uterine incision do I have? A transverse (lower segment) incision or a vertical (classical or lower segment) incision? The transverse incision is safer for future vaginal births, since it does not weaken the body of the uterus.

2. What about future births? Am I a good candidate for a vaginal birth? Be sure you know the reason for your caesarean and whether that reason is likely to be a problem next time. Most women can have vaginal births in the future. You should find out right away so that you do not go home assuming that you are unable to give birth vaginally.

Such a belief is difficult for some women to reverse in a future pregnancy. If your doctor does not recommend a future vaginal birth, be sure to ask why, and consider seeking a second opinion if your caregiver's reasons do not seem well-founded.

Later, if you still have doubts or feelings of disappointment, your childbirth educator, a counsellor and other women who have had similar experiences may be able to help you and your partner review the birth and come to terms with persistent feelings of sadness or anger. Many women find it helpful to go over their hospital chart with their caregiver.

Vaginal Birth after a Previous Caesarean (VBAC)

Most women who have had caesareans can have vaginal births with future pregnancies. The caesarean surgery, as it is now performed, almost always leaves a strong, healthy uterus with a scar that heals well—a condition that means a future labour and vaginal birth is less likely to cause scar separation. Now that doctors and midwives have gained experience managing VBAC labours, they find the risk of scar separation for most women to be minimal. Their experience agrees with the numerous medical reports that document the safety and benefits of VBACs over repeat caesareans. These benefits include reduction in post-operative complications, shortened hospital stay and other economic benefits, ability to resume normal activity more quickly and psychological benefits.[3]

There are some situations in which a VBAC may be impossible or unwise (for example, if the reason for the first caesarean still exists). If you have a chronic illness or a physical condition that makes a vaginal birth unsafe or impossible, you should have another caesarean. In most cases, however, the reasons for the first cesarean do not recur. The most common indications for the first caesarean—failure to progress, foetal distress, mal-position, mal-presentation, or even cephalo-pelvic disproportion (CPD)—rarely come up again in future pregnancies.

If the caesarean incision in the uterus was high and vertical (a classical incision), there is a higher risk that the scar will separate during labour than if the incision was low and transverse. Most physicians support VBACs only with a low transverse scar; few would support a VBAC for a woman with a classical incision.

A fear of scar separation (sometimes called *uterine rupture*) is the main reason why both caregivers and parents are sometimes reluctant to plan a VBAC. The likelihood of uterine rupture is somewhat higher (0.5–1.0 percent) with a VBAC than when there is no scar on the uterus. Uterine rupture can be diagnosed by evaluation of the foetal heart rate pattern, observation of the shape of the abdomen and monitoring of the mother's blood pressure. If the scar separates during labour, you will have another caesarean delivery and the separation will be repaired. Under these circumstances, the caesarean may have to be performed quite suddenly because of possible foetal distress and excessive bleeding from the uterus. Sometimes (about 0.7 percent of births following a previous caesarean) the scar weakens, causing a window effect (called *uterine dehiscence*) but not a true separation. Though the scar has thinned, it does not adversely affect the mother or foetus, and it heals itself as the uterus returns to its non-pregnant size. Although vaginal delivery after a previous caesarean is generally considered safe it is associated with an increased risk to the baby. A recent study suggested that the risk of a baby dying as a result of scar rupture is 1 in every 775 labours after a caesarean. Although uncommon, this represents over a ten-fold risk compared with elective caesarean. It is necessary for you as parents to assess the potential risks and benefits.

In Australia, conventional practice is to offer an elective repeat caesarean in the event of you having had two or more caesareans. This is because the rupture rate may be as high as 3 percent.

VBAC Preparation

You may need to prepare differently for a VBAC than you would if you had had a previous vaginal birth. Besides the recommendations on page 319 ('To Improve Your Chances for a Vaginal Birth'), you may find it helpful to address any negative feelings leftover from your caesarean that could interfere with your self-confidence and optimism for a VBAC.

Some communities have caesarean and VBAC support groups where women meet, share their stories and concerns, and support each other in coping with the emotional issues surrounding caesareans and VBACs. Some communities also have special childbirth preparation classes for women and couples planning VBACs. Other communities include VBAC information in a childbirth review course. When you research classes, ask about their content on VBAC preparation. Find out if they address the emotional aspects of VBACs and possible differences in the medical management of the labour, along with the knowledge and skills necessary to prepare for childbirth.

For some women, the previous labour that ended in caesarean delivery was profoundly difficult or even traumatic. If this is true for you, it is important to talk with a knowledgeable counsellor who can help you make plans that are best for you and not based on fear.

Emotional Reactions Associated with VBAC

As you review the circumstances of your caesarean, you may explore any deep-seated feelings in yourself that may have come up during the course of your labour. Sometimes, the nature of labour itself evokes emotional responses (fear, a need to protect yourself and so on) that you may have felt in other painful or uncontrollable situations such as sexual, physical or emotional abuse; loneliness; or helplessness. (See page 42 for more information on these experiences.) Anyone who has experienced difficulties like these may find them coming up unexpectedly in the psychologically stressful circumstances of pregnancy or labour. If, as you read this, you feel that you have had some experiences that have left you with unresolved or disturbing psychological issues, it may help to address them and deal with them. Good books are available that explore the psychological aspects of pregnancy and birth. (See Recommended Resources.) A counsellor or psychotherapist may also be able to facilitate your resolution of these issues. Ask your childbirth educator, public health nurse or caregiver for referrals.

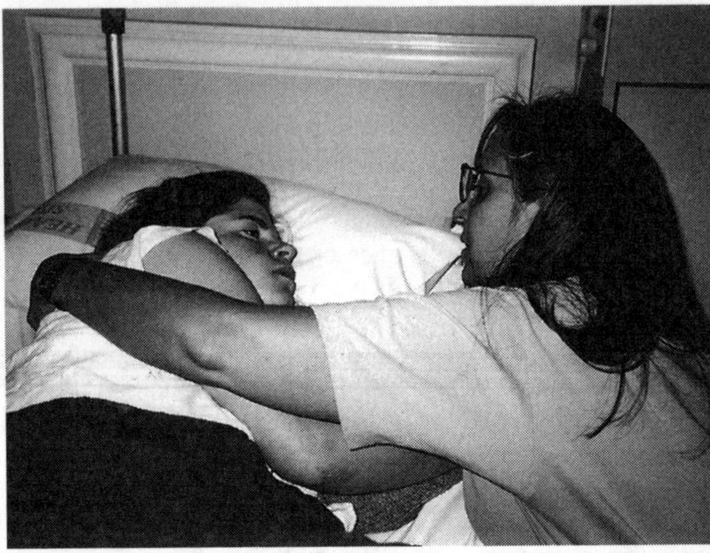

Photograph by Penny Simkin

A midwife provides encouragement and helps you overcome your fears.

The greater challenge for the VBAC woman in labour seems to be emotional rather than physical. The following emotional challenges have been described by women who have anticipated and experienced a VBAC. You may or may not encounter these. They are perfectly normal reactions, but you will need to understand how to deal with them.

Fears. You may fear pain, a long labour, a scar separation, complications, another caesarean, 'failure' or 'the unknown'. The list goes on and on, and sometimes the thought of labouring again is more frightening than the risks of major surgery. It may seem easier to plan another caesarean. If you disclose such fears to your caregiver, childbirth educator or support group, you will probably receive considerable reassurance and support. These people can help you identify the most distressing parts of your previous birth experience, and they can help you set limits to help ensure that your next birth will not be as difficult. For example, you and your caregiver could plan that if a long, non-progressing labour recurs, you will not wait for hours before having the caesarean.

Lack of confidence. You may doubt your ability to give birth vaginally. You may hesitate to invest much time and effort in a VBAC because you do not want to be disappointed again. Because you did not give birth vaginally before, you may lack hope or confidence that you can this time. It helps to acknowledge the differences between last time and this; this is a different pregnancy, a different birth. Get to know people who have had VBACs. You may find out that they also lacked confidence and hope beforehand. Ask them what helped them deal with those feelings. Be sure you know what to expect and ways to cope with labour pain, and surround yourself with people who can give you confidence. A midwife or your childbirth educator can encourage both you and your partner if you begin doubting your abilities. She or he can also suggest comfort measures and labour promoting measures and can help you deal with medical decisions, if they arise.

Stress in labour. In addition to the emotional hurdles that come up in most labours (see Chapter 9), there are specific events in a VBAC labour that may raise your anxiety level:

- Getting into early labour may be your 'moment of truth'. As you really get going, you may suddenly wonder if a VBAC is such a good idea after all. Be prepared for this, and have ideas for dealing with it. You may find yourself tensing and overreacting to early labour contractions, which will increase your pain. (Review Chapters 8 and 9 for suggested ways to handle the discomforts and emotional hurdles of early labour.)
- Flashbacks to your previous labour may be triggered by particular events that remind you of your last labour (for example, starting labour the same way or having the same hospital room or nurse). Such events may elicit unpleasant associations or memories. Do not suppress these flashbacks. Acknowledge them openly and figure out how the circumstances are different this time. If your partner has similar flashbacks, it is better that he or she not mention them to you. Your partner should discuss them with your nurse or caregiver.
- Approaching the point in labour (in hours of labour or centimetres of dilation) where you had a previous caesarean may loom as a large hurdle for you. Until you pass that point, you may continue to question your ability to have a VBAC. Once you have passed it, however, you may heave a sigh of relief and feel a boost of optimism.

Improving Your Chances of Having a VBAC

As a woman who has had a caesarean, you know that you could have another. Preparing psychologically for both a vaginal birth and caesarean birth is challenging. To improve your chances of having a VBAC, your preparation should be realistic and include the following:

- Learning the reasons for the previous caesarean
- Changing caregivers and hospitals if their policies led to your first caesarean or if they do not support VBACs
- Improving your eating and health habits if they contributed to your need for the caesarean
- Exploring any negative or destructive emotions that may have contributed to or resulted from the caesarean
- Taking childbirth classes and mastering coping skills and comfort measures
- Planning to use medications and interventions only if necessary
- Having caring, supportive people to help during labour

By following these suggestions, you will have done all you can do to ensure a vaginal birth. However, there is no guarantee of a reasonably normal labour in which the baby and mother remain healthy throughout. Therefore, you have to keep the caesarean option open. It is a wise solution when serious problems arise.

Remember, you will likely feel happy and fulfilled when you know you were well cared for and when you did a good job—no matter how you gave birth.

Chapter 12

Pain Medications during Labour, Birth and Post Partum

Every culture throughout history has had its childbirth experts (midwives, priests, shamans, medicine men and doctors) who established dietary, spiritual and behavioural guidelines to ease the birth process and improve outcomes. These experts also used drugs during childbirth for various purposes, most commonly to ease labour pain or to bring on strong labour contractions. In earlier times and in other cultures, these 'drugs' were extracts from plants such as poppies (opium and laudanum), fruits (wine and brandy), willow bark (aspirin), rye fungus (ergot, which caused uterine contractions) and many others. At this time, pain medications for relief of childbirth pain include sedatives, tranquillisers, narcotics, narcotic-like drugs and anaesthetic agents. (For more information, see page 340.)

Pregnancy, birth and breastfeeding pose a unique challenge in the search for safe, effective drugs. Both the mother and baby are affected when the mother takes medication—something you and your caregiver must think about when considering the use of medication. Your caregiver should evaluate all the possible effects of a drug when considering how to treat a particular problem, and you should know the possible disadvantages and risks as well as the benefits of any medication that may be used. You should also be informed of other measures, interventions or precautions used along with a particular medication to ensure safety, and whether there are other acceptable ways of addressing the problem.

Try to learn about pain medications before labour. Then, when the need for medication arises in labour, you already have some knowledge. This chapter provides general information on the variety of pain relief medications used in labour, birth and post partum. It includes those that are widely used as well as many less common ones. Charts in chapter 10 discuss medications used in labour for purposes other than pain relief (for example, cervical ripening and labour induction agents, page 272; drugs to contract the uterus after birth, page 275; drugs to slow or stop premature contractions, page 299; drugs to hasten foetal lung maturity, page 301; and drugs to manage pre-eclampsia or control high blood pressure, page 302).

Considering Medication for Pain Relief in Childbirth

Some women want very much to have a natural childbirth (give birth without using medications), while others cannot imagine themselves going without pain medications. Most women's desires, however, fall somewhere in between. While these women would like to minimise their use of strong pain medications, they do not want to suffer. The information in this chapter will help you form your own opinions and preferences regarding the use of pain medications.

The following factors play a major role in whether you will use pain medications in childbirth:

1. *Your prior wishes.* Do you have a strong preference for an unmedicated birth ('natural childbirth'), or do you prefer to use pain medications? How strongly do you feel about this preference? Your wishes should be clearly stated in your birth plan.

2. *Childbirth preparation classes.* If your class offers thorough discussion of all available options for pain relief (medical and non-medical) and provides opportunities for you and your partner to master self-help comfort measures, you will be better able to cope with labour pain effectively. If, on the other hand, your class is brief or based on the assumption that you will not be using self-help measures, you are more likely to require pain medications.

3. *The degree and quality of support you will have from your partner, midwife and caregiver.* You are more likely to avoid, postpone or minimise the use of pain medications if your partner plays a continuous active role in encouraging and helping you with self-help comfort measures and if your doctor or midwife is confident and encouraging of self-help efforts. If that kind of support is lacking, if you do not want that kind of support or if the custom in your hospital is to use pain medication, then you are more likely to use it.

4. *The nature of your labour.* The more straightforward and uncomplicated your labour is, the better your chances are for an unmedicated birth. If your labour is prolonged, complicated or includes the use of painful interventions, you are more likely to need pain medications. If you have a caesarean birth, you will, of course, require pain medications in the form of anaesthesia.

General Considerations

As you consider the pros and cons of labouring with or without pain medications, keep these factors in mind:

- Labour often hurts more than you may have anticipated.
- Medications can relieve some or all of your labour pain.
- Although many new techniques and medications are available today, a perfect method for abolishing the pain of labour and childbirth has not yet been achieved.

Pain Medication Preference Scale (PMPS)

Before selecting your preferences on pain medications, learn about the labour process, comfort measures, self-help techniques and the various medications available to you and their benefits and risks.

Use this scale to find the approach to pain relief that best suits you and to discover the kind of assistance you will need. Positive (+) numbers indicate a desire to use pain medications, and negative (–) ones indicate a desire to avoid them.

Ask your partner to use this scale to express his or her preferences regarding your use of pain medications in labour. If the two of you do not agree, your wishes should prevail. You will need to discuss ways to make sure that you get the support you need and that you will be working together.

No one knows in advance how long or how painful labour will be or if there will be complications. Despite these unknowns, your preferences about the use of pain medications (as expressed before labour) are a helpful guide to those who are with you during labour.

Rating	Your Preference	Ways Your Partner Can Help You (Some of these measures can also be done by the midwife or caregiver.)
+10	I do not want to feel any pain. I prefer to be numb and to get anaesthesia before labour begins. *(an impossible extreme)*	• Discussing your wishes and fears with you • Explaining that you will have some pain, even with anaesthesia • Making sure the staff knows that you want medication as soon as possible in labour • Promising to help you get medication
+9	I want as much pain medication as I can have. I fear labour pain and believe I cannot deal with the pain and stress.	• Doing the same as for +10 above • Helping you write a birth plan that clearly expresses your preferences on pain medication • Helping you use relaxation and comfort measures for coping in early labour • Ensuring that someone will always be there to help you and provide emotional support
+7	I want anaesthesia in labour as soon as the doctor/midwife will allow it, preferably before labour becomes painful.	• Doing the same as for +9 above • Helping you learn your caregivers' policies on pain medication (timing and drugs used) • Helping you learn any factors that might delay anaesthesia
+5	I want epidural anaesthesia in active labour (4–5 cm). I will try to cope until then, perhaps with narcotic medications.	• Doing the same as for +7 above • Encouraging your breathing and relaxation • Knowing and using a variety of comfort measures prior to active labour • Suggesting the use of medications when you are in active labour
+3	I want to use some pain medication, but as little as possible. I plan to use self-help comfort measures until I receive medication.	• Doing the same as for +5 above • Helping you reduce medication use • Helping you get medications when you decide you want them • Suggesting half doses of narcotics or a 'light and late' epidural
0	I have no opinion or preference. *(a rare attitude among pregnant women)*	• Helping you become informed about labour pain, comfort measures and medications • Following your wishes during labour

Pain Medication Preference Scale (PMPS)

Rating	Your Preference	Ways Your Partner Can Help You (Some of these measures can also be done by the midwife or caregiver.)
-3	I would like to avoid pain medications if I can. If coping becomes difficult, I will not feel guilty taking them.	• Helping you write a birth plan that expresses your preferences • Emphasising coping techniques • Not suggesting that you take pain medication • Not trying to talk you out of pain medications if you request them
-5	I have a strong desire to avoid pain medications because of the side effects to me, my labour and my baby. I will accept medications if labour is difficult or very long.	• Preparing for a very active support role • Practising comfort measures with you in class and at home • Helping you write a birth plan that expresses your preferences • Not suggesting medications; if you ask for them, suggesting different comfort measures and providing more intensive labour support • Helping you accept pain medications if you become exhausted or are not benefiting from support techniques and comfort measures
-7	I strongly desire a natural childbirth because of the benefits to my baby and to my labour as well as the gratification of meeting the personal challenge. I will be disappointed if I use pain medications.	• Doing the same as for –5 above • Helping you enlist the support of your caregiver and request a nurse who will help with natural birth • Planning and rehearsing ways to get through painful or discouraging periods in labour • Prearranging a plan for letting others know if you truly want medication (for example, a 'last resort' code word)
-9	I definitely do not want pain medications. I want my support team and the staff to refuse my requests for medication.	• Exploring with you the reasons for your feelings • Helping you see that the staff cannot deny you requested medications • Promising to help as much as possible but leaving the decision about medication up to you
-10	I want no medication, even for caesarean delivery. *(an impossible extreme)*	• Doing the same as for –9 above • Helping you gain a realistic understanding of the risks and benefits of pain medications

Total absence of pain from the beginning to the end of labour is not safe or possible, even with the best pain medications.

- Absence of pain in late labour is possible with anaesthesia. Sometimes, however, the labouring woman continues to feel some pain due to problems with administration or her individual reaction.
- Drugs and anaesthetics affect your labour. Sometimes, they promote relaxation and speed labour progress; sometimes, they slow labour progress and increase your need for other medical interventions such as Syntocinon, forceps, vacuum extraction or caesarean delivery.
- When you request pain medication, there may be a delay before the anaesthesia staff can respond (for example, when they must complete a more pressing task). Also, once administered, some medications take more time to take effect than others.

- Most physicians and midwives discourage heavy or unlimited use of pain medications throughout labour and during childbirth.
- Any medication you receive affects your baby directly or indirectly.
- The specific effects of medication on you and your baby depend on the particular drug, the amount received, how and when in labour it is given, individual reactions to the drug and other factors. When you receive medication, the medical staff watches for negative effects and takes appropriate action.
- The choice of medication is influenced by such factors as allergies you may have, other medications you may be using regularly, unusual anatomical conditions of your spine, some medical conditions and others.
- Special precautions and added interventions are needed with most pain medications to prevent, minimise or treat side effects that may interfere with labour progress or harm you or your baby. For example, precautions such as restriction to bed, restriction of fluids by mouth, intravenous (IV) fluids, Syntocinon augmentation, oxygen, frequent checks of your blood pressure and blood oxygen levels, vaginal exams, catheterisation of your bladder, and continuous electronic foetal monitoring are more often necessary if you have pain medications than if you do not.
- Because the immature liver and kidneys of the newborn are unable to rapidly detoxify, metabolise or excrete medications, the effects of some drugs last longer for the baby than they do for the mother.
- Pain medications or anaesthetics are often used when birth requires painful interventions or surgical assistance—such as Syntocinon augmentation, forceps, vacuum extraction or an episiotomy—and are always used for caesarean births.

Weighing the Benefits and Risks of Pain Medications

In most labours, if pain medications are used judiciously with up-to-date methods, the benefits to the mother are relaxation or sleep and reduction of or total relief from pain. The risks are slight, subtle and probably temporary. Occasionally, however, even with excellent care, medications cause more serious and longer direct or indirect effects. One of your caregiver's goals is to be aware of all potential risks and to be ready to deal with them.

The choice is not always an easy one. With the help of your caregiver, you must weigh the expected physical or psychological benefits of a particular medication against its possible risks.

One factor that cannot be predicted or controlled is the nature of the labour itself. It is wise to remain flexible when considering the use of medication. Most labours are uncomplicated and, if you so desire, can be handled without pain medications. In such cases, the benefits of pain medications do not clearly outweigh the possible risks. Other labours are more difficult. Some are very long and exhausting, and some may require medical or surgical procedures that increase pain. In such cases, the benefits of medication more clearly outweigh the potential risks. Since you may have a difficult labour that requires pain medications, your birth preparations should include an understanding of medications and the circumstances in which they might be used.

Ideally, you and your caregiver should discuss the following questions before labour. If you try to discuss these questions during labour when you are in great pain or if there is an emergency, calm discussion may be impossible.

1. What medications are most commonly used for pain relief in your caregiver's practice?

2. How does each medication relieve pain? What is the mechanism through which it reduces pain awareness?

3. Have you ever had an adverse reaction (allergy or side effect) to this or a similar drug? Have you told your caregiver and the anaesthesiologist about any drug reactions you have had and any other medications you are taking?

4. What are the potential risks or undesirable side effects of the drug on the mother, foetus/newborn or labour progress?

5. How is the medication given (for example, by mouth, injection, IV drip or another way)?

6. What precautions does your caregiver take to prevent, control or treat undesirable side effects?

Once you have the answers to these questions, you will know what to expect and be better able to make an informed decision. Then, if you need or want medication, you can choose thoughtfully and appropriately. Later, when you look back on your labour, you will feel satisfied that you handled a difficult situation well.

Pain Medications Used in Labour and Birth

Each drug and anaesthetic has specific characteristics that make it inappropriate to use during particular phases of labour. Some medications should not be given too early because they may interfere with the progress of labour. Others should only be given early because they can have harmful effects on the newborn if they remain in effect at birth; with these drugs, much of the drug is excreted from the baby's system before birth, if there is enough time. Because of the different drug effects, you may be offered one medication during the latent phase of labour and a different medication during the active phase or later. The goal of using medications is to relieve some or all of the pain while not seriously compromising the wellbeing of your baby or the progress of your labour.

Medications that are used for pain relief in labour and birth cause either *analgesia* (pain relief) or *anaesthesia* (loss of sensation). These medications can be classified as *systemic medications* and as *regional* and *local* anaesthetics.

Systemic Medications

Systemic means 'affecting your whole body'. Systemic medications come in many forms (pills, liquids, injections into muscle or vein, suppositories, or gases). All are absorbed into your bloodstream and, because they go wherever your blood goes, they exert effects throughout your entire body or system (hence the name *systemic*). The desired effect is to reduce your pain, but there may be other effects—some desirable, some undesirable.

Because systemic medications are carried throughout your body, including your placenta, they cross over to your baby and may cause side effects in the baby as well as in you. The magnitude of these effects in your baby depends on the amount of medication used, the number of doses, and the amount of time between the last dose and the delivery of your baby. Other important factors are the baby's maturity, health and response during labour. With the same amount of medication, a healthy, full-term baby will probably show fewer side effects than a premature, ill or distressed baby. The medication or its metabolic by-products may not completely disappear from the baby's bloodstream for hours or days after birth, and obvious or subtle neuro-behavioural changes (described in the 'Systemic Medications' chart) may be present during the first few days after birth. These changes may be so subtle that they are obvious only to professionals who examine your baby with very sensitive tests such as the Brazelton Neonatal Neurobehavioural Assessment Scale.

Systemic Medications

Systemic medications are listed here with their *generic* (chemical) names first and their *brand* names in parentheses. Effects and side effects vary, depending on the drug used, total dosage, timing, foetal condition and the mother's individual response.

Type	Drugs Used (listed by frequency of use)	Benefits and/or Purposes	Possible Risks and/or Disadvantages	Additional Precautions/ Procedures/Interventions to Ensure Safety
Sedatives and hypnotics	*Barbiturates:* • pentobarbital (Nembutal) • secobarbital (Seconal) • amobarbital (Amytal) • phenobarbital (Luminal)	Sedatives (which reduce anxiety, irritability and excitement) or hypnotics (which induce rest, relaxation or sleep) are administered only in early labour. Sedatives are smaller doses and hypnotics are larger doses of the same drugs. They may be used to give the mother a rest by decreasing contractions in a slow, painful pre-labour.	• *To mother:* Hypnotic doses may cause dizziness and disorientation and can prolong labour by impairing uterine activity. • *To baby:* Barbiturates may accumulate in foetal tissue and cause respiratory depression (very slow breathing), decreased responsiveness and impaired sucking ability in the newborn.	• Should be discontinued before active labour to reduce effects on newborn • Oxygen and resuscitation equipment on hand if baby is born soon after barbiturates are given *Note:* Rarely used today because of undesirable side effects

Systemic Medications

Type	Drugs Used (listed by frequency of use)	Benefits and/or Purposes	Possible Risks and/or Disadvantages	Additional Precautions/ Procedures/Interventions to Ensure Safety
Tranquillisers	*Phenothiazines:* • promethazine (Phenergan) • prochlorperazine (Compazine) *Other:* • hydroxyzine (Vistaril or Atarax)	Tranquillisers are used to reduce tension, apprehension and anxiety. If used in labour, the dosage is timed to wear off before birth. The phenothiazines and hydroxyzine are also used to reduce nausea and vomiting. They are sometimes combined with narcotics to increase the effects of lower doses of narcotics.	• *To mother:* Tranquillisers may cause drowsiness, dizziness, blurred vision, confusion, dry mouth, and changes in blood pressure and heart rate. When given with barbiturates or narcotics, tranquillisers may increase their sedative and depressant effects. • *To baby:* Use of phenothiazines near term can inhibit newborn reflexes and cause jaundice.	• Should be discontinued before active labour to reduce effects on newborn • Oxygen and resuscitation equipment on hand if baby is born soon after tranquillisers are given • Observation for and treatment of jaundice
Inhalation analgesia	• nitrous oxide (Entonox)	Nitrous oxide rapidly reduces pain awareness and in low concentration may be used during normal labour. The mother, using a hand-held mask, administers the drug as needed. In higher concentrations, it is a general anaesthetic and causes loss of consciousness. (See page 344.)	• Reduces mother's ability to use upright positions and to push effectively	• Confinement to bed • Mixed with oxygen to ensure adequate blood oxygen levels

Systemic Medications

Type	Drugs Used (listed by frequency of use)	Benefits and/or Purposes	Possible Risks and/or Disadvantages	Additional Precautions/ Procedures/Interventions to Ensure Safety
Narcotic or narcotic-like analgesics *Note:* These are given intravenously, either by direct injection or injection into an intravenous line. Sometimes, a patient-controlled analgesia (PCA) device is used in labour, but more often after a caesarean. The woman presses a button when she needs medication, causing release of the narcotic into her IV.	• pethidine • morphine • fentanyl (Sublimaze)	Narcotic analgesics, usually given during active labour, reduce pain awareness and promote relaxation between contractions. Some may indirectly speed a labour that has been slowed by tension and stress. Large doses of narcotics (especially morphine) are sometimes used in a prolonged pre-labour in hopes of stopping contractions and giving the mother a rest. They may also be used in post partum.	• *To mother:* Narcotic analgesics may cause drowsiness, hallucinations, dizziness, euphoria, respiratory depression, nausea, vomiting and slowing of digestion. They may lower blood pressure. They often interfere with mental activities and the use of self-help comfort measures. Narcotics may temporarily slow labour progress, especially if the medication is given before the active phase of labour. • *To baby:* Narcotic analgesics may make the foetal heart rate readings appear abnormal, depress the newborn's respiration and alter the infant's behavioural responses (for example, breastfeeding) for several days or weeks.	• Restriction to bed • Continuous monitoring of foetal heart rate (FHR) • Reminders to mother to breathe deeply • Maternal position changes or oxygen to improve FHR abnormalities • Should be discontinued before active labour to reduce effects on newborn • Oxygen and resuscitation equipment on hand if baby is born soon (within 4 hours) after narcotics are given • Availability of narcotic antagonist for mother or baby, if necessary, to reverse side effects • Patient-controlled analgesia devices, which are designed to maintain adequate pain relief and protect against an overdose
Narcotic antagonists	• naloxone (Narcan)	Narcotic antagonists reduce narcotic effects such as hallucinations, respiratory depression (very slow breathing), sedation and hypotension (low blood pressure). Narcan is given by injection to the labouring woman if there is narcotic toxicity, or to the newborn when there are respiratory problems caused by narcotics.	• *To mother and baby:* Abrupt reversal of narcotic depression may result in rapid heart rate, increased blood pressure, nausea, vomiting, sweating, trembling and the return of pain awareness to the mother. The effects of narcotics may return if the narcotic antagonist wears off before the narcotic.	• Continued observation of mother or baby for return of narcotic side effects • Repeated dose of narcotic antagonist as needed

General Anaesthesia (A Two-Step Process)

Type	Drugs Used (listed by frequency of use)	Benefits and/or Purposes	Possible Risks and/or Disadvantages	Additional Precautions/ Procedures/Interventions to Ensure Safety
STEP 1: **Pre-anaesthesia drugs (induction agents)**	• thiopental sodium (Pentothal) • methohexital sodium (Brevital) • thiamylal sodium (Surital) • ketamine (Ketalar)	Pre-anaesthesia drugs (induction agents) are given intravenously before administration of inhalation agents. They are usually very short-acting barbiturates that produce drowsiness and semi-consciousness.	• *To mother:* Induction agents cause respiratory depression (very slow breathing), lower blood pressure and may change heart rate. Large doses may reduce uterine activity. • *To baby:* Large doses may result in respiratory depression and poor muscle tone.	• Monitoring of mother's breathing, pulse, heart function (on electrocardiogram, or EKG), blood pressure and blood oxygen levels (with pulse oximeter) • Monitoring of baby and resuscitation, if needed
STEP 2: **Inhalation agents**	• isoflurane (Forane) • nitrous oxide (Entonox) • enflurane (Ethrane) • halothane (Fluothane)	Inhalation agents rapidly provide loss of sensation and consciousness. They may be used for caesarean birth when speed is important.	• *To mother:* Inhalation agents may cause nausea, respiratory depression, changes in blood pressure and heart rate, and elevated temperature. They may increase the incidence of post-partum haemorrhage. The most serious, though rare, risk is inhalation of vomited material, which can cause pneumonia and possibly death. Modern anaesthesia technique minimises these risks. • *To baby:* Inhalation agents may cause respiratory depression, drowsiness, poor muscle tone and low Apgar scores.	• Monitoring of mother's breathing, pulse, heart function (on electrocardiogram, or EKG), blood pressure and blood oxygen levels (with pulse oximeter) • Mixed with oxygen to ensure adequate blood oxygen levels • Antacid to mother before receiving anaesthetic • Intubation (tube in mother's windpipe) to protect against inhalation of vomited material • Anaesthesia administration close to the start of surgery to minimise effects on baby • Monitoring of baby and skilled staff available for resuscitation, if needed

General Analgesia and General Anaesthesia

General analgesia refers to a reduction of pain and awareness without a total loss of consciousness. For labour or a post-partum procedure, it is achieved by inhalation of a gas. A general analgesic takes effect almost immediately. In fact, it acts more quickly than any other form of systemic medication. *General anaesthesia* refers to a total loss of both sensation and consciousness. A general anaesthetic is used on rare occasions for caesarean delivery.

The main difference between general analgesics and general anaesthetics is in the concentration of the gas used (percent of drug and percent of air). A lower concentration reduces pain awareness but does not remove it completely. For example, with one particular inhalation agent, nitrous oxide, the mother sometimes holds the mask to her face and inhales the gas. As she loses awareness, the mask falls away and she regains awareness.

General anaesthetics, which involve higher concentrations of the gas, are always administered by an anaesthetist or anaesthesiologist. Under general anaesthesia, the mother is somewhat more likely to vomit, breathe in the vomited material and develop pneumonia. Anaesthesia practitioners are trained to prevent such a complication if general anaesthesia has been used. General anaesthetics may be used in the following situations:

- Emergency caesareans, when a rapid loss of sensation is required for delivery within minutes
- For caesareans in small or rural hospitals that do not have round-the-clock regional anaesthesia services (described at right)
- In the rare instance that an epidural or spinal block (described below) cannot be placed successfully
- When the woman cannot tolerate a regional anaesthetic
- If the woman has a bleeding tendency or has a low platelet count

General analgesia is achieved through a two-step process. First, an anaesthesia 'induction agent' is given intravenously. This quickly makes the woman very relaxed and unconscious. Then she inhales a gas that continues loss of consciousness until the end of surgery. A tube is inserted through the woman's mouth into her trachea (windpipe) to keep her airway open and to allow administration of the anaesthetic. Because an unconscious person may vomit, the tube helps prevent her from inhaling the vomited material. After general anaesthesia, a woman may have a mild sore throat and hoarseness for a day or two. Only when the benefits of general anaesthesia outweigh its risks will it be used. Otherwise, regional anaesthesia is preferred. (See page 344 for the risks and disadvantages of general anaesthesia.)

Regional and Local Analgesia and Anaesthesia

The placement of the anaesthetic or analgesic determines the area where sensation is reduced and pain is relieved. The anaesthetic is usually one of the 'caine' drugs—bupivacaine (Marcaine or Sensorcaine) or lidocaine (Xylocaine). The narcotics or narcotic-like drugs that may be used include morphine (Duramorph), fentanyl (Sublimaze) and others. The amount of pain relief and extent of side effects depend on the timing of administration, duration of the block, and concentration and total dose of the medication.

Placement of Anaesthetic, Nature of Pain Relief	When Given	Benefits and/or Purposes	Possible Risks and/or Side Effects	Additional Precautions/ Procedures/Interventions to Ensure Safety
Standard Epidural Block (with a relatively high concentration of 'caine' drugs)				
• A catheter is placed in the epidural space between the vertebrae in the lower back. • During placement of the catheter, the mother lies on her side or sits up and curls forward. • Medicine is given by continuous drip or repeat injections into the catheter. • Pain relief: loss of sensation (numbness) in lower half of body	• Prior to a caesarean • Other epidural blocks (see following pages) can be changed to a standard block if a caesarean becomes necessary. • Until recently, the standard block was used for both vaginal and caesarean birth, but today it is seldom used if a vaginal birth is expected.	• Provides excellent pain relief without impairing mental awareness • Allows rest and sleep for an exhausted mother • Fewer side effects for newborn than systemic narcotics	*To mother:* • Inability to move lower half of body • Fever (chances increase with duration of epidural) • Drop in blood pressure • Impaired labour progress • Inability to urinate • Decreased bearing-down reflex and effectiveness in pushing • Delay in foetal rotation and descent • Spinal headache if the epidural needle goes in too far • Side effects from the procedures used to ensure safety (see next column) • Post-partum backache *To foetus/newborn:* • Foetal/newborn fever • Foetal distress (from drop in mother's blood pressure) • Some diminished newborn reflexes and responses may last for days.[1]	*Routine:* • Restriction of food and fluids by mouth • IV fluids before anaesthetic is given • Restriction to bed • Various devices to closely monitor mother's blood pressure, blood oxygen levels, heart function, temperature, contractions and foetal heart rate *Used as needed:* • Oxygen by mask • Syntocinon to speed labour • Bladder catheter • Forceps, vacuum extractor, episiotomy, caesarean delivery *For newborn if mother had fever in labour:* • In special care nursery for 48 hours for observation and antibiotics • Septic work up looking for infection (includes blood culture and spinal tap)

Regional and Local Analgesia and Anaesthesia

Placement of Drug, Nature of Pain Relief	When Given	Benefits and/or Purposes	Possible Risks and/or Side Effects	Additional Precautions/ Procedures/Interventions to Ensure Safety
Segmental ('Light') Epidural Block **(with a relatively low concentration of 'caine' drugs or a mix of narcotic with a 'caine' drug)**				
• Same placement as for standard epidural (above); weaker concentration of drug • Pain relief: loss of sensation (numbness) in abdomen and back, with partial awareness in perineum and legs	• As early as 2 cm dilation, though many caregivers prefer to wait until 5 cm or later (the 'light and late' epidural) to avoid slowing labour progress	• Same as above • Allows more movement of legs and trunk (even squatting with assistance) than the standard block	• Same as above, except more freedom to move • Side effects are less frequent than with standard block, especially if epidural is both 'light' and 'late'.	• Same as above

Regional and Local Analgesia and Anaesthesia

Placement of Drug, Nature of Pain Relief	When Given	Benefits and/or Purposes	Possible Risks and/or Side Effects	Additional Precautions/ Procedures/Interventions to Ensure Safety
Epidural or Spinal (Intrathecal) Analgesia with Narcotic or Narcotic-like Drugs				
• For epidural (sometimes called a 'walking epidural'), placement is similar to standard epidural. (See page 346.) • For spinal, single injection between vertebrae in lower back through dura into intrathecal space of spinal canal • Pain relief: good for contraction pain and back pain until late first stage; usually inadequate for transition and second stage. Spinal effects last for a few hours in labour up to 24 hours after a caesarean (if a long-lasting narcotic is given).	• As early in labour as 2 cm • Not usually helpful if given in late first stage (Other anaesthetics can be used at this time.) • After caesarean delivery • Some hospitals offer patient-controlled epidural analgesia; the mother can release small amounts of medication into the epidural catheter whenever her pain returns; the device prevents an overdose.	• Good relief of labour pain until 6–8 cm • Good relief of post-caesarean pain up to 24 hours • Ability to move freely in bed remains. Some women can stand or even walk a bit, with assistance. • Sensation other than pain (touch, pressure, temperature) remains. • When compared to systemic narcotics, more pain relief with less medication	*To mother:* • Usually causes itching all over body • Frequently, nausea and vomiting • Inability to urinate • Weakness in legs or loss of balance while walking • Cold sores, if morphine is used in a woman with a history of oral herpes[2] • Side effects of epidural and spinal narcotics have not been studied as extensively as the 'caine' drugs, though caesarean rates remain similar.[3] • Spinal headache (rare) *To foetus/newborn:* • Unknown, though fentanyl does reach the foetus and is present in newborn for at least 24 hours.[4] • Effects on newborn are less than with systemic narcotics, probably because of lower dosage.	*Routine:* • Restriction of food and fluids by mouth • IV fluids • Assistance while walking • Checking muscle strength in legs before walking • Various machines for close monitoring of mother's blood pressure, blood oxygen levels, heart function, temperature, contractions and foetal heart rate *Used as needed:* • Additional medications to control itching and nausea (Some of these make the mother sleepy; others decrease pain relief.) • Bladder catheter • Additional anaesthesia late in labour for 'breakthrough pain' • If spinal headache occurs, 'blood patch' (see page 356) and lying flat for hours or days

Regional and Local Analgesia and Anaesthesia

Placement of Drug, Nature of Pain Relief	When Given	Benefits and/or Purposes	Possible Risks and/or Side Effects	Additional Precautions/ Procedures/Interventions to Ensure Safety
Epidural or Spinal (Intrathecal) Narcotics Followed by Epidural Anaesthetic ('caine' drug)				
• A narcotic may be used early, followed by an anaesthetic later, both given in the epidural space. • The 'needle through needle' technique, a combined spinal-epidural (CSE): A needle is first placed in the epidural space, with a thinner needle inserted through it into the intrathecal (subarachnoid) space to create a spinal. A narcotic is injected and the thin needle removed. A thin tube (epidural catheter) is run through the epidural needle into the epidural space. The epidural needle is then removed. Later in laboor, with 'breakthrough pain', an anaesthetic is dripped into the epidural space through the catheter. • Pain relief: Narcotic in early labour is good for contraction pain and back pain. With epidural, numbness in trunk.	• Mixture: as early as 2 cm, but most wait until 4–5 cm • Narcotic alone: as early as 2 cm • Anaesthetic addition: 6–8 cm when 'breakthrough' pain occurs	• Same as above for epidural or intrathecal narcotics and for segmental epidural block with anaesthetic, except that: • Combining narcotics with anaesthetic allows for lower drug concentrations than if either is used alone. • The 'needle through needle' technique, though complex, allows for a postponement of use of anaesthetic until late labour, and a rapid response when 'breakthrough pain' occurs.	• Same as above for epidural or intrathecal narcotics and for segmental epidural block with anaesthetic	• Same as above for epidural or intrathecal narcotics and for segmental epidural block with anesthetic

Regional and Local Analgesia and Anaesthesia

Placement of Drug, Nature of Pain Relief	When Given	Benefits and/or Purposes	Possible Risks and/or Side Effects	Additional Precautions/ Procedures/Interventions to Ensure Safety
Spinal (Intrathecal) Block (with 'caine' drug)				
• Usually between third and fourth lumbar vertebrae through the dura into the subarachnoid space • Given as a single injection while mother sits up or lies on side, curling forward as for an epidural (See page 355.) • Pain relief: complete numbness in lower half of body	• Almost exclusively for a caesarean delivery • Occasionally, in late labour, for vaginal birth (may be referred to as a 'saddle' block)	• Nearly 100 percent of women receive good anaesthesia. • Administration is usually quick and medication takes effect almost immediately—both important if a rapid caesarean is necessary.	*To mother:* • Occasionally, feeling of being unable to breathe because chest becomes anaesthetised • Drop in blood pressure • Spinal headache (1 percent) *To foetus/newborn:* • Foetal distress • Subtle neuro-behavioural effects for days	*Routine:* • Restriction of food and fluids by mouth • Large amount of IV fluids • Restriction to bed • Various machines for close monitoring of mother's blood pressure, blood oxygen levels, heart function, contractions and foetal heart rate • Bladder catheter *Used as needed:* • Oxygen by mask • Syntocinon to promote uterine contractions • Forceps, vacuum extractor, episiotomy *If spinal headache occurs:* • Lie flat in bed for several days • 'Blood patch' *If breathing difficulties arise:* • Assisted ventilation

Local Blocks

Placement of Drug, Nature of Pain Relief	When Given	Benefits and/or Purposes	Possible Risks and/or Side Effects	Additional Precautions/ Procedures/Interventions to Ensure Safety
Pudendal Block				
• Injections into both sides of vagina to block pudendal nerves • Pain relief: loss of sensation (numbness) in vagina and perineum	• Second stage • Third stage (rarely)	• Reduces pain during delivery, especially if forceps or vacuum extractor is used • Sometimes used for episiotomy and/or repair of episiotomy	*To mother:* • May impede bearing-down reflex and effectiveness in pushing • May relax muscle tone in perineum enough to impede foetal rotation *To foetus/newborn:* • Foetal distress (drop in FHR) • Medication reaches foetus and remains in newborn circulation; may cause short-term neurobehavioural changes. • Though area affected is small, a relatively large amount of medication is needed.	*Routine:* • Foetal monitoring *As needed:* • Syntocinon to speed labour • Episiotomy • Forceps or vacuum extractor
'Local' Perineal Block				
• Several injections around the vaginal opening • Pain relief: loss of sensation (numbness) in perineum	• Second stage, before episiotomy • Third stage for repair of episiotomy or tear	• Relief of pain of crowning or episiotomy • Relief of pain during stitching after birth	*To mother:* • If given during second stage, may increase swelling in perineum and likelihood of tears *To foetus/newborn:* • If given long before birth, foetal distress or altered newborn reflexes may occur.	• Postpone until after birth; use if stitches are necessary

Local and Regional Anaesthesia

Local or *regional* anaesthetics cause a decrease or total loss of sensation (numbness) in a specific area or region of the body. Such anaesthesia is often referred to as a *block*. Most anaesthetic drug names end with *caine* (Xylocaine, bupivacaine, ropivacaine and so on). Injected near specific nerves, the anaesthetic blocks the transmission of impulses over those nerves. The major functions of nerves are to conduct sensations (including pain) to your brain and to control your muscle activity, organ function, blood flow and temperature in the area affected. These functions are diminished by regional or local anaesthetics.

Lower doses of an anaesthetic take away pain and other sensations without taking away all muscle control. Higher doses remove both sensation and the ability to use your muscles. Higher doses are also likely to affect your baby more than lower doses. Other factors also influence your response or your baby's: the medications selected, the area injected, the technique of administration, your individual response and your baby's condition during labour. Local and regional anaesthetics do not affect your mental state. You do not become groggy, sleepy or confused as you do with most systemic pain medications. To minimise the side effects of regional blocks, various additional precautions and interventions must be employed to maintain safety; some of these may be irritating, uncomfortable or confining. (See chart on page 346.)

Local Anaesthesia

The difference between local and regional anaesthesia is in the location of the injection. Local anaesthetics are injected into the skin, muscle or cervix. They block sensation in a small, local area near nerve endings. The rarely used paracervical block numbs the cervix, the pudendal block numbs the vagina and the perineal block numbs the perineum.

Regional Anaesthesia

Regional anaesthetics are given in the lower back near nerve roots in the spinal column. The anaesthetic affects the region of the body to which these nerves and their branches go; the region can be as small as the abdomen and lower back only, or as large as the entire body below the chest. Regional blocks provide pain relief in a

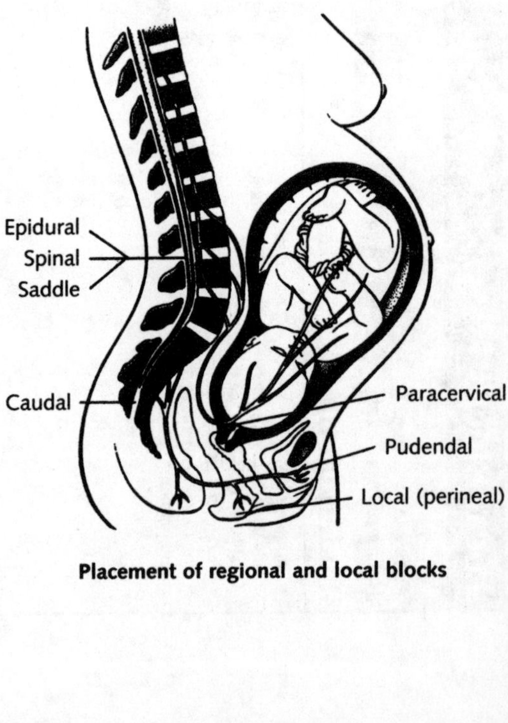

Placement of regional and local blocks

much larger area than local blocks, while using smaller amounts of medication. Today, spinal and epidural blocks are the most commonly used regional blocks for childbirth.

Current methods of epidural analgesia and anaesthesia focus on reducing side effects while maintaining some sensation and function in the lower two thirds of the body. This differs from the total loss of feeling and function that accompanied regional blocks until the late 1980s. Today, the epidural can be tailored to the individual circumstances, desires, and needs of each labouring woman in the following ways:

- Delaying the epidural until active labour
- Lowering the concentration of the anaesthetic (the 'caine' drug)
- Using narcotics or narcotic-like drugs alone or in combination with a lower anaesthetic concentration (often referred to as epidural analgesia, since sensation remains in the lower body)
- Using a continuous infusion (drip) of these lower concentrations (as opposed to periodic injections, or 'top-ups', of the higher concentrations)
- Using patient-controlled epidural analgesia (PCEA) that allows the labouring woman some control over the flow of medication (within safe limits)
- Combining the spinal and epidural, with the narcotics in the spinal (or intrathecal) space and the 'caine' drug in the epidural space, or with a mixture of narcotic and 'caine' drugs in both spaces
- Slowing or stopping the epidural infusion at the beginning of the second stage of labour, to allow the epidural to wear off so that the mother can bear down more effectively
- Having the mother delay pushing until the baby's head is visible at the vaginal outlet (sometimes referred to as 'passive descent' and 'labouring down') in order to reduce the need for forceps, vacuum extraction or a caesarean[5]

With these changes, the incidence of some side effects is reduced. However, because some side effects still occur, all precautions and procedures that accompany the epidural must still be employed.

Procedure for Epidural and Spinal Blocks

The procedures for epidural and spinal blocks are as follows:

1. The mother is given IV fluids to help reduce the chance of a drop in blood pressure and to enable administration of drugs, if necessary.

2. The mother lies on her side with her body curled, or she sits up, leaning forward. The anaesthesiologist cleans her lower back (the antiseptic often feels cold) and numbs her skin with a local anaesthetic.

3. If she is getting an epidural, a needle is inserted into the epidural space. A thin plastic tube (a catheter) is threaded through the needle, the needle is removed, and the catheter is taped to the mother's back. (See the illustration on page 353 for the exact location.) Then the anaesthesiologist injects the anaesthetic and/or analgesic. The catheter is attached to a device that steadily releases small amounts of the drug into the

epidural space. Within a few minutes, the mother begins to notice the effects (tingling, numbness), and within fifteen to twenty minutes, she will probably experience good pain relief. It sometimes takes longer or another catheter placement to achieve good anaesthesia.

4. If the mother is getting a spinal, a needle is inserted through the dura (the tough membrane that surrounds the spinal cord and cerebrospinal fluid). A single injection of anaesthetic or narcotic is given into the fluid in the intrathecal space of the spinal canal.

5. The mother's blood pressure, pulse and blood oxygen levels are checked frequently, and labour contractions and the foetal heart rate are closely monitored. If the mother's blood pressure drops, the anaesthesiologist may give her medications or more IV fluids to raise it. If her blood oxygen levels decrease, she may be given oxygen to breathe via a mask. If her contractions slow down, the caregiver may use Syntocinon to augment them.

Other Factors to Consider

- Midwives administer only the perineal (local) block.
- General practitioners and obstetricians administer pudendal and perineal blocks and in some settings give intrathecal (spinal) narcotics.
- Usually, an anaesthesiologist or nurse anaesthetist administers epidural, spinal and general anaesthesia. Depending on your health insurance, there may be an additional fee for the services of these specialists. Some small or rural hospitals do

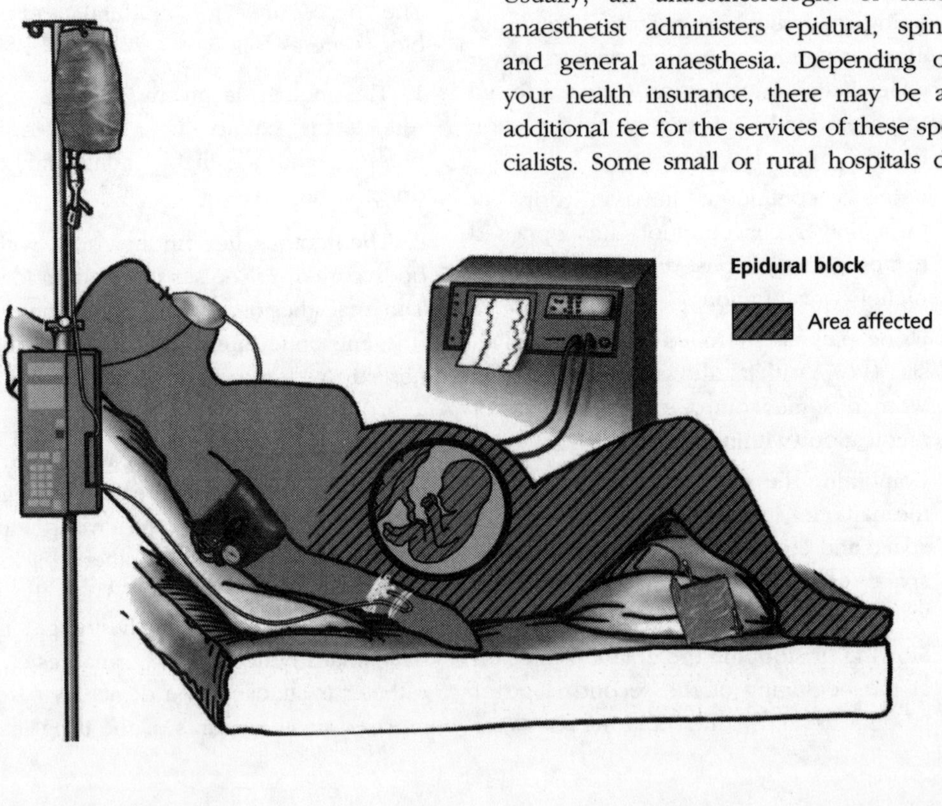

not have enough staff to provide twenty-four-hour obstetrical anaesthesia services. When anaesthesia personnel are not available, the staff relies on simpler methods—such as systemic medications, local blocks and intrathecal narcotics—for relief of labour pain.

- Where available, regional anaesthesia (epidural or spinal) is preferred for caesarean birth rather than general anaesthesia, because it has fewer side effects and allows the mother to be fully conscious. For planned caesareans, spinal anaesthesia is generally preferred over an epidural because of its ease of administration and rapid onset. If the need for a caesarean arises in labour for a woman who has had no previous anaesthesia, a spinal is also preferred.
- Spinal anaesthesia requires puncture of the dura. Rarely, a spinal headache may result (the mother has a headache when her head is elevated but not when she lies flat). The pain is thought to be caused by a leak of cerebrospinal fluid (the fluid surrounding the spinal cord and brain) through the puncture site in the dura. The occurrence of spinal headache is much less likely than in the past, since the needles now used are designed to prevent this problem. Treatment may include bed rest, increased fluids and other measures. The headache usually disappears as the dura heals and closes the puncture site. If the headache lingers more than a few days, a *blood patch* may be made by injecting a small amount of the mother's blood into the epidural space near the puncture site. A clot then forms and seals

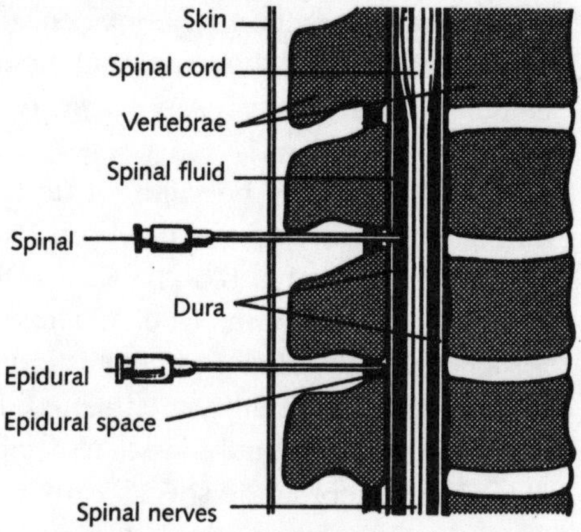

Placement of spinal and epidural blocks

the puncture. This technique is usually effective for immediate and permanent relief of spinal headache.

- With epidural anaesthesia, the anaesthetic is injected outside the dura in the epidural or extradural space. A spinal headache does not occur with this type of injection, except in the rare situation when the dura is penetrated unintentionally. If this happens, the spinal headache is, unfortunately, more likely than with spinal anaesthesia, because the needle used for an epidural is much larger than for a spinal and causes a larger hole in the dura.
- Epidural narcotics take effect more quickly than epidural anaesthetics.
- Compared to spinal blocks, epidural blocks require more expertise to administer and are slower to take effect.
- Incidence of maternal fever increases when a labouring woman has epidural anaesthesia or analgesia, because temperature regulation is altered along with

awareness of sensation. The incidence of fever increases with the length of time the epidural is in place. Any time fever occurs, infection is suspected; the mother's blood may be cultured (tested) during labour and, if the newborn baby also has a fever, his blood will also be tested soon after birth. Until the results are known (this takes forty-eight hours), both mother and baby are treated for infection with IV antibiotics. The baby may also be kept in the special care nursery for observation until the culture results are known. The mother can visit and feed her baby. In a few hospitals, the baby also undergoes a septic work up, which includes blood studies, a spinal tap and culture of spinal fluid. Thus, even though epidurals do not cause infection, the epidural fever may lead to testing, possible unneeded treatment, separation of mother and baby, and worry for the parents while they wait to learn whether their baby has an infection.

Post-partum Medications

While you may need no pain medications at all after the baby is born, they are available for 'afterpains' (see page 363) and perineal or post-caesarean pain. In the past, a nurse gave prescribed medications at designated times as well as when the mother requested medication for pain relief or other discomforts. Today, caregivers recognise that most mothers are able to determine their own medication needs. Caregivers have developed self-administered medication (SAM) programs that give women more responsibility for their own use of medications and that help prepare them to use medications safely at home.

Epidural or spinal narcotics may provide effective pain relief without causing drowsiness for the first day after a caesarean delivery. These methods of pain relief make it relatively easy to get out of bed and move around. However, itching and nausea are frequent side effects of epidural or spinal narcotics. There are medications to counteract these side effects, though these medications may cause drowsiness or diminish pain relief. An outbreak of cold sores (oral herpes) may occur if a woman who is prone to cold sores receives epidural or spinal morphine. After the epidural or spinal narcotic wears off (between several hours and up to twenty-four hours after the injection), the mother usually takes oral pain medications until she does not need them.

Some hospitals offer patient-controlled analgesia (PCA) for mothers following a caesarean birth. With PCA, you have an IV drip in place. Whenever you need pain relief, you can press a button to release a small dose of narcotic into the IV fluid. You have greater control over your comfort and more rapid pain relief. The PCA unit is used for approximately twenty-four hours following a caesarean birth. Mothers on PCA often have better pain relief, use less total medication, and are usually less groggy than those who are given injected or oral narcotics on a schedule. PCA has the disadvantage of requiring an IV in place, which might be unnecessary otherwise. An IV makes movement in and out of bed and baby care more awkward and cumbersome.

When a mother uses oral narcotic medications in post partum, the dosage depends on her need for pain relief and her need to be able to care for herself and her baby. Though small amounts of the pain medication reach your baby via your breast milk, the advantages of a better start with breastfeeding and self-care must be balanced against that disadvantage. Since narcotics do cause drowsiness, most women use them only as long as needed and switch to less powerful medications as healing occurs. After a caesarean birth, use of oral pain medications may make it easier for you to move around, feed and care for your baby. At first, use the pain medications that you take home from the hospital as directed. As the pain subsides, reduce the dosage. If you do not need pain relief, you may stop using them, even if you have not used all of them.

Chapter 13

Post-partum Period

The post-partum (after birth) period is a time of physical and emotional readjustment. The mother's reproductive organs return to their pre-pregnant state, usually within six weeks. The family incorporates and accepts a new person into the home, and the role of each parent within the family changes to meet the needs of the new baby.

Every family's adjustment is unique. Some families find a comfortable new balance within weeks. Most spend the first year adjusting to the arrival of a new baby. Numerous factors influence the family's experience—some of which ease and some of which slow the adjustment process.

Influences on Adjustment

Some of these influences may have occurred earlier in your life. Others may arise during pregnancy. The birth itself may influence the speed and smoothness of your recovery. In addition, factors in the early post-partum period and during the months following the birth may speed or slow your physical recovery and affect the time it takes to adjust to having a new baby and to find a comfortable balance in your new lifestyle.

- *Pre-pregnancy* factors include the parenting you received; your mental health and that of your family; your physical health and wellbeing; previous exposure to trauma; and experience with previous pregnancies, births and baby care.
- Factors *during pregnancy* include the presence or absence of pregnancy complications, prolonged bed rest or treatment for a high-risk pregnancy, financial worries, a physically demanding job, lack of sleep, presence or lack of supportive people in your life, and the quality of your relationship with the baby's father.
- Factors *during the birth* include a normal birth versus a complicated or caesarean birth and the presence or absence of

continuous, competent, caring support during labour.

- *Early post-partum* factors include immediate contact with your baby (including breastfeeding) versus separation from your baby, the presence or absence of post-partum pain, and the health and wellbeing of both you and your baby.
- *Later post-partum* factors include the timing of your return to employment; the baby's temperament; the baby's continuing health and wellbeing; the presence or absence of later feeding problems; sufficient sleep for both parents; your emotional state; and continuing supportive and caring relationships with your partner, family and friends.

Discharge from the Hospital or Birth Centre

The length of your hospital stay after birth varies from one to two days after a vaginal birth and from two to four days after a caesarean, unless there is a medical reason to stay longer. If you give birth in an out-of-hospital birth centre, you will go home three to six hours after the birth. With a home birth, the midwife usually leaves three or four hours after the birth.

How long you can or should stay in the hospital or birth centre can be confusing for new parents (and for their parents who experienced much longer hospital stays). In general, the post-partum care setting after the first day has changed from inside to outside the hospital. The wellbeing of new mothers and their infants should be assessed when the baby is three to four days old. This assessment takes place in a post-partum follow-up clinic, in the health care provider's office, or in the home. Such an assessment is necessary to detect jaundice, dehydration and excessive weight loss in the infant and to help mothers with feeding challenges, evaluation of pain or infant care questions. The assessment can also provide assurance about what you are doing well.

Ask your health care provider about your plan for care during pregnancy, childbirth and the first several days after birth. Make your hospital and post-partum plans with this knowledge in mind. (See pages 155–159 for information on post-partum planning.)

If you and your baby are doing well, you may have the option of leaving the hospital before twenty-four hours after the birth. You might prefer a 'shortened stay' to save money or to get back to your other children and to the comforts of home (your own food, your own bed and your familiar surroundings). If you choose a shortened stay, you will have less time to learn about baby care and breastfeeding from the nurses. If at all possible, have help at home during at least the first few days. You will need to learn what observations to make of yourself and your newborn for problems that require medical attention. You will also need resources you can call upon if you have any concerns. Many hospitals offer classes and educational materials. You might be able to return to the hospital the next day to attend baby care classes, if they are offered. Some hospitals provide a clinic visit or home visit by one of their nurses to check on you and your baby, to answer questions and to offer practical advice. Within a few days after you come home, plan to contact your health care provider or a public health nurse for a check-up and a chance to ask questions.

Post-partum Physical Recovery

Your body makes many physical adjustments in the first days and weeks after childbirth. You may feel uplifted and energetic immediately after the birth and for the next few days or weeks. This feeling is often called the 'birth high'. On the other hand, you may feel exhausted, let-down or even disappointed. Most women experience sudden changes in their moods, and all new mothers get tired and need rest.

Beginning with birth, your body undergoes rapid physical and hormonal changes. These changes are normal but can be positively or negatively affected by the factors listed on pages 359–360. In addition, fathers and partners often experience some adjustment problems. For example, their moods fluctuate, and they feel tired. You may all benefit from the assistance of family and friends. Plan ahead for this possibility.

Early Recovery Period

Immediately after the birth, your health care providers closely observe your physical condition to assess your recovery. They frequently check your temperature, pulse, respiratory rate and blood pressure. They also monitor the amount and character of your lochia (bloody discharge); the size, firmness and position of your uterus; and the functioning of your bladder and bowel. If you have had anaesthesia, they assess the return of feeling and movement in your legs.

Uterus

Involution. Through a process called 'involution', the uterus returns to its non-pregnant size five or six weeks after the birth. Immediately after the birth of the placenta, the uterus weighs between 1 and 1.4 kilograms, and the top of the uterus (fundus) can be felt at the navel. During the next two days, the uterus remains approximately the same size (about the size of a grapefruit) and feels firm and tight. To help maintain the firmness of the uterus and to prevent heavy blood loss from the placental site, you or your nurse massages your uterus, stimulating it to contract. (See page 246 for instructions.)

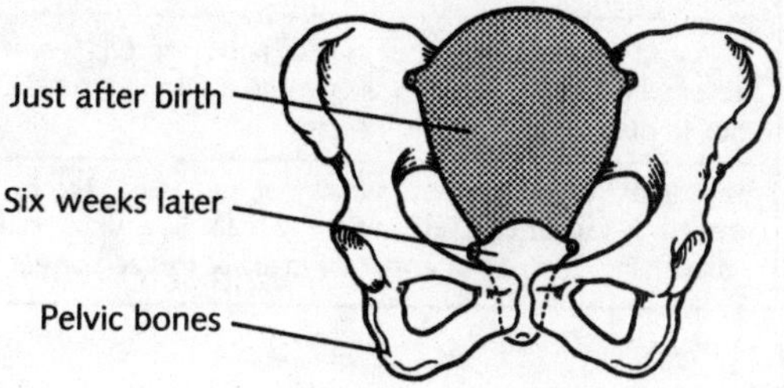

Involution of the uterus

Warning Signs during Post Partum

Report to your caregiver any of the following signs, which may indicate a problem requiring treatment:

Warning Signs	Possible Problems
Fever (temperature of 38°C or greater)	• Uterine infection • Bladder or kidney infection • Breast infection (mastitis) • Infection of caesarean incision • Infection of episiotomy or tear • Other illness
Burning with urination, or blood in urine	• Bladder or kidney infection
Inability to urinate	• Swelling or trauma of the urethral sphincter
Swollen, red, painful area on the leg (especially the calf) that is hot and tender to the touch	• Thrombophlebitis (blood clot in the blood vessel); do not rub or massage the area
Sore, reddened, hot, painful area on breast(s), along with fever and flu-like symptoms	• Breast infection (mastitis)
Passage of blood clot larger than a lemon followed by heavy bleeding, or any bleeding heavy enough to soak a large sanitary pad in an hour or less	• Passage of some (but not all) of the retained placenta • Uterine infection
Extremely foul or fish-like odour to vaginal discharge; vaginal soreness or itching	• Uterine infection • Vaginal infection
Increased pain at site of episiotomy or tear; may be accompanied by foul-smelling or pus-like discharge	• Infection of episiotomy or tear • Reopening of incision or tear
Opening of caesarean incision; may be accompanied by pus-like discharge or blood	• Infection of caesarean incision
Appearance of rash or hives; may be accompanied by itching	• Allergic reaction to medication
Severe headache that begins at birth and is worse when upright	• Spinal headache following regional anaesthesia
Any sudden onset of pain that is new, such as abdominal tenderness or burning near perineal stitches when urinating	• Uterine infection • Reopening of perineal tear or incision
Pain and tenderness in front and/or back of pelvis, accompanied by difficulty walking and a 'grating' sensation in pubic joint	• Separation of pubic symphysis (cartilage between the pubic bones)
Feeling extremely anxious, panicky or depressed; accompanied by rapid heart rate, difficulty breathing, uncontrollable crying, feelings of anger, or inability to sleep or eat	• Post-partum mood disorders, including anxiety and panic attacks, obsessive thinking or worrying, or depression

Nursing your baby also helps keep your uterus firm.

A week after the baby's birth, your uterus weighs 450–675 grams. After two weeks, the uterus lies within the pelvis and weighs about 225 grams. By the end of five or six weeks, the uterus weighs 50–100 grams, and it has nearly returned to its pre-pregnant size.

During involution, *lochia* (bloody discharge) flows from the uterus and out the vagina. For the first few days after the birth, the red lochia flow is heavy. It is normal to pass jelly-like clots, especially in the first days after the birth. Lochia often has a strong 'fleshy' odour. The amount of flow may change with your activity or body position. Lochia is generally heavier when you change positions such as standing or sitting up after lying down, when you breastfeed or when you have a bowel movement. It will also be heavier with overexertion. Use this symptom to remind yourself to slow down and rest. Within ten days, lochia diminishes and becomes pale pink or rust in colour. During the next several weeks, it becomes yellowish white, white or tan. Lochia may continue for as long as six to eight weeks. (See the chart on page 362 for warning signs regarding lochia.)

Afterpains. These are the uncomfortable and sometimes painful contractions of the uterus after the birth, which often occur during breastfeeding and are more common if you have had a child before. To ease the pain, relax and use slow breathing patterns. Ibuprofen or other medications prescribed by your health care provider may also help. Afterpains usually disappear after the first week.

Return of menstruation. If you are not breastfeeding, you will probably begin menstruating again four to eight weeks after the birth. If you are breastfeeding, you may not menstruate for several months or until you wean, though ovulation can occur during this time. Your first few menstrual periods following delivery may be heavier and longer than usual, but they will return to normal.

Cervix and Vagina

With the completion of involution, the cervix will have returned almost to its pre-pregnant size. (The outer opening of the cervix remains somewhat wider.) The vagina will gradually regain its tone, and the labia will remain somewhat looser, larger and darker than before pregnancy.

Breasts

Breastfeeding mothers. For the first twenty-four to seventy-two hours after birth, the breasts secrete *colostrum*, a clear yellow fluid that is the baby's first milk. More mature breast milk appears between the second and fifth day. At this time, breasts may be engorged (full, hard, hot and painful), which may present some feeding challenges. Frequent nursing may prevent this initial engorgement or help it subside. (See Chapter 15 for more information on breastfeeding.)

Non-breastfeeding mothers. The breasts of non-breastfeeding mothers will probably have the same initial changes as those in breastfeeding mothers. Binding your breasts, applying ice packs and avoiding breast stimulation are effective ways to diminish milk production and increase comfort. These measures are as

To Bind and Ice Your Breasts

If you are not going to breastfeed, binding your breasts will help decrease painful engorgement when your milk comes in. Use an extra wide elastic (Ace) bandage or a tightly woven band of cloth about 30 centimetres by 1.8 metres. Wrap it snugly around your chest two or three times. This will compress your breasts and decrease the amount of swelling that occurs as your milk comes in. Rewrap every few hours and wear the binding for twenty-four to forty-eight hours starting on the second or third day after you have given birth.

Once your milk comes in, ice your breasts every four hours or so for twenty minutes during the daytime. This will decrease the pain from the tissue inflammation and swelling that accompany engorgement. Use a sports ice bag or several bags of frozen peas over your bra or T-shirt and hold in place with binding material. You may refreeze the bags for repeated use.

Your caregiver may suggest ibuprofen or acetaminophen for pain relief.

helpful as the milk-suppressing medications used in the past, which were discontinued because of their serious side effects.

Hormonal Changes

After delivery, your body undergoes sudden and dramatic changes in hormone production. When the placenta is delivered, oestrogen and progesterone levels drop abruptly and remain low until your ovaries begin producing these hormones again. If you breastfeed, your production of other hormones (for example, prolactin and oxytocin) increases and remains high while your oestrogen and progesterone levels remain low, until you wean your baby.

Circulatory Changes

Some blood loss is a natural result of childbirth. Average blood loss during an uncomplicated vaginal birth amounts to about 1 cup. If you have had an episiotomy or a sizable tear, you may lose more. You will continue to lose blood in your lochia for a few weeks, but do not be alarmed. During pregnancy, you accumulated extra blood and fluid, so the blood loss during and after birth is not harmful.

In the early post-partum period, you will lose the extra fluid accumulated during pregnancy by urinating large quantities during the day and perspiring heavily, especially at night. As a result, you will lose as much as 2.3 kilograms of fluid during the first week after birth.

Abdominal and Skin Changes

After birth, your abdominal muscles are lax and it takes six weeks or more for them to regain their tone. Exercise speeds the process. Your stretch marks fade but do not completely disappear. If you have had an increase in skin pigmentation, it will fade. Any increased hair growth on your abdomen also disappears gradually.

If you pushed very hard for a long time during delivery, you may have broken blood vessels in your eyes and on your face and neck. These broken vessels (called 'petechial haemorrhages') are the result of rapid and large changes in blood pressure during and between pushing efforts. They are not serious and will disappear with time, usually within a week or two.

Back and Hip Pain

Many women experience lower back pain after birth. Women who have injured or broken their tail bones (coccyx) prior to birth or whose babies were quite large may experience pain or a tender, bruised feeling in that area after birth. The passage of the baby through the pelvis may have caused the tail bone to flex or even re-break. Taking ibuprofen recommended by the caregiver, applying heat or cold packs to the area, and sitting on a partially inflated donut-shaped pillow can help. The tail bone will reset itself, but it may take weeks to several months.

Women who have had epidural or spinal anaesthesia may have a lingering backache for the first few days or weeks following birth. Their hips may hurt, too. This may have resulted from twisting the lower back or over-stretching the pelvic and hip joints during labour and birth (while the woman was numb). Ibuprofen recommended by the caregiver can help. If you have pain that interferes with your ability to walk or roll over, call your caregiver.

Self-Care after Birth

Rest and Sleep

Fatigue and sleep deprivation present a great challenge to your physical and emotional recovery. Finding time to sleep may seem an impossible task. Let your need for sleep and rest take precedence over non-essential household chores. Take every opportunity to rest or nap. Even if you cannot sleep, simply resting is restoring. Rest will give you energy to meet your baby's often unpredictable needs to be fed and cared for throughout the day and night. If you have other children at home, meeting their needs for attention and care will also be easier.

Many parents notice that their babies seem to sleep better during the day than at night. Newborn night wakefulness is common and temporary. Gradually, newborns assume the wake-sleep cycles of their families. In the meantime, you may wonder if

Recipe for Sleep in the First Weeks after Birth

To succeed in getting enough sleep, you must take your need for sleep seriously. Many first-time parents use and appreciate the following approach to obtain an adequate amount of sleep. (It does not work as well if you have other children.)

- Ask yourself how many hours of sleep you regularly needed before pregnancy in order to function well. Six hours? Eight hours? That is the amount of sleep you now owe yourself every day.
- Since you cannot get this amount of sleep in one stretch because of interruptions for feedings and baby care, you will require more hours in bed to get your allotted amount of sleep.
- Plan to stay in bed or keep going back to bed until you have slept your allotted number of hours. This means that, with the exception of meals and trips to the bathroom, you do not get up, shower and dress in the early morning. You can keep a mental note of approximately how much time you have slept at each stretch. You stay in your nightclothes until you have slept the set number of hours. You may have to stay in bed from 10 P.M. until noon the next day to get eight hours of sleep! If that's what it takes, do it. Then brush your teeth, take a showe, and dress.
- Many parents find it easier to follow this recipe if their baby sleeps with them or nearby.
- As your baby grows and begins to sleep for longer stretches, it will take you less time to get enough sleep.

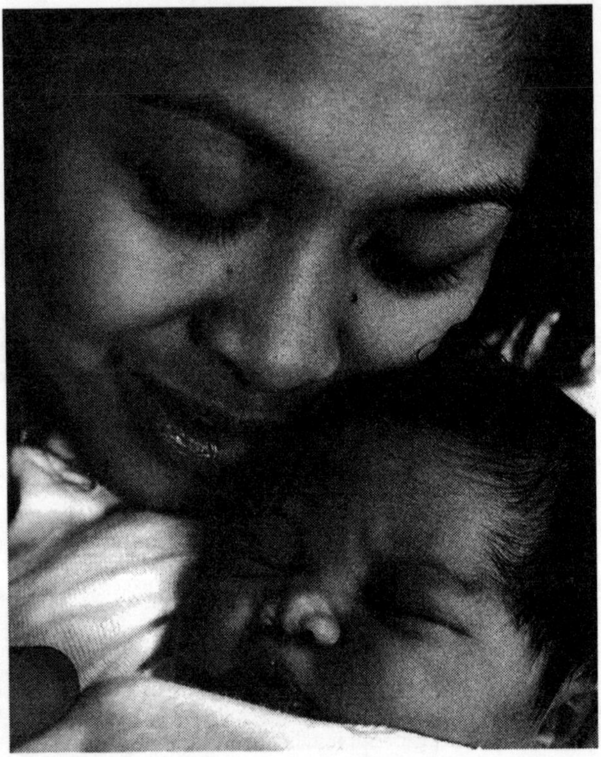

Savour the quiet moments with your baby.

you will ever sleep at night again.

The advice to 'sleep when your baby sleeps' can be frustrating for parents who are accustomed to sleeping only at night. In addition, many new mothers feel 'wired' and hyper-alert as they listen for their baby's mews and cries. So what can new parents do to reduce their fatigue?

- First, acknowledge your need for rest and commit yourselves (both parents) to giving this a high priority (right after meeting your baby's needs for food and comfort). Laundry and dishes can be done by someone else or can wait until you have had a nap.
  - If you have trouble falling asleep, even when your baby is asleep, rest and try the relaxation countdown. (See page 183.)
  - You may find it easier to sleep if your baby is close to you. If your baby is some distance away from you, you may strain to listen for your baby's sounds, which could interfere with your ability to rest or sleep.
  - Some mothers find that their baby's sounds increase their anxiety and restlessness. If that is true for you, let others hold your baby while you rest.
  - Give yourself permission to do whatever you need to do to rest, including turning off the phone, limiting visitors, sitting outside, taking short walks, nurturing yourself with food and beverages, having a foot massage or taking pain medication if you need it.
- You will learn, as all parents do, to rest and sleep when you can. It takes time to adjust to night wakefulness and to learn how to nap.

Activity

If your labour and birth were normal, it is safe to begin mild post-partum exercises within a day or two. (See pages 138–143.) It is also all right to wait a few weeks. Start gradually and do what makes you feel good. You are overdoing it if the exercises tire you, cause stress or increase your bleeding. Follow your caregiver's guidelines about exercise and other activities such as driving, stair climbing and lifting.

Perineal Care

Special care of the perineum is suggested, especially if you have had stitches for an episiotomy or a tear, or are very bruised or swollen. The basic goals of perineal care are to relieve pain, promote healing and prevent infection. Your stitches dissolve in two to four weeks and the tissue is usually healed within four to six weeks, though you may feel discomfort for some time. Discomfort during intercourse may persist for several months. See your health care provider if the discomfort persists. It may be treatable.

- Your nurse or midwife will apply an ice pack to your perineum as soon after birth as possible to reduce pain and swelling. Use ice intermittently for the next several days. You can put crushed ice or a frozen wet washcloth in a zip-lock bag and wrap it in several layers of paper towels. Hold it in place with your perineal pad. Or, you can dampen your clean pad with witch hazel and freeze it before use. Frozen witch hazel pads provide soothing pain relief to a tear site, an episiotomy site and haemorrhoids. Witch hazel can be purchased from a pharmacy.
- Frequent pelvic floor contraction exercises (Kegels and Super Kegels) increase circulation in your perineum, promote healing and reduce swelling. They also help restore strength and muscle tone in your pelvic floor. You may begin to do Kegels immediately after birth. Do not be discouraged if you cannot do Kegels as well as you could before birth. The strength of your pelvic floor usually improves quickly.
- After you urinate, clean yourself by pouring warm water over your perineum from the front towards your rectum. 'Peri bottles' are often provided in the hospital for this purpose. Remember to take yours home with you.
- Do not use tampons before your post-partum check-up.
- Do not douche.
- Always pat or wipe yourself from front to back, to prevent infection of the perineum from organisms in the rectal area.
- Your health care provider may prescribe or give you preparations to apply to your perineum to increase comfort.
- A *sitz bath* can help relieve perineal soreness. Sit in a clean tub of warm water for ten to twenty minutes. You may receive a portable sitz-bath basin from the hospital. After your bath, lie down for fifteen minutes or more to decrease perineal swelling caused by the warm water. If you desire, use cold water in your sitz bath. It is soothing and does not increase swelling.
- You may be given a plastic donut pillow to sit on. The donut lifts your perineum off the surface you are sitting on. You can make your own donut pillow by rolling a bath towel lengthwise and shaping the rolled coil in the shape of a horseshoe. Sit with both buttocks supported by the towel. Sitting on a pillow designed for nursing or baby support may also help to increase your comfort.

- Sitting is sometimes painful if you have stitches. Though it may seem surprising, some women find sitting on a firm surface more comfortable than sitting on a soft one or a donut (both tend to separate the edges of the incision). When sitting on a firm surface, sit on one side of your buttocks first; then ease onto both sides. This helps press your incision together and is less painful. Try both firm and soft surfaces and use the more comfortable option.
- Lie down and rest as often as you can in the first week or two after birth. When you sit or stand, gravity works to increase swelling.

Bowel and Bladder Function

- At first, urination may be difficult because of slack abdominal tone or soreness and swelling around your urethra, which result from bruising during birth or having had a catheter in your bladder. If you have trouble, relax, drink lots of liquids, pour warm water over your perineum to help start your flow, or try to urinate in the shower or bathtub. If you are unable to urinate, you may need to be catheterised by your nurse to empty your bladder.
- You may become constipated after delivery because of lax abdominal muscles or the soreness of the perineum, episiotomy or haemorrhoids. Iron supplements and narcotic pain medications may also contribute to constipation. You can avoid constipation by eating fresh and dried fruits, vegetables, and whole-grain cereals and by drinking plenty of water. Walking, exercising your abdominal muscles, and responding when you have the urge to move your bowels rather than postponing it will help restore normal bowel function. If you are sent home with a stool softener, follow your health care provider's instructions for its use.
- Supporting your perineum by gently pressing toilet tissue against your stitches can help relieve soreness when you bear down for a bowel movement. Using such support may also help allay fears of hurting yourself while straining.

If these suggestions do not help and you remain uncomfortable, your physician or midwife may prescribe a laxative, suppositories or an enema.

Haemorrhoids

Haemorrhoids are common during pregnancy and even more common in early post partum. They almost always go away within a month or so after birth. There are several ways to reduce the discomfort of haemorrhoids and promote healing:

- Avoid constipation.
- Try the pelvic floor contraction, or Kegel, exercise (see page 130), with emphasis on the muscles around the anus.
- Modify for home use any hospital procedure that helped, such as witch hazel and sitz baths. (See page 367.)
- Your physician or midwife may prescribe medication. Surgical treatment of haemorrhoids is sometimes necessary in extreme cases.

Nutrition

- Continue eating healthfully as you did during pregnancy. (See Chapter 4 for more information.)
- To lose any extra pounds remaining after birth, do not go on an extreme diet. Most new mothers lose weight gradually over a period of several months with no special effort. If you choose to reduce in a more intentional way, a weight loss of 450–900 grams per week is the maximum suggested for most mothers.
- Make sure your diet contains plenty of roughage so you will not become constipated.
- Your physician or midwife may recommend that you continue your prenatal vitamins and iron supplement.
- See page 441 for specific suggestions for nutrition while breastfeeding.

Practical Help

After the birth, the reality of being unable to do everything as before can be upsetting. Some women who take pride in their independence find it difficult to ask for help. Accepting help, however, can speed recovery by providing you with more opportunities to rest and sleep. Since getting enough rest is essential but also very difficult at this time, think of creative ways to minimise your household tasks and to get help and constructive advice. Accept all comfortable and convenient offers of help and direct them to meet your needs. Perhaps your mother or another relative will stay for a week or two. Ask someone to cook (and perhaps freeze) a few meals, do the dishes and laundry, do the grocery shopping and other errands, vacuum and dust, or simply keep an eye on the baby while you get a bath or rest. If friends or family are wearing you out, tell them you are exhausted, excuse yourself with your baby if you prefer, and retire to the bedroom. Limit visitors if you are tired. This is no time to take on the role of perfect hostess. Many families hire part-time household help for a few weeks after the birth. Agencies specialising in post-partum home care exist in many communities.

Later Recovery Period

Post-partum Examination

It is important that you have a post-partum check-up within three to eight weeks after delivery. A general physical examination, which includes a pelvic exam, will be done to assess your recovery; it will also give you a chance to discuss with your midwife or doctor any physical or emotional problems, your out-of-the-home work schedule and your preferences for family planning. (If, however, you notice any of the warning signs listed in the chart on page 362, call your health care provider right away rather than waiting for your scheduled post-partum visit.) Your physician or midwife will recommend Pap tests on a regular schedule. This almost painless test effectively detects the early symptoms of cervical cancer.

Breast Self-Examination

Your caregiver will also recommend monthly breast self-examination. The best time to check your breasts is right after your menstrual period. If you are breastfeeding, check on the first day of each month after a feeding. While only a small percentage of breast changes indicate cancer, you should tell your physician about any thickening, lumps that do not go away after feeding or within a day or two, or non-milk discharge. Here is how to check your breasts:

- You can examine your breasts while bathing or showering. Wet, soapy skin allows your fingers to slide easily over your skin. Flatten your fingers and move them gently over every part of each breast, feeling for any lump or thickening.
- Standing in front of a mirror, look at your breasts with your arms at your sides, and then with your arms raised over your head. Look for changes in contour, swelling, dimpling of the skin or changes in the nipple. Compare one breast to the other. They should look similar.

You should also examine your breasts while lying down. To check your right breast, put a pillow under your right shoulder and place your right hand under your head. With your left hand (fingers flat), press gently around your breast in a circular motion. Making smaller circles, gradually move in towards the nipple until you have examined your entire breast (including the nipple). Repeat this procedure on your left breast after switching the pillow and placing your left hand behind your head. There are also other correct techniques of breast examination that follow the same key concepts (systematic, thorough and regularly done).

Post-partum Adaptation

The birth of your baby represents a sudden disruption in the usual balance of your life—both physically and emotionally. Your basic needs for food, sleep, and physical comfort and for emotional wellbeing, independence, and relative predictability suddenly are pushed aside by the basic needs of your baby. Your well-ordered life is temporarily thrown into disorder.

Post-partum adaptation (also called post-partum recovery) means that your life is returning to more predictable patterns. You can take care of life's daily demands, you feel rested most of the time, and you are beginning to enjoy some of your previous interests again. In addition, your body is healing and you feel competent in understanding and meeting your baby's needs.

When Will I Get Back to 'Normal'?

As new parents, you may wonder if life will ever be as it was before. You may yearn for the simpler, more predictable lives you had before your baby was born. It takes time for you to physically recover from the birth and to achieve a comfortable and rewarding new lifestyle that balances the interests and demands of your former life with the joys and needs of your new life with your baby. How long this takes depends on a number of influential factors, each of which may either ease or slow your recovery and adaptation. For example, your comfort with and knowledge of newborns, your physical and mental health, your financial state, your baby's health and temperament, and the amount of support you have from family and friends all play a role in the speed of your recovery. (See page 359 for a fuller description of these factors.) When all or most of these factors are positive, your physical recovery and emotional adjustment after childbirth will probably take four to twelve weeks. If you find it is taking longer for you to feel like yourself again, think about the factors influencing your recovery. You may recognise one or more negative factors that explain why your recovery is delayed. It may be that some of these negative factors are not under your control. Consult your caregiver or your childbirth educator for resources that may assist you in your recovery.

The figure below shows a typical time frame that begins with the birth of your baby, continues with the associated disruption of physical and emotional wellbeing, and ends with the establishment of a new balance in your life. Just as labour progresses in a fairly predictable or 'typical' pattern (see figure on page 224), so does the post-partum recovery period.

Sexual Adjustments

Some women and men want to resume intercourse as soon as possible after the birth. Others may prefer to wait or may even feel afraid. Obviously, a sore perineum, a demanding baby, lack of help and extreme fatigue will affect your ability to relax and enjoy making love. You still need to feel

Time Frame for Post-partum Adaptation

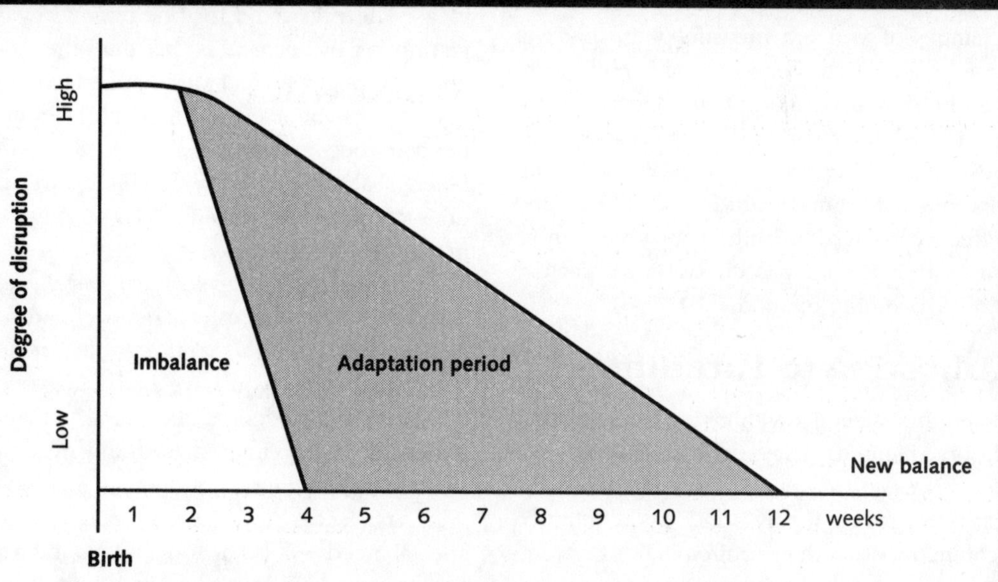

loved, however. If you are not ready to resume intercourse, cuddling and 'pleasuring' (touching and enjoying each other's bodies sensually with or without orgasm and without pressure to have intercourse) can help you both relax and show your love. Keep your sense of humour and be honest with each other about your feelings. Many new mothers are not interested in sex or even being touched or caressed, but their partner's interest in sex may be unchanged. Recognising this difference is the first step in finding ways to accommodate each other.

Doctors sometimes routinely recommend that new mothers refrain from intercourse for six weeks, but this is a somewhat arbitrary suggestion. It is probably safe to have intercourse when your stitches heal, your vaginal discharge declines and you feel like it. But be gentle. You may be sore at first. After birth, you will have a decrease in vaginal lubrication because of hormonal changes; if you are breastfeeding, this will continue. Any sterile, water-soluble lubricant can help. Keep in mind that conception can occur whether or not menstruation has resumed. A condom in combination with spermicidal foam, cream or jelly is safe and effective soon after birth. Your physician or midwife can help you choose a satisfactory family planning method.

Adjusting to Parenthood

Parenthood begins with giving birth and will last a lifetime. The early weeks are not always easy. However, a good start sets the stage for strong family bonds and continued commitment to the requirements of parenting. And, if you and your partner are nurtured and helped at the beginning, you will have more time and energy to give to your baby and to your new roles as parents.

Parenting

Each of you needs to develop your own comfortable relationship with your new baby. Try not to interfere with each other or protect each other from the realities of baby care (like nappy changing and crying). Support each other. You do not have to do things the same way to appreciate each other as parents. Distinguish between small problems and large ones. Let the small problems (nappies on backwards, pyjamas inside out) go, so you can work out the large ones together. If you have different approaches to the baby's crying, try to discuss your views and arrive at a comfortable solution. Consult your baby's health care provider, a parent educator or a good newborn care book for ideas. The price paid for one parent always getting his or her way is that the other parent may begin to feel discouraged, incompetent, less involved and resentful. Parents need to become aware of their goals and feelings about parenthood. This awareness does not happen overnight; it is an ongoing process.

Parenting is not an instinctive skill; it is learned. Your ability as a parent depends on several factors: how your parents treated you; experiences you have had with young children; knowledge of the physical, emotional and intellectual abilities and needs of infants and children; examples of parenting you have seen; and the temperament and special needs of both you and your baby. Even if you have not had much experience caring for babies and young children, you can learn about your baby's abilities, needs and development by reading, attending parenting classes, or observing your baby's behaviour and her responses to your care. Your baby is your best teacher as long as you are open to learning from your little one.

A Note to Fathers and Partners

Once your baby is several days old and the newness and lustre of a brand new baby has worn off, the constant demands and frequent crying of a newborn begin to tax everyone's endurance and patience. It may seem to you that the baby's mother is better able than you to soothe your baby and meet her needs, especially if she is breastfeeding. But if this is her first baby, she is as new at parenthood as you are. In addition, no matter how many children you have, she needs your daily support and participation in baby care.

This early time with your new baby is important for both of you. Despite the baby's crying and your frustration at not always knowing what your baby needs, spending time caring for your baby during these early months will provide you with lifelong memories as you watch her personality emerge and unfold. Acknowledging that both of you are under a lot of stress and then sharing the work and joy of parenting will strengthen your relationship and your family.

A Note to Parents Having Another Baby

Sometimes new parents feel guilty when another child comes into the family. These feelings are normal. If you are having another baby, you may feel like you are abandoning your first-born. You may feel that you cannot give your second child what you gave your first, in terms of undivided attention. Of course, the exclusive relationship that you had with your older child will inevitably change. However, try to see the positive influences a sibling will eventually bring to the family. Your first child will enrich the new child's life, and the new baby will enrich the lives of the whole family. Every child has a different experience with the parents—not necessarily better or worse, just different. (For more on preparing a sibling for the birth of another baby, see Chapter 16.)

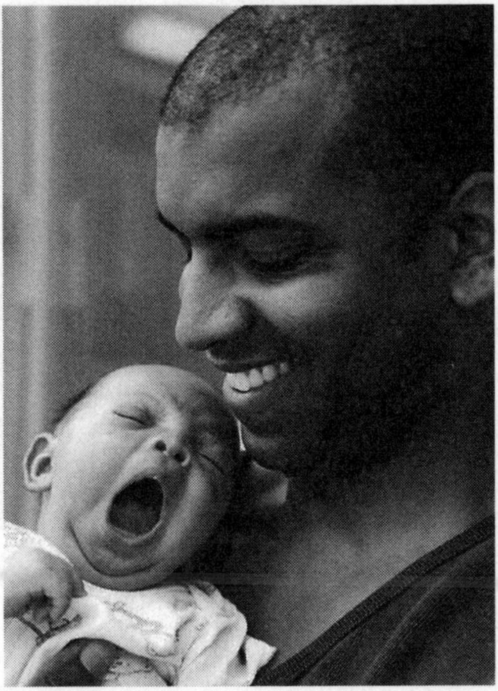

Photograph by Patti Ramos

You cannot take your eyes off your amazing newborn.

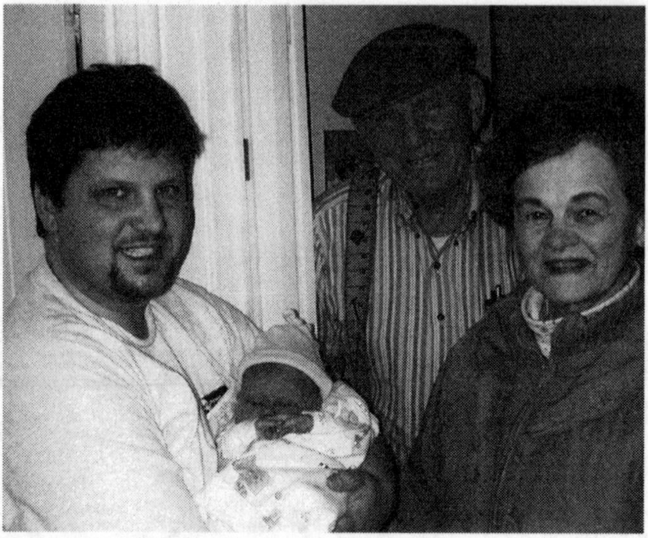

The baby's proud grandparents eagerly greet their new grandchild.

For families in which the marriage or partnership was healthy before the baby arrived, the addition of a new baby brings new and unexpected demands, some of which are stressful. Fatigue, loss of sleep and finding time to eat and care for yourself are often huge issues. With the arrival of a new baby, most families find that the amount of work increases dramatically and the family budget may be strained. In a marriage or partnership that was tense or shaky, the addition of a new baby can threaten or even lead to the end of the relationship if the partners do not get help and support. Many communities have excellent programs available to families to strengthen relationships and preserve marriages or partnerships. Check with your childbirth educator, health care provider, hospital or health department for information about classes and counselling.

The challenges of parenting increase for the single parent. The time, energy and emotional demands are much greater. Parent support groups and parent-infant classes can be very helpful. Other single parents and friends may also be a source of support and help.

Family Relationships Change

The first weeks after the birth present a sudden leap into parenthood. The birth of a new baby, especially the first baby, brings many emotional, physical and social changes to the primary people involved. Women become mothers, men become fathers and their parents become grandparents. There are shifts—some supportive, some stressful—in established family relationships.

Grandparents and other extended family members are usually eager to be a part of your baby's life. To help make their involvement rewarding to everyone, think about the role you would like them to play and the role they wish to play. Try to discuss these ideas and expectations with them. You may want to use the 'Letter to Grandparents' on page 375 as a guide.

Returning to Employment

For many new mothers, returning to work after childbirth is a financial necessity. For others, returning to work is necessary for career development or because they love their job. In some families, the mother returns

A Letter to Grandparents

Dear Grandparents,

Congratulations on the birth of your new grandchild! This birth marks the continuation of your family into a new generation. Your support and love can ease your own child's transition into parenthood.

The new parents need to hear from you that you think they are wonderful parents—the very best parents your grandchild could have. They need to hear from you that parenthood is challenging, tiring and yet one of the most important and rewarding roles they will ever have. Let them know you have confidence in them.

What your grandchild needs most from you is your nurturing support of his or her parents. You need to honour their thoughtful decisions and their style of parenting, even if they are different from yours. You will find that some things have changed since you had children, and some have remained the same. Please respect their parenting choices, offer advice if asked and help them find up-to-date answers to their questions. It may help if you read the same books they are reading about newborn care and feeding.

The new parents need you to support them as they learn about and care for their new baby. They need to have hands-on experience with their baby to learn the skills that all parents need to develop. So, while it is tempting to hold and care for your grandchild all day, let them care for their baby. If your children invite you to come and help, recognise it as an honour. Ask them how you can help prepare meals, do laundry, shop and clean the house. You will work hard, sleep little and leave tired and appreciated.

If you are unable to be with the new family or if your relationship is strained or difficult for you or them, think of what you can do to support them. You could send help in the form of household help, nappy service, meals or presence of another family member. Reaching out in this way would be appreciated and could go a long way towards healing your troubled relationship with them.

Remember your own first weeks as new parents and try to have realistic expectations of the new parents by forgiving them if they forget to thank you for your help and your gifts. Memories—ones that are never forgotten—are made in these first weeks following birth. Your care and concern at this time will also enhance your relationship with your grandchild. Your children will always remember your love and acceptance.

With best wishes for joyful grandparenting,

Penny Simkin
Janet Whalley
Ann Keppler

Authors, *Pregnancy, Childbirth and the Newborn* © 2001

to work and the father or partner stays home to parent. The decision to return to work is usually made before the birth. This timing means the woman and her partner cannot know how attached they will become to their baby and how much they will miss her while away.

If you are wavering about your decision for both parents to return to work and have the option of making other plans, consider the following:

- Can you or your partner delay returning to work until your baby is older?
- Can you or your partner work part-time or job-share?
- Can either of you work at home?
- What are the costs of returning to work? (These may include clothing, transportation, day care, convenience foods and more trips to the doctor with an ill child.) Will your income equal the total costs of working outside the home or exceed these costs by enough to make working worthwhile?
- How would you and your partner feel about one of you not working?
- Could you or would you want to simplify your lifestyle to allow one of you to stay home?

Once you have carefully considered your options, you will make the best choice for each of you and your family. Whether you stay home with your baby or work outside the home, life is more challenging with a baby. You and your partner will need to support each other to accommodate the change.

When both parents plan on returning to work, finding affordable, safe and dependable child care becomes the foremost priority. Ideally, arrangements for child care are made during pregnancy. If this was not possible for you, give yourself a week or two to recover from birth and to get to know your baby. Then begin your search. You might start by talking to fellow employees about their day-care arrangements. Contact local agencies to find licenced facilities, homes or other providers (such as nannies). Consider the possibility of using family members to babysit. And, consider the possibilities of changing work schedules, working part-time so you and your partner can provide child care, or bringing your small infant to work with you.

Next, begin interviewing day-care providers. Visit day-care facilities and homes. Check their licences. Take your baby with you. Pay attention to the responses of the day-care providers to you and your baby. How do they respond to the babies already in their care? With respect and kindness, or with impatience and detachment? Ask questions about how they support breastfeeding mothers, how they feel about your visiting when you are able, how they deal with crying babies and what they will do if your child becomes ill. Find out about their hours of operation and their holiday and vacation schedule. Trust your instincts about the home or facility.

If you are choosing an in-home provider, interview potential providers in your home. Observe how they interact with your baby. Ask the same questions you would ask at a day-care facility or home. Also, ask about backup plans if they should become ill or go on vacation. Request references and contact them.

Post-partum Emotional Challenges

After childbirth, you will experience emotional ups and downs. These emotional fluctuations may be partly due to the extreme changes in hormone levels (for example, oestrogen, progesterone, oxytocin, prolactin and thyroid hormone) that occur after birth. Emotional changes may also be partly due to fatigue, inexperience or lack of confidence in caring for a newborn baby, loneliness or isolation from supportive adults, and/or the round-the-clock demands from your baby. These changes may also be partly due to a disappointing or very difficult birth experience; an unexpected illness or condition in the baby; personally stressful situations (social, financial, physical and so on); or a personal or family history of mood disorders including depression, anxiety and panic attacks, or bipolar illness. For some women, these emotional fluctuations are mild and decrease within a few weeks. For others, they are overwhelming, long-lasting and may require treatment.

Baby Blues

'Baby blues' affect about 80 percent of all new mothers. The blues generally occur within the first week after birth and often begin about the time milk comes in. Symptoms include crying easily; feeling overwhelmed; feeling a loss of control; feeling exhausted, anxious or sad; and feeling a lack of confidence about being a parent. The blues are temporary and rarely last longer than a week. They are relieved by getting more rest and sleep; by reducing the pain of sore breasts, perineum or incision; and by being surrounded by supportive family and friends.

Post-partum Mood Disorders

Post-partum mood disorders (PPMD) is the term used to describe four emotional conditions occurring in the first year after giving birth. These four conditions include anxiety and panic disorder, obsessive-compulsive disorder, post-partum depression and post-traumatic stress disorder. About 20 percent of women will have PPMD following birth, and they may experience one or more of these conditions. PPMD usually occurs within two months after giving birth, though it may occur anytime in the first year following childbirth.

1. Post-partum Anxiety and Panic Disorder

A woman may experience symptoms of anxiety and panic, which include shortness of breath, sensations of choking, light-headedness, faintness, rapid heart rate or chest pain. She may feel nauseated and may have diarrhoea. She may have an immobilising fear of being alone, of dying, of her baby dying or of leaving the house.

2. Post-partum Obsessive-Compulsive Disorder (OCD)

Post-partum OCD is characterised by obsessive (recurring over and over) thoughts and by compulsive rituals (acts and mannerisms repeated over and over). Obsessive thoughts cannot be controlled. They repeat themselves again and again and may include the fear of being a 'bad' mother, the fear of hurting the baby in some way or the fear of germs. Compulsive rituals can include constant hand washing (perhaps hundreds of times each day), frequent house cleaning, compulsive and excessive checking on the baby, or constantly making sure that the doors are locked. These rituals interfere with normal daily living.

3. Post-partum Depression

Post-partum depression varies in its degree of seriousness and symptoms from woman to woman. It generally occurs between two weeks after birth up to one year, with most depression beginning between the sixth week and the sixth month. Common symptoms include feelings of hopelessness, despair, exhaustion, lack of energy and loss of interest in anything. A woman suffering post-partum depression may experience extreme feelings of inadequacy or low self-esteem; surprising and frightening outbursts of anger at her spouse, partner or other children; and recurring thoughts about hurting herself (even suicide) or her baby. She may be unable to sleep even when she has the opportunity, she may forget to eat (or she may overeat), and she may find herself crying constantly.

4. Post-partum Post-Traumatic Stress Disorder

Post-partum post-traumatic stress disorder may result from the trauma of a difficult or frightening childbirth or from traumatic situations surrounding pregnancy or birth, such as an unexpected illness, unexpected problems for the baby, or insensitive or hurtful care. This disorder can also occur when childbirth triggers memories of a past trauma such as a frightening hospital experience, physical or sexual abuse, or rape. Common symptoms include preoccupation with or memories ('flashbacks') of the trauma, recurrent nightmares, anger and rage, and extreme protectiveness of self or baby. Anxiety and panic attacks may accompany the flashbacks or nightmares.

Risk Factors for Post-partum Mood Disorders

- History or presence of emotional problems, panic disorder, obsessive-compulsive disorder (OCD), or depression in self or immediate family member
- Traumatic pregnancy or childbirth experience
- Recent major stresses such as miscarriage(s), death in the family, a move, change or loss of job, marriage, separation, or divorce
- Unsupportive spouse or partner, or no partner
- Lack of supportive friends or family
- History of severe premenstrual symptoms such as depression, irritability and anger

Myths and Facts about Post-partum Mood Disorder (PPMD)

- Myth: It will go away if I just 'tough it out' or ignore/deny it.
- Fact: *Acknowledging the way you feel and getting help will speed your recovery.*

- Myth: Having PPMD means I am a weak person.
- Fact: *Strong, intelligent women have PPMD. You did nothing wrong and you did not cause it.*

- Myth: Having PPMD means I am a 'bad' mother.
- Fact: *Many women with PPMD feel they are 'bad' mothers because of the thoughts or feelings they have. They think only 'bad' mothers ever get angry or have thoughts about hurting themselves or their baby. It is helpful to know that women with PPMD who recognise that their thoughts are harmful will not act on these thoughts. Good mothers do the best they are able to do.*

- Myth: If I take medication for PPMD, I cannot breastfeed.
- Fact: *There are medications used to treat PPMD that are compatible with breastfeeding. Check with your caregiver or therapist.*

- History of physical, emotional or sexual abuse
- History of substance abuse or living with someone who is abusing drugs or alcohol
- History of or current eating disorder
- Unplanned and unwanted pregnancy
- Low self-esteem
- Poor or absent mother-daughter relationship
- Financial pressures
- High expectations of self with a personal need to be 'perfect' and 'in control'
- Having a 'high-need' infant or an infant with a chronic medical condition
- History of infertility
- Thyroid disease
- Excessive sleep deprivation

Treatment for Post-partum Mood Disorder

Appropriate treatment for PPMD depends on the severity of the symptoms and may range from lifestyle changes to therapy and medication. Lifestyle changes that can help women who have PPMD include:

- Eating well
- Avoiding alcohol, caffeine and over-the-counter sleep medications
- Getting regular exercise (such as walking)
- Being in sunlight or its equivalent often enough to make you feel good and to decrease the possibility of suffering from seasonal affective disorder (SAD)
- Having time for yourself with a break from responsibility
- Getting adequate rest and sleep

Attending a PPMD support group helps women and their families understand the condition, recognise some of the causes, realise they are not alone, and learn about resources for support. (See Recommended Resources, page 490, for PPMD contacts.) Your childbirth educator, local hospital, health department or caregiver can also tell you about local support groups.

Counselling and therapy can be very helpful in treating PPMD. Choose a knowledgeable therapist or psychiatrist who specialises in this disorder. Medication for depression, OCD and anxiety can be quite effective in treating PPMD. Counselling along with medication (rather than medication alone) leads to more rapid recovery.

PPMD affects not only the mother but the whole family. It can also affect the mother's relationship with and attachment to her baby. Women with PPMD often worry about their inability to be physically and emotionally available to their babies during the important early weeks and months. Fathers and other family members also worry. The best way the father and family can help a woman with PPMD is by encouraging her to get treatment, by finding ways to make sure she gets rest and sleep, by helping with housework, and by providing supportive and loving care.

Post-partum Psychosis

Post-partum psychosis is rare, occurring in about one in one thousand women after childbirth. It usually occurs soon after birth and is characterised by severe agitation, mood swings, depression and delusions. Women with post-partum psychosis need immediate care and treatment from a psychiatrist. They are given medications to treat their symptoms and are often hospitalised at the beginning of their illness. Once home, medications are monitored by the psychiatrist and arrangements are made for ongoing psychotherapy.

A Baby Changes Your Life

Parenting an infant interrupts the usual flow or equilibrium in a person's life. To keep this period of your life in perspective, take a look at the 'Pie of Life' chart on page 381. While you will be a parent for the rest of your life, the time spent with your infant is brief and represents only a small portion of your life. Enjoy it!

The 'Pie of Life' chart illustrates the predictable phases in your life. Roughly one third is spent before you have a child. During this time, you develop as an individual and form a relationship (marriage or other) that leads to the decision to bear a child. Another third is spent bearing and rearing a child or children. The last third is spent with an 'empty nest'. The children have left, and you and your partner find yourselves in yet another phase of your lives with reduced parenting responsibilities and more freedom to pursue other interests. Once again you are a couple. It is possible that a woman will spend the very last years of her life as a widow, since women usually live longer than men.

Pie of Life

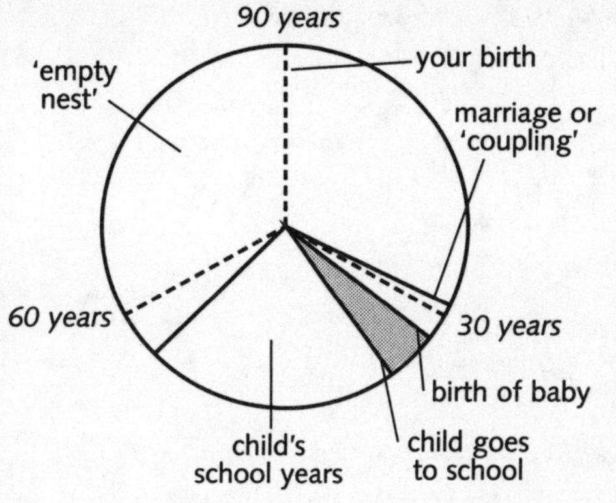

In proportion to the rest of your life, the time you spend bearing children and caring for them before they enter school is short. Although this time is brief, it is probably the most demanding and stressful of your life, for you both as individuals and as a couple. It is during this period that many couples, so caught up in caring for children and pursuing one or two careers, neglect the little things that keep them close together. To avoid this, be sure to make time for conversation and shared fun and activities.

In addition, it is important not to neglect your individual interests, even though they must take a lower priority when your baby and young child need so much of your attention. Even if it must be on a smaller scale, pursuing individual interests keeps you growing as a person and, in the process, as a parent and partner. Later in life, you will probably find that what you did during this brief childbearing period played a significant role in your individual growth and the development of your family.

Chapter 14

Caring for Your Baby

New parents are often surprised at the physical appearance of their newborn. The size and shape of the head, the baby's initial dusky blue colour, the presence of vernix and streaks of blood, the beautiful hands and feet, the enlarged reddened genitals and the baby's size make a strong first impression. You will probably find that you cannot take your eyes off your new baby.

Your Newborn's Appearance

Body

The average full-term baby weighs 3–3.4 kilograms and measures about 50 centimetres. A newborn baby's shoulders are narrow, his abdomen protrudes, his hips are small, and his arms and legs are relatively short, thin and flexed.

Head

Your baby's head is large in proportion to the rest of his body. Your baby's head may be elongated or moulded from pressures within your pelvis during labour and birth. This condition is called *moulding*. The head returns to a normal round shape within a few days. Occasionally, the scalp or face is bruised and swollen, but this will disappear in time.

Babies are born with two *soft spots* or *fontanels* (areas where the bones of the skull have not completely fused). There is a large, diamond-shaped soft spot on the top front portion of the head, while a smaller, triangle-shaped spot lies at the back. The larger one usually closes by eighteen months; the smaller one by two to six months. The membrane covering the fontanels is thick and tough, so brushing or washing the scalp will not hurt your baby.

Hair

Some babies are born with full heads of hair, while others are virtually bald. Fine, downy body hair, called *lanugo,* may be noticeable on your baby's back, shoulders, forehead, ears and face. It is most pronounced in premature babies. Lanugo usually disappears during the first few weeks.

Eyes

Fair-skinned babies usually have grey-blue eyes; dark-skinned babies have brown or dark grey eyes. If the eye colour is going to change, it usually does so by six months. The tear glands of most newborns do not produce many tears until about three weeks of age.

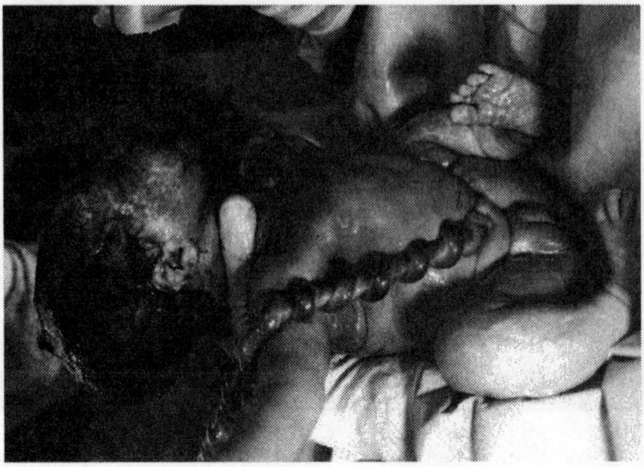

Photograph by Marilyn Nolt

Seconds after birth, the baby is soaking wet, streaked with vernix and blood, and her cord is still pulsating.

Blister on the Lip

Intense sucking often causes a painless blister on the centre of your baby's upper lip. Sometimes the sucking blister peels. It needs no treatment and disappears gradually as the lip toughens.

Skin

At birth, your baby's skin is greyish-blue, wet, and streaked with blood and varying amounts of vernix, a white creamy substance. Within a minute or two after your baby begins breathing well, the skin colour changes to normal tones, beginning with his face and trunk and soon reaching his fingers and toes.

Obstructed sweat and oil glands cause small white spots, called *milia,* on your baby's nose, cheeks and chin. When the glands begin to function, which may take several weeks, the milia disappear. You do not need to treat the condition or try to remove the whiteheads; simply wash his face with water.

Fair-skinned newborn babies often look blotchy, with areas of redness and paleness. After a few weeks, the baby's skin has a more even colour, although it becomes more mottled-looking when he is cold.

Many babies have peeling skin, particularly at the wrists, hands, ankles and feet. Overdue babies peel more than term babies. This is normal and no treatment is usually necessary. If there are cracks on the wrists or ankles that bleed, apply moisturiser.

Vernix caseosa, the white creamy substance that protected your baby's skin before birth, often remains in skin creases even after bathing. There is no need to remove the vernix. Gently rub it into your baby's skin.

Stork bites and *angel kisses,* red areas on the skin formed by the collection of tiny superficial blood vessels, often appear on the back of the baby's neck, eyelids, nose or forehead. They redden when the baby cries. Most are not permanent birthmarks and are not caused by injury during birth. Although they usually fade or disappear within six to nine months, some, especially those on the neck, may remain longer or may be permanent.

Mongolian spots, areas of dark pigment, commonly appear on the lower back and buttocks and occasionally on the thighs or arms of some babies, usually of Native American, Asian, African or southern European descent. The spots look like black-and-blue marks or bruises, but they are not bruises. They gradually fade and usually disappear by age four. It is important that day-care providers and others who care for your baby know these spots are not bruises.

Breasts

Due to maternal hormones, which reached the baby in utero, both male and female babies may have swollen breasts. Some babies even leak milk from their nipples. This swelling and leaking is normal and needs no treatment. Do not try to express milk from your baby's nipples, as this may cause infection. The condition will disappear within a week or two.

Umbilical Cord

A newborn baby's umbilical cord is bluish-white in colour and 2.5–5 centimetres long immediately after it is cut. A plastic cord clamp applied to the cord stops bleeding. The cord clamp is removed when the cord is dry, usually before discharge from a hospital or within twenty-four to forty-eight hours after birth. The umbilical cord usually falls off within two weeks after birth.

The goal of cord care is to prevent infection and to promote cord separation from the abdomen. In an effort to prevent infection and hasten separation, many different substances and rituals have been used for cord care. Only a few of these have been well studied.

Substances such as triple dye, alcohol and chlorhexidine solution were once thought to prevent infection but have not been found to do so. In addition, when mothers keep their infants in their rooms rather than in nurseries, the lowest rates of cord infection occur.[1] In a randomised, controlled trial comparing cleaning the cord with alcohol at each nappy change and allowing the cord to dry naturally without treatment, researchers found neither group developed a cord infection. In addition, the cord came off a day earlier in the group in which the cord was allowed to dry naturally.[2]

What recommendations can be made for cord care today?

- Anyone caring for infants and their cords must wash their hands very well before touching the infant.
- Use baby soap or no soap while bathing newborns, to maintain the acid pH of the infant's skin and to reduce the growth of bacteria.
- To keep the cord dry and clean, place the nappy, nappy wrap and plastic pants below the cord until it comes off.
- Clean the cord daily, or when it is soiled, with warm water or alcohol and let it dry thoroughly. Or, allow the cord to dry naturally without treatment.
- Report to the baby's care provider any redness of the skin surrounding the cord,

any strong foul odour, or any presence of pus or bright red blood oozing from the cord. It is normal to see dark red blood or clear yellow sticky fluid as the cord falls off.

- If your infant has been discharged with the cord clamp still on, let your care provider or hospital remove the clamp later. You may remove it if you have very clear directions and feel comfortable removing it. Never cut the cord clamp off.

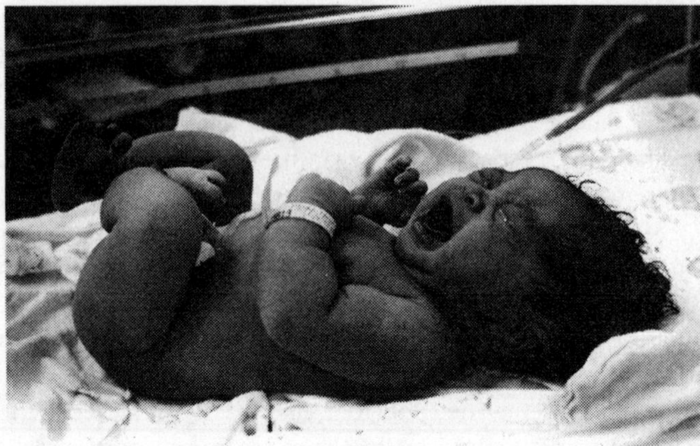

Photograph by Marilyn Nolt

An hour later with her ID bracelet on, the baby has received a vitamin K injection and seems to want to be with her mother.

Genitals

Maternal hormones may cause swollen genitals in both male and female newborns. Female infants may have a milky or bloody discharge from the vagina called a 'pseudo menstrual period'. This discharge indicates your baby's uterus has responded in a healthy way to your hormones and is now shedding its first lining. Male infants may have an unusually large, red scrotum. These conditions are normal, temporary and do not require treatment.

Bathing Your Baby

Newborns can be given sponge baths or tub baths right from birth. Tub baths do not cause increased infection of cords or circumcisions. Infants are usually more comfortable in a warm tub bath than being washed with a wet cloth. In fact, babies stay warmer and calmer when immersed in warm water. Newborns do not need to be bathed more often than once or twice a week.[3]

If you choose to give your baby a sponge bath, lay the baby on a soft towel on a firm surface. Fill the sink or small tub with warm water. Without undressing your baby, first wash her eyes with water. Next, wash her face with warm water and dry. Then dampen her hair with water. Apply a little soap to her scalp and rub gently. Rinse her hair and head and dry her. If it is cool, put a hat on her head. Next, undress her, but cover her with a warm receiving blanket or towel to avoid chilling her. Put a little mild liquid soap on a wet, warm washcloth and wash her upper body. Rinse and dry her. Next, wash and dry her back, and then her lower body, making sure to get the nappy area clean. Finally, dress her warmly.

To give your baby a tub bath, fill a sink or baby bathtub with comfortably warm water. Hold the baby securely with her head resting in the crook of your arm and with your hand gently grasping her arm. Lower her into the tub so that the water covers all of her body, and her head and neck are above the water. Use water to clean her eyes and face. Next, wash her hair with mild soap, massaging her head with your fingers or a soft brush. Then, add a little mild baby soap and wash her body. Let her enjoy the warmth of the water. Once you have finished her bath, take her out and dry her with a towel you have warmed in the dryer. Be sure that her skin and hair are very dry before you put her clothes on, to avoid chilling her.

Many parents enjoy bathing with their baby. Not only is it a pleasurable experience, it saves time, too. Fill the tub with comfortably warm water. Get in the tub first and have someone hand you the baby, or pick your baby up from a car seat you have placed next to the tub. Enjoy relaxing in the water together. Fussy babies may be calmed during a bath. Use just a little mild baby soap to clean the baby. Once you have finished cleaning the baby, hand her to someone who can dry her and dress her, or wrap her in a warm towel and place her in the car seat until you have finished your bath.

Nappies for Your Baby

You can nappy your baby using cloth or disposable nappies. Cloth nappies can be purchased and washed at home or you can use a baby nappy service. Disposable nappies come in a variety of sizes and styles and, though convenient, may be much more expensive and need to be properly disposed of following the directions on the package.

Disposable nappies usually have adhesive tabs that hold the nappy in place. Be sure the top of the nappy is below the cord until the cord is off.

Cloth nappies are often used with plastic pants or nappy wraps. You will have many choices of size of nappy, type of fabric, style of plastic pants, and type of nappy wrap.

Nappies may be held in place with pins or by the nappy wrap. Be sure the nappy and nappy wrap or plastic pants are below the cord until the cord is off. You will become more adept at folding and using nappies with practise. Your childbirth educator, nurse or nappy service can teach you how to nappy and to know how many nappies to get for your newborn.

Your Baby's Layette

Use the following guide in getting what you need for your newborn baby:

Bed	Crib Bassinette (optional) 2–4 sets of bed linens for crib or bassinette 3–6 receiving blankets 1–2 blankets for warmth 2–4 waterproof pads for crib, lap and nappy-changing areas
Diapers	4 dozen cloth nappies, nappy service or disposable nappies (newborns use about 90 nappies per week) 6–8 waterproof wraps or pants for use with cloth nappies 3–6 washcloths to clean baby when nappying Nappy wipes Nappy pail (if using cloth nappies) Nappy rash ointment (ask caregiver about what to use) Changing table (optional)
Bath	2–4 hooded towels or soft towels 6–8 baby washcloths Baby soap and shampoo Baby bathtub (optional) Cotton swabs for umbilical cord
Baby clothing (Some large babies are born too big for newborn-size clothing.)	4–8 undershirts or 'onesies' 3–6 gowns or stretch suits with feet 2 blanket sleepers (depends on season) 1–2 jumpers (depends on season) 1–3 pairs of booties or socks Hats: 1 knit hat for newborn, 1 appropriate for season (sun hat, warm hat for outdoors) Dresser (optional)
Travel	Car seat (mandatory in all states, ACT and Northern Territory) Nappy bag
Baby equipment (These are optional, but come in very handy.)	Thermometer (blunt-tipped or one designed for babies) Baby sling or front pack Carriage or stroller Baby swing Large exercise ball (birth ball) Blunt-tipped nail scissors or baby nail clippers Massage oil Mobile

Newborn Tests and Procedures

Routine care of the newborn includes many tests and procedures. These vary somewhat among health care providers and institutions. The following table describes many newborn routines and tests. Try to find out which ones are used by your health care provider and what choices you have.

Test or Procedure	Where Required or When Indicated	What It Is	Comments
Infant vital signs	In all settings, the baby's heart rate, respiratory rate and temperature will be assessed frequently in the first few hours after birth, and then every several hours thereafter.	Your nurse or midwife will assess your baby's vital signs to be sure your baby is adjusting to life as a newborn and to detect problems with the heart, lungs or need for warming.	The normal infant heart rate is 90–160 beats per minute with a regular rate and rhythm and with no audible heart murmurs. Infants breathe 30–60 times per minute. The infant should appear pink and breathe easily without grunting, flaring nostrils or retracting her chest (pulling in her chest under her ribs). Normal underarm temperature is between 36.5°C and 37.5°C. If the heart rate or rhythm is cause for concern, or if there is a breathing problem, the baby will be assessed by her health care provider or admitted to the nursery. If she has a fever, she will be admitted to the nursery and may have a septic work up (see page 390) and intravenous (IV) antibiotics. If she is too cool, she will warm up quickly if placed skin-to-skin with her mother and covered with warmed blankets. If she is still cool after 20 or 30 minutes, she may be wrapped warmly in several blankets and placed under a special radiant warming light or admitted to the nursery and placed in a special bed or isolette for warming.
Vitamin K	Required and recommended in all states, ACT and Northern Territory	Vitamin K is injected into the baby's thigh or possibly administered orally. Vitamin K given soon after birth enhances blood clotting and may prevent a bleeding disorder of the newborn called haemorrhagic disease.*‡	The Therapeutic Drugs Administration (TDA) has approved both injectable and oral forms. If injected, the infant receives one dose of 1 mg of vitamin K1 (Konakion) into the thigh muscle. If given orally, the infant receives 2 mg of vitamin K1 at birth, another 2 mg dose at 1–2 weeks of age, and a final dose of 2 mg at 4 weeks of age. Over-the-counter preparations have not been shown to be effective. Breastfed babies are slower to produce adequate amounts of vitamin K than those fed formula. Formula contains small amounts of vitamin K.*‡

Newborn Tests and Procedures

Test or Procedure	Where Required or When Indicated	What It Is	Comments
Septic work up	When medically indicated	Blood is drawn and cerebrospinal fluid may be obtained by spinal tap; they are sent to the laboratory to be tested for bacteria that cause illness and disease.	Baby is admitted to the nursery for IV antibiotics. If the blood and cerebrospinal fluid are found to be normal, antibiotics will be discontinued. If the tests show the presence of bacteria, the baby will stay in the nursery for a full course of antibiotic therapy.
Test for jaundice	If the baby's skin and whites of his eyes are yellowish, an elevated bilirubin level is suspected.	Blood taken by pricking the baby's heel is sent to a laboratory, where the bilirubin level is determined. If high, the baby has significant jaundice. Sometimes, a special instrument, such as a jaundice metre, is used to estimate the blood levels of bilirubin by flashing a light over the skin of the sternum.	Jaundice may result from prematurity, bruising of the baby during labour or birth, blood incompatibilities (Rh and ABO), sepsis (infection), exposure to certain drugs given to the mother in labour, or liver or intestinal problems. Most jaundice is not harmful. (See page 401 for a more detailed discussion of jaundice and its treatment.)

Newborn Tests and Procedures

Test or Procedure	Where Required or When Indicated	What It Is	Comments
Test for hypoglycemia	• If baby is large (over 4 kilograms) or small (under 2.3 kilograms) • If baby is thought to have low blood sugar • If baby becomes chilled • If baby is preterm	Blood obtained by a heel prick is tested for hypoglycemia (low blood sugar).	Hypoglycemia can lead to respiratory distress, lethargy, slow heart rate, seizures and (in the most severe cases) death. Treatment includes frequent breastfeeding or formula feeding and/or feedings of sugar water (5 or 10 percent dextrose solution). In more serious cases, the baby may be admitted to the nursery and given IV dextrose. Low blood sugar can occur in babies when the mother is diabetic or when the mother has received large amounts of IV fluids with dextrose and water (a sugar solution).
Infant security	Essential for all facilities providing maternity care	All hospitals and large birth centres should have a policy in place to prevent kidnapping, to ensure that all babies are properly identified, and to safeguard against confusing or switching infants.	Learn about the infant security policy at your hospital or birth centre. All babies should be given wrist and ankle bands at birth that match their mothers. All staff providing care for babies should wear easy-to-read identification badges. And there should be a written plan for how the facility would respond if an infant were missing. Many facilities have video surveillance and sensors that lock doors and units immediately when a baby is missing. Having your baby in your room with you at the hospital (or birth centre) and being sure that you never leave her unattended at the birth facility or after you go home are the best ways to keep your baby safe.
Newborn hearing screening	Variable; some hospitals test only infants at high risk for hearing deficits or deafness, while other hospitals screen all newborn babies.	Newborn hearing is assessed in the first days after birth using one of several devices for a period of about 10 minutes while the infant is sleeping.	Infants who are born prematurely, who have a family history of hearing deficits or deafness, or who have been exposed to pathogens or medications that put them at risk for hearing loss or deafness are tested. Universal hearing screening is being considered as a standard for all babies, since 50 percent of infants with hearing deficits have no risk factors.

* American Academy of Pediatrics, 'Vitamin K Ad Hoc Task Force', *Pediatrics* 91(5) (1993): 1001–2.
† American Academy of Pediatrics and American College of Obstetricians and Gynecologists, 'Guidelines for Perinatal Care', 1997.
‡ F. I. Clark and E. J. P. Janes, 'Twenty-Seven Years of Experience with Oral Vitamin K1 Therapy in Neonates', *Journal of Pediatrics* 127 (1995): 301–04.

Newborn Blood Tests to Screen for Congenital Disorders

Newborn babies are screened for a variety of treatable conditions including PKU (phenylketonuria), congenital hypothyroidism, galactosemia, cystic fibrosis, sickle cell anaemia and beta thalassaemia. In all the following screening tests, a blood sample, ususally on Day 3, is obtained from a small prick on your baby's heel and sent to the laboratory for testing. Usually, only one heel prick is necessary to obtain blood for these tests.

Test or Procedure	Where Required or When Indicated	What It Is	Comments
Test for PKU (phenylketonuria)	In all states, ACT and Northern Territory	Blood is obtained by a heel prick and tested for elevated phenylalanine levels. For greater accuracy, this procedure may be repeated at 7–14 days. The test is 95 percent accurate.	PKU is an inherited metabolic disease occurring in 1 infant in every 10,000–25,000 in Australia. With this disease, the infant is unable to digest phenylalanine (an amino acid), which builds up in the blood. If untreated, PKU causes mental retardation. It is treated by diet. A low phenylalanine formula or combining breastfeeding with a low phenylalanine formula is used during infancy. Once solid foods are introduced, a special diet followed through adolescence is very effective in preventing retardation.*
Test for hypothyroidism	In all states, ACT and Northern Territory	Blood obtained after 12 hours of age is tested for T_4 thyroid hormone and TSH (thyroid stimulating hormone) levels. Re-testing a second time between 2 and 6 weeks identifies 10 percent more infants missed by the first screening.	Hypothyroidism (low production of thyroid hormone) occurs in 1 in every 3600–5000 newborns in Australia. There is a higher incidence among females, offspring of mothers with thyroid disorders and those who have other children with thyroid disorders. The condition can be transient or long-term. Treatment with replacement hormone avoids serious long-term effects, including mental retardation, growth failure, deafness and neurological abnormalities.*†

Newborn Blood Tests to Screen for Congenital Disorders

Test or Procedure	Where Required or When Indicated	What It Is	Comments
Test for galactosemia	Variable; required in most states, ACT and Northern Territory; always performed if medically indicated	Blood is obtained after breastfeeding or formula feeding and is tested for elevated galactose content, which indicates an inability to digest and utilise galactose (milk sugar).	Galactosemia (inability to digest galactose, a sugar in milk) is a hereditary disorder and occurs in 1 in 60,000–80,000 infants. Without treatment, galactosemia is fatal. Symptoms include vomiting, diarrhoea, jaundice and poor weight gain. Treatment includes a diet that is galactose free.*
Test for sickle cell anaemia and beta thalassaemia	Variable; performed if medically indicated	Blood is obtained any time after birth and tested for the presence of abnormally shaped red blood cells.	Sickle cell anaemia and beta thalassaemia are inherited disorders resulting in the production of abnormal red blood cells. In the United States, sickle cell anaemia occurs in 1 in 375 people of African descent. Less severe forms occur in people of Arabic, East Indian, Middle Eastern and southern European descent. Screening is nearly 100 percent accurate using the isoelectric focusing method. These disorders cause anaemia, severe joint pain, bone deterioration, serious infections and death. Treatment for sickle cell anaemia includes antibiotics; immunisations to prevent or treat infection; and avoidance of high altitudes, dehydration, exposure to cold and excessive exertion. Beta thalassaemia occurs less frequently than sickle cell anaemia and may be treated with supportive measures (as with sickle cell anaemia) and with blood transfusions.

*American Academy of Pediatrics Committee on Genetics, 'Newborn Screening Fact Sheets', *Pediatrics* 98 (1996): 473–501.
†J. H. Dussault, 'Screening for Congenital Hypothyroidism', *Clinical Obstetrics and Gynecology*, 40(1) (March 1997): 117–23.

Your Newborn's Senses

Until recently, we believed that new babies were extremely limited in their range of responses. We thought that a wet nappy, hunger or colic were the only things that brought out a response in a new baby. We believed that babies could not see at birth, and when they finally did see, they could not discern colour. We also believed that babies could not hear at birth because their ears were full of mucus and fluid. And we thought that babies could be spoiled if they were picked up every time they cried. How we underestimated babies, for all these beliefs are myths! After years of study, we now recognise the newborn's amazing capabilities, some of which are described as follows.[4]

Vision

When he is quiet and alert, your baby can focus on objects 18–46 centimetres away. His vision at birth is about 20/200 and will be about 20/20 by six months.[5] He prefers to look at human faces (especially the eyes), round shapes, high contrast of dark and light colours, complex patterns and slowly moving objects—particularly shiny ones. Your newborn can follow a slowly moving object in a 180° arc above his head (if the object catches his attention). Some infants are sensitive to bright lights and will open their eyes wider when the lights are dimmed.

Hearing

Infants hear from birth and react to sound. They respond to voices, especially higher pitched voices (which is why people often unconsciously raise the pitch of their voices when talking to babies). Your baby heard your heartbeat, your voice, your partner's voice, and other internal and external noises while inside you. He may become calm or alert when he hears these familiar voices or sounds (when you hold him close or talk to him) or when he hears similar sounds such as a dishwasher, a washing machine or certain music. He will also startle at sudden, loud noises.

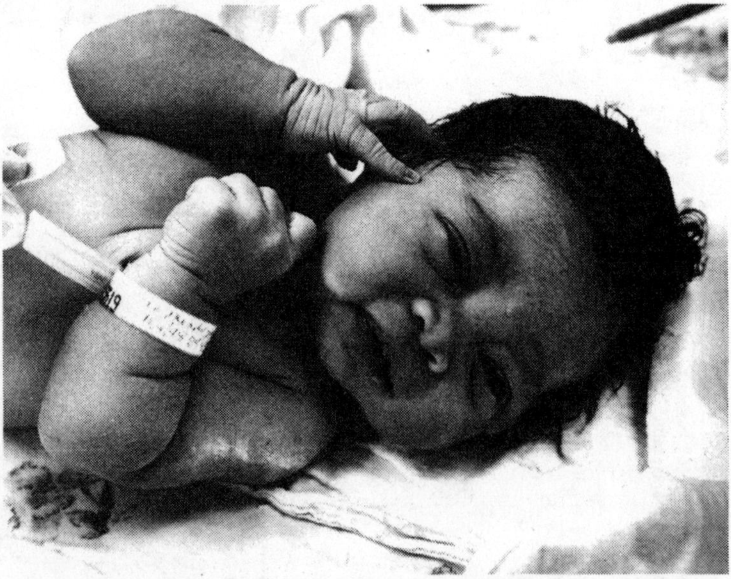

Photograph by Marilyn Nolt

Your baby sees clearly at close range and prefers looking at faces.

Smell

Your baby has a refined sense of smell. Within the first week, he recognises differences in smells and can even tell the difference between his mother's milk and another mother's milk. In fact, the smell of your milk when you hold him may excite him to root and suckle.

Taste

Babies may react to sweet, sour, salty and bitter tastes, and often prefer sweet substances.

Touch

Your baby enjoys being stroked, rocked, caressed, gently jiggled or bounced, and allowed to nestle and mould to your body while being held. He also likes comfort and warmth—not too hot or too cold.

Infant Cues

From birth, your baby has the ability to let you know a lot about what she wants, likes and does not like. The efforts she makes to communicate with you are called *infant cues*. As you get to know your baby better, you will be able to interpret her cues more easily.

Although a newborn baby cannot smile or talk, she has other ways to communicate with you. Of course, fussing and crying are ways to tell you she is hungry, lonely or uncomfortable. Rooting, wakefulness or sucking her hand tells you that she is hungry. Crying is a late hunger cue. Waiting until your baby cries before you feed her makes feeding more difficult. (See Chapter 15.) Heavy eyelids tell you she is sleepy. But when your baby is in a calm, quiet alert state, she uses all kinds of subtle ways to get your attention and keep it. As you begin to recognise these cues, you will be impressed by how much your baby can tell you.

Your baby uses her eyes to capture your attention and get you to look at her and talk to her. Her eyes brighten and open wide, and she stares at you intently. She explores your face, which she finds especially appealing. If you ignore this cue or look away, she may vocalise or move her arms to catch your attention. And as you return her gaze, a quiet dialogue begins. She may interrupt the dialogue by turning or looking away when she needs a rest and time to process what she has seen. After a brief rest, she may return her gaze to you. By returning her gaze when she wants to explore your face, and by giving her a chance to turn away and rest without coaxing her to look back at you, you are showing your sensitivity to her needs. Your baby is actually capable of engaging you in an interaction. She may open her eyes wide, look at you and study your face. Right from birth, she is able to imitate some of your facial expressions. Shape your mouth into an O. If she is in a quiet alert state and can see you clearly, she will shape her mouth into an O. If you stick out your tongue, she will copy you. When she is older (six weeks or more), she will smile at you and will respond to your smile by smiling and cooing. Babies have the amazing ability to help their parents fall in love with them by their endearing facial expressions and interactions.

Developmental Milestones

Here is a list of developmental characteristics and behaviours and the approximate ages at which your baby is most likely to begin to show them. If your baby is premature, these milestones may occur somewhat later.

Behaviour or Characteristic	Approximate Age
Looks or stares at your face	Birth to 4 weeks
Holds her head off the bed for a few moments while lying on her stomach	Birth to 4 weeks
Pays attention to sound by becoming alert or by turning towards it	Birth to 6 weeks
Smiles or coos when you smile, talk or play with her	3 weeks to 2 months
Holds her head upright while lying on her stomach	5 weeks to 3 months
Holds her head steady when upright	6 weeks to 4 months
Brings her hands together in front of herself	6 weeks to 3½ months
Laughs and squeals	6 weeks to 4½ months
Rolls over from front to back or back to front	2 months to 5 months
Grasps a rattle placed in her hand	2½ months to 4½ months

Your infant is the best person to teach you what calms her and what stimulates or agitates her. When your soothing efforts are effective, her fussiness lessens, she becomes calmer, and she relaxes and moulds to your body as you hold her. If your jiggling, attempts to feed or efforts to burp agitate her, she becomes more active and fussy and she stiffens. Coping with crying is one of the greatest challenges of parenthood, but in time you will figure out what soothes your baby. (See page 406 for more on crying.)

Parent-infant classes can help you learn more about your baby's cues and talents, as can your baby's health care provider or nurse, your childbirth educator or other experienced parents. The books *Your Amazing Newborn, Touchpoints,* and *Nighttime Parenting* (listed in the Recommended Resources) are excellent sources of information on newborns. Take advantage of these and other resources; they can help you enjoy and understand your baby better.

Development and Growth

Each baby is an individual with a unique temperament and personality. Your newborn differs from others in his appearance; activity level; response to pain, hunger or boredom; and sleeping and eating patterns. Your child is like a puzzle; it will take time for you to figure him out. If you remember that your child is an individual, not a reflection of you, it will make the job of parenting easier. Some babies are more difficult to live with than others. An infant who has a combination of intense reactions, irregularity, slow adaptability and a high activity level is a challenge to care for; you will need to be more patient and flexible. As you get to know your baby, you will learn about his temperament and learn to care for him in a more effective or satisfying way.

While your baby's temperament tends to change little over time, his abilities and size will change rapidly. Remember that normal patterns of development vary widely from one baby to the next. Do not feel anxious if your baby takes a developmental step later or earlier than someone else's infant. His developmental pattern is uniquely his own. If, however, you notice that your baby misses some of the developmental steps listed on the previous page or is consistently behind in the age when he begins to do them, bring it to the attention of the baby's doctor or nurse practitioner. Early detection and treatment may improve long-term development.

Your Newborn's Reflexes

Your baby is born with many normal reflexes. As he matures, many of these early reflexes or reactions will disappear. In the newborn exam, a nurse or doctor checks these reflexes, which are a sign of his good neurological health.

Awake or asleep, your baby yawns, quivers, hiccups, stretches and cries out without apparent reason. Many of these behaviours are reflexive in nature; he cannot control most of his movements. Hiccups are common in newborns and can occur soon after feeding. Hiccups usually bother parents more than the baby. They go away without treatment.

Other reflexes are protective. Coughing helps move mucus or fluid from his airway and relieves irritation. A new baby sneezes when he needs to clear his nose, when his nose is irritated or when a bright light shines in his eyes. He blinks if his eyelashes are touched, and he pulls away from a painful stimulus such as a blood draw from his heel. If he is lying on his stomach, he lifts his head and turns it to the side to avoid smothering. If you place an object over his nose and mouth, he twists away from it, mouths it vigorously or attempts to knock it off with his arms. A newborn is not helpless.

Some reflexes have specific names. The *Moro* or 'startle' reflex occurs when your baby is alarmed or surprised by a noise, bright light or quick movement. He is more likely to startle when he lies on his back. He suddenly flings his arms and legs out and straightens his body. The *grasp* reflex occurs when you place your finger in his palm; he responds by firmly grasping your finger. The *automatic walking* or *stepping* reflex occurs when the baby feels pressure on the bottoms of his feet. If you support him upright with his feet bearing some weight, he will alternately move his feet as if walking. Your baby is born with well developed *sucking* and *swallowing* reflexes; these survival reflexes enable him to eat and thrive. He eagerly suckles on a breast or bottle nipple and swallows the milk. When in need of soothing himself, he suckles on your breast, or sucks on his fingers or yours. The *rooting* reflex is especially pronounced when he is hungry. Stroke his cheek with your finger and he turns towards the touch with his mouth open and searching. Tickle his lips and he will open his mouth wide. These reflexes are but a few your baby has to help him adapt and live outside your uterus.

Sleeping and Waking

After an initial period of wakefulness after birth, many babies sleep a lot during the first day. They rouse only briefly and may not be very interested in feeding; others are just the opposite—waking, fussing and feeding frequently. Both are normal. Your baby's sleep cycle is closely related to how often she eats. After adjusting to her new environment, a baby will sleep twelve to twenty hours in a twenty-four-hour period. Early on, her sleeping periods may be short but frequent. As long as she feeds well, how long she sleeps is very individual and is not a concern.

When your baby is older, she may awaken at night and then settle back to sleep. However, a newborn may need to be fed, walked, rocked, changed, sung to, massaged or otherwise soothed before going back to sleep. Many new parents wonder when to feed their baby. When your infant is hungry, she will awaken, root and suck at anything close by, and she will wave her arms and legs vigorously to tell you she is hungry. If you wait, she will finally cry. (For more on feeding your baby, see Chapter 15.)

Where your baby sleeps is a personal decision. Many parents of newborns find they get more sleep if they tuck the baby in bed with them. The newborn is still making the transition from being a foetus wrapped snugly and warmly in her mother's uterus, hearing the sounds of her mother's body. The newborn has long wakeful periods at night just as she did in her mother's body during pregnancy. At night, the foetus is not rocked in the amniotic fluid as she was when her mother moved about during the day. Being in bed with her parents, she stays warm and hears the reassuring sounds of her parents' breathing. Also, parents find it easier to meet her night-time needs when she is close by. Having your newborn in bed with you does not mean she will stay there for life. As she grows older and needs you less at night, she can be moved to a crib or bed of her own. You will know the right time to move her there.

If having your baby in bed with you is uncomfortable, placing her in a 'sidecar' (an extender beside your bed) or a basket or bed near your bed will allow her to be near you and be comforted by your breathing sounds and will allow you to respond quickly to her needs.

Wherever she sleeps, she needs to be positioned on a firm surface on her back to reduce the risk of sudden infant death syndrome (SIDS). Being placed face down on a lambskin, soft mattress or quilt has been associated with death from suffocation. (See discussion on SIDS on page 419.)

Periodically, place your baby on her tummy when she is awake to prevent the development of a misshapen head and to give her an opportunity to lift her head and strengthen her neck muscles. Holding your baby in your arms or in a front pack also provides these benefits.

Sleep-Activity States

Six infant states of sleep and wakefulness have been identified: deep sleep, light sleep, drowsiness, quiet alert, active alert and crying. While each state has specific characteristics, the way babies change from state to state varies. Some move gradually from one state to another, while others make abrupt transitions. Some spend more time asleep or quiet alert or crying than others. You cannot completely control your infant's states; they are somewhat determined by personality.

Being able to identify the state your baby is in helps you give appropriate care. The following descriptions of each state explain their implications for parenting.[6]

Sleep States

Deep sleep. In this state your baby is very still and relaxed; her breathing is rhythmic. She occasionally jerks or makes sucking movements with her lips, but rarely awakens. You cannot feed or play with your baby in this state. If you manage to rouse her at all, she will stay awake only for a moment, then resume a state of deep sleep. Take this opportunity to rest, sleep, eat, make a phone call, take a bath, spend some time with your partner and so on.

Light sleep. This state of sleep is the most common in newborns. Your baby's eyes are closed, but they may move behind her lids. In light sleep she moves, makes momentary crying sounds, sucks, grimaces or smiles. She breathes irregularly. She responds to noises and efforts to arouse or stimulate her. Sometimes, she awakens to a drowsy state or remains in this state and falls into a deep sleep.

Many parents rush to care for a baby who moves and makes mewing or crying sounds. Often, however, the baby is not ready to wake up. Wait a few moments to see if the baby is entering the drowsy state and needs care or is falling back to sleep.

Awake States

Drowsy. In this state your baby appears sleepy, her activity level varies and she may startle occasionally. Her heavy-lidded eyes, opening and closing for brief periods, lose focus or appear cross-eyed. She breathes irregularly and reacts to sensory stimuli in a drowsy way. She either returns to sleep or becomes more alert. If you want your baby to return to sleep, avoid stimulating her. If you want her to wake up, talk to her, pick her up, massage her, or give her something to suck on or look at.

Quiet alert. This state, which usually precedes a long sleeping period, is pleasing and rewarding for parents. Your baby lies still and looks at you calmly with bright, wide eyes. She breathes with regularity and focuses attentively on what she sees and hears. By providing something for her to look at, listen to or suck on, you will encourage her to stay in this state. You can sing and talk to your baby and enjoy these moments of eye contact, alertness and calm.

Active alert. In this state hunger, fatigue, noises and too much handling readily affect your baby. She cannot lie still; she may be fussy. Her eyes are open but do not appear as bright and attentive as in the quiet alert state. She breathes irregularly and makes faces.

When your baby reaches the active alert state, it is time to either feed or comfort her. If she is not hungry, she probably needs less stimulation. If you act immediately, you may bring her to a calmer state before she enters the crying state.

Crying. A crying baby is difficult for every parent. Keep in mind that your baby has only one way of telling you she cannot cope anymore. If she is hungry, overstimulated, tired, sick, gassy, frustrated, wet, cold, too warm or lonely, she says so by crying. She also moves her body actively, opens or closes her eyes, makes unhappy faces and breathes irregularly. Sometimes, crying is a release, a self-comforting mechanism that enables her to enter another state. More often, she needs you to feed or comfort her. (See page 406 for more on crying.)

Recording Your Baby's Sleep and Activity

Sometimes, parents are puzzled by their baby's apparent unpredictability and are unaware of any consistency in the daily pattern. If that is true for you, make a chart like the one below to record your baby's activities and sleep periods for a week. This chart will show you how long and when your baby sleeps, is awake and content, or is awake and crying. You will also see the large amount of time you spend nappying, feeding, and caring for your baby. After using the chart for a week, you can often see that your

Sample Sleep and Activity Chart

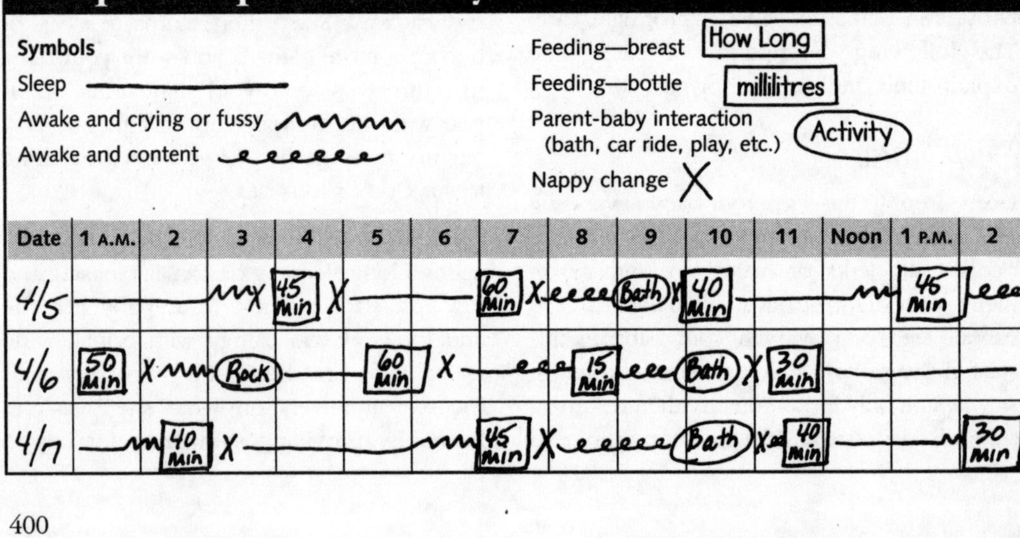

baby does follow a fairly consistent pattern. As your baby matures, the sleep and activity patterns will undergo further changes.

Common Concerns about Newborns

Newborn Jaundice

A yellow tint to the baby's skin or the whites of the eyes is called *jaundice,* which is caused by a high level of bilirubin in the baby's blood. Bilirubin results from the breakdown of unneeded red blood cells that occurs normally in newborns. Bilirubin is excreted from the baby's body in his bowel movements. Until it is excreted, bilirubin may cause jaundice. About 50 percent of newborns have some mild yellowness in their faces and necks by the third or fourth day of life. This condition, called physiological jaundice, disappears without treatment. Occasionally, however, the jaundice is more of a concern. Your baby's health care provider should check him if the whites of his eyes or the skin of his chest below his nipple line is yellow. This more pronounced jaundice usually shows up on the third or fourth day of life and is often associated with poor feeding, prematurity or bruising that occurred during birth.

The level of bilirubin is measured by a blood test in which blood is taken from the baby's heel. If the concentration of bilirubin is high enough to warrant treatment, the baby's health care provider will make sure the baby gets adequate feedings, and the baby will be given phototherapy at home or in the hospital until further blood tests show improvement. *Phototherapy* (or light therapy) provides a special type of cool light to the baby's skin, causing the bilirubin level to drop. Light therapy can be given in three ways. Usually in the hospital, special overhead bank lights (called 'bili lights') shine on the infant's naked chest or back. Soft pads cover the infant's eyes and protect them from the light. At home and in many hospitals, a special blanket wrapped around the infant can deliver light therapy. Light is emitted from fibre-optic filaments to the baby's back or chest. A third method is a special bed in which the baby lies on his back on a net hammock over a light-therapy source. Use of the blanket or hammock does not require eye protection. Phototherapy usually lasts two to four days.

Jaundice that appears on the first or second day of life is even more serious and may require intensive treatment. This early jaundice may result from infection or from certain blood incompatibilities such as Rh incompatibility or ABO incompatibility. Rh incompatibility may occur when the mother's blood is Rh negative and the baby's blood is Rh positive. (See page 76.) ABO incompatibility may occur when the mother's blood type is O and the father's is A, B or AB. Phototherapy may be used with these conditions, but on the rare occasions when the level of bilirubin becomes very high, a blood exchange transfusion may be needed. The baby's blood is replaced with new blood to lower the level of bilirubin to a safe level, preventing possible hearing loss or more severe neurological damage.

Jaundice that becomes apparent more than a week after birth is uncommon. This type of jaundice might be related to being breastfed (and usually does not require treatment), or it might be caused by some other condition. You may be the first to notice jaundice in your baby. If you are concerned, call your baby's health care provider.

Circumcision

Circumcision, the removal of the foreskin covering the head (glans) of the penis, is probably the oldest surgical operation known, dating back some six thousand years. It is a ritual of the Jewish and Islamic religions. The rate of circumcision today varies geographically. It is uncommon in Latin America, Europe, China and the Far East, but is commonly performed in North America. Circumcision is a surgical procedure that requires written consent from the parents. Since the decision about circumcision is up to you and your partner, discuss the subject during pregnancy when you have more time to gather information.

Facts to Consider

- There are no legal and few medical reasons for circumcising the male newborn.
- The Australian College of Paediatricians has not taken a stand for or against circumcision but recommends that parents be well informed before making the decision.
- Circumcision should not be done if an infant is sick, has a bleeding disorder, has not yet received vitamin K or has hypospadius, a defect in which the urethral opening is on the underside of the head of the penis.
- The procedure usually takes less than thirty minutes. Healing takes seven to ten days.
- The newborn will feel pain.
- Local anaesthesia, by injection of lidocaine at the base of the penis or at the midshaft, is available to reduce the pain associated with circumcision. Complications from anaesthesia are rare and consist of tissue injury or bruising at the site of injection. Application of local anaesthetic creams to the penis one hour or so before circumcision has also been shown to decrease pain, though less effectively.[7] Sucking on a pacifier that delivers a small amount of sugar water during the procedure has also been shown to reduce the pain response.
- Complications from the circumcision procedure itself occur in 2–6 per 1000 circumcisions. Complications range from minor to serious and include irritation of the head of the penis from the friction of wet nappies, pain on urination, bleeding, infection and scarring of the urinary outlet.
- There may be a fee for hospital equipment and a doctor's fee, both of which may or may not be covered by health insurance.
- Many public hospitals no longer offer circumcision.
- Some studies note a slightly increased incidence of cancer of the penis in elderly uncircumcised males, while others report the opposite findings.[8] Those that show an increase in penile cancer note that it is associated with two factors: being

uncircumcised and having poor long-term hygienic care of the penis. It is recommended that parents and the older child make a lifetime commitment to careful hygienic care of the uncircumcised penis.[9]

- Some studies have found an association between not being circumcised and urinary tract infection in the first year of life. The risk of developing a urinary tract infection is low (about 1 percent).[10] Exclusive breastfeeding, which reduces the incidence of urinary tract infections three-fold, may reduce this possibility.[11]
- Contrary to previous reports, there is no evidence that circumcision prevents cancer of the prostate gland, nor does it prevent sexually transmitted diseases.
- There is conflicting evidence about whether newborn circumcision or non-circumcision affects adult sexual performance.

The Circumcision Procedure

Parents who decide to have their son circumcised should discuss the method of circumcision, the use of anaesthesia, and potential risks and benefits with their infant's care provider. They will be asked to sign a consent form. Sometimes, parents are allowed to be with their son during the procedure, if they wish.

The doctor carefully inspects the penis to be sure no conditions exist, such as hypospadius, that would make circumcision contraindicated. The baby is placed on his back in a special plastic bed with his body held firmly in place by Velcro straps. Babies are generally more comfortable if their arms are swaddled across their chests. Their upper body is kept warm with a blanket or by a radiant heater. The penis is washed with an antiseptic liquid. A sterile sheet is placed over the lower body with a hole in the centre to reveal the penis and scrotum. The baby is given a teat to suck on that delivers a small amount of sugar water during the procedure.

There are different methods used to circumcise male infants: Gomco clamp, Plastibell device and Mogen clamp. In all methods, the foreskin must be separated from the glans (head). In 90 percent of newborn boys, the foreskin adheres to the glans. With some devices, the foreskin is held in place with special surgical clamps, and a small, vertical incision is made in the foreskin. The foreskin is then peeled away from the glans of the penis.

Care of the Circumcised Penis

If you choose to have your son circumcised, ask the medical staff about the care of the penis. Care of the circumcised penis varies depending on the circumcision technique used. Infants who have the foreskin removed using the Mogen clamp or Gomco clamp usually have Vaseline gauze applied to the circumcision site for twenty-four hours following the circumcision. You will be instructed to watch for bleeding, lack of urination or swelling. If you observe any of these signs, call your baby's health care provider. The Vaseline gauze usually falls off in twenty-four hours. If it does not, soak it off in a bath or by wrapping the area in a warm, moist nappy or washcloth. Gently remove the gauze. If you cannot get it off, call your baby's caregiver or the hospital. Once the gauze is off, put some Vaseline over the site and on the nappy to keep the nappy from irritating the circumcised area.

If a Plastibell device was used, a small plastic ring will be left on your baby's penis following circumcision, and it will be tied in place with a suture thread. The Plastibell will usually fall off seven to ten days after the circumcision. Never pull the ring off; let it fall off on its own. As it begins to fall off, you may see small patches of yellow or white, which are normal signs of healing tissue. Any swelling, bleeding, inability to urinate or pus-like discharge needs to be reported to your baby's health care provider.

Care of the Intact (Uncircumcised) Penis

The intact foreskin of a newborn does not usually retract (pull back). It is joined to the glans, so do not force it back over the end of the penis. It will gradually become looser, and between four and eight years of age most boys' foreskins are fully retractable. Normal bathing provides adequate cleansing during infancy. Once the foreskin can be naturally drawn back, cleaning the glans with soap and water is all that is necessary.

Spitting Up

Many babies spit up milk during or after a feeding. Some babies spit up more than others. Your baby is more likely to spit up if she cries hard before a feeding, eats too much too quickly or swallows air during the feeding. If you have a large milk supply, she may swallow too much too quickly and spit up some of it. Babies have an immature sphincter muscle at the entrance to their stomachs, which allows milk to come up with air bubbles. Spitting up is usually not harmful, but you may reduce it in the following ways. Burp your baby during and after feedings (burp newborns after each breast or after every 50 millilitres of formula). Do not overfeed her with formula. Handle her gently and, after feeding, position her either on her side or sitting in an infant car seat with her head elevated. Babies generally outgrow the tendency to spit up by five to nine months of age.

If spitting up seems to be associated with pain, call your baby's health care provider. Continuous or frequent forceful (projectile) vomiting is more serious and can lead to dehydration. If your infant vomits after each of two or three consecutive feedings and seems sick or weak, consult your baby's health care provider.

Bowel Movements

A newborn's stool pattern is different from an adult's. Your baby's first bowel movements will consist of *meconium,* a sticky, green-black substance present in the intestine before birth. By two to three days of age, he will have brown, brown-green or brown-yellow stools the consistency of cake batter. After your milk comes in, or by three to four days of age, your baby will have more liquid yellow, green or brown stools with or without curds. The frequency and consistency of stools depend on the individual baby and on the food he is fed. Breastfed newborns usually have a stool after each feeding or at least two large runny stools a day once your milk is in. Formula-fed babies have frequent stools in the first several days after birth. By a week, they may have one or two putty-like stools a day.

Constipation (hard, dry stools that are difficult to pass) rarely occurs in breastfed babies, but is a more common concern in formula-fed babies. Some breastfed babies (older than one month) may have only one bowel movement a day or one per week. This normal shift in stool patterns may concern parents. These babies are not constipated; their more mature digestive systems are efficiently using more of their mothers' milk. Call your baby's health care provider, however, if your baby seems constipated or if you are concerned.

Your baby may have *diarrhoea* if his stools are mucousy, foul smelling, much more frequent than usual, blood-tinged, or when he appears ill and listless. When in doubt, note the colour, consistency and frequency of your baby's stool; then call your baby's health care provider. Though diarrhoea and vomiting are rare in the exclusively breastfed infant, they are serious conditions, especially for the very young infant.

Nappy Rash

Many substances can irritate your baby's skin, including urine and stool, some laundry products, inadequate nappy washing or chemicals used in some disposable nappies. To prevent or treat nappy rash caused by urine, change nappies frequently, rinse the nappy area with water at each change and avoid plastic pants, which retain moisture. If you wash your own nappies, you can reduce irritation from laundry detergents by running the nappies through an extra rinse cycle or by changing to a milder detergent. To reduce the amount of ammonia retained in the nappies, add half a cup of vinegar to the nappy pail or rinse water.

Other treatments for nappy rash include switching to a different type of nappy, blow-drying your baby's clean bottom with a hair dryer set at medium heat, or applying a commercial ointment to the clean, dry, irritated skin. Avoid nappy rash preparations containing zinc oxide, which mask the nappy rash with a white covering. If nappy rash persists, consult your baby's health care provider.

Other Rashes

Newborn rash. Some newborns develop a characteristic rash in the first week. You will see red blotches with waxy yellow or white pimples in the middle. The rash (erythema toxicum) appears on the trunk, arms and legs and disappears without treatment.

Facial rashes. Mild rashes on the face commonly occur in the first months of life. The rashes (smooth pimples, small red spots or rough red spots) come and go and rarely require treatment.

Prickly heat. This common warm-weather rash appears on overdressed or overwrapped babies. Found most often in the shoulder and neck regions, prickly heat looks like clusters of tiny pink pimples surrounded by pink skin. As it dries, the rash becomes slightly tan. Prickly heat may look worse than it apparently feels to your baby. To avoid this rash, keep her from becoming overheated.

Cradle Cap

Cradle cap is a yellowish, scaly, patchy condition found on the scalp or sometimes behind the ears. Daily washing or brushing of the scalp may prevent cradle cap and will help treat it if it does appear. Gently comb or brush out the scales using a baby comb, fingernail brush or soft toothbrush; then wash with mild soap. Continue this procedure every day or two until the scales are gone.

Newborn Breathing Pattern

Periods of irregular breathing are normal in newborns but may be worrisome to new parents. When your baby is sleeping, he will snort, squeak, pant, groan and even occasionally pause in his breathing. He breathes more rapidly (with a rate between 30 and 60 breaths per minute) than you do. These irregularities usually disappear in a month or two.

If you are worried whether your baby's breathing patterns are normal, observe your baby when he is sleeping. If you note the signs above, you should not be concerned. If you observe signs of respiratory distress (blue lips, struggling to breathe, flaring nostrils or deep indentation of the chest with each breath), call your health care provider immediately.

Crying

A newborn may spend a lot of time crying, and most parents feel frustrated when they cannot understand why their baby cries. This is a natural reaction. Try to respond quickly, before the baby gets so upset that she cannot calm herself easily. Try to stay as calm as possible by taking some deep breaths and talking quietly to the baby and yourself. Your tension is contagious; move slowly and calmly around a crying infant.

All babies have fussy times. Very often these fussy, sometimes gassy times occur in the evening and have been called 'the arsenic hours'. Use the suggestions for comforting a crying baby on page 407 or ask someone knowledgeable for advice on how to soothe your baby and how to cope during this stressful time. As with most parenting challenges, time, your increasing confidence as a parent and the maturation of your baby bring an end to the newborn fussy time. If you are spending many hours a day soothing your baby, it can be very stressful. You may need to take a break now and then. Some parents fear that if they give their babies too much attention, they will spoil them. A newborn, however, cannot be spoiled. She needs feeding, attention, cuddling and handling to develop a trust in your ability to meet her needs. Enjoying and responding to your baby is not spoiling her. When your infant cries, she needs more care, not less. Your newborn infant is not 'manipulating' you when she cries for your attention; she simply has no other way to tell you she needs soothing. You might have trouble figuring out exactly what she wants, but pick her up, cuddle her, and trust your instincts and feelings.

Newborn babies cry when they are hungry, overstimulated, tired or uncomfortable. They may cry because they have a gas bubble in their stomach and need to burp, or because they need to be held and rocked.

They may cry because they have an uncomfortable nappy rash or their circumcision site may be sore. They may cry if they have a wet or dirty nappy, though that usually does not bother newborns unless they are cold. And they may cry if they are ill. If you know the reason your baby is crying, soothing her will be easier. If you do not know why she is crying, try comforting her with the following suggestions:

- First consider hunger. Some babies need to nurse frequently for several feedings in a row before settling in for a longer (over one hour) rest between feedings. You may need to calm her by holding her and letting her suck on your finger before she is able to feed again.
- Try calming her by cuddling and holding her against your chest. Talking or singing to her may help.
- Find ways to use repetitive motion, which often helps soothe babies. For example:
  - Hold her in your arms, a front pack or a sling as you rock from side to side.
  - Hold her in your arms as you gently bounce on the bed for several minutes. (Birth balls are wonderful for such bouncing.)
  - Make a hammock out of a blanket by holding two corners of the blanket while someone else holds the other two corners. With your baby resting on her back, gently swing her side-to-side in the hammock.
  - Put her in a baby swing, which can both comfort her and give you a chance to eat a meal or rest.
  - Take her outside for a stroller ride.
  - Take her on a car ride—car rides put most babies to sleep!
- Some newborns enjoy being swaddled snugly in a receiving blanket, which helps them feel more secure and, in turn, more calm.
- Change her nappy if it is wet or dirty and check to see that she is not over- or underdressed.
- Try taking her into a warm bath with you. She may calm in the warm water and may even breastfeed there.
- Some babies calm to the humming sound of appliances. Place her safely in an infant seat on or near a running clothes dryer, dishwasher or washing machine. The repetitive sound and vibration may be soothing. Do not leave her unattended there. The vibrations can cause the seat to slide.
- Try a soothing massage focusing on the tummy or head.

Give each calming technique some time to work, being careful in your distress not to overstimulate her. If nothing seems to calm her and you are losing your temper, you may need to put your baby safely in her bed or car seat and take a short break. In five or ten minutes, your baby may have settled down and you may feel less frustrated. If not, never shake or roughly handle your baby. Call someone to help you. In time, with practice and patience, you will become more comfortable in your ability to settle your baby.

Colic

Colic is a condition in which the infant cries inconsolably after most feedings. Colic is different from the expected and normal evening fussy time. Colicky babies seem especially gassy. If you think your baby has colic, talk with his health care provider. Colicky symptoms can sometimes be mistaken for another condition called *gastroesophageal reflux* (GER) that causes pain for the infant. With GER, some of the acidic stomach contents flow up into the oesophagus, causing the tissue to become inflamed and painful. GER can be treated with medication and by positioning the baby in an upright position.

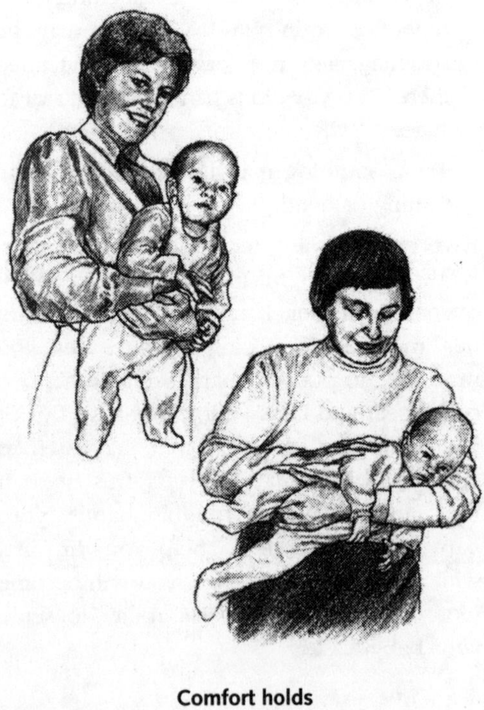

Comfort holds

If your baby has colic, some of the following techniques may be helpful:

- Use a comfort hold that provides pressure against his abdomen. While he is awake, you can lay him on his abdomen across your lap or on a hot water bottle filled with warm water and wrapped in a towel. You can also lay him on your arm looking away from you.
- Try all the techniques used to soothe a crying baby.
- Talk with a breastfeeding counsellor (see page 428) if you are breastfeeding, or with your baby's health care provider if you are formula feeding, to determine whether food sensitivities might be contributing to the problem.
- Try abdominal massage by writing 'I love you' on your baby's abdomen. Start on the left side, stroking the letter *I*. Next, stroke down the left side and across his lower abdomen, making the letter *L*. Finally, stroke down the left side of his abdomen across his lower abdomen, and up the right side to make the letter *U*.
- Proprietary preparations, frequently recommended as a colic remedy, have been found to be no more effective than a placebo in the treatment of colic.

Try to keep in mind that colic does not produce any lasting harmful effects, and it usually disappears by the third or fourth month. Consult your baby's health care provider if constant crying is associated with vomiting, spitting up, a cold, a fever or hard stools.

Special Babies

Premature Babies

An infant born before thirty-seven weeks and weighing less than 2.5 kilograms is considered *premature*. Some babies born as early as twenty-four weeks gestation live and grow to be healthy infants. Advances in the care of preterm infants have increased the survival of very tiny babies and have greatly reduced the long-term respiratory and neurological problems that preterm infants born even a decade ago had. However, every day in the womb improves your baby's chances of survival and normal development. Her appearance and physical abilities depend to some extent on just how early she was born. A premature infant looks different from a full-term infant: The premature infant is small, limp and frail; her skin is reddish and appears tissue-paper thin, and she has little or no fat or muscle. Her head appears disproportionately large. Vernix and lanugo are abundant, fingernails and toenails have not grown out, and her tiny ears are soft and hug her head. Her cry is more feeble, and she may be more difficult to soothe than a full-term infant.

A premature infant is physically vulnerable until she grows older. She sucks weakly, and her swallow and gag reflexes are unreliable. Tube feeding is sometimes necessary. Because her body temperature is unstable (often below normal), she is usually kept in a temperature-controlled isolette. Breathing may be more difficult; her respirations are irregular, rapid and often shallow because her lungs are immature. She may need oxygen and help with breathing. Her ability to absorb food is less efficient than that of a full-term infant, although her need for nutrients—especially calories, protein, iron, calcium, zinc and vitamin E—may be greater.

Giving birth to a premature infant may be upsetting and frightening. Your premature baby needs special medical attention that may separate her from you, but she also needs to be touched and talked to even while inside the isolette. Your baby's nurse may encourage you to hold your preterm infant next to your bare chest, skin-to-skin. Your closeness, breathing movements and warmth will help her regulate her respirations, keep her warm, and comfort her (and you). If this close physical holding is done regularly, premature babies have been found to grow faster. This skin-to-skin contact is called *Kangaroo care*. Because it is so beneficial, if you are at risk for preterm labour, you may want to learn more about it. Speak to the nurse manager of the newborn nursery, and find out about its policies on Kangaroo care and how to arrange it.

If your baby is too immature to suckle at your breast, you can express milk, which can be fed to her through a tube passed from her mouth to her stomach. Your milk is different from the milk of a mother of a full-term baby, and is better suited to the nutritional needs of your premature infant. Your milk also contains antibodies and immune factors that help protect her from infection and disease. By feeding, touching and caring for her, you help your baby and yourself through this difficult time.

Parent support groups provide information, assistance and emotional support to the parents of a premature infant. In addition to listening with understanding and giving practical suggestions, members of a support group may have a lending library of books and may even supply you with clothing or patterns for clothing small enough for your baby. If you would like more information about premature babies, check with your local childbirth education group, caregiver or hospital. (For more on preterm labour, see pages 60–63; for preterm birth and Kangaroo care, see pages 303–304.)

Small-for-Gestational-Age Babies

In the past, some full-term babies who weighed less than 2.5 kilograms were wrongly called premature. Babies who are small in size and weight for the length of pregnancy are more appropriately called *small for gestational age (SGA)*. This condition may have any of several possible causes: an inadequate transfer of nutrients across the placenta to the baby; the effects of some drugs, such as tobacco, taken during pregnancy; some congenital and genetic malformations; and certain infections of the foetus, such as toxoplasmosis. Sometimes the cause is unknown.

The SGA baby presents special challenges to the parents, similar to those presented by a premature baby. These babies do not move easily from state to state (for example, from active to quiet alert or from drowsy to deep sleep). They are often fussy and more difficult to soothe than other infants. Parents of SGA babies have to spend a great deal of time calming and quieting their babies. Techniques that seem to work include frequent feeding, gentle rocking, talking quietly and maintaining a calm environment. These parents soon learn that their babies can handle only one source of stimulation at a time. Too much stimulation—such as talking to the baby while feeding, making eye contact or jiggling her while talking—overwhelms this intense baby and causes her to cry or become agitated. Over time, the SGA baby matures and becomes less intense and fussy. Your sensitivity to her special needs helps her while she matures.

Playing with Your Baby

Play is more important to babies than it is to adults. For an adult, play is usually a form of recreation; for a baby, it is a valuable form of exercise and is a means of learning about himself and the world around him. When he grabs and shakes a rattle, gums and chews a teething

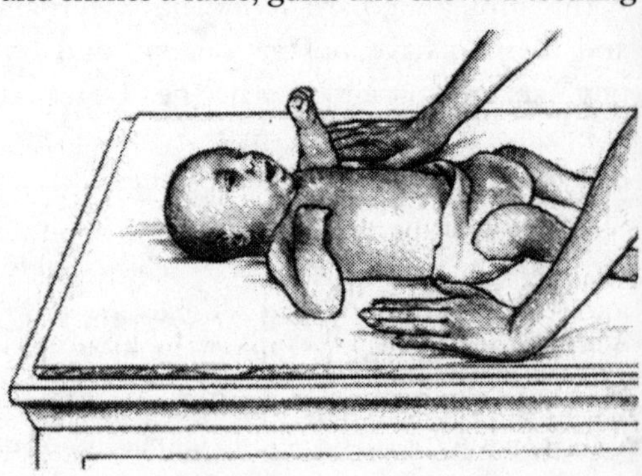

Talk to your baby and then watch for his response.

ring, squashes and squeaks a rubber duck, he is learning that he can make things happen.

When you talk, coo, laugh, hug and kiss your baby, he learns that certain things he does make an impact on you. Learning activities (play) for a baby during an average day may include singing, talking and dancing; caressing, touching and cuddling when changing or feeding him; a massage; baby exercises; moving to different rooms; games such as peek-a-boo; and playing with appropriate toys. (See page 142 for mother-baby exercises.)

Baby Massage

Massage is the language of touch. With a massage, you can calm and soothe your baby and communicate your love and care. During massage, keep the following points in mind. A nice way to start is with a bath. Then, after making sure the room is warm, remove the towel or receiving blanket and put your baby on the floor. (You can also sit with the baby on your lap or kneel in front of her.) Baby lotion and baby oil soak into the skin too fast, so use vegetable oil or massage oil. Put the oil on your hands first, and then rub your hands together to warm them. Tell your baby what you are doing, or sing a song. Rub gently during the first month; as the baby gets older, you can exert more pressure. Once you have touched the baby, keep at least one hand in contact with her until the massage is over. Don't massage your baby's trunk if her stomach is full. Be sensitive and responsive to her reactions; stop if she is not enjoying herself.

If she is enjoying herself, and she probably is, here are some motions you can try:

- Stroking with your open palms
- Stroking with your thumbs or fingers
- 'Raking' with the tips of your fingers
- Tapping lightly with the tips of your fingers
- Massaging arms or legs with a gentle wringing motion
- Doing whatever feels good to you and makes the baby happy

Car Safety

In Australia, law requires that every baby needs to be restrained in a car seat that meets current motor vehicle safety standards. The car seat needs to be the right size for the infant, needs to be correctly fastened to the car and needs to be installed according to the manufacturer's instructions. Newborns are placed in rear-facing car seats, while infants who are over 9 kilograms and are at least one year of age face forward. Rolled up towels or receiving blankets may be tucked in around the infant's head for support. For newborns, shoulder straps need to be in the lowest slots. The harness should be snug and the harness retainer clip positioned at the level of the nipples. Be sure that the shoulder straps are snug against the baby's shoulders. Avoid wrapping the baby in blankets that pad his shoulders, and do not use add-on car seat pads (unless they have slits for harness straps) so there will be no thick padding over the shoulders, which makes the car seat unsafe.[12]

Never place infants riding in rear-facing seats in the passenger side of the front seat that has an airbag. In a crash, the airbag would hit the back of the car seat and could cause serious injury.

Premature and small babies weighing 2.5 kilograms or less may need special arrangements for travelling in a vehicle. Before discharge from the hospital, premature and small infants will be placed in their car seats and monitored for an hour to assess their ability to breathe adequately. If the baby is unable to breathe well, adjustments will be made to the car seat, or a special car bed will be used to ensure safe transport.

Medical Care

Infants should be scheduled to receive routine examinations and care by their health care providers. A check-up at three to four days after birth includes such things as assessing the baby's feeding, checking for jaundice and discussing any parent concerns. Another check may be scheduled between seven and fourteen days of age to assess the baby's weight and feeding, answer parents' questions and possibly repeat newborn blood-screening tests. (See the chart on page 392 for more on these tests.) The infant will continue to be seen on a routine schedule. Your baby's health care provider will let you know when your baby needs to be seen.

Immunisations

Infants and children are given immunisations at their routine examinations to protect them from acquiring certain potentially serious diseases. (See 'Recommended Childhood Immunisation Schedule' on page 413.) The ability to immunise infants and others against such diseases as polio and diphtheria has been one of the most important contributions to public health in the last century. Because most new parents have never known anyone who had polio or diphtheria or even measles, it might be difficult to understand why immunising themselves and their children is so important.

Many expectant and new parents have become informed health care consumers. They know that despite the benefits of immunisation, there are risks and side effects with each vaccine. Immunisations prevent specific diseases and their common complications—including death. The risk of vaccine side effects is extremely low. Still, the concerns about a few of the publicised risks of immunisation for infants can be alarming to new parents. Some parents, in an effort to protect their children from the side effects and risks of the vaccine, decide not to have their children immunised. They would rather take the chance of having their child get the illness than take the chance of having their child suffer the side effects of the vaccine. The weight of accurate, carefully researched evidence shows this would be a poor decision, as the risk from the disease is far greater than any slight risk from immunisation.

Recommendations on immunisations change periodically as new vaccines become

Recommended Childhood Immunisation Schedule*
Australia, 2002

Children born on or after 1 May 2000 will be immunised according to this schedule. The vaccines are listed under routinely recommended ages.

Hepatitis B vaccine (hep B) should be given to all infants at birth and should not be delayed beyond 7 days after birth. Infants whose mothers are hepatitis B surface antigen positive (HBsAg+ve) should also be given hepatitis B immunoglobulin (HBIG) within 12 hours of birth.

In the Northern Territory, all Aboriginal children aged 2–14 years in Central Australia are recommended to have 23 valent polysaccharide pneumococcal vaccination every five years.

Vaccine	Birth	2 mos	4 mos	6 mos	12 mos	18 mos	4 yrs
Hepatitis B	**Hep B**	**Hep B**	**Hep B**	**Hep B (For NSW, QLD, SA, ACT, NT only)**	**Hep B (For VIC, WA, Tas only)**		
Diptheria, tetanus, acellular pertussis		**DTPa**	**DTPa**	**DTPa**		**DTPa**	**DTPa**
H. influenza type b		**Hib**	**Hib**		**Hib**		
Polio		**OVP**	**OPV**	**OPV**			**OPV**
Measles, mumps, rubella					**MMR**		**MMR**

* Approved by the National Health and Medical Research Council. For further information or to order a copy of the Australian Immunisation Handbook (7th edition) phone the Immunisation Infoline on 1800 671 811 (free call). Further information can also be found at the Immunise Australia website: www.immunise.health.gov.au

Childhood Immunisations

Immunisation and Effects of Disease	Vaccine: How and When	Side Effects of Vaccine	Comments
DTPa (diphtheria, tetanus, acellular pertussis) **Diphtheria** Infection affecting the throat, nose and skin; can lead to kidney or heart damage and is fatal in 10 percent of cases **Tetanus** Severe spasm of the neck and jaw muscles (lockjaw), which can lead to death in 50 percent of cases **Pertussis (acellular)** Long and severe bouts of coughing (whooping cough); 70 percent of pertussis deaths occur in children under one year of age.	Combined immunisation Given at 2, 4 and 6 months by injection in thigh Booster shots at 18 months and 4 years	Local pain and tenderness at the injection site, mild fever and irritability, all of which might last a day or two Serious side effects: • Crying lasting over 3 hours (11 in 10,000 immunisations) • Convulsions (3 in 100,000 immunisations) • Floppiness (limp or pale) (5 in 100,000 immunisations)	DTPa replaces the old DPT vaccine, and its use has greatly reduced the risk of serious side effects. (For example, the risk of convulsions is 20 percent less.)
Hib (H. influenza type b) **Haemophilus influenza type b** Respiratory infection with cold-like symptoms and muscle aches and pains; Hib disease is the most common cause of bacterial meningitis. In 25 percent of cases, this type of meningitis can result in permanent brain damage.	Given at 2, 4 and 12 months by injection in thigh	Redness at injection site and mild fever that might last a day or two High fever (over 38.5°C) occurs with 1 in 100 immunisations. Rarely, allergic reactions have been reported.	The most serious infections occur in the first 4 years of life.

Childhood Immunisations

Immunisation and Effects of Disease	Vaccine: How and When	Side Effects of Vaccine	Comments
Hep B (hepatitis B) **Hepatitis B** Infection of the liver with symptoms of nausea, weakness and jaundice (yellowing of the skin and the white part of the eyes); can lead to chronic liver infection, which is associated with cirrhosis and liver cancer	Given soon after birth by injection in thigh Three more injections in the series are given over the next twelve months.	Side effects are rare. Localised pain and tenderness at injection site	
OPV (poliomyelitis vaccine) **Polio** Viral infection with fever, headache, loss of appetite, vomiting and sore throat; can lead to muscle weakness and paralysis; 10 percent of cases are fatal.	Given at 2, 4 and 6 months of age and again at 4 years of age by injection	OPV may cause pain and tenderness at the injection site, but it does not cause paralytic polio.	

Childhood Immunisations

Immunisation and Effects of Disease	Vaccine: How and When	Side Effects of Vaccine	Comments
MMR (measles, mumps, rubella) **Measles** Rash and fever; can possibly result in hearing loss, encephalitis, mental retardation or death **Mumps** Infection of the salivary glands; can result in infection of testicles, possibly leading to sterility or (in meningitis) possibly leading to deafness or death **Rubella** (German measles) Not serious for children; for pregnant women, can cause miscarriage, stillbirth or birth defects affecting the eyes, ears, heart and neurological system of the baby	Given by injection at 12 months of age Booster shot at 4 years of age	Possible tenderness at the injection site and mild fever 5–12 days later, may develop a rash and fever that might last a day or two May develop mild, temporary joint pain 2 weeks or more after vaccine; the pain may cause your child to limp. Very rarely, a high fever or convulsions occur.	Report a high fever or convulsion to your baby's health care provider.

available. Check with your baby's caregiver to get the latest information. Many day-care centres, preschools and schools now require proof of immunisation against certain illnesses before admitting a child. To find out what is required where you live, ask your baby's health care provider.

Your baby's health care provider will supply you with an immunisation form or infant health care record upon which you can record the dates of completed immunisations and any reactions your child may have had. It is important to maintain this written record for proof of immunisation and as a reminder of when immunisations are due. If the schedule for a series of immunisations is interrupted, resume it where you left off in the series rather than beginning again. Be sure to inform your baby's health care provider of any reactions your baby has to immunisations.

When to Call for Medical Help

If you are worried about illness in your baby, call her physician or health care provider. Before you call, however, note on paper your baby's temperature (see page 418) and all the symptoms that worry you. Here are some things your baby's health care provider may wish to know:

- **Physical symptoms.** Abnormal temperature, breathing difficulties, coughing, vomiting, diarrhoea, constipation, fewer wet nappies, rash.
- **Behavioural symptoms.** Listlessness, loss of appetite, unusual fussiness or irritability, change in typical behaviour and activity level (for example, if your baby loses interest in her surroundings or is unable to muster a quiet smile).
- **Newborn warning signs.** If your baby has any of the warning signs in the chart on page 418.
- **Home treatment.** What have you done to treat the illness or condition, and how has your child responded? Have you given your child any medications? What and when?
- **General considerations.** Has there been recent exposure to illness? Is anyone at home or at the day-care centre sick?

Have a paper and pencil handy to write down the health care provider's suggestions. Also, know your pharmacist's phone number, as the health care provider may want to call in a prescription.

Taking Your Baby's Temperature

If your baby seems sick (listless, unusually fussy, no appetite, runny nose), take his temperature. To quickly assess whether your baby has a fever, feel the back of your neck and compare that warmth to the warmth of your baby's chest, abdomen or back. Remember that a newborn's hands and feet are often cold even though his body is warm.

If your baby feels hot, you can take his temperature under his arm (axillary temperature) using an oral or digital thermometer. Ask your health care provider to show you how to take your baby's temperature under the arm.. Ear probe thermometers are not as accurate as axillary temperatures[15] and are not considered to be accurate in newborns. Likewise, temperature strips that may be placed on the forehead and pacifier thermometers are not as accurate as axillary temperatures. Call your baby's health care provider if your baby's temperature is above 37.5°C or below 36.5°C.

Newborn Warning Signs

If any of the following signs appear in the first month, call your baby's health care provider:

- Any axillary temperature above 37.5°C or below 36.5°C
- Possibility of jaundice if your baby's face, trunk and the whites of his eyes are yellowish
- Changes in your baby's behaviour, such as listlessness or unusual fussiness or irritability
- Problems with the cord, including bright red bleeding that makes a spot (larger than a twenty-cent coin) on the nappy or singlet, redness of the skin around the cord, or a foul odour or pus-like discharge
- Problems with the circumcision, including bright red bleeding (more than a small spot), swelling, foul discharge or an inability to urinate
- Problems with feeding, including a breastfed newborn baby who feeds less than seven or eight times in twenty-four hours, or any baby who feeds ineffectively
- Too few wet nappies (fewer than one wet cloth nappy a day for each day of age, until the mother's milk comes in; at three or four days after birth, fewer than six or more wet cloth nappies in twenty-four hours). If you are using disposable nappies, place a facial tissue in the nappy to detect wetness.
- Problems with bowel movements, including no bowel movement in the first day of life or in any forty-eight-hour period thereafter. (See page 404 for a description of normal bowel movements in newborns.)
- Problems with breathing, including signs such as blue lips, struggling to breathe, flaring nostrils or deep indentations of the chest when breathing

Colds

It is normal for some babies to have a slight stuffy, rattly noise in their noses. Your infant probably has a cold, however, if she has a very runny nose, is fussier than usual, has trouble eating and sleeping and perhaps has a slight fever.

To lessen the chance of a cold, minimise the number of visitors (adults and children) when the baby is very young. People with colds should stay away. Make sure all those who want to touch the baby wash their hands thoroughly first. You will probably want to consult your baby's health care provider during your baby's first cold. He or she may suggest clearing the nostrils gently with saline nose drops. Antibiotics have no role in treating colds.

Medications

Use the following guidelines if your baby's health care provider prescribes medications or vitamins for your baby:

- Give only the medication your baby's health care provider specifies. Aspirin, even baby aspirin, is no longer recommended for infants and children because of its association with Reye's syndrome, a very serious disease.
- Use a medicine dropper placed between the baby's cheek and gum. Hold the infant in a semi-upright position and let the infant suck the medication as you gently squirt it in. You might try placing the dropper next to a pacifier or your finger.

- Pour medication into an empty bottle teat and have the baby take it all; fill the emptied teat with water and have the baby take all that too, to ensure that the baby has received a full dose.
- Do not put medication in formula, juice or water. You will not be sure how much your baby has received if he refuses to finish it.

Sudden Infant Death Syndrome (SIDS)

Sudden infant death syndrome (SIDS) refers to the unexpected death of an apparently healthy infant, usually while asleep or in bed. The cause is not fully understood.

Almost every parent worries about SIDS at some time. You may know someone whose baby died of SIDS, or you may have read about it. There is no way to minimise the loss and grief caused by SIDS, but the following facts may help you put your fears and worries into perspective:

- A baby's parents do not cause SIDS; it cannot be predicted and it cannot be prevented. SIDS occurs even in the hospital.
- Less than one death per thousand live births in Australia is caused by SIDS.
- Ninety percent of SIDS deaths occur between two and six months of age.
- Death occurs quickly and painlessly and is not the result of suffocation, asphyxiation or regurgitation.
- SIDS is not caused by immunisations; in fact, SIDS deaths occur more commonly in infants who have not been immunised.
- Families who have lost a previous baby to SIDS are no more likely to lose subsequent babies to SIDS than any other family.
- SIDS is not contagious.
- No one is to blame for SIDS.

It is helpful to remember that SIDS occurs rarely. Also, there are some things you can do to lower your baby's risk for SIDS:

- During pregnancy, do not smoke and avoid exposure to second-hand smoke. Once your baby is born, do not expose your baby to tobacco smoke.
- **Always place your baby on her back to sleep.** Placing her on her tummy (or side) to sleep increases her risk for SIDS. If she seems unhappy on her back or wakens easily, swaddling her in a blanket may help.
- Be sure that anyone who cares for your baby (relatives or day-care workers) knows that your baby needs to sleep on her back.
- Avoid overdressing your infant. Dress her as you are dressed, with perhaps one more layer of clothing or a light blanket.
- Remove soft toys, pillows and bedding from her bed. Also, never place her on a lambskin, even on her back.
- Breastfeed. Breastfeeding is associated with a lower risk of SIDS.

Placing your baby on her back can dramatically reduce her risk of SIDS. When she is awake, however, place her on her tummy to play and interact with you.

SIDS support groups are available to

help parents cope with their loss. Your SIDS association can be contacted via the state or territory offices. They will also provide more information about sleeping position, support services, monitors or any other matter relating to SIDS.

State and Territory SIDS Offices

SIDS and Kids ACT
PO Box 3118
Weston, ACT 2611
ph: (02) 6287 4255
email: canberra@sidsandkids.org

SIDS and Kids Hunter Region
PO Box 64
The Junction, NSW 2291
ph: (02) 4969 3171 AH: 0438 693 176
email: hunterregion@sidsandkids.org

SIDSnew south wales
PO Box 379
Guilford, NSW 2161
ph: (02) 9681 4500 or 1800 651 186
email: sydney@sidsaustralia.org.au

SIDS and Kids Northern Territory
GPO Box 3414
Darwin, NT 0801
ph: (08) 8948 5311
email: darwin@sidsandkids.org

SIDS and Kids Queensland
PO Box 241
Mt Gravatt, QLD 4122
ph: (07) 3849 7122 or 1800 628 648
email: brisbane@sidsandkids.org

SIDS and Kids South Australia
301 Payneham Road
Royston Park, SA 5070
ph: (08) 8363 1963 or 1800 656 566
email: adelaide@sidsandkids.org

SIDStasmania
2 Spring Street
Burnie, Tas 7320
ph: (03) 6431 9488 or 1800 625 675
email: tasmania@sidsandkids.org

SIDS and Kids Victoria
1227 Malvern Road
Malvern, VIC 3144
ph: (03) 9822 9611 or 1800 240 400
email: melbourne@sidsandkids.org

SIDS and Kids Western Australia
33 Sixth Avenue
Kensington, WA 6151
ph: (08) 9474 3544 or 1800 199 466
email: perth@sidsandkids.org

National website for SIDS:
www.sidsaustralia.org.au

Chapter 15

Breastfeeding and Formula Feeding

During pregnancy, your baby grows rapidly from a fertilised egg to a mature baby weighing around 3 kilograms. All your baby's nutritional needs are met by your body via the placenta. For the newborn, growth continues at a rapid rate, and all his nutritional needs are still met by your body via milk from your breasts (or alternatively, by formula). The extraordinary growth occurring in the first months of life after birth is illustrated by the fact that the full-term infant generally doubles his birth weight by four to five months and triples it by one year. He also grows 25–30 centimetres longer in the first year of life.

Breast milk and formula provide nutrients for the baby's gain in weight and length. Breast milk, however, is the only source of nutrients that also contribute to the rapid and healthy growth of the baby's brain and nervous system, the maturation of his digestive system and the development of his immune system.

In addition, the manner in which a baby's nutritional needs are met greatly influences his physical, social and emotional wellbeing. Feeding your baby in a caring and loving way is just as important as providing nourishment that promotes your baby's healthy growth.

History of Infant Feeding

Infant feeding practices have changed markedly in the past one hundred years and even since you were a baby. You may wonder why you were fed water as a newborn and cereal in the first months of life, when your baby's doctor now encourages you to avoid water feedings in the early months of newborn life and to delay starting cereal and other solid foods until your baby is about six months old. In the early 1900s, most babies were breastfed. Other foods were seldom offered, except cod liver oil to prevent rickets and orange juice to prevent scurvy. From about 1920 through 1970, solid foods were offered earlier and earlier (even in the first week of life) to supply the baby with iron, vitamins and a more varied diet. Parents and their doctors believed that introducing solid foods early would not only improve infant nutrition, but would also help babies sleep through the night sooner (a myth). Breastfeeding declined during this time because it was thought to be old-fashioned, and formula feeding, thought to be a more scientific approach to infant feeding, became highly popular. In 1940, fewer than half of all babies in Australia were breastfed; by the late 1960s, the number declined to less than one fourth.

By 1975, however, another change was in place. Breastfeeding was becoming increasingly popular, partly because it reflected the 'back to nature' movement of the time and partly because it was discovered to have previously unrecognised emotional and health benefits for baby and mother. In 1979, over 50 percent of Australian mothers breastfed their babies. Today, about 80 percent of mothers breastfeed their newborns and about 22 percent are still breastfeeding at six months.

Obstacles to breastfeeding have been identified. These include factors such as lack of information or apathy on the part of health care providers; disruptive hospital practices such as giving water and supplements to babies without medical need; lack of follow-up care in the early post-partum period; maternal employment; lack of broad societal support; and commercial promotion of infant formula through distribution of hospital discharge packs, baby gifts from formula companies distributed by the maternity caregivers during pregnancy, and television and general magazine advertising.[1]

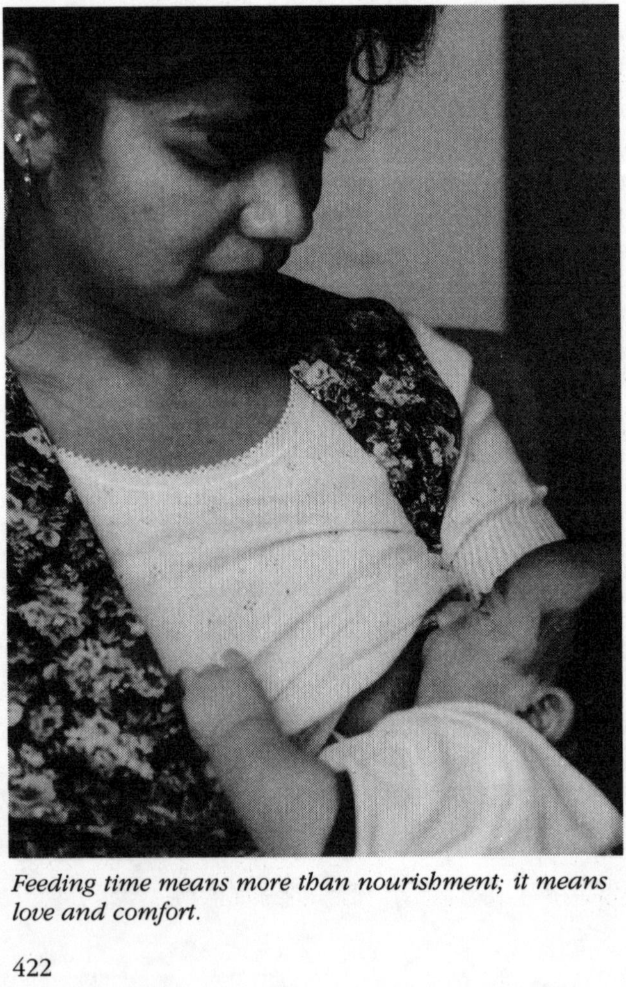

Photograph by David Stein

Feeding time means more than nourishment; it means love and comfort.

There are three overlapping feeding periods in the first year of life and optimal feeding guidelines for each: the *nursing period,* during which breast milk or an iron-fortified formula is the only food in the infant's diet; the *transitional period,* during which solid foods are offered in addition to breast milk or formula; and the *modified adult period,* during which most of the infant's food comes from the family table, along with breast milk or formula.[2]

Breast Milk or Formula?

Deciding whether to breastfeed or formula feed is an important and personal choice. Before making up your mind, try to become well informed about each method of feeding. Almost all health care providers acknowledge that breastfeeding is the best way to feed babies because of the health benefits for both babies and their mothers. Except in certain rare instances, breastfeeding is recommended.

Despite these endorsements of breastfeeding, you may have some doubts or some reasons not to breastfeed. For example, you may be concerned about a medical condition you have or worried that breastfeeding might be less convenient than formula feeding. Your partner may be concerned that he or she will be left out of the feeding experience, or you may be concerned that returning to work will make it difficult for you to breastfeed. Or, you may have had a previous difficulty or disappointment with breastfeeding. Your individual circumstances need to be thoughtfully considered as you make your choice. Use your various resources (your caregiver, a breastfeeding expert or counsellor, your baby's doctor, breastfeeding support groups) as you consider your options. The following three sections may also assist you in your decision-making; they describe why breast milk is recommended by health care professionals, challenging situations in which breastfeeding should be considered and situations in which formula is recommended.

Why Breast Milk Is Recommended

- The nutritional composition of breast milk is ideal for human infants.
- As your baby grows and his nutritional needs change, your milk adapts to meet these needs.
- Breast milk is easily digested.
- Breastfeeding is both economical and convenient.
- Breastfeeding promotes attachment and a close, nurturing relationship between mother and baby.
- Breastfeeding reduces the incidence and severity of diseases and infections such as ear infection, respiratory infection, meningitis and urinary tract infections. It also reduces symptoms such as diarrhoea and vomiting.
- Infants exclusively breastfed through three months of age are nine times less likely to be hospitalised for infections compared to formula-fed infants.[3]

- Breastfed infants have a reduced incidence of some chronic conditions and diseases that occur later in life, such as insulin-dependent diabetes mellitus, Crohn's disease, ulcerative colitis and multiple sclerosis.[4]
- Breastfed infants have lower rates of lymphoma than formula-fed infants.[5]
- Breastfed infants have fewer and less severe allergies compared to formula-fed infants.[6]
- Breastfeeding enhances the development of the brain and is associated with higher cognitive test scores than feeding formula to a baby.[7]
- Breastfeeding has been shown to have a protective effect that helps reduce the possibility of sudden infant death syndrome (SIDS).[8]
- Breastfeeding reduces post-partum bleeding and aids involution (the return of the uterus to its normal size).
- Breastfeeding reduces the risk of some diseases for the mother, including pre-menopausal breast cancer and ovarian cancer.[9]
- Breastfeeding mothers have fewer hip fractures in the post-menopausal period than women who never breastfed.[10]

Challenging Situations in Which Breastfeeding Should Be Considered

- If your husband or partner (or another family member) is concerned about not being able to feed your breastfed baby, it is helpful to recognise that he or she can still be actively involved in baby care and parenting. In addition to nourishment, babies need cuddling, soothing, bathing and social interaction. Fathers and partners can be experts in these aspects of baby care. Your partner can also support you by assisting and encouraging your efforts to breastfeed your baby. Although you are the one who produces milk and feeds your baby, your partner's and family's support and encouragement are often the key factors in keeping you going if difficulties arise. The newborn period is short, and as your baby grows older his need for social interaction and play increases dramatically, giving his father or other family members many more opportunities (other than feeding) to get to know and parent him.
- Breastfeeding is more challenging when a mother returns to employment. (See page 459 for more information on breastfeeding and working outside the home.)
- Breastfeeding is also more difficult with a baby who is born prematurely or has a physically limiting condition such as Down syndrome or cleft lip and palate. However, in these instances breastfeeding or providing the baby with pumped breast milk can still be an excellent way to help your baby grow and stay healthy. There are special techniques for holding and feeding babies with unique physical challenges. A breastfeeding counsellor can be of great help.
- If you have had a previous unhappy breastfeeding experience, talk with a breastfeeding counsellor during your pregnancy to discuss how or if breast-

feeding can be different this time. If you remain unsure right up to the time you give birth, give breastfeeding a try. It is easier to stop breastfeeding than to try to begin when your baby is a week or two old.

If you have made a firm decision not to breastfeed or find you cannot breastfeed, this chapter will provide you with helpful information about formula feeding. (See pages 461–463.) Mothers who have tried hard to breastfeed and have not been able to make it work often feel sad about their loss. Seek the support of a breastfeeding counsellor or your care provider as you adjust to a different method of feeding.

When Formula Feeding Is Recommended

There are a few instances in which breastfeeding is not recommended:

- When the mother is HIV positive (and lives in a developed country)[11]
- When the mother has untreated tuberculosis
- When the mother takes certain drugs that could harm the baby, such as lithium or radioactive medications for medical studies or treatment
- When the mother uses street drugs such as heroin, cocaine or methamphetamines
- When the mother has had extensive breast surgery, making it nearly impossible for the baby to breastfeed
- When the baby has galactosemia, a rare condition in which the baby is unable to digest the sugar in milk
- When the mother would be uncomfortable, resentful or unhappy breastfeeding

Some Concerns about the Use of Formula

- Formula has no capacity to enhance the development of the baby's immune system.
- The earlier the introduction of formula, the greater the risk for the development of severe allergy (asthma and eczema) and infection in the infant.
- Manufacturers of formula include at least minimum levels of twenty-nine nutrients and maximum levels of nine nutrients in their formula. However, there are over two hundred nutrients and components in breast milk; most of these components are not present in formula.
- Babies fed low-iron formula have a higher incidence of anaemia and lower cognitive test scores compared to breastfed infants or infants fed iron-fortified formula.[12]
- Soy formula has been associated with a higher incidence of auto-immune thyroid disease than either breast milk or cow milk formula.[13]
- Occasionally, formula is recalled because of manufacturing errors. Such formula puts the baby at risk and causes anguish in parents.

Breastfeeding

Breastfeeding describes the interaction between mother and baby as the baby nurses from her mother's breast. Preparation for breastfeeding begins during the early teen years when the ductal system within female breasts grows in response to increasing amounts of oestrogen. During pregnancy, the breasts prepare for *lactation* (milk production and secretion) through a complex interplay of hormones that together cause accelerated growth of the ductal and lobular systems within the breasts. The blood supply to the breasts supports this growth and, later, supplies the nutrients in breast milk.

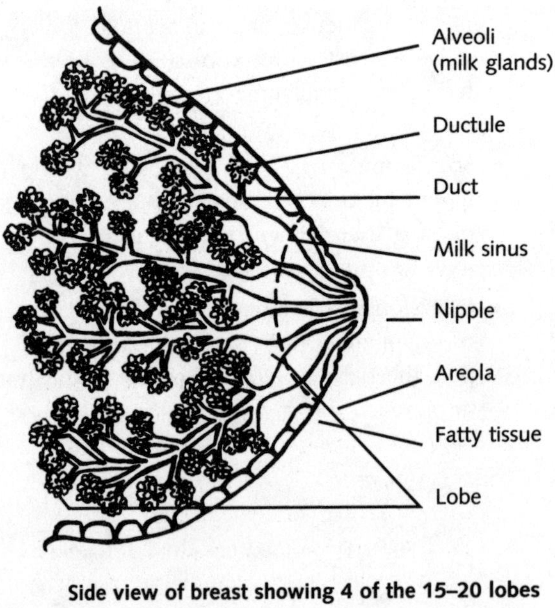

Side view of breast showing 4 of the 15–20 lobes

During the second trimester and as early as sixteen weeks gestation, prolactin (a hormone from the anterior pituitary gland) stimulates the production of *colostrum* (the first milk); placental lactogen stimulates the breasts to secrete colostrum. Some women leak colostrum from their breasts during pregnancy; many do not. After birth, blood levels of progesterone fall and prolactin levels increase, causing the production of breast milk. These amazing changes in the breasts that lead to milk production are a natural outcome of pregnancy.

Anatomy of the Breast

The breasts are well designed to make milk. The illustration at left shows a cross section of a breast. Each breast contains fifteen to twenty *lobes,* or milk-producing units, arranged like spokes of a wheel around the nipple. Each lobe has approximately twenty to forty *lobules;* within each lobule are numerous *alveoli* that contain the milk-producing cells. Milk flows from the alveoli through *ductules* into longer *lactiferous ducts.* The milk then enters the *milk sinuses* (located under the areola) and leaves the breast through many *nipple openings.* The *areola* is the darker area around each nipple. As the infant compresses the sinuses with her lips and gums and massages the extended areola with her tongue, she draws milk into her mouth. *Montgomery glands,* the small bumps on the areola, secrete a lubricating substance that keeps the nipple supple and helps prevent infection. (Use only water to clean your breasts, as soap removes the special lubrication provided by the Montgomery glands.)

You will probably notice some external breast changes during pregnancy. Your breasts are probably larger and their veins more visible. You may have developed stretch marks as your breasts have grown. Your areolae may have enlarged and darkened in colour. This change will help make your breasts easily visible to your newborn and help her direct her mouth towards your nipple. The Montgomery glands are also larger. Colostrum, which has been present in your breasts since the middle of pregnancy, may leak from your breasts or appear as a dried crust on your nipples. All these changes are positive physical signs that your breasts are responding to the hormones of pregnancy and are preparing to make milk for your baby.

Between two and six percent of women have *accessory mammary tissue,* which is extra breast tissue under the arm or below the breast that is sometimes accompanied by a nipple. Accessory mammary tissue may swell with the hormones of pregnancy and may enlarge as milk comes in. If left alone, it will diminish in size and not cause a problem during breastfeeding. Cold packs placed over the area may increase your comfort.

Breasts, areolae and nipples normally vary in size and shape from one woman to another. The size of the breast is related to the amount of fatty tissue surrounding the milk-producing structures; breast size has nothing to do with the amount of milk produced. With rare exceptions, breasts of all sizes and shapes are perfect for breastfeeding.

Prenatal Preparation for Breastfeeding

You can take some steps during pregnancy to get yourself ready for the early days of breastfeeding. First, learn as much as you can about breastfeeding. Read books, attend a breastfeeding class, and seek the support of groups such as Breastfeeding Australia, Tresillian or new mothers' groups. If possible, be around women who are nursing so you can see and learn how they hold their infants for feeding and how they fit breastfeeding into their busy lives.

Choose caregivers for yourself and your baby who are committed to supporting breastfeeding. During pregnancy, ask your caregiver to assess your breasts for breastfeeding. Since many caregivers never received training in this skill, you may need to be assessed by a breastfeeding expert. The assessor will note the changes that have occurred in your breasts, look for the presence of scar tissue from biopsies or breast surgeries, and carefully evaluate your nipples.

If you have specific concerns about your health, your nipples or breast anatomy, past breast surgeries, a previous unhappy breastfeeding experience, or if you know you are expecting more than one baby, make an appointment to have a prenatal visit with a knowledgeable breastfeeding expert in your community. Together, you can determine any steps that should be taken during pregnancy or in the early post-partum period to improve your breastfeeding experience.

Finally, arrange for help during the first weeks at home. Enlist the support of family

Breastfeeding Help-lines

The Australian Breastfeeding Association, formerly known as Nursing Mothers, has help-lines across Australia that will refer you to a trained volunteer breastfeeding counsellor:

- Victoria 03 9885 0653
- New South Wales 02 9639 8686
- Queensland 07 3844 8977 or 07 3844 8166
- South Australia and Northern Territory 08 8411 0050
- Western Australia 08 9340 1200
- ACT 02 6258 8928
- Tasmania 03 6223 2609
- North Tasmania 03 6331 2799

General breastfeeding information and details on the association can be found on their website: www.breastfeeding.asn.au

and friends to help you with meals and household tasks so you can focus on feeding and caring for your baby and yourself. Have the phone numbers of a breastfeeding counsellor and/or breastfeeding help-lines readily available. The first few weeks are generally the most challenging for new breastfeeding mothers; later, breastfeeding becomes much easier, more convenient and enjoyable.

How Milk Is Made

Two hormones, prolactin and oxytocin, play a significant role in milk production and milk ejection (flow). The infant's suckling at your breast stimulates the anterior pituitary gland, located in your brain, to release prolactin into your bloodstream. *Prolactin* causes the cells in the alveoli to draw water and nutrients from your blood to make milk. *Oxytocin* is released into your bloodstream by the posterior pituitary gland in response to the infant's suckling and in response to hearing your baby awaken, fuss or cry. Oxytocin causes the small muscles around the milk-producing cells to contract and expel the milk. It also causes the ducts to widen and shorten, facilitating milk flow. This process is called the *let-down reflex.*

You will probably not feel your let-down until your mature milk is in. You may feel the let-down as a tingling, itching or burning sensation in your breasts, or you may have no sensation even though your baby is getting your milk. When your milk lets down, you will probably hear your baby swallow, see milk in his mouth or feel uterine cramping, especially if this is your second baby or more. The sensations of let-down vary widely. While the first let-down is the most noticeable, you will have many let-downs during each feeding.

The amount of milk you produce is generally affected by the frequency and duration of breastfeedings. The more your baby suckles at your breast, the more milk you produce. Delaying or limiting feedings, using a pacifier, offering supplements (formula, water or other liquids), or attempting

Nipple Types

Nipples can be placed into one of three broad categories, based on how they respond to being compressed between a thumb and fingers at the base of the nipple (the 'pinch test').[14] If you know the type of nipple you have, you will know what (if anything) you should do during your pregnancy or breastfeeding to help make breastfeeding go more smoothly.

1. **Typical nipples.** Nipples that elongate or protrude when compressed are most common. No special prenatal preparation is necessary.

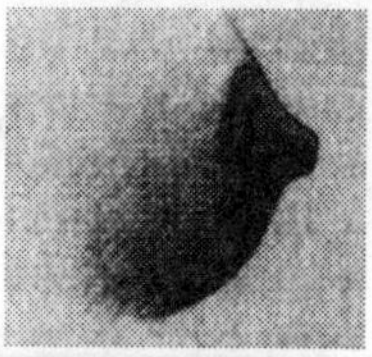

Typical nipple

2. **Flat nipples.** Some nipples flatten or move inwards (retract) when compressed. For some women, this may change during pregnancy as the size of the nipple increases and its ability to protrude improves in response to hormonal changes. In the beginning of your breastfeeding experience, you may need help to shape your nipple in a way that allows your baby to latch onto your breast effectively.

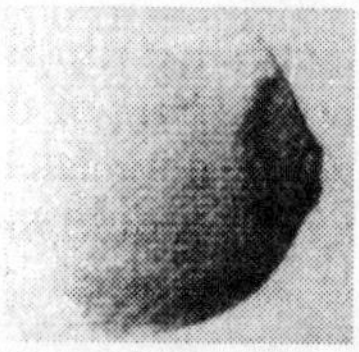

Flat nipple

3. **Inverted nipples.** Some nipples are tucked into the areola (inverted). When compressed, some of these nipples will protrude while others remain tucked in, probably because the tissue is bound inwards by tiny bands (adhesions).

Treatment for Flat or Inverted Nipples

If you have the type of nipple that remains flat or inverted when compressed, getting started with breastfeeding will be a challenge for you. Here are a few suggestions to help you breastfeed:

1. Learn about ways to treat flat or inverted nipples before your baby is born.

2. Contact a breastfeeding expert who can help with early breastfeeding.

3. Some women benefit from the use of *breast shells* in pregnancy. A breast shell is a two-part plastic shell with an opening in an inner ring and small holes in the outer dome for air circulation. The opening is placed over your areola with your nipple centred. Shells are worn inside your bra for several hours a day in the beginning and later all day (removing them at night). They are thought to be helpful in promoting flat or inverted nipples to protrude. You may continue to use the shells after birth, wearing them fifteen to thirty minutes before a feeding to help your nipples protrude. You can purchase breast shells at stores specialising in breastfeeding supplies. Breast shells need to be washed in hot soapy water and rinsed with hot water between uses.

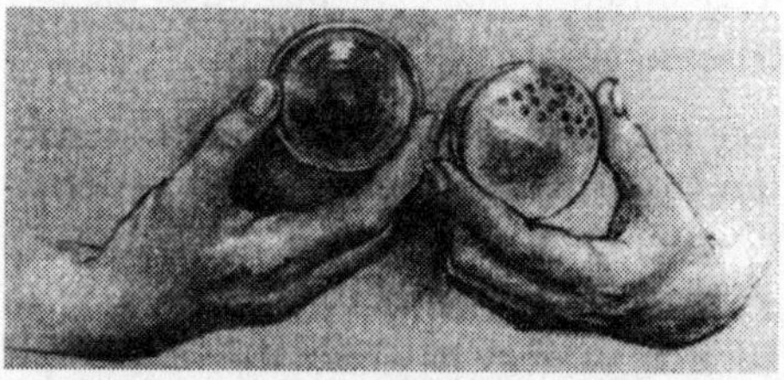

Breast shell

4. After the birth, you may need to use a breast pump to draw out your nipples or to express milk until your baby can feed at the breast. The hospital nurses can help you with this and with other ways to make breastfeeding easier.

to place your baby on a three- or four-hour feeding schedule will delay your milk coming in and decrease your milk production. Feeding frequently, in response to your baby's hunger cues, and letting your baby feed as long as he wants to feed will help you develop a good milk supply.

Composition of Breast Milk

The first milk produced by the breasts, *colostrum,* is a yellowish or clear syrupy fluid that is higher in protein and lower in fat than mature milk. Colostrum is ideally suited to the newborn's needs: It provides a laxative effect that helps to speed the passage of meconium; it helps establish the proper balance of bacteria in the infant's digestive tract; and, because colostrum is rich in antibodies, it protects the infant from infection. *Transitional milk* (milk with a yellowish tint) is produced next. It is higher in fat and calories and lower in protein than colostrum. Usually by the end of the first week of breastfeeding, the *mature milk* comes in. Mature milk is bluish white (like skim milk) and contains more calories than colostrum or transitional milk.

Mature breast milk varies in composition during each single feeding. The small amount of milk produced early in the feeding is called *foremilk.* The larger portion of milk releases with the let-down reflex and is called *hindmilk.* Hindmilk contains more fat and protein than foremilk and provides more of the calories your infant needs to thrive. As your infant grows, her requirements for nutrients change and the composition of your breast milk changes further according to her needs.

Some of the components of breast milk include the following:

Water. Water is the largest constituent of breast milk (about 87 percent). Water helps newborns maintain their body temperature. Even in very hot climates, breast milk contains all the water a baby needs.

Fats. Fats account for about half of the calories in breast milk. One of these fats, cholesterol, is necessary for normal development of the infant's nervous system, which includes the brain. Cholesterol enhances the growth of a special coating on nerves as they grow and mature (myelinisation). Fatty acids, which are richly present in breast milk, also contribute to the healthy growth of the brain and nerves. Polyunsaturated fatty acids, such as docosahexanoic acid (DHA), in breast milk aid visual development.[15]

Carbohydrates. Lactose (milk sugar) is the primary form of carbohydrate in breast milk, where it is present in proportionally greater quantities than in cow milk. Lactose helps the infant absorb calcium and is easily metabolised into the two simple sugars (galactose and glucose) necessary for the rapid brain growth occurring in infancy.

Proteins. The primary protein in breast milk is whey. Easily digested, whey becomes a soft curd from which nutrients are readily absorbed into the baby's bloodstream. By contrast, casein is the primary protein in cow milk. When cow milk or cow milk formula is fed to a baby, the casein forms a rubbery curd that is less easily digested, sometimes contributing to constipation. Some components of the proteins in breast milk play an important role in protecting the infant from disease and infection.

Vitamins and minerals. Some of the many vitamins and minerals present in breast milk deserve special attention because, due to inadequate quantities, they are unable to meet the baby's needs as she grows and develops.

Iron, though present in human milk only in small quantities, comes in a highly absorbable form. A full-term, healthy, breastfed baby rarely needs iron supplementation or a dietary source of iron before six months of age.[16]

Vitamin D is essential for the absorption of calcium into the bones. Though rare, rickets (a disease that causes bone deformities) has occurred in breastfed infants whose mothers were vitamin D deficient and in infants who had little exposure to sunlight due to climate or clothing. Breastfed infants in those circumstances should be given supplemental vitamin D.[17]

Fluoride is a mineral that strengthens tooth enamel, protecting against tooth decay. Only small amounts of fluoride are present in breast milk. Fluoride is contained in the natural water resources in some regions of Australia, but not in all. Some communities add fluoride to their water supply if it has none of the mineral; other communities do not. The fluoride in a mother's drinking water, however, has minimal effect on the fluoride levels in her breast milk. If the baby is not drinking water or if the water supply is severely deficient in fluoride, check with your health care provider if a fluoride supplement is needed. Remember that distilled water has no minerals, including fluoride (unless it is added). If you are using bottled water, check with the manufacturer to determine the fluoride content.

Breastfeeding Basics

First Feedings

Right after birth, you can help establish your milk supply and avoid some early breastfeeding problems by keeping your baby with you (preferably skin-to-skin) so that he has total access to your breasts, by nursing as soon as possible and by allowing your baby to suckle frequently. Most newborns are alert and interested in feeding or nuzzling in the first hour after birth. Take advantage of this time to begin breastfeeding. Research has shown that frequent and unrestricted feedings help prevent painful engorgement[18] and lead to the development of an abundant milk supply.[19]

The first feeding is special. You and your baby get to know each other and begin the beautiful, synchronous interaction that characterises breastfeeding. If you have never breastfed before, the techniques of feeding may seem awkward and cumbersome at first. Be reassured that the skill of breastfeeding improves with experience and time. Here are some suggestions:

- Breastfeed your baby as soon as possible after birth. Most babies are alert and interested in feeding in the first hour after birth, more so than in the next eight to twenty-four hours.
- Nurse your newborn in an atmosphere of calm and tranquillity, if possible; doing this helps you relax and allows you and your baby to focus on the feeding.

- For the first feeding, surround yourself with only family members and friends with whom you feel very comfortable. Have your husband or partner request that other visitors leave during the feeding so you can have some privacy as you begin to learn to breastfeed.
- Use the help of experienced staff; or, request some private moments alone if you feel confident about breastfeeding without help.
- Get into a comfortable position with your back well supported. Use pillows to support your arms and the baby. If you have had a caesarean, your first feeding may be delayed beyond the first hour after birth, and you will need extra help. (See page 328.)

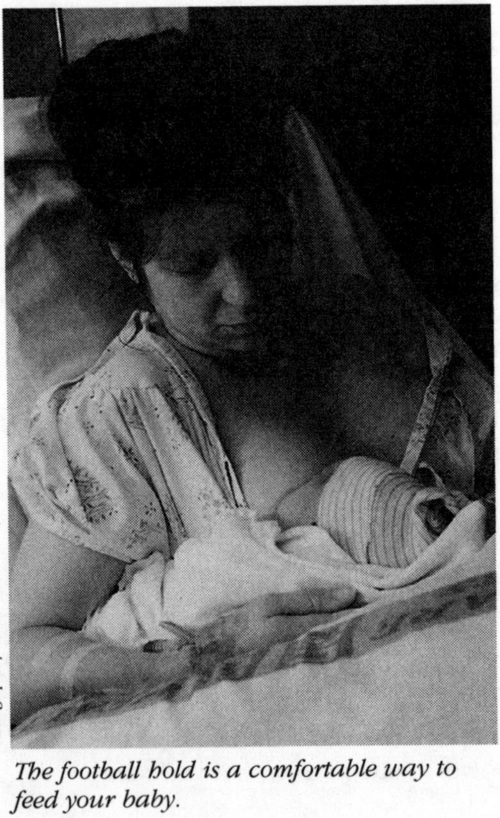

Photograph by David Swain

The football hold is a comfortable way to feed your baby.

Helping Your Baby Latch onto Your Breast

1. Make yourself comfortable in one of the positions described on page 435.

2. Hold your breast with your free hand behind but not touching your areola. Place your thumb above and your fingers below the areola. (See illustration.) Compress your breast with your thumb and fingers, centring your baby's mouth on your nipple.

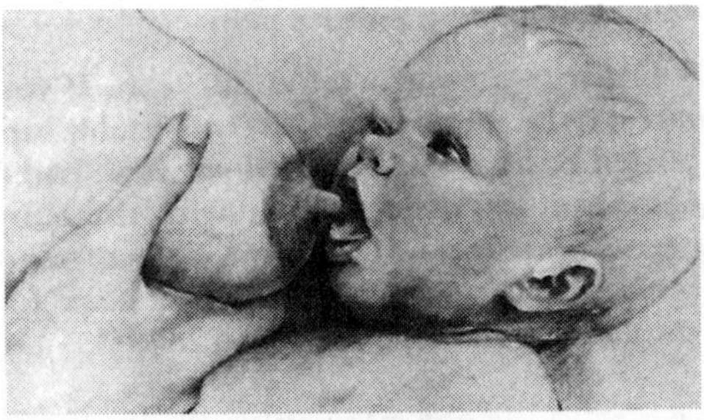

Mouth open wide

3. Stroke your baby's lower lip with your nipple to get him to open his mouth. Once his mouth opens wide (as wide as a yawn), pull or roll him gently towards you and hold him close, so his open mouth latches onto your breast and his tummy is against your chest or abdomen. Be patient. It sometimes takes many attempts before your baby opens his mouth wide enough to latch onto your breast. Just keep lightly stroking his lower lip. Expressing some colostrum and rubbing it

over your nipple may increase his interest in feeding. Bring your baby to your breast rather than bringing your breast to your baby.

4. Make sure to get as much of your areola as possible into your baby's mouth, to ensure a good latch. His nose will be touching your breast. Unless your breasts are quite large, he can still breathe. He will not allow himself to smother. If you feel you need to help him breathe more easily, lift your whole breast a little and bring his buttocks in closer, to rearrange his position and give him more breathing space. Doing this is preferable to pressing the breast away from his nose, which may interfere with his latch.

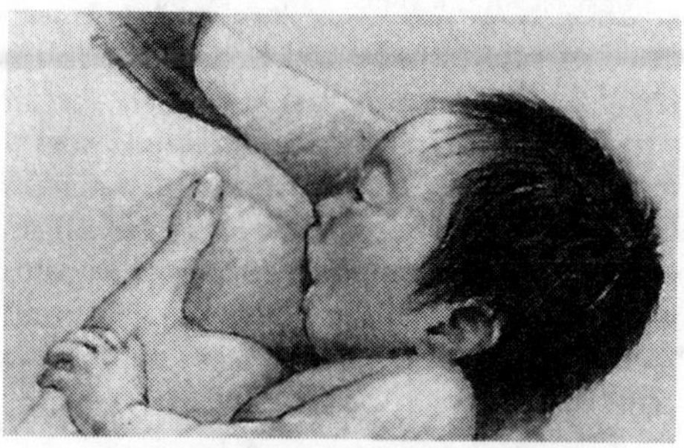

Good latch using the cradle hold

5. Let your baby suckle at the first breast for as long as he wishes (ten to thirty minutes is common), and then offer the other breast. He may feed from one breast or both. Avoid watching the clock. Instead, watch your baby. He will let you know when he is done feeding by drifting off to sleep and/or slipping off your breast.

6. Contrary to a popular myth, limiting feeding time does not prevent sore nipples. The best way to prevent sore nipples is to be sure the baby has a good latch for feeding. (See page 434 for information on evaluating latch.) If you try to stop his feeding after five to ten minutes to get him to feed from the other breast, you may find he does not latch well and the feeding ends. If he feeds from one breast only, begin feeding on the other breast next time.

7. During the first week or two after birth, the let-down reflex may occur within several minutes or more after your baby begins suckling. Once breastfeeding is established, let-down occurs within seconds after the baby begins to suckle. You will know your milk has let down when you hear your baby swallowing.

8. Some babies seem to know how to feed right from the start, while others seem sleepy or uninterested or have difficulty latching onto the breast. If you have difficulty getting started because your baby is drowsy, the suggestions in the box on page 434 may help. Remember that after the first two to three hours, many normal babies show little interest in suckling until they are about twenty-four hours of age. By the second day, most babies perk up and become eager to nurse.

9. Ask for help from an experienced nurse or a knowledgeable caregiver. It is important to get breastfeeding off to a good start.

The early feedings may be different from what you expected. Your baby may tentatively lick and mouth your breast. He may struggle to get a good latch. Or, he might immediately latch onto your breast, tug and suck vigorously. Energetic nursers sometimes grasp and pull on the nipple so firmly they surprise you and cause some pain. You may experience painful uterine contractions (afterpains) with feeding, especially if this is your second baby or more. Relaxation and breathing (as you did in labour) may help.

Do not despair if your baby does not nurse on the first try or if every feeding seems to take a lot of work and many attempts before he latches well. Whether he suckles or not, the stimulation of his nuzzling, licking and being close to your body encourages milk production. Sometimes, babies are tired from a long labour or are drowsy from the effects of some medications. Sometimes, they need time and practice to become organised for efficient nursing. You may also be tired following a long, difficult labour. Rest and nourishment will relieve your fatigue, just as rest and time will help your baby. With patience, perseverance and perhaps the help of knowledgeable breastfeeding experts, both you and your baby will almost certainly learn to nurse quite efficiently.

How to Know If Your Baby Is Latching Well

When the baby latches well onto the breast, she will be able to get the milk she needs more easily. Following are two lists (signs of an effective latch and signs of an ineffective one) that will help you know if your baby is latching well.[20]

How to Wake a Sleepy Baby

After the first day or so, newborn babies need to feed at least eight times in a twenty-four hour period. If your baby does not awaken to feed, try to wake him when he is in a light sleep state. You can use the following techniques to help you wake the baby or to keep him awake while feeding:

- Unwrap him and take off his clothes (leaving him in just a nappy).
- Dim the lights so he can open his eyes. Talk to him.
- Try holding him in a supported standing or sitting position.
- Try massaging his arms, legs and chest while he is at the breast.
- Express some colostrum or milk from your breast and rub it onto his lips. Be patient. If he only nuzzles on the first day, that is a good start.
- Massage your breast to enhance milk flow and to entice him to suckle more vigorously. (See page 439.)
- Try burping him or changing his nappy.
- Change his position for feeding or switch him to the other breast.
- Be sure he is not drowsy from wearing too much clothing.
- If he does not feed after you have tried to interest him for ten to fifteen minutes, let him sleep and try again when you see him start to rouse.
- If you continue to have a problem feeding a sleepy baby, get the help of a knowledgeable breastfeeding expert.

Signs of an Effective Latch

- Your baby opens her mouth as wide as a yawn with her tongue down and forward just before she latches onto your breast.
- She draws the nipple and much of your areola into her mouth.

- Her chin indents your breast and her nose touches your breast.
- Her lips are flanged out ('fish mouth') and her tongue is extended over her lower gum.
- Her jaw moves rhythmically as she suckles.
- She begins the feeding with short, rapid sucks. Once the milk lets down, she settles into a slower pattern with bursts of sucking and short pauses.
- You will be able to hear her swallow. In the first days before the milk comes in, she may need to suckle five to ten times before she has enough milk to swallow. Once the milk has come in, you can hear her swallow each time she suckles.

Signs of an Ineffective Latch

- Your baby's lips are pursed as though she is sucking on a straw.
- Her cheeks appear sunken, as there is not enough breast tissue to fill her mouth.
- You hear clicking noises during a feeding.
- You do not hear her swallow.
- She slips off the breast and roots frantically.
- You feel nipple pain that continues after the first minute or so.

Positions for Breastfeeding

The same principles of good latch apply for every position used for breastfeeding. Have the baby face the breast with his chin and the tip of his nose touching the breast. If needed in the beginning, hold the breast and shape the nipple by compressing the breast with your fingers behind the areola. Use pillows to support your arm and your baby's body.

Each position has special advantages. Use the one that is most comfortable and effective for feeding.

Cradle hold. The baby's head is cradled in the crook of your arm. Your forearm supports his body and your hand supports his buttocks or upper legs. He faces your breast with his chin touching your breast and his tummy and chest turned towards your chest or abdomen. Your other hand supports your breast with your thumb above and your fingers below your areola. Your fingers slightly compress the breast behind the areola.

Advantages:

- Usually the easiest position to learn
- Position most mothers use most frequently

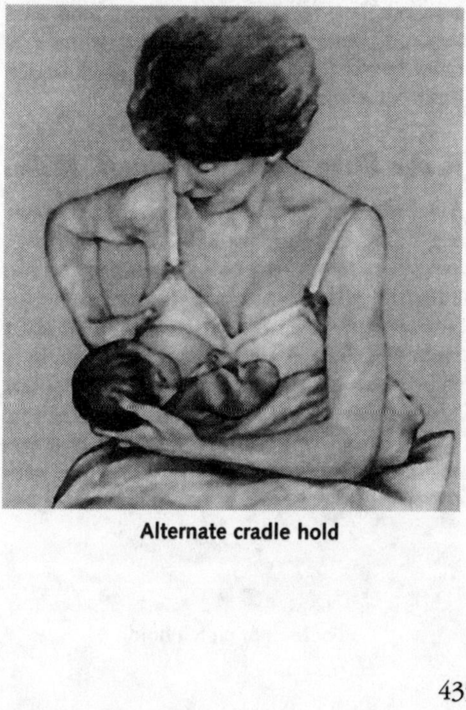

Alternate cradle hold

Cross or alternate cradle hold. In this position, the hand nearest the breast from which you are feeding supports and shapes the breast. Your other hand supports the nape of the baby's neck with fingers below the baby's ears. Avoid cupping the baby's head in your hands, as this may cause your baby to rear his head back from your breast. Your forearm supports your baby's trunk.

Advantages:

- Supporting the nape of the neck using your hand provides better control of the baby's head than using your forearm.
- Especially helpful when feeding a premature infant or an infant who is having difficulty latching onto the breast

Football or clutch hold. The hand nearest your feeding breast cradles the nape of your baby's neck. His body is tucked beside your body, under your arm. He rests on his back or slightly tipped on his side. Your other hand supports your breast and shapes your nipple. To assist the latch, move his head and chest towards your breast. Avoid flexing his chin onto his chest, as this makes it difficult for him to swallow and even to breathe. Also, avoid cupping his head in your hand.

Advantages:

- Easy to see that the baby has latched onto the breast effectively
- May be more comfortable for mother who has had a caesarean birth, as the baby is held away from the incision
- Comfortable for a mother with large breasts, as the baby's chest helps support the weight of the breast
- When the breast is very full, it may be easier to shape the breast in this position.

Lying down. Lie on your side with your lower arm tucked around your baby, who lies on his side facing your lower breast. You may also lie on your side with your lower arm tucked under your head. Try each position to determine which is more comfortable. Place a pillow between your knees and behind your

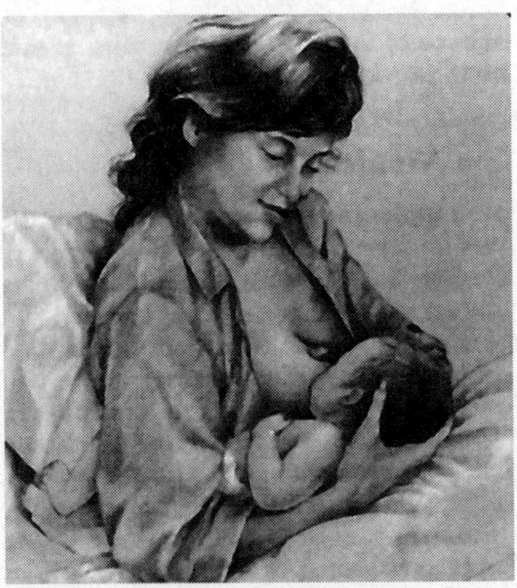

Football or clutch hold

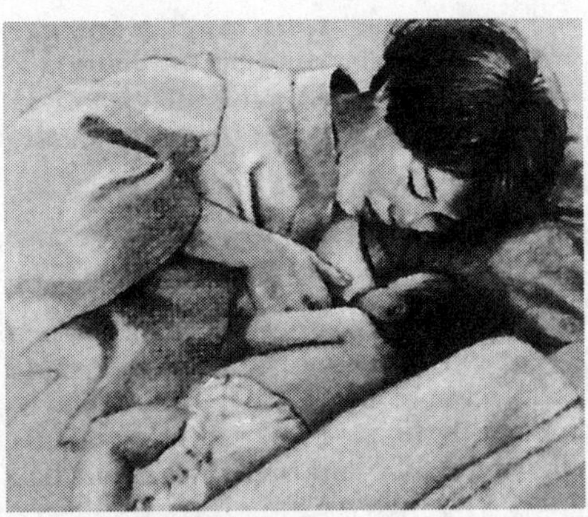

Lying on your side

baby's back to increase your comfort. In this position, it is possible to tip your body over slightly and feed from the top breast, too.

Advantages:

- Easy to rest during feedings
- Most comfortable for women who have painful perineal incisions or tears or who have painful haemorrhoids

Disadvantages:

- This position often takes some practice to learn.
- This position may be difficult for women who have large breasts.

Baby sits to feed. This position is similar to the football position. Your baby sits on your lap or on a pillow on your lap with his legs straddling the side of your body nearest the breast from which he is feeding. Your forearm supports his back and your hand supports the nape of his neck. Your other hand holds the breast and shapes the nipple.

Advantages:

- Easy to see if the baby has a good latch
- Especially helpful for babies whose mothers have large volumes of milk that let down rapidly (Sitting decreases the effect of gravity and helps the baby to swallow the rapid milk flow, to continue breathing and to avoid possible choking.)

How to Know When to Feed Your Baby

Feeding Cues

Breastfeed your baby in response to her feeding cues. She lets you know she wants to feed when she wakes from a drowsy state, roots towards anything that touches her cheeks or lips, or brings her hand up towards her mouth. Fussing and crying are late feeding cues. Respond to the early cues for feeding.

The First Days

Trying to feed a fussy or crying infant is difficult. On the first day of life, most babies are interested and eager to feed in the first two or three hours following birth. Then the baby becomes sleepy until she is about twenty to twenty-four hours of age.[21] If she has fed well soon after birth, breastfeeding has gotten off to a good start. Continue to offer her opportunities to feed when she indicates she is hungry, or at least every three hours. If she has not fed well before you both are discharged from the hospital or after the first day following a home birth, arrange to get some breastfeeding support the next day.

When your baby is one day of age, she becomes more wakeful. Many babies want to feed constantly. They may cluster their feedings (feeding five or more times in three hours followed by a period of deep sleep), or they may want to feed constantly until your milk comes in. Feeding your baby as often as she gives hunger cues helps ensure that your milk will come in soon and in abundance. Babies need to feed at least eight times in twenty-four hours, and some may feed as often as fifteen to eighteen times.

Begin each feeding with the breast opposite the one you began with at the previous feeding. Babies usually nurse most vigorously at the first breast. By alternating breasts, you make sure both breasts are stimulated to make milk. If you forget which breast you began with last time, press your fingertips against your breasts and begin with the one that feels more full. Feed from the first breast for as long as your baby is interested (ten to twenty minutes on average during the first few days). She will slide off the breast on her own. Then offer her the other breast, which she may or may not take.

If your baby remains with you in your hospital room, or if she is with you at home, you will know when she needs to be fed. However, if she spends some or most of her time in the nursery, you will want to ask the nursing staff to bring your baby to you when she is hungry—day or night. Also, keep in mind that full-term, healthy babies do not need supplemental bottles of formula, sugar water or water if they are breastfed frequently in response to feeding cues. Their requirements for nourishment and fluids are met as long as breastfeeding is not limited.

Using Bottles and Pacifiers in the First Days

Supplemental bottles of formula, sugar water and water are not only unnecessary, they have several disadvantages. Formula and sugar water diminish your baby's hunger and interfere with her desire to nurse. Furthermore, sucking on a bottle teat is entirely different from suckling at your breast. A newborn may have some difficulty adapting to different sucking patterns and differences in flow in the early weeks. This difficulty is sometimes called 'nipple confusion'. Also, if the baby has trouble breastfeeding, she may find bottle-feeding easier and begin to refuse the breast. This refusal can be devastating to the mother who wishes to breastfeed.[22]

Avoid the use of pacifiers to delay feedings in the early weeks. Delaying feedings postpones your milk coming in. Also, using a pacifier may satisfy your baby's sucking needs enough to interfere with breastfeeding, which may lead to poor weight gain. On the other hand, those few babies who nurse almost constantly without giving their mothers a rest may be able to use a pacifier without having it interfere with breastfeeding.

First Weeks

Over the next few weeks after birth, your baby will nurse every one to three hours. Over time, your baby will take in more milk at each feeding, reduce the total number of feedings, and feed more during the day and evening than at night. Babies do not always nurse on a regular schedule. Sometimes, they cluster their feedings, nursing four or five times in five or six hours and then sleeping for several hours.

Growth Spurts

At about three weeks, six weeks, three months and six months, your baby may suddenly change her feeding pattern and return to more frequent nursing. She may be fretful, irritable, and more sensitive to stimuli during this time and may seem to need to nurse almost constantly. She is probably experiencing a growth and developmental spurt; nursing frequently is her way of stimulating your breasts to make more milk to meet her greater need. Do not be troubled by her increased demands. Usually within a few days or a week, when your milk supply increases, your baby's need for more milk will be satisfied and she will return to a more predictable pattern of breastfeeding.

When Your Milk Comes In

With frequent and unlimited nursing, you can expect your milk to come in between the second and fourth day after birth. Your breasts become heavy, full and tender. You may even feel swollen in your armpits, because breast tissue extends to the armpit. Your nipple may appear flattened because of the swelling. When your milk comes in, the blood flow to your breast also increases and there is some degree of oedema (fluid retention) in your breast tissue. Both these factors contribute to the temporary discomfort and swelling that often accompany the sudden increase in milk production. The normal discomfort and swelling that occur when the milk comes in is sometimes called 'engorgement', but the term *engorgement* is reserved for a more serious condition caused by unrelieved breast fullness. True engorgement may be associated with a fever above 38.3°C, acute continuing pain, tingling and numbness in the mother's arm and fingers,[23] and difficulty removing milk from the breast even with a pump.

Relief of Breast Fullness

The best way to relieve breast fullness and tenderness is to nurse frequently. It may be difficult for your baby to latch onto your swollen, flattened nipple. You can soften your nipple and areola by hand-expressing a few drops of milk to make the areola more compressible. (See page 451 for information about hand expression.) Applying warm packs or standing in a warm shower may start the flow of milk, making the areola softer and easier for your baby to latch onto. Once your baby is feeding, massage your breasts (see below) to enhance milk flow. Let your baby feed as long as he wishes on the first breast. If he does not feed from the other breast, hand-express or use a commercial rented pump to reduce the fullness in the other breast.

After feeding, apply a cool, moist pack or an ice pack to your breast to reduce tenderness. If you use an ice pack, wrap it in a tea towel or apply it over light clothing. Some women have found that cool cabbage leaves applied to their swollen breasts reduce tenderness and swelling. Though their effectiveness is not scientifically proven, the leaves do no harm and may be soothing.[24] You may use the pain-relieving medications, such as ibuprofen, that were given to you after birth to reduce discomfort and relieve the inflammation that accompany swollen breasts. The feelings of fullness and tenderness usually do not last longer than a day or two. If your baby is unable to nurse even after you express some milk from your breast, seek help and support from a person knowledgeable about breastfeeding.

Enhancing Milk Flow

Breast massage during a feeding enhances the flow of milk from your milk-producing glands. The massage helps relieve breast fullness, helps to empty plugged ducts and makes more high-calorie hindmilk available to the baby.[25] This technique is especially

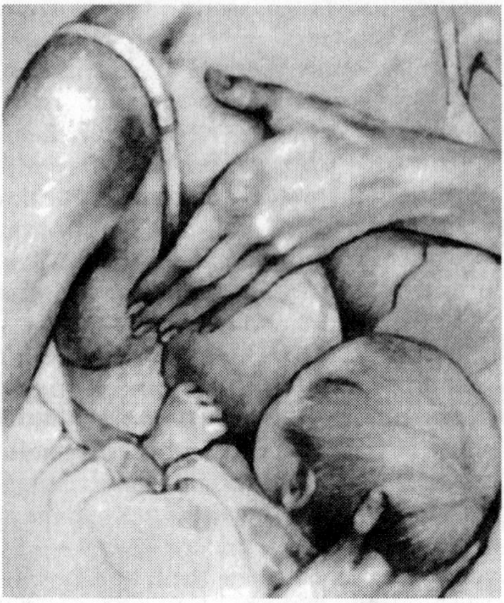

Massage during a feeding

useful for sleepy babies (to entice them to continue feeding) and for babies who are gaining weight slowly.

Once the baby has latched well, pay attention to her pauses in suckling. When she pauses, gently press your fingertips against the milk-producing glands located in the upper outer portion of your breast, near your arm. You will notice a burst of suckling as milk is pressed towards the milk sinuses and into your baby's mouth. If your baby pauses again, rotate the position of your fingertips and press on another portion of your breast. Be careful not to press too close to your areola, as this can interfere with your baby's latch.

Is Your Baby Getting Enough Milk?

Once your milk has come in, a number of signs can tell you if your baby is getting enough milk. Most babies who are getting enough breast milk show these positive signs:

- Feed vigorously at least eight to twelve times in twenty-four hours
- Have six or more wet cloth nappies in a twenty-four hour period. If you are using disposable nappies, it is difficult to tell how often your baby is urinating because the moisture is absorbed away from the surface. Place a tissue or a small piece of paper towel in the nappy. The tissue or towelling will remain wet if your baby has urinated.
- Have two or more loose stools in twenty-four hours once your milk has come in. It is common for your baby to have a stool after almost every feeding in the first month or so. Later, the number of stools usually decreases.
- Seem content after feedings

If your baby is not getting enough milk, he will show other signs and may have problems with weight gain. (For more information, see page 444.)

Burping Your Baby

Some babies swallow air when they cry or gulp milk while feeding. Swallowed air can make the baby feel full and uncomfortable. Try burping the baby during and after feeding. Try each of the following burping methods to find the one that is most effective for your baby. If after a minute or two she has not burped, stop trying. She probably does not need to burp.

- **Over-the-shoulder.** Place your baby high on your chest with her head peeking over your shoulder. Support her well across her back and buttocks. Gently pat or rub her back until you hear a burp.
- **Over-the-lap.** Place your baby on her tummy across your lap. Gently rub or pat her back until you hear a burp.
- **Sitting and rocking.** Sit your baby sideways on your lap. Place your thumb and first finger under her chin with your palm supporting her chest and your other hand supporting her back. Gently rock her forwards and back. You may lightly rub or pat her back until you hear a burp.

Maternal Nutrition While Breastfeeding

During pregnancy, your body prepared for lactation by storing energy in the form of 2.3–3 kilograms of extra fat that is not lost immediately after birth. This fat provides some of the extra calories necessary for milk production in the early months.

Your body also draws on your vitamin and mineral reserves to make milk. What you eat has very little effect on your being able to produce enough healthy breast milk. While you do not have to have a perfect diet to

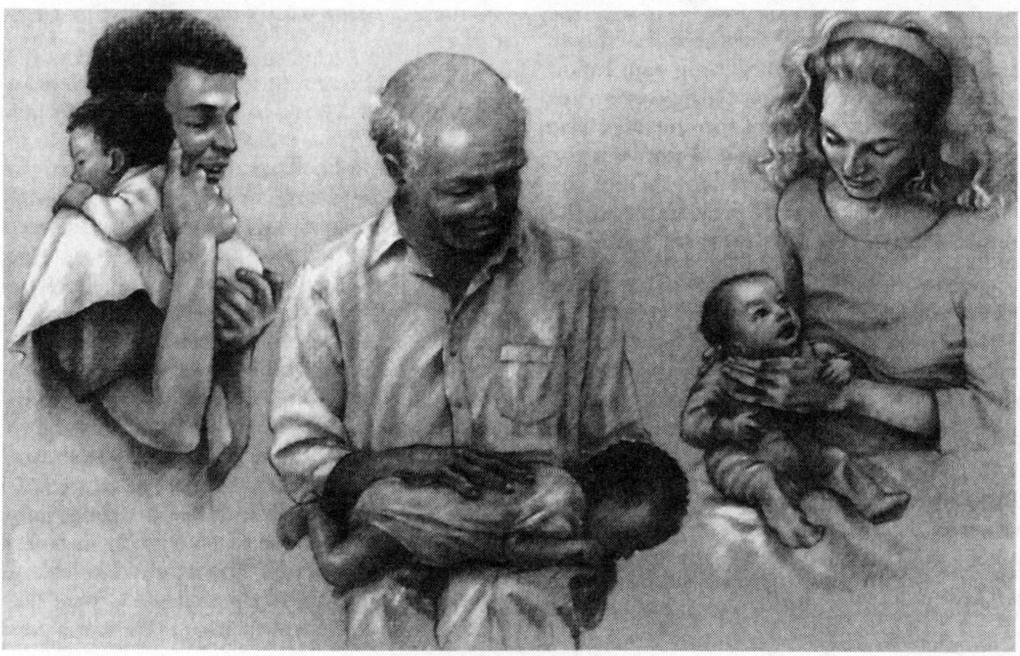

Burping positions

make nutritious breast milk, your diet will affect how you feel. With a poor diet, over time your nutritional stores may be depleted. To maintain these stores, eat a variety of healthy foods just as you did during pregnancy. You will have an initial large weight loss in the first month or so following birth. During that first month, some women have an increase in appetite, while others are not hungry. Baby care and feeding fill the hours of the day, so finding time to eat may become a challenge for you. If you have help at home, let others prepare your meals. Eat what tastes good and drink plenty of fluids.

After the first month, consume enough calories to maintain your weight. If you are breastfeeding twins, triplets, or a newborn and a toddler, you need more calories than mothers with one breastfeeding baby. If you want to lose weight, limit your weight loss to 450 grams per week. Be sure your diet contains over 1500 calories and avoid liquid diets and diet medications. Losing more than 450 grams per week and severely restricting calories will compromise your nutritional wellbeing and your health and may cause you to produce less breast milk.[26]

Your diet while nursing should include some extra protein, more calcium-containing foods, more vitamins and more fluids than your normal diet. (See Chapter 4 for lactation requirements.) A vitamin and mineral supplement is recommended if the foods you eat do not contain adequate amounts of vitamins and minerals for lactation. The vitamins and minerals most likely to be deficient in the diet include vitamin B_6, thiamine, folic acid, calcium, zinc and magnesium.[27] Levels of vitamin B_6, thiamine and folic acid in breast milk are directly related to the mother's dietary or supplemental intake. Inadequate intake of these vitamins reduces maternal stores and poses health risks for mother and baby.[28] If you are a vegan, you need vitamin B_{12} supplementation.

Drink enough fluids to keep yourself well hydrated. You know you are getting enough fluid if your urine is light straw-coloured. Adequate fluids keep you from feeling thirsty but (contrary to a popular myth) are not associated with increased milk production.

You may wonder if certain foods should be avoided or could cause problems for your baby. You may be told to avoid cabbage, broccoli and spicy foods because they are thought to cause colic. There is no evidence to support these claims. Generally, all the foods you would normally include in your diet are fine for breastfeeding. In fact, the foods you eat flavour your breast milk and introduce your baby to the foods he will eventually get from the family table. Breastfed babies have been shown to like the taste of garlic. Researchers found that babies drank more breast milk when their mothers took garlic capsules than when their mothers had no garlic. Breastfed babies were also found to accept peas and beans from the family table more readily than formula-fed infants.[29]

Less than one percent of the caffeine a breastfeeding mother consumes appears in her breast milk. A serving or two a day does not have an effect on her infant. However, many women who eliminate or limit caffeine during pregnancy find they are sensitive to it when they add it to their diet in post partum.

A chemical similar to caffeine is found in chocolate; as with caffeine-containing beverages, a little chocolate will not bother the baby.

The alcohol content in breast milk is approximately equal to the concentration in your blood. Therefore, the effects on the baby correspond to the amount you have consumed. Though an occasional drink has not been proven harmful, it is probably wise to eliminate alcohol consumption, especially during the early months of breastfeeding. If you drink alcohol, do not drink more than 3 glasses of wine, two beers or 55 millilitres of liquor in any single day.[30] Researchers compared breastfeeding when mothers drank alcohol to when they did not. They found that infants took in less breast milk in the three to four hours after their mothers drank alcohol than when they did not.[31] Breastfeeding before drinking alcohol reduces the amount of alcohol the baby gets from breast milk.

Food Sensitivity

There may be rare instances in which a food you have eaten adversely affects your baby, and she develops a rash, a chronic runny nose, diarrhoea or excessive fussiness. A baby who has a strong family history of food allergies may react to some of the foods, food preservatives, food dyes and food additives her mother eats. The most common foods having the potential to cause these reactions include cow milk, eggs, fish, shellfish and nuts.

Some babies react to the sheer quantity of a certain food a mother eats, such as a large bowl of cherries, large volumes of juice or enormous amounts of chocolate. If you think a certain food is bothering your infant, eliminate it from your diet and see if it makes a difference. If you eliminate milk, you need to be sure you are getting adequate amounts of calcium through your diet or a dietary supplement. Discuss your concerns with a breastfeeding expert or your baby's doctor. They may be able to help you identify the food causing your baby's problem and provide you with nutritional guidelines.

Some foods can tint breast milk slightly, although it is not a problem for the baby. There are reports of breast milk becoming more orange or pink if mothers drink orange soft drink or certain red fruit drinks, or if they eat gelatin containing red or orange dyes. Breast milk may become greenish if a mother drinks Gatorade or eats kelp and other forms of seaweed. Some women have noticed a greenish tint to breast milk after taking a vitamin supplement; others have observed a slight greyish colour to their milk after having taken iron supplements.

Some Early Breastfeeding Challenges

Almost every woman has questions about or challenges with breastfeeding in the first weeks and months following birth. Some of these are common and predictable and can be handled quite easily. Others are more serious and require more information and assistance. Following are some of the more common breastfeeding problems and suggestions for resolution.

When Your Baby Is Not Getting Enough Milk

A number of signs can tell you that your baby is not getting enough milk. If your baby feeds less than eight times in twenty-four hours, has few wet nappies, has urine that appears to have reddish 'brick dust' in it, or has fewer than one stool in a day after your milk is in, there is an increased risk that your baby may have problems with dehydration or weight gain. If you notice the signs listed above, call your baby's caregiver and request to have your baby assessed and weighed. Take your baby to be seen by his caregiver immediately if any of the following happen:

- Your baby seems constantly hungry and is seldom content after feedings.
- He is lethargic and not interested in feeding at all.
- He has dry mucous membranes in his mouth (the mouth does not glisten with a moist appearance).
- His skin stays 'tented' when you gently pinch the skin of his arm, leg or abdomen and then let go.
- His eyes, face, chest and abdomen are yellow in colour.
- You are worried and concerned.

Most babies lose from 5 to 10 percent of their birth weight by the third or fourth day of life. Once transitional milk is in, babies steadily gain weight. Term infants usually regain their birth weight by ten to fourteen days.

If your baby's weight gain does not follow these guidelines, you may not be producing enough milk and you will need to take measures to increase your milk supply. (See page 446.) Sometimes, weight gain problems are not due to inadequate milk production, but to the baby's inability to take enough milk. Insufficient breast milk production by the mother or insufficient intake by the baby could be due to any of the following factors:

Ineffective latch. When the baby is unable to latch well onto the breast, he will not get enough milk. One sign of a poor latch is that you may have very sore or cracked nipples. A poor latch may occur when the breast is engorged; when the baby is premature, ill or has a neurological condition that impairs his ability to suckle; when the baby latches onto only the nipple; or when there is something about the baby's mouth anatomy, such as a tight frenulum ('tongue tie'), that makes it difficult for him to suckle. If you are not able to help your baby achieve an effective latch, get help from someone who is knowledgeable about breastfeeding. Most of the factors causing a poor latch can be remedied; the sooner you get help, the sooner the problem is resolved.

Scheduled feedings. A newborn breastfed baby, especially a slow-gaining baby, needs to be fed more frequently than every three or four hours. All newborns need to be fed at night. Do not postpone feedings. Feed him whenever he indicates an interest in nursing (see page 437 for feeding cues), and make sure he nurses for as long as he wants to feed.

Limiting feedings to one breast. Offering only one breast at each feeding may result in inadequate milk production and may limit the amount of milk a baby gets. Switch to the other breast after your baby finishes feeding at the first breast. The baby may nurse very little on the second breast in the first week or so, but he will probably want to nurse from both breasts as he grows.

Pacifiers. Use of pacifiers has been associated with the development or reinforcement of faulty sucking patterns and shorter duration of breastfeeding.[32] When the baby is not able to suckle effectively or when the frequency of feedings is delayed by soothing a baby with a pacifier, the baby gains weight more slowly. The best advice is to avoid using pacifiers.

Sleepy baby. Most parents appreciate a baby who sleeps a lot, but if your baby goes for long stretches without feeding, he may not be getting enough milk. Try waking him every two to three hours during the day and every three to four hours at night. If your baby is not gaining weight, it is even more important to feed him often. If he is sleeping so soundly that you simply cannot rouse him, it is better to wait a half hour and try again than to continue the frustrating and futile effort of waking a baby who is deeply asleep. If your baby is very drowsy during feedings, pauses for long intervals, or even falls asleep even though he spends a long time at the breast, he may not get much milk. If he remains sleepy or lethargic and you cannot get him to nurse, call his caregiver. (See page 434 for suggestions on how to wake a sleepy baby.)

Jaundice. Inadequate milk intake increases the incidence of jaundice, which is caused by a high level of bilirubin in the blood. Bilirubin is excreted from the baby's body in his bowel movements. Because babies who feed poorly have fewer stools, they are not able to rid their bodies of bilirubin, and they become jaundiced. (See page 401 for discussion of jaundice.) Babies who are jaundiced are often sleepy and uninterested in feeding. If your baby's face, the whites of his eyes, chest and tummy seem yellow, call his caregiver so he can be assessed for jaundice. Once the jaundice is treated, a healthy baby usually becomes more interested in feeding.

Breastfeeding does not have to be interrupted to treat jaundice. Bottles of water should be avoided, as bilirubin is not excreted in urine, and water supplements may reduce the amount of milk a baby takes.

Prolonged or late-onset jaundice occurs in some breastfed babies. In the past, this was called 'breast milk jaundice' and was thought to be caused by a substance in the mother's milk interfering with the liver's ability to process bilirubin. However, there is no research to support this theory. Instead, breast milk has been shown to increase the absorption of bilirubin from stool through the intestines, which leads to a slower drop in bilirubin or prolonged jaundice.

Prolonged jaundice should be evaluated by the baby's caregiver and treated when indicated. Prolonged jaundice is associated with infection, hypothyroidism and intestinal obstruction.

Problems with the let-down reflex. Extreme stress, inadequate nipple stimulation and excessive amounts of alcohol, caffeine and tobacco all may delay or inhibit the let-down reflex.[33] Eliminate or limit your intake of alcohol and caffeine, and reduce as much as possible the number of cigarettes you smoke.

To reduce your stress and increase the stimulation to your breasts, spend a day in bed with your baby to help increase your milk supply. Pick a day when you have help with meals, household chores and your other children. Spend the day nursing your baby as often as possible, eating and drinking well, sleeping, nurturing yourself and letting others nurture you. Besides helping to restore your milk supply and helping you catch up on needed rest, this specifically focused day can help a baby with suckling at the breast, can improve your baby's weight gain, and can provide a wonderful opportunity to learn more about your baby.

Inadequate milk supply. Sometimes, the baby does not get enough milk because the mother is not producing enough milk to meet the baby's current needs for milk. If you feel that your milk supply is inadequate, try the following suggestions:

Ways to Increase Your Breast Milk Supply

1. Feed frequently, at least eight to twelve times in twenty-four hours.

2. Never limit feedings. Let your baby feed for as long as he needs to feed. (Usually, a feeding lasts ten to thirty minutes on each breast.)

3. Make sure your baby is latched well onto the breast and that you are able to hear him swallow as he suckles. Otherwise, try again until he is latched well and you hear him swallow.

4. Take your baby to bed with you and feed him skin-to-skin. Stay in bed as long as you are able. This gives you time to rest and pay close attention to your baby's feeding cues. Nuzzling and feeding frequently enhance milk production.

5. Get help from a breastfeeding expert who may encourage you to:

- Rent a commercial electric double pump. Pump after each of eight feedings for ten to fifteen minutes. If your baby is not able to nurse, pump whenever your baby feeds, to build your milk supply.
- If you need to supplement your baby, feed your baby your expressed breast milk (or prescribed formula, if you do not have enough expressed breast milk) via a tube attached to your breast, using a syringe or bottle-feeding device to hold the milk. In this way, your baby receives all his milk from your breast and stimulates you to make more milk.

When a good milk supply dwindles. If you have had an adequate milk supply and your baby has gained weight well, but now your milk supply has decreased, consider the following possibilities:

- Have you begun to take birth control pills containing oestrogen? This type of birth control pill can decrease your milk supply.
- Have you recently returned to employment or another time-consuming activity? Feeding less frequently can affect milk supply.
- Are you offering more supplemental bottles and not breastfeeding as often? This situation decreases breast milk supply.

If you can determine the reason, take the steps listed above to increase your supply. If you do not produce more milk, seek the help of a breastfeeding expert.

Spitting Up or Vomiting

Spitting up some milk after feeding is not unusual for breastfeeding babies. Some babies seem to spit up more than others, and it often occurs while burping or following a feeding. Usually, the amount of milk spit up ranges from a dribble to 2–3 tablespoons. If your baby regularly or occasionally spits up and is otherwise healthy and growing well, do not worry. Spitting up is really more an inconvenience than a concern.

Spitting up is more common when a mother has a strong let-down reflex and an abundant milk supply. It may also occur because your baby gulps air while feeding. Try sitting your baby up for feedings to help her with the rapid flow of milk. (See page 437.)

If your baby vomits frequently after feedings, is not growing well, does not have frequent bowel movements and wet nappies, or seems sick, she should be seen by her care provider. He or she can determine if your baby has a condition that must be treated.

Sore Nipples

Sore nipples may occur at any time but are most common during the first weeks of breastfeeding. Soreness may range from discomfort only when the infant first grasps the nipple to pain that continues throughout and between feedings. Sore nipples can almost always be treated successfully. In severe cases, the nipples may crack and bleed, but even these cases can be successfully treated without stopping breastfeeding. A description of the common causes for sore nipples follows. In cases in which the cause is not easily determined and treated, see your caregiver for help.

Early tenderness. Research has shown that most women have some degree of tenderness at the beginning of the first feedings. This type of pain usually lasts a week or less.[34] The tenderness probably results from the physical tugging, compressing and rubbing of the baby's mouth on the nipple and areola that occurs as babies learn to breastfeed. The nipples may appear a little reddened, bruised or swollen. Mothers feel a burning sensation that causes them to grimace and breathe rapidly. As the feeding progresses, the pain subsides. To help reduce some of the pain, hand express a few drops of milk to soften the areola before feeding, and focus on helping your baby latch well. Some women find the use of special breast creams to be soothing, but they are not necessary to resolve the discomfort.

Nipple soreness related to poor latch. A poor latch is the most common cause of nipples that remain sore throughout the feeding. Maternal factors associated with poor latch include breast fullness, engorgement, or flat or inverted nipples. Infant factors associated with poor latch include latching with a slightly open (not wide open) mouth, a tight frenulum ('tongue tie'), biting with feeding or tucking the lower lip inwards during feedings. One or both nipples may crack and bleed. Pain may continue between feedings. This type of nipple soreness makes mothers dread feeding. Following are some suggestions for prevention and treatment:

- Correct the latch. Shape the nipple and areola so your baby can get more than the nipple in his mouth. Try compressing the areola to fit the angle of the baby's mouth. Try not compressing while holding the areola and centring the baby's mouth on your nipple. Use the method (or a variation of one) that works. If a poor latch is the problem, correcting it will result in instant relief of most of the soreness, even if your nipple is cracked and bleeding.
- Feed frequently. If you put off feeding, your breasts become fuller, making it more difficult for your baby to latch on.
- Begin feeding on the least sore side, since babies feed most vigorously at the beginning of a feeding.
- Hand express some milk before feeding, to soften the areola and make latching on easier.
- If your soreness is located where your baby's bottom lip has been positioned, your baby may have tucked his lower lip inwards over his gum. Gently pull his lip out and your pain should lessen.
- If you need to take him off the breast to reposition him, before pulling him away slip your finger into his mouth and break the suction so your nipple comes out easily.
- If you use breast pads, change them when they become wet. Cloth pads are often less irritating than paper.
- Breast shells can help a flat nipple protrude (see page 429) and they keep clothing from rubbing against a sore nipple.
- Take the pain relief medications, such as ibuprofen, that were given to you after birth.
- Be seen by a breastfeeding expert who can help you with latch and can suggest treatments that aid healing. She may suggest the use of special nipple creams or a hydrogel dressing (a gel-like circular dressing that has been shown to increase comfort and speed healing). If infection or allergy is suspected to be a problem, she may encourage you to see your caregiver or a dermatologist. In rare instances, she may suggest you pump your breasts for a day or two to give your nipples a rest from the baby's suckling.

Nipple soreness due to over-vigorous or incorrect pumping. If you need to pump milk (see page 451), choose a good quality manual or electric pump. Commercial electric pumps are the most efficient and effective. Such pumps can be rented. Be sure to read or listen to directions for use. Centre your nipple in the breast pump cup. When the nipple is not centred, friction is applied unevenly to the areola and the nipple becomes sore. Use only enough suction to cause milk to flow well. Too much suction stretches the areola too deep into the pump cup and may injure the tissue.

Nipple soreness due to infection. Nipple soreness can be caused by infection of the nipple, including bacterial infections (most often caused by *Staphylococcus aureus*), fungal (yeast) infections and viral infections (such as a herpes sore). If you have a herpes sore on your nipple, you will have to discontinue breastfeeding on that side until it heals.

Bacterial infections often accompany cracked, bleeding nipples that remain sore for a long time. Your care provider may suggest the use of an antibiotic cream for your nipples and may prescribe a topical cream to reduce inflammation.

If both nipples are painful during and between feedings and the pain is sharp, deep and searing into the breast, you may have a *yeast infection*. Your nipples may appear pink and irritated, or they may appear normal. Occasionally, white yeast patches are present. Yeast infections are most common following antibiotic therapy or when the mother has a vaginal yeast infection. They also occur when the baby has a yeast nappy rash or has a yeast infection of his mouth (thrush). Both mother and baby should be treated to prevent one passing the infection to the other.

If you have a yeast infection of your breast, both you and your baby need to be treated whether he has any visible symptoms of a yeast infection or not. Consult your care provider or a breastfeeding expert for treatment suggestions. He or she may suggest a topical over-the-counter anti-fungal cream, such as miconazole, to treat your nipples and your baby's nappy rash, or you may take a prescribed oral medication. Your baby's caregiver may prescribe a liquid medication, such as nystatin suspension, to apply to the mucous membranes of your baby's mouth. If these treatments do not work, gentian violet (a dark purple liquid) applied to your nipples and your baby's mouth may be suggested.

Breast Pain on Let-Down

Some women experience a sharp, deep pain behind the areola at the beginning of each feeding. The pain, which subsides when the milk is flowing, does not indicate a problem and usually goes away in time without treatment. The pain is probably caused by the release of oxytocin, which shortens and widens the ductules and ducts, thereby increasing the pressure of the milk flow through them. Or, if you have had surgery on your breast in the past, such pain may be due to the stretching of scar tissue.

Leaking

Milk often leaks from the breasts in the first few weeks or months of nursing. The leaking usually subsides as your breasts become more finely tuned and 'learn' how much milk to make and when to let it down. Leaking between feedings usually occurs when your breasts are very full, when you hear your baby (or any baby) cry or when you are sexually aroused. Following are some suggestions for your comfort:

- When you start to feel the milk let down, press your hands or forearms firmly against your breasts to slow the flow of milk. This action can be done discreetly in public places.
- Compress your nipple between your thumb and forefinger to stop the flow of milk.
- To prevent soaking your clothes, wear washable cotton breast pads and change them when they become damp. Avoid the use of breast pads with plastic liners, as they retain moisture, which contributes to nipple soreness.

Plugged Ducts

The gradual development of a tender, swollen lump in the breast, not accompanied by a fever, is usually a *plugged duct*. The plugged duct may feel sore and lumpy and may be reddened. The following steps help to relieve the discomfort:

- Apply a warm, moist compress to the sore area before and during feedings.
- Feed from the affected breast first.
- Massage the area towards the nipple during feedings.
- While showering, massage your breast with your fingers pressing from the plugged duct towards the nipple.
- Avoid poorly fitting bras; they may obstruct milk ducts. Also, check the fit of your baby carrier. In some carriers, the straps press on the breasts. If worn for several hours, this prolonged pressure may lead to a plugged duct.

Any lump that does not go away within a week or two needs to be evaluated by your care provider.

Mastitis

Mastitis is an infection of the breast, which can occur at any time while you are nursing. Mastitis comes on suddenly. The breast may have a tender, reddened area or the whole breast may be involved. Symptoms include fever, chills, fatigue, headache, and sometimes nausea and vomiting. Many women feel as though they have a severe flu. If you have these symptoms, call your caregiver. Your caregiver will probably prescribe antibiotics, advise you to continue nursing, and encourage you to drink fluids and spend as much time resting as possible.

- Continue to nurse from both breasts. The milk is not harmful to your baby.
- Take all the prescribed antibiotics. If you stop taking the antibiotics when you start to feel better, the infection will return.
- If you are not feeling better within twenty-four hours after starting antibiotic treatment, call your caregiver. You may need a different antibiotic.
- Rest and stay in bed until you feel better.
- Apply a warm wet compress over the painful area to help increase circulation to the breast.
- Take ibuprofen or acetaminophen to reduce fever, pain and inflammation.
- Avoid constricting bras and clothing so that milk may flow easily. During feedings, massage your breasts if massage feels comfortable.

Expressing and Storing Breast Milk

Collecting your milk using hand expression or a pump becomes easier with practice. You need clean hands, clean equipment, and clean bottles or disposable bottle liners, or any clean container meant for food storage.

Hand Expression

Expressing by hand is effective, inexpensive and always available. To hand express your breast milk, place your thumb on the top of your areola and your fingers below.

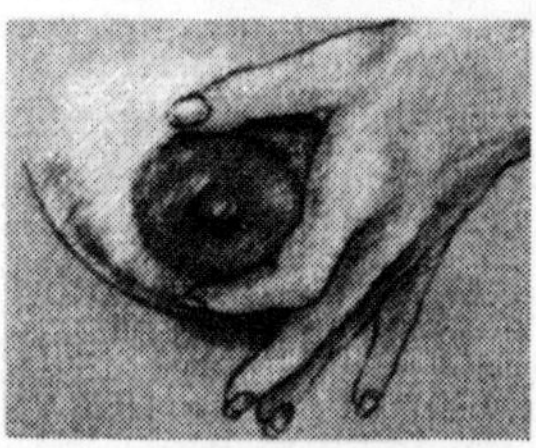

Finger placement for hand expression

Lift your breast and gently press it against your chest wall with your hand. Compress your milk sinuses between the pads of your thumb and fingers. Continue pressing your fingers together and pressing your breast against your body until the flow of milk stops. Repeat this process until the flow of milk slows and you have the milk you need. Collect your milk in a measuring cup or special collecting device available at breastfeeding stores. At first, you may get only drops of milk, but with practice you will get a steady spray.

Circumstances in Which Pumping Is Helpful or Necessary

Sometimes, it is more efficient and desirable to use a pump to express your milk, as in the following circumstances:

- Your baby is in the neonatal intensive care unit and unable to breastfeed.
- Your baby is in the special care nursery and is not yet able to feed frequently or vigorously.
- You are trying to build or rebuild a milk supply.
- You need to express breast milk to supplement the milk that your baby receives by breastfeeding.
- You must leave your baby because of employment outside the home.
- You must leave your baby to travel.
- You are having a medical procedure or taking a medication that is unsafe for your baby. In this case, you can temporarily stop breastfeeding and still maintain your milk supply by pumping until it is safe to resume breastfeeding.

Pumping Your Milk

To pump your milk, you can buy or rent a pump. A breastfeeding expert, midwife or doctor may help you select a pump. If only an occasional bottle is needed, hand expression or a manual pump is sufficient. If you need to pump several bottles or more a day, or if you are pumping to build or maintain your milk supply, you may need to rent or buy an electric breast pump with a double pumping setup. The following suggestions may be helpful:

- Find a private, uninterrupted, warm environment for pumping. Take your phone off the hook or let your answering machine pick up messages. If you have older children, find an activity they can enjoy while you are pumping.
- If you have time, massage your breasts before pumping. To massage your breasts, cup your hands around your breasts and stroke gently but firmly from the chest wall towards the areola, or jiggle or gently shake your breasts. You can also stroke your breasts lightly with your fingertips to simulate the sensations of a let-down.
- Develop a ritual such as having a glass of water or cup of tea. Listen to familiar music or a relaxation tape while you pump.
- If you are separated from your baby while pumping, imagine you are nursing your baby or look at pictures of your baby and visualise your milk flowing.

Breast Milk Storage

The following guidelines are for milk storage for healthy, term infants; if your baby is in a neonatal intensive care unit or special care nursery, you may be given other guidelines. Fresh breast milk can be stored for ten hours in a room with temperatures ranging between 19°C and 22°C, and in a refrigerator kept at 0–2°C for eight days. It can be safely stored in the freezer (set at the lowest setting) of a combination refrigerator-freezer for three to four months. Place the milk at the back of the freezer away from the door, where the temperature remains coldest. Breast milk can also be stored in a deep freeze with a constant temperature of -18°C for six months or longer. Milk frozen for six months or longer remains an excellent source of nutrition for your infant.[35]

Breast milk can be stored in clean glass or plastic bottles or feeding bags designed for breast milk storage. If bottle liner bags are used, it is best to double-bag the milk, as these bags are less durable than those designed for breast milk storage. Always leave room at the top of the bag or bottle for expansion of the milk as it freezes. Label the container with the date the milk was collected. Use the oldest milk first. Breast milk loses some (not all) of its anti-infective and nutritional properties over time and with freezing and heating. Still, it is far more nutritious than formula.

To thaw frozen breast milk, place the milk container in warm water. As the water cools, exchange it with more warm water. Breast milk can be fed to the baby at room temperature or slightly warmer. Never thaw breast milk in the microwave or in a pan on the stove. Many important anti-infective properties can be destroyed, and there is a risk the baby could be burned with unevenly heated milk. Breast milk should be gently shaken to mix the fat (which rises to the top during storage) back into the milk. Once breast milk is thawed, it can be safely kept in the refrigerator up to twenty-four hours. It should not be refrozen.[36]

Feeding Your Baby Expressed Breast Milk or Supplemental Formula

When your baby needs your expressed milk or supplemental formula, there are many ways she can be fed. The method you use depends on many factors, including your baby's age and maturity, how long you are apart from her, and if the supplementation is permanent or temporary. In complicated situations, a breastfeeding expert can assist you with a feeding plan.

Whenever a breastfed baby is unable to feed at the breast or when she needs extra milk, providing expressed breast milk is best. When that is not possible, an appropriate formula can be used. Following are some methods for feeding your baby with expressed milk or supplemental formula:

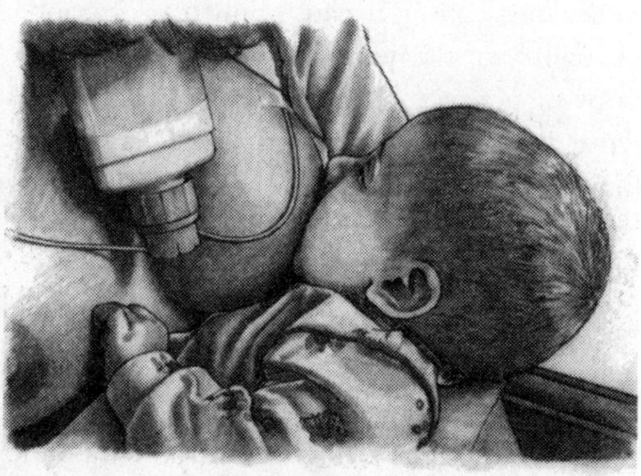

Supply Line system

Droppers, spoons and cups. Droppers, spoons and small medicine cups can be used to feed breastfed babies small amounts of supplemental milk. These devices provide a temporary solution for supplementation and have the advantage of avoiding the early introduction to bottle teats.

Tubes. Tubes can be attached to the breast to deliver milk from syringes or from commercial bottles and bags. The baby can receive the extra milk she needs while breastfeeding by means of a tube that is connected to a container (syringe, bottle or bag) filled with milk. The tube is placed next to the nipple and attached to the breast with paper tape. The container of milk may either be hung by a cord around your neck or pinned to your shirt, depending on the device used. The syringe and tube device is intended for temporary use. The tube and bottle or bag device can be used for the entire time you are breastfeeding, if you are unable to produce enough milk for total breastfeeding. The Supply Line system (available from your pharmacy) is a bottle with two tubes that can be attached to each breast. A breastfeeding expert can show you how to supplement in this way. This methods has the advantage of providing all the baby's nutrition while she suckles at her mother's breast.

Bottles. Bottles can be used to feed babies or provide supplemental milk. If possible, wait to use bottles until the baby is breastfeeding reliably (usually after several weeks). Bottles have the advantage of being easy to use. Because of the ease of feeding, however, they have the possible disadvantage of teaching a breastfed baby to prefer the bottle to breastfeeding. If you are introducing a bottle because you must be away for an extended time or you are returning to work, the first bottle-feeding may be a challenge for the baby's father, friend or day-care provider. If you know you will want your baby to use a bottle, offer the bottle between four and eight weeks of age and give it regularly, but only after the baby latches onto the breast quickly and easily with every breastfeeding. Waiting until the baby is several months old may make it more difficult to introduce the bottle, because as time passes many babies become reluctant to take the bottle. If the baby is older or is reluctant to take the bottle right away, consider these suggestions:

- Sucking from a bottle is a new experience for a breastfed baby. Babies are able to learn something new most easily when they are calm. Offer 15–30 millilitres of milk after a breastfeeding. The goal is to acquaint your baby with a bottle before she is expected to take an entire feeding from it.
- Some babies do well with a bottle if they are distracted by your talking or singing and not focused on the fact that they are not breastfeeding.
- If your baby absolutely refuses the bottle, do not push her to continue trying. Have her caretaker use a dropper, cup or spoon to feed her enough milk to take the edge off her hunger. Then try later with the bottle. Eventually, she will accept this method of feeding.
- There is no perfect bottle or teat and none are like the breast. So choose a teat and brand that looks durable and easy-to-clean and stick with it until your baby becomes familiar with it.
- If your goal is to continue breastfeeding, make sure your baby has more opportunities to breastfeed than bottle-feed.

Special Situations

Under certain circumstances such as the ones described below, breastfeeding mothers and their babies need more support and persistence than usual to establish lactation or to continue breastfeeding. A breastfeeding expert from your hospital or a baby health centre can help you in these challenging situations. Your childbirth educator or baby's care provider can make a referral.

Caesarean Birth

If you have had a caesarean, recovering from childbirth and from the surgery is challenging. You need help with household chores so you can concentrate on rest, comfort and feeding your baby. Try feeding lying down or sitting upright with your back supported and a pillow on your lap. Choose the position that is most comfortable for you. Take your pain relief medication, because only trace amounts actually get into your breast milk. With time, moving about and taking care of yourself and your baby will become easier. Women who have had caesareans are just as successful at starting and continuing to breastfeed as women who have given birth vaginally.

Premature Infants

It is both possible and desirable to breastfeed if your baby is premature. At a time when you may feel sad and worried about her wellbeing, it helps to know that you can do something important for your baby that no one else can do. If your baby is not yet able to suckle well, express your colostrum with a pump. Many hospitals have efficient electric breast pumps. As soon as your baby is able to take oral feedings, this expressed colostrum and milk can be fed to your baby by tube or dropper until she is able to suckle at your breast. You will need the continuing support of your partner, the nursing staff, a breastfeeding expert, and/or a support group to establish and maintain your breast milk supply and to overcome some of the obstacles you may encounter in the process. A support group can help immensely with advice, not only on breastfeeding but also on practical matters such as where to get tiny baby clothes and how to juggle time with your hospitalised baby with the other demands of your life.

Mothers who give birth to premature infants produce milk that is different from the milk produced by the mother of a full-term infant. Especially well suited to the unique nutritional needs of the premature baby, the mother's milk is higher in protein, nitrogen, sodium, calcium, fat and calories. Also, because hospitalised premature infants are at risk for infection, the protective components of breast milk are especially important. Breastfed premature infants have lower rates of infection and serious bowel problems than formula-fed premature infants.[37] Also, breastfed premature infants have been found to have higher IQ scores at seven and one-half to eight years of age compared to formula-fed premature infants.[38]

Spending time in the nursery with your premature baby exposes you to some of the organisms that can cause infection in your baby. Because you have a mature immune system, your body makes antibodies to protect you from these organisms. The antibodies are present in your breast milk, and when your premature baby gets your milk, she is protected from infection. Your ability to make these antibodies is enhanced when you hold your baby skin-to-skin as with kangaroo care. (See pages 304 and 409.)

Tandem Nursing

Mothers who breastfeed their newborn and their older child at the same time are *tandem nursing*. Tandem nursing allows the mother to maintain a nursing relationship with her older child and at the same time develop a nursing relationship with her baby. Because the newborn's needs for colostrum and breast milk are important, the baby is fed first. Toddlers can be encouraged to wait until the baby has finished feeding. As the baby grows older, both baby and older sibling can be nursed at the same time. Sometimes, the older child's desire to nurse is temporary as she adjusts to the new baby, and sometimes she just wants to nurse occasionally. In these situations, tandem nursing provides an opportunity for the mother, older child and baby to have special moments breastfeeding, and helps the mother and older child adjust to the changes in the family.

Tandem nursing is more challenging when the older child nurses very frequently and cannot wait to feed. In this instance, getting support from a breastfeeding expert or your childbirth educator can be very helpful and reassuring.

Nursing While Pregnant

If you become pregnant while you are still nursing a toddler or older child, you will face the decision of whether to continue breastfeeding or to wean that child. This can be a difficult decision to make. You may want to continue breastfeeding but may find that one of the earliest symptoms of pregnancy is sore nipples and fatigue. In addition, your older child may become less interested in nursing as the flavour of the milk changes and there is a decrease in volume due to the hormones of pregnancy. However, if you are healthy and well nourished and have a nursing child (older than one year) when you become pregnant, you will probably have no difficulty nursing through your pregnancy.

Babies whose mothers nursed through a pregnancy were similar in size when compared to babies born to mothers who weaned six months before becoming pregnant. Also, breastfeeding while pregnant did not adversely affect the pregnancy.[39]

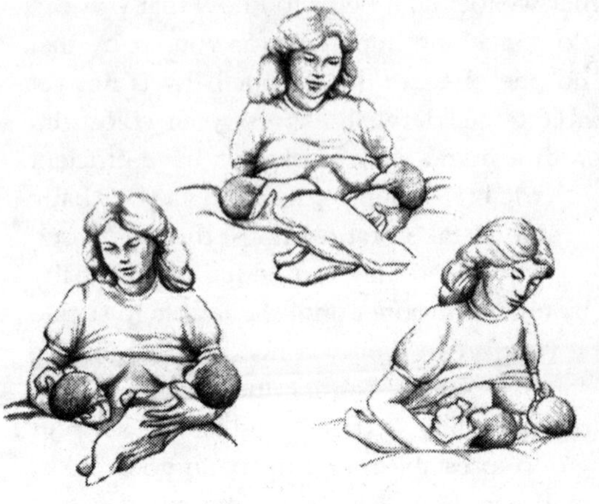

Ways to feed two babies at the same time

Breastfeeding Multiples

It is possible for you to exclusively breastfeed twins and triplets. In the beginning, though, it is more difficult than feeding one baby. Also, because there is a higher incidence of prematurity with multiples, the challenge of feeding multiples may be further complicated.

Soon after you discover you are expecting more than one baby, begin lining up the support and help you will need once the babies are born. Make contact with a support group for parents of multiples. Such groups help parents prepare for the extra work and offer suggestions about the best ways to cope. Contact a breastfeeding expert to learn about the special challenges of feeding multiples and to learn about useful equipment such as breastfeeding pillows that make feeding easier. The breastfeeding expert can provide you with breastfeeding help and support in the early days and weeks. Family, friends and possibly hired help can assist you with baby care and household chores. This will also make sure you have many opportunities for rest and sleep.

In the beginning, you may find it easier to feed one baby at a time. As time passes and you become familiar with each baby and comfortable with breastfeeding, feeding two babies at the same time (if they are willing) saves you time. Your need for calories and nourishment is greater than for mothers feeding one baby. Have a friend or relative make you some nutritious muffins filled with dried fruit, whole grains and nuts. You can freeze them and, when you need a snack, defrost one and eat it along with a glass of water or milk for a quick, tasty snack.

Breastfeeding When the Mother or Baby Is Ill or Hospitalised

If you are hospitalised soon after birth or later, you may have several options for baby care and feeding depending on your condition and the treatments you are receiving. Many hospitals allow your partner to stay in your room with you and care for your baby there. You can breastfeed your baby or pump your milk for your baby and have a chance to cuddle and be near him. If you are separated from your baby, you may be able to pump your milk so your baby can have it at home. Hospital breastfeeding experts do visit surgical and medical floors and can assist you in person or by phone.

If your baby is ill or hospitalised, your presence is essential to his wellbeing. Your breast milk helps protect him from infections and helps bolster his immune system, and breastfeeding gives him the closeness and comfort he needs. If he is unable to nurse, pump and save your milk until he is able to take oral feedings. Having an ill or hospitalised baby is very upsetting. Being able to breastfeed or provide your baby with your expressed milk is a personal way to contribute to his recovery.

Use of Medications and Drugs during Breastfeeding

You may wonder whether the drugs and medications you take appear in your breast milk and have an effect on your baby. With few exceptions, any medication or drug you take will be present to some degree in your breast milk. Most medications do not present a problem for your baby, but there are some that do.

Some practical considerations. Always consult your caregiver and your baby's caregiver or a breastfeeding expert about *any* medication you plan to take while breastfeeding. This includes prescription medications, over-the-counter medications and herbal remedies. Street drugs such as cocaine, heroin, methamphetamines and so forth pose serious risks for you and your baby and should not be used during breastfeeding.

Ask the following questions:

- Do I absolutely need this medication now?
- Could the medication be delayed until the baby is more mature and better able to handle the medication?
- Is there a safer alternative? (For example, could an antibiotic be chosen for the mother that could be safely given to the infant, or could the dosage of the medication be reduced and still be therapeutic?)
- Could the medication be given topically (rubbed on the skin) rather than taken orally? Topical preparations usually result in lower levels of medication in breast milk.
- Could the timing of the medication or the feedings be scheduled so the smallest amount is in the breast milk? (Remember that time-release medications and some drugs take a long time to clear the body.)
- Should breastfeeding be temporarily interrupted when medications considered unsafe for breastfeeding are given? The mother would pump and discard her milk

until the treatment is complete and the medication is out of her system.

- What symptoms that could be side effects of using maternal medication should parents watch for in their infants?
- Does the caregiver or breastfeeding expert with whom you consult have access to the most accurate data and books about medication use during breastfeeding? (See Recommended Resources for current books on medication use during lactation.)

Medications used for pain relief following childbirth are generally safe for breastfeeding. Do take the pain medication you need to remain comfortable. Your care provider knows which medications are safe for breastfeeding infants. Stool softeners and haemorrhoid medications will not bother your baby.

No vaccinations are contraindicated for the breastfeeding mother. So, if you need to have the mumps, measles and rubella (MMR) vaccination after birth or you want to have a flu shot, it is safe to do so.[40]

Birth control pills containing oestrogen should not be taken during breastfeeding, as this can decrease your milk supply. 'Progestin only' types of contraception, including the 'mini pill' and Depo-Provera, are considered compatible with breastfeeding.

When a mother smokes, her baby is exposed to second-hand smoke. In addition, nicotine and other chemicals in the tobacco get into the breast milk. If you smoke, avoid smoking in the presence of your baby. Exposure to cigarette smoke increases the incidence of sudden infant death, respiratory infections and ear infections. Try to cut down on the number of cigarettes you smoke a day, to reduce the effect on your baby and improve your health. Smoking is associated with increased fussiness in the baby.[41] However, it is still better for an infant to be breastfed than formula-fed when the mother smokes. Formula-fed infants of smoking mothers are seven times more likely to develop respiratory illnesses than breastfed infants of mothers who smoke.[42]

When You Need to Wean

Sometimes, due to unexpected circumstances such as the death of a baby or a serious medical condition for the mother, women need help with unanticipated weaning. Sometimes, a woman must wean to qualify for acceptance into an infertility treatment program. In each of these instances, there is sadness, grieving and uncertainty. If you are weaning because of a medical reason, you may be able to wean gradually over several days.

If your baby has died, it is not necessary to immediately and actively begin to suppress your milk production. Some women have found comfort in expressing their milk for donation to a milk bank in remembrance of their baby. If you want to comfortably suppress milk production, wear a snug-fitting supportive bra to provide comfort as your breasts swell. Ice packs applied to your breasts over your bra or light clothing and taking ibuprofen to reduce inflammation help. The soreness of full breasts may last a day or two. You make leak milk for a week or more.

If you are weaning in an attempt to become pregnant again or for personal reasons, you may want to take several days or more to gradually wean your baby. You may want to have a weaning ritual in which you celebrate the time you had together breastfeeding. Throwing a party or reading a meaningful poem or letter can be satisfying and helpful. Eliminate feedings gradually, leaving the most important feedings (morning and night-time) for last. Gradually replace feedings with formula from a bottle or cup, as appropriate. Use the comfort measures described above if your breasts become swollen and sore.

Working Outside the Home

It is possible to breastfeed exclusively and to work outside the home by expressing and storing milk to be fed to your baby while you are away. The more flexible your job and the longer your maternity leave, the easier it will be for you to combine breastfeeding and work. You might consider switching to part-time employment, establishing a work schedule of longer days with an opportunity to take one or two long feeding breaks during the day, or choosing a daycare setting near or at your workplace so you can nurse your baby during your breaks and at lunch time. You might also discuss with your employer the possibility of telecommuting full-time or part-time. You could then feed your baby regularly during the workday. If feeding your baby during the workday is not an option, make arrangements for time and privacy to express or pump milk at work. Follow the storage guidelines on page 452 for your milk. Mothers who are not able to pump at work can still breastfeed. This requires feeding frequently when at home. Many babies go on a 'reverse feeding schedule', feeding in the evenings and at night and taking few, if any, supplements at day care.

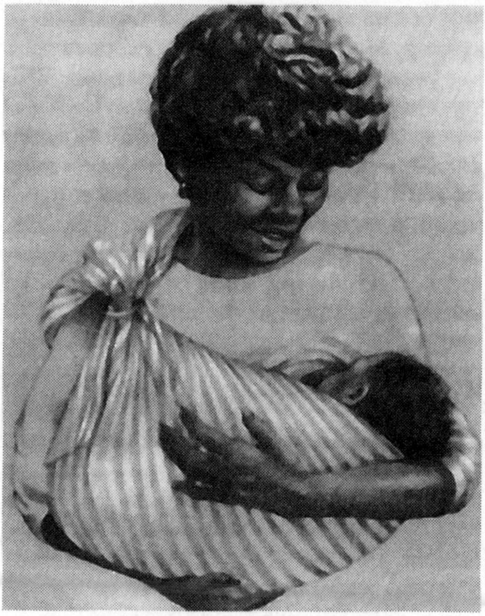

Breastfeed whenever possible

The longer you are able to wait to return to work, the easier it is. If you are able to extend your maternity leave until your baby feeds less frequently, is taking solid foods and is on a more predictable schedule, breastfeeding will be easier.

Some working mothers decide to breastfeed while at home and supplement with formula while they are away. The breasts are amazingly cooperative in producing enough milk as long as you continue to nurse frequently when you are with your baby. If your milk supply begins to dwindle, nurse frequently during the evening and on days off to stimulate your milk production. The extra work it takes to continue breastfeeding and to provide your baby with expressed milk pays off in many ways, especially in protecting your baby from infections he is exposed to in a day-care setting.

Re-lactation

It may be possible to re-establish lactation after you have stopped nursing or after you have been separated from your baby. However, it requires persistence and commitment to succeed on your part (as well as an interested baby). Frequent, round-the-clock nursing is the most effective method. You may use a Supply Line system. This device encourages the baby to suckle at an empty or near-empty breast while receiving supplemental formula. The suckling stimulates milk production while the device provides your baby with enough milk for growth. Your milk supply may be increased by using an electric pump following feeding. A breastfeeding expert who is knowledgeable about re-lactation can support and advise you if you decide to re-establish breastfeeding.

Mothers who wish to breastfeed their adopted babies can use these same methods. Even though they may never have had a pregnancy or nursed a baby, these mothers can sometimes produce breast milk (though usually not a full supply) and have the experience of breastfeeding. Often, even a small amount of breast milk reduces problems with constipation that are common with formula-fed infants.

Breastfeeding and Fertility

Exclusive breastfeeding greatly reduces the chance of becoming pregnant. You have less than a 2 percent chance of becoming pregnant if:

- Your baby is less than six months of age.
- You have not had a period until after fifty-six days post partum.
- You are nursing frequently (at least every four hours during the day and every six hours at night).
- You rarely supplement, giving tastes of foods or fluids only occasionally.[43]

After you begin giving solid foods, you can extend some of the protection breastfeeding provides to prevent pregnancy by breastfeeding before solid foods are offered at each meal and by continuing to breastfeed during the day and night. It is important to know that you can ovulate before you have a period. Therefore, talk to your midwife or doctor about appropriate methods of contraception while you are breastfeeding. Barrier methods (such as condoms and diaphragms), intrauterine devices (IUDs), and progestin-only pills ('mini pill') and injections (Depo-Provera) are considered compatible with breastfeeding. Birth control pills containing oestrogen are associated with a reduced milk supply and shorter duration of breastfeeding, especially when they are begun in the early weeks of breastfeeding.[44]

Formula Feeding

An iron-fortified, commercially prepared formula is recommended for infants under a year who are fully or partially formula-fed. Evaporated milk formulas are not well suited to your baby's nutritional needs. Whole, 2 percent, 1 percent or fat-free cow milk and goat milk are not good choices for infants under one year of age; they are difficult for babies to digest and they lack many important and necessary nutrients. Your baby's doctor can recommend a formula for your baby and give you guidelines on how much to feed your baby. Because commercial formulas are fortified with vitamins and minerals, your baby will not require a vitamin supplement. So, if you change from breastfeeding to formula feeding, discontinue any vitamins you gave your baby while nursing. An exception might be a fluoride supplement after six months of age, if your water supply does not contain fluoride.

Infant Formulas

Most infant formulas are made from cow milk or soybeans. Except in extremely rare instances, an iron-fortified formula is best. Low-iron formula is recommended in rare medical conditions such as hyperferrenaemia (excessive iron stores). Contrary to a common belief, low-iron formula does not decrease colic, constipation, diarrhoea, fussiness or vomiting. When infants are fed low-iron formula, their risk for becoming anaemic (having low iron) is greatly increased. Also, the use of low-iron formula is associated with lower cognitive test scores at age five.[45]

The best choice of formula for a healthy infant with no cow milk allergy is an iron-fortified cow-milk-based formula. Soymilk formulas are recommended only when a baby is unable to digest milk sugar (such as a baby with a rare condition called galactosemia) or when the family chooses to have a vegetarian-based diet with no animal protein. In those cases, select a soymilk formula that is iron-fortified. Contrary to a popular belief, infants can be allergic to soymilk. Up to 25 percent of babies with a milk allergy are also allergic to soy.[46] When allergy is a concern, your baby's caregiver may suggest a hypo-allergenic (does not cause allergy) formula. These formulas are more expensive than the more commonly used formulas. Choose a brand of formula you like and your baby tolerates, and stick with it. All babies, whether breast- or formula-fed, get gassy. Switching formulas does not decrease gas or reduce constipation.

Formulas are available in ready-to-feed preparations, canned liquid concentrates and a powdered form. They are all equal in their nutritive value. The powdered formula is least expensive, while the ready-to-feed is slightly more expensive than the concentrate. The ready-to-feed formula might be useful for trips or during the early days of post partum, to save you time.

When preparing formula, carefully follow the directions on the can or package. If your water supply is safe for drinking, you may use tap water to mix formula. If you are using water from a well or source that may not be safe for drinking, boil the water before using it to mix formula. You can use bottled water and water from a water-filter container; do not use distilled water, as it lacks some of the beneficial minerals found in water. Always use the correct amount of water to mix formula. If you use too little water with the concentrate or powder, you can cause diarrhoea, dehydration and other problems for your baby. If you use too much water, your baby will not receive enough calories and nutrients to thrive.

Equipment: Bottles and Teats

There are many choices of bottles. Glass bottles are easy to clean and do not become stained by formula, but they are heavy and can break. Plastic bottles are lightweight and do not crack or break easily. Some feeding units use a disposable plastic bag for the formula inside a rigid plastic container. The feeding bag system reduces the work of cleaning bottles, but it is not as easy to mix formula in a bag as it is in a bottle.

There are also a variety of teats to choose from. Select one your baby likes and then stay with that type of teat. Before feeding, check the teat to be sure formula drips from the bottle. If it comes out in a stream, the teat hole is too big and your baby will get too much too fast and she may spit up. If the milk drips very slowly or not at all, your baby may tire and not get enough (or any) milk. If the teat hole is too large, discard the teat. If it is too small, check to be sure old formula is not clogging the hole, or pierce the hole with the tip of a clean needle and check it again.

If your water supply is safe for drinking, then bottles and teats do not need to be sterilised. Bottles may be washed by hand or in the dishwasher. Teats can be cleaned with a teat brush using hot soapy water, rinsed with hot water and dried thoroughly.

Tips for Formula Feeding

Feeding your baby can be a wonderful and enjoyable experience. Cuddling your baby during feedings and even holding your baby skin-to-skin gives your baby the closeness she needs. The cuddling and feeding promote bonding and provide you with some wonderful memories.

You can make your baby's feedings consistently successful and happy by remembering to do a few simple things:

- Hold your baby in a semi-reclining position rather than flat on her back. She will be more comfortable for feeding and will swallow less air.
- Hold your baby sometimes in your right arm and sometimes in your left, to promote normal eye muscle development and symmetrical neck muscle development. Your baby will gaze at you as she feeds.
- In the beginning, burp your baby about halfway through the feedings. Babies that gulp air often need to burp more. As she grows older, she does not need your help to burp; she will burp any accumulated air on her own.
- In the first few days of life, full-term babies feed from eight to twelve times in twenty-four hours. As they grow older, they take more at each feeding and eat less often.

- Trust your baby to let you know how much she needs to eat. She may not always be interested in taking the same amount at each feeding. Do not coax her to empty the bottle if she seems satisfied. When she rapidly and consistently finishes each feeding, it is time to add another 30 millilitres of formula to her bottle.
- Offering your baby warmed milk is a way of making feeding more comfortable. Always check to be sure the milk is comfortably warm and not hot. As she grows older, she may prefer room temperature or cool formula.
- Never prop a bottle and leave your baby alone for feedings. Interacting with a loving person during feeding helps her thrive emotionally and develop trust in you and those who care for her.
- Babies do not need extra water or water bottles until they begin taking solid foods. Never mix honey in the baby's water or dip pacifiers in honey. Feeding honey (cooked or uncooked) to a baby less than one year of age has been associated with infant botulism.

Conclusion

Feeding your baby has far greater significance than simply providing nutrients and calories for physical growth. A baby whose feeding cues are consistently responded to develops a sense of trust, security and well-being. A baby who is smiled at, talked to and cuddled develops a sense of emotional security. And holding your baby close stimulates the senses of touch, smell and taste. All these things occur during feeding. Feeding also provides many opportunities for your baby to express affection towards and appreciation of you—by cooing, grinning, patting and other endearing behaviours. Feeding time is an important catalyst for the emotional development of the infant and the strengthening of family ties.

Chapter 16

Preparing Other Children for Birth and the Baby

If you are expecting your second child (or third or more), you will want to prepare your older child for the birth of a sibling—a baby brother or sister. You will need to teach your child in a realistic and age-appropriate manner about pregnancy, birth and life with a newborn. This chapter offers a variety of suggestions for preparing your child. Some will be more appropriate than others, depending on the age and maturity of your child and your plans and desires. Several books listed in the Recommended Resources can also help prepare you and your child for another baby. (For additional information, see the sections on 'When You Are Pregnant Again' on page 37 and 'Note to Parents Having Another Baby' on page 373.)

Preparations before the Birth

When to Announce the Pregnancy

When is it best to tell your child you are pregnant? If you are especially tired or are vomiting each morning, you might announce the pregnancy early in order to relieve a child who may be worried that you are ill. On the other hand, announcing it very early means a long waiting period for a young child who has little, if any, concept of time. Some parents prefer to announce the pregnancy after the first trimester, when the likelihood of miscarriage is reduced. Others put it off until later, when the pregnancy becomes obvious. Linking the expected birth date to a special event or season makes the wait more understandable. Making a special calendar together helps the child who repeatedly asks when the baby will come.

Some parents feel reluctant to announce the pregnancy because they worry about displacing the older child; however, waiting does not diminish these feelings of displacement. In addition, waiting too long risks your child's hearing about your pregnancy from someone else. Try to announce the pregnancy early enough to allow time to ease your child's adjustments by including her in the preparations and providing her an opportunity to develop positive feelings and realistic expectations about the new baby.

Involving Your Child during the Pregnancy

The following suggestions will help involve and prepare your child before the birth:

- Discuss with your young child what 'baby', 'brother' and 'sister' mean. Give examples of families you know who have more than one child.
- Talk to your child about pregnancy and birth. Find out what your child already knows, correct any misconceptions, fill in the gaps and answer questions. Use appropriate terms or examples such as the baby is in the 'uterus' ('a special place where babies grow') not in the 'stomach'

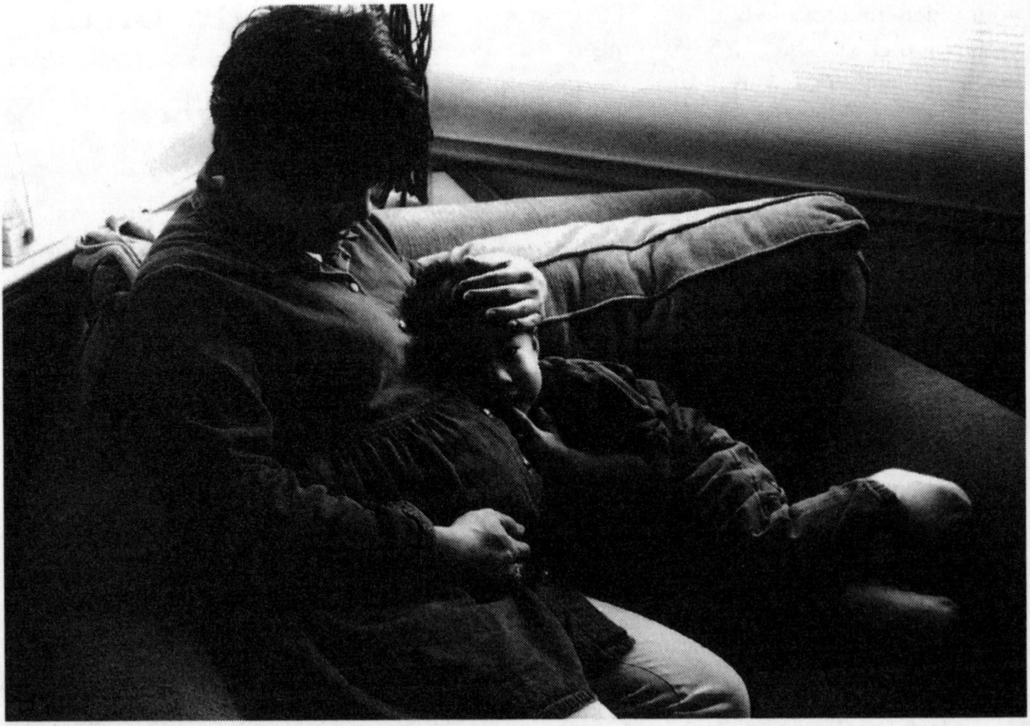

Photograph by Bruce Miyake

Your child will enjoy feeling the baby move, especially when the baby hiccups.

or 'tummy'. However, you will want to avoid overwhelming a small child with too much information.

- Read books to your child about pregnancy, birth, new babies and feelings about being a big brother or sister.
- Arrange to bring your child to one or more prenatal visits to meet your doctor or midwife.
- Let your child hear the baby's heartbeat and feel the baby move. Talk about foetal development with your child. Tell your child what the foetus can do (hiccup, suck his thumb, hear, wiggle and kick, for example).
- Attend a sibling preparation class if one is available in your area. Let your child see films, slides or pictures of births and newborns. A demonstration of a birth with a doll can also be helpful.
- Practise prenatal exercises with your child. Explain that these exercises help you feel better during pregnancy and afterwards.
- Take your child on a hospital tour, if possible. Talk about her coming to visit you there when the baby is born.
- Help your child make a picture book about pregnancy, birth, babies, big brothers and sisters, and families.
- Show your child photographs or videotapes of herself as a baby—especially ones showing you or her father caring for her as a newborn.
- Have your child see and interact with a friend's baby. Let her see how small and sometimes unplayful a baby is.
- Have your child help you pack your suitcase or the baby's bag for the hospital. If she will be staying with someone while you are in the hospital, have her pack her bag, including special gifts for those who will care for her.
- Make changes in room or sleeping arrangements several months before the birth, to prevent your child from feeling suddenly displaced by the baby. Talk with your child about where the baby will sleep. Tell your child the baby will be sleeping in your room. Set up the new baby's sleeping area to give your child time to become accustomed to where the new baby will be.
- Safety-proof your home if you have not already done so, since accidents can happen when you are busy with the new baby.

Follow your child's lead about how much and when to discuss birth and the baby. Be sensitive to the possibility of overloading your child with talk of a new baby.

Should Your Other Child Be Present When You Give Birth?

Many hospitals and birth centres today welcome children to be present at birth, and most invite children to visit their mother and baby sister or brother very soon after birth. They leave the decision to you. Caregivers and psychologists disagree in their opinions regarding children attending birth.[1] Most agree, however, that if a child spends time with his mother and the new baby soon after birth, it reduces separation anxiety and helps the child adjust to life with a new baby.

Some parents feel that it is too complicated and possibly disturbing to have their other child attend the birth. They are concerned about the logistics of caring for the child during labour, the gamble that the child will be in good health and the possibility of having to interrupt the child's sleep. Or, they are concerned about the child's reactions to his mother's pain and possible crying out, and to the presence of blood and possible use of instruments. They may feel their child is too young or will turn only to his mother for attention during labour, or may distract or disturb his mother or the staff.

Other parents feel that birth is a family event, and that if their child is well prepared and well cared for at the time, being at the birth will be a joyful and healthy experience. They feel a bond between the children will be created, and that positive, healthy attitudes about birth will be encouraged.

Assess your child's physical health and emotional readiness. The personality and maturity of your child are important considerations. If your child is ill and feels sick, he may not tolerate the birth experience well. If your child has had a recent painful, traumatic, or frightening experience involving his own body, doctors or hospitals, he may not be ready to attend a birth.

Obviously, you (and your child, if he is old enough to make such a decision) must want him to be present. Do not allow yourself to be talked into it if you are uncomfortable with the idea.

The decision is a personal one, best made by you, your partner and your child.

Guidelines for Having a Child Present at Birth

If you decide your child will be present, the following guidelines will help ensure that it will be a positive experience for everyone, especially your child:

- Education for everyone involved is essential in providing understanding, accurate interpretation and constructive responses.
- As parents, you must be prepared. Take childbirth classes or review what you learned in previous classes. You need to feel comfortable about birth and know how to relax and respond appropriately to contractions.
- Plan favourite toys and comfort items, such as a special blanket, to have available for your child during labour and birth.
- Arrange for a support person for your child—someone different from the mother's support person. A relative, a close friend or sometimes the child's father can be there to look after the child's needs and help interpret and explain what is going on.

Preparing Your Child

In some areas, classes are available for children. Many books, films and teaching aids are available, and family discussions are essential.

Familiarise your child with the following:

- The birth setting, equipment and caregivers. A tour of the hospital and visit to the doctor's or midwife's office are a good idea.
- The sights and sounds of labour and birth: his mother unclothed; her face red with effort; the presence of blood; the baby's initial wetness, vernix and dusky colour; moaning, grunting, crying out or straining by the mother; the baby's crying; the painless cutting of the cord; and so on
- The appearance of a newborn, placenta and umbilical cord
- The duties of the mother, father, your child's support person and your birth attendants
- The tasks your child can perform: bringing a cool cloth for mum, giving back rubs, walking with mum, bringing fluids, taking pictures, playing music, being quiet when mum asks and so on
- What labour and birth is like (long, boring and exciting at times)
- The possible interactions between the older child and the newborn (touching and holding)

At the Birth Setting

- Provide an environment for the birth that makes your child's participation feasible and stress-free (room for your child, flexibility to come and go, and clear guidelines).
- Make sure the labour and delivery staff (nurses, midwives and doctors) are supportive and will not be upset at having a child present. Find out in advance the hospital's policies regarding children's attendance at birth.
- Have an alternative plan to use if your child is sick, asleep (and does not want to wake up) or bored; if he changes his mind; or if labour complications develop and require that you transfer from the alternative setting to a standard labour ward or delivery room. Before your labour, explain these possibilities to your child, and prepare a plan for his care under such circumstances.
- Have realistic expectations of your child. One does not expect a two- or four-year-old to be transformed during labour. He will not suddenly become calmer, ask fewer questions or begin to perceive birth as a transcendental experience. Children still fuss, need to go to the bathroom, say 'no', argue, need cuddling, want to know where their toys are and so on.

The point of all this is that children are children; they will not suddenly step out of character during labour or after the birth of a new baby. Children take birth in stride, responding as they would to any long-awaited, exciting event. With preparation and good support at the time, the birth of a new sibling can be a positive experience for your child. And with it exists the potential for developing long-term, healthy attitudes about birth.

Guidelines for Care of a Child Who Will Not Be Present at the Birth

If you are planning a hospital birth with a typical one- or two-day stay after a vaginal birth, or especially after a two- or three-day stay following a caesarean, consider the possibility of separation anxiety, which sometimes occurs when a child is separated from one or both parents. When you leave to have your baby, your child's ability to tolerate the separation will vary depending on your child's age, how long the separation lasts, how comfortable she is with her caregiver and setting, how well she understands what is happening, how often she has been separated from you before and how much contact she has with you while you are in the hospital.

Most young children experience some degree of separation anxiety, including such reactions as fretting or crying for mother, sadness, clinging, irritability, sleeping difficulties and tantrums. When they are reunited with their mothers, some children react in a positive way, while others continue to react negatively and may even ignore their mothers. These reactions are the child's way of expressing her dismay at being left.

Suggestions

You can do several things to ease a child's anxiety over being left at home:

- At some point during the last weeks of your pregnancy, let your child know you will be leaving to go to the hospital for the birth. Tour the hospital with your child, if possible. Tell your child where she will be (at home or visiting someone) and who will care for her while you are away. Your child will be less anxious if she is familiar with the person who will care for her during your absence. A close friend, relative or a favourite babysitter can make theseparation less traumatic. When labour begins, tell your child when you are leaving and where you are going.
- Before the birth, increase the father's or other loved one's role as caregiver, if he or she is not already responsible for much of your child's daily care such as giving baths and putting the child to bed. Try to establish a routine that is not greatly disrupted by your hospitalisation or the arrival of the new baby.
- Plan to have your child visit you and the new baby in the hospital. Sibling visitation has become recognised as valuable to the emotional wellbeing of the family, and most hospitals allow children to visit their mothers after the birth of a baby. Learn about the policies at your hospital. May you see your older child in your room, the hallway or a visitor's lounge? Many hospitals welcome siblings in the room immediately after birth to see both mother and newborn.
- What can you realistically expect when your child visits you in the hospital? She will probably be reassured by seeing you and the baby, responding in a positive way to the opportunity to visit. It is possible, however, that she may ignore you and the baby, cling excessively or cry uncontrollably when it is time to leave. You may feel that it would have been easier on both of you to avoid the visit entirely. However, as difficult as it may be for a young child to see you for short periods and not be able to stay with you, it is healthier for your child to see you, even if only briefly, than to be separated for a longer period. The negative reaction shows that the child is under stress; the visit provides her with an opportunity to express her anger or frustration.

If your hospital stay is prolonged and your child cannot visit you, you might try a 'long-distance' visit with her; talk on the phone or send home Polaroid pictures, notes and gifts.

Adjusting to the New Baby

Besides the possible separation from his mother, an older sibling feels another traumatic change: the constant presence of a helpless, crying newborn who requires almost continuous care. Life is never the same for the older child after the arrival of a baby. Parents who once provided total attention and care for the older child are suddenly less available—all because of the new baby!

Your child may react in a variety of ways: temper tantrums; attention-seeking behaviour; return to outgrown behaviour such as thumb-sucking, wanting a pacifier, feeding from bottle or breast, or wetting his pants; excessive preoccupation with the baby; withdrawal; aggression towards parents or baby (hitting, biting, throwing things); and changes in eating and sleeping patterns. Some parents have never seen such behaviour in their child before and are caught by surprise.

Suggestions

Perhaps the most important way you can help your older child adjust to the newborn is to accept whatever reaction he displays. Try not to be disappointed in him. Accept the behaviour as a normal reaction to the stress and changes in his life brought on by the arrival of the new baby. The age of your child has much to do with how and when he will react to the baby. Some children, particularly those three to four years old or older, recognise immediately the impact the new baby has on their relationship with their parents. Younger children tend not to recognise the threat for several months, until the baby begins crawling, interfering in play and getting into things. Even children eight to ten years old feel resentment towards the baby, although it is usually accompanied by guilt and may be successfully hidden from the parents. The following suggestions may also help ease your child's adjustment to a new baby in the family:

- Before and after the birth, read books to your child about living with a new baby.
- Give your child a doll so he has a 'baby' to care for.
- Plan for time alone with your older child to do what he wants to do. This could be when the baby is asleep or when someone can watch the baby.
- Respond to your child's requests, comments and actions. Ignoring him when you are busy may diminish his sense of self-worth at this vulnerable time.[2]
- When your child behaves negatively, correct his behaviour as you always have. If you feel guilty over bringing this 'rival' into your child's life, you may find yourself letting him break family rules or overstep the boundaries he has always had. This is not a good solution for either of you. Young children, especially two- to four-year-olds, are reassured by

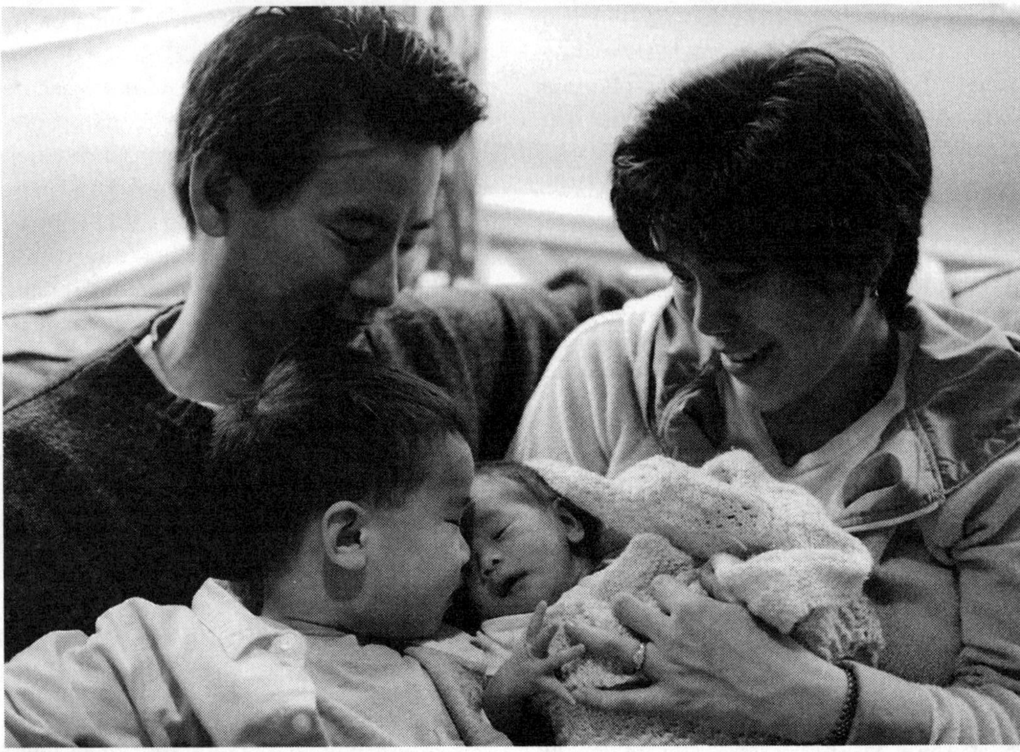

The big boy gets to know his baby brother.

familiar structure, rules and routines. Your child may be troubled if you suddenly become permissive.

- Help your child express his feelings in words: 'New babies sure make a lot of noise'. 'Sometimes it seems that the baby never wants to sleep. It makes it hard for us to have our special time together, doesn't it?' 'Sometimes it's hard to have a tiny baby around all the time'.
- Have a birthday party after the birth with cake for everyone. Give a gift to your older child and encourage your child to make or buy a gift for the baby.
- When visitors bring presents for the baby, your older child may feel left out. It may help to have him open them, to have special treats or gifts ready for him, or to delay opening them until he is not around.
- If he wants to help, include your child in baby-care activities that are appropriate to his age: holding the baby; helping with nappying, dressing or bathing the baby; helping feed and burp the baby; and entertaining the baby with smiles, singing or talk.
- Allow your child to have nothing to do with the baby, if that is what he wants.

- Think of activities that you and your child can do together that will help him feel good about himself. Spend time on useful tasks (even small ones) that allow you to work together and that allow him to feel successful.
- Use the time you spend feeding the baby to read, talk, play or share a snack with your older child. Have special toys or books that are saved for use only during feeding times.
- Avoid statements like 'You now have a new playmate' or 'You're going to love the baby' when these are not very likely to occur.
- Provide new and stimulating activities or experiences that reinforce your child's awareness of his capabilities in comparison with the new baby (for example, planting seeds, blowing bubbles, making biscuits or washing dishes).
- Tell the baby about her special older sibling while he is with you and listening. For example, 'Today, Sara Jane (baby), Peter (older child) and I are going to take you to the grocery store. We're going to pick out something good to eat for dinner and maybe some of Peter's favourite animal crackers. I always like going to the store with your big brother, don't you?'
- Take care of yourself. Try to rest when possible. This may not decrease your child's resentment or jealousy, but you will be able to cope better.

Remember that although adjusting to a new baby may be difficult, even traumatic, for a child, it is one of life's normal growth experiences. Your goal is not to have your child feel no displacement, but to have him adjust in a healthy and positive way. With time and your help, your child will find ways to adjust to the baby. A lasting bond between the siblings will eventually develop.

Appendix I

Ten Steps of the Mother-Friendly Childbirth Initiative

A mother-friendly hospital, birth centre or home-birth service:

1. Offers all birthing mothers:
   - Unrestricted access to the birth companions of her choice, including fathers, partners, children, family members and friends;
   - Access to professional midwifery care.

2. Provides accurate descriptive and statistical information to the public about its practices and procedures for birth care, including measures of interventions and outcomes.

3. Provides culturally competent care—that is, care that is sensitive and responsive to the specific beliefs, values and customs of the mother's ethnicity and religion.

4. Provides the birthing woman with the freedom to walk, move about, and assume the positions of her choice during labour and birth (unless restriction is specifically required to correct a complication), and discourages the use of the lithotomy position (flat on back with legs elevated).

5. Has clearly defined policies and procedures for:
   - Collaborating and consulting throughout the perinatal period with other maternity services, including communicating with the original caregiver when transfer from one birth site to another is necessary;
   - Linking the mother and baby to appropriate community resources including prenatal and post-discharge follow-up and breastfeeding support.

6. Does not routinely employ practices and procedures that are unsupported by scientific evidence, including but not limited to the following:
   - Shaving;
   - Enemas;
   - IVs (intravenous drip);
   - Withholding nourishment;
   - Early rupture of membranes;
   - Electronic foetal monitoring.

   Other interventions are limited as follows:
   - Has an oxytocin use rate of 10 percent or less for induction and augmentation;*
   - Has an episiotomy rate of 20 percent or less, with a goal of 5 percent or less;
   - Has a total caesarean rate of 10 percent or less in community hospitals, and 15 percent or less in tertiary care (high-risk) hospitals;
   - Has a VBAC (vaginal birth after caesarean) rate of 60 percent or more with a goal of 75 percent or more.

7. Educates staff in non-drug methods of pain relief, and does not promote the use of analgesic or anaesthetic drugs not specifically required to correct a complication.

8. Encourages all mothers and families, including those with sick or premature newborns or infants with congenital problems, to touch, hold, breastfeed and care for their babies to the extent compatible with their conditions.

9. Discourages non-religious circumcision of the newborn.

10. Strives to achieve the WHO-UNICEF 'Ten Steps of the Baby-Friendly Initiative' (see page 475) to promote successful breastfeeding.

* This criteria is currently under review.

Source: The Coalition for the Improvement of Maternity Services.

Appendix II

Ten Steps of the Baby-Friendly Initiative

To promote successful breastfeeding, a hospital will:

1. Have a written breastfeeding policy that is routinely communicated to all health care staff.

2. Train all health care staff in skills necessary to implement this policy.

3. Inform all pregnant women about the benefits and management of breastfeeding.

4. Help mothers initiate breastfeeding within an hour of birth.

5. Show mothers how to breastfeed and how to maintain lactation even if they should be separated from their infants.

6. Give newborn infants no food or drink other than breast milk, unless medically indicated.

7. Encourage rooming-in and allow mothers and infants to remain together twenty-four hours a day.

8. Encourage breastfeeding on demand.

9. Give no artificial teats or pacifiers (also called dummies or soothers) to breastfeeding infants.

10. Foster the establishment of breastfeeding support groups and refer mothers to them on discharge from hospitals or clinics.

Source: The United Nations and the World Health Organisation.

References

CHAPTER 1:

1. P. Simkin, 'Just Another Day in a Woman's Life?' *Birth* 18 (December 1991): 203–10; P. Simkin, 'Just Another Day in a Woman's Life? Part II: Nature and Consistency of Women's Long-Term Memories of Their First Birth Experiences', *Birth* 19 (June 1992): 64–81.

2. A. B. Bennetts and R. W. Lubic, 'The Free-Standing Birth Centre', *Lancet* 8268 (13 February 1982): 378; J. P. Rooks et al., 'Outcomes of Care in Birth Centres', *New England Journal of Medicine* 321 (28 December 1989): 1804.

CHAPTER 2:

1. D. Gordon et al., 'Advanced Maternal Age As a Risk Factor for Cesarean Delivery', *Obstetrics and Gynecology* 77 (April 1991): 493; S. Ziadeh and A. Yahaya, 'Pregnancy Outcome at Age 40 and Older', *Arch Gynecol Obstet* 265(1) (March 2001): 30–33; P. Murgis, V. Camemi and G. Cadili, 'Pregnancy and Delivery After 40 Years of Age', *Minerva Ginicol* 49(9) (September 1997): 377–81.

2. Jack Heinowitz, *Pregnant Fathers: Entering Parenthood Together* Parents As Partners Press (1995).

CHAPTER 3:

1. R. Romero, H. Munoz, R. Gomez et al., 'Does Infection Cause Premature Labor and Delivery?' *Semin Reprod Endocrinol* 12 (1994): 227–39; R. F. Lamont, 'The Prevention of Preterm Birth with the Use of Antibiotics', *Eur Journal of Pediatrics* 158 Supl 1 (December 1999): S2–4.

2. American College of Obstetricians and Gynecologists (ACOG), *Technical Bulletin on Preterm Labor* 206 (June 1995): 3.

3. American College of Obstetricians and Gynecologists (ACOG), *Technical Bulletin on Preterm Labor* 206 (June 1995): 7; J. E. Harding et al., 'Do Antenatal Corticosteroids Help in the Setting of Preterm Rupture of Membranes?' *American Journal of Obstetrics and Gynecology* 184(2) (January 2001): 131–39.

4. L. A. Green and R. D. Froman, 'Blood Pressure Measurement during Pregnancy: Auscultation Versus Oscillatory Methods', *Journal of Obstetric, Gynecologic and Neonatal Nursing* (February 1996): 155–59.

CHAPTER 4:

1. The Food Guide Pyramid Booklet, 'How to Make the Pyramid Work for You', U.S. Department of Agriculture (1996): 8–9.

2. Food and Nutrition Board, *Nutrition during Pregnancy and Lactation: An Implementation Guide*, National Academy Press (1992): 35.

3. N. Satter, C. Berry and I. A. Greer, 'Essential Fatty Acids in Relation to Pregnancy Complications and Fetal Development', *British Journal of Obstetrics and Gynaecology* 105 (December 1998): 1248–55.

4. B. Abrams and J. Parker, 'Maternal Weight Gain in Women with Good Pregnancy Outcome', *Obstetrics and Gynecology* 76 (July 1990): 1; B. Worthington-Roberts, 'Maternal Nutrition and the Outcome of Pregnancy', *Obstet Gynecol* 112.

5. M. M. Weigel and R. M. Weigel, 'Nausea and Vomiting of Early Pregnancy and Pregnancy Outcome: An Epidemiological Study', *British Journal of Obstetrics and Gynaecology* 96 (November 1989): 1304.

6. T. Vutyavanich et al., 'Pyridoxine for Nausea and Vomiting of Pregnancy: A Randomized, Double Blind, Placebo-Controlled Trial', *American Journal of Obstetrics and Gynecology* 173 (1995): 881–84.

7. D. deAloysio and P. Penacchioni, 'Morning Sickness Control in Early Pregnancy by Neignan Point Acupressure', *Obstetrics and Gynecology* 80

(1992): 852–54; J. Belluomini et al., 'Acupressure for Nausea and Vomiting of Pregnancy: A Randomized, Blinded Study', *Obstetrics and Gynecology* 84 (1994): 245–48.

8. N. R. Cooksey, 'Pica and Olfactory Craving of Pregnancy: How Deep Are the Secrets?' *Birth* 22(3) (September 1995): 129–37.

9. N. C. Rose and M. T. Mennuti, 'Periconceptional Folate Supplementation and Neural Tube Defects', *Clinical Obstetrics and Gynecology* 37(3) (1994): 605–20; L. E. Daley et al., 'Folate Levels and Neural Tube Defects: Implications for Prevention', *Journal of the American Medical Association* 274 (1995): 1698–1702.

10. G. M. Shaw et al., 'Risks of Orofacial Clefts in Children Born to Women Using Multivitamins Containing Folic Acid Periconceptionally', *Lancet* 345 (1995): 393–96.

11. K. J. Rothman et al., 'Teratogenicity of High Vitamin A Intake', *New England Journal of Medicine* 333 (1995): 1369–73.

CHAPTER 5:

1. O. Fernandes et al., 'Moderate to Heavy Caffeine Consumption during Pregnancy and Relationship to Spontaneous Abortion and Abnormal Fetal Growth: A Meta-Analysis', *Reproductive Toxicology* 12(4) (July-August 1998): 435–44.

2. B. Eskenazi, 'Associations between Maternal Decaffeinated and Caffeinated Coffee Consumption and Fetal Growth and Gestational Duration', *Epidemiology* 10(3) (May 1999): 242–49.

3. J. W. Scanlon, 'A Cup of Coffee and a Cigarette: Prolonged Caffeine Blood Levels in Healthy Babies', *Perinatal Press* 5 (July/August 1981): 87.

4. S. Schenker et al., 'Fetal Alcohol Syndrome: Current Status of Pathogenesis', *Alcoholism: Clinical and Experimental Research* 14 (September/October 1990): 635; J. D. Chaudhuri, 'An Analysis of the Teratogenic Effects That Could Possibly Be Due to Alcohol Consumption by Pregnant Mothers', *Indian Journal of Medical Science* 54(10) (October 2000): 425–31.

5. G. R. Bunin et al., 'Risk Factors for Astrocytic Glioma and Primitive Neuroetodermal Tumor of the Brain in Young Children: A Report from the Children's Cancer Group', *Cancer Epidemiology, Biomarkers & Prevention* 3 (1994): 197–204.

6. N. R. Shah and M. B. Bracken, 'A Systemic Review and Meta-Analysis of Prospective Studies on the Association between Maternal Cigarette Smoking and Preterm Delivery', *American Journal of Obstetrics and Gynecology* 182(2) (February 2000): 465–72; R. L. Andres and M. C. Day, 'Perinatal Complications Associated with Maternal Tobacco Use', *Semin Neonatal* 5(3) (August 2000): 231–41.

7. N. R. Butler and H. Goldstein, 'Smoking in Pregnancy and Subsequent Child Development', *British Medical Journal* 4 (8 December 1973): 573.

8. B. B. Little et al., 'Methamphetamine Abuse during Pregnancy: Outcomes and Fetal Effects', *Obstetrics and Gynecology* 72 (October 1988): 541; M. D. Anglin et al., 'History of Methamphetamine Problems', *Journal of Psychoactive Drugs* 32(2) (April-June 2000): 137–41.

9. J. A. Duke, *The Green Pharmacy Herbal Handbook: Your Comprehensive Reference to the Best Herbs for Healing*, Rodale Press (2000).

10. Ibid.

11. A. K. Henry and J. Feldhausen, *Drugs, Vitamins, Minerals, Pregnancy*, Fisher Books (1989): 40.

12. *Sumatriptan in Pregnancy Registry, Interim Report* (1 January 1996 through 30 April 1997) Glaxco Wellcome (1997).

13. G. Shaw, 'Adverse Human Reproductive Outcomes and Electromagnetic Fields: Brief Summary of the Epidemiologic Literature', *Bioelectromagnetics* Supplement 5 (2001): S5–18; J. Stellman and M. S. Henifin, 'Video Display Terminals', *Office Work Can Be Dangerous to Your Health*, 2nd ed., Fawcett Crest (1989): 71.

14. A. Milunsky et al., 'Maternal Heat Exposure and Neural Tube Defects', *Journal of American Medical Association* 268(7) (Aug 1992): 882–85; M. A. S.

Harvey et al., 'Suggested Limits to the Use of the Hot Tub and Sauna by Pregnant Women', *Canadian Medical Association Journal* 125 (1 July 1981): 50.

15. N. Roeleveld et al., 'Occupational Exposure and Defects of the Central Nervous System in Offspring: Review', *British Journal of Industrial Medicine* 47 (1990): 580; G. P. Giacoia, 'Reproductive Hazards in the Workplace', *Obstet Gynecol Surv* 47(10) (Oct 1992): 679–87.

16. J. P. Zhang et al., 'Effect of Smoking on Semen Quality of Infertile Men in Shandong, China', *Asian J Androl* 2(2) (June 2000): 143–46.

17. P. B. Marshburn et al., 'Semen Quality and Association with Coffee Drinking, Cigarette Smoking, and Ethanol Consumption', *Fertility and Sterility* 52 (July 1989): 162.

CHAPTER 6:

1. P. Horns et al., 'Pregnancy Outcomes among Active and Sedentary Women', *Journal of Obstetrical, Gynecological and Neonatal Nursing* (January 1996): 49.

2. American College of Obstetricians and Gynecologists (ACOG), 'Exercise and Fitness: A Guide for Women', Number 173 ACOG (May 1998).

3. ACOG, 'Exercise in Pregnancy', Number 180 ACOG (May 1998).

4. C. M. Samselle et al., 'Effect of Pelvic Muscle Exercise on Transient Incontinence during Pregnancy and after Birth', *Obstetrics and Gynecology* 91 (March 1998): 406–12.

CHAPTER 7:

1. J. Green, V. Coupland, J. Kitzinger, *Great Expectations: A Prospective Study of Women's Expectations and Experiences of Childbirth*, 2nd ed., (Books for Midwives Press (1998).

2. Ibid.; M. Sandelowski, 'Expectations for Childbirth versus Actual Experiences: The Gap Widens', *Mat Child Nurs* 9 (1984): 237–39.

CHAPTER 8:

1. J. J. Bonica, 'The Nature of the Pain of Parturition', *Principles and Practices of Obstetrics Analgesia and Anesthesia*, 2nd ed., Williams and Wilkins (1995).

2. P. Simkin, 'Stress, Pain and Catecholamines in Labor, Part I: A Review', *Birth* 13(4) (December 1986): 227–33; L. Ginesi and R. Niescierowicz, 'Neuroendocrinology and Birth 1: Stress', *British Journal of Midwifery* 6(10) (October 1998): 659–63; A. Robertson, 'The Pain of Labour', *Midwifery Today* 37 (1996): 19–21, 40–42.

3. S. Kitzinger, 'Pain in Childbirth', *Journal of Medical Ethics* 4 (1978): 119.

4. P. Simkin, 'Stress, Pain and Catecholamines in Labor, Part I: A Review', *Birth:* 13(4) (December 1986): 227–33.

5. M. Eriksson et al., 'Warm Tub Bath during Labor: A Study of 1385 Women with Prelabor Rupture of the Membranes after 34 Weeks of Gestation', *Acta Obstet Gynecol Scand* 75 (August 1996): 642–44.

6. M. Eriksson et al., 'Early or Late Bath during the First Stage of Labour: A Randomised Study of 200 Women', *Midwifery* 13 (1997): 146–48; P. Simkin and M. A. O'Hara, 'Selected Non-pharmacologic Methods of Pain Relief in Labor: A Systematic Review', *American Journal of Obstetrics and Gynecolocogy*, in press.

7. C. S. Mahan and S. McKay, 'Are We Overmanaging Second-Stage Labor?' *Contemporary OBGYN* (December 1984): 37.

8. J. Roberts and D. Wooley, 'A Second Look at the Second Stage of Labor', *Journal of Obstetrical, Gynecological and Neonatal Nursing* 25 (June 1996): 415–23.

9. M. Labrecque et al., 'Randomized Controlled Trial of Prevention of Perineal Trauma by Perineal Massage during Pregnancy', *American Journal of Obstetrics and Gynecolocogy* 180(3 1) (March 1999): 593–600; M. Labrecque et al., 'Randomized Trial of Perineal Massage during Pregnancy: Perineal

Symptoms Three Months after Delivery', *American Journal of Obstetrics and Gynecolocogy* 182(1, part 1) (January 2000): 76–80; E. Eason et al., 'Preventing Perineal Trauma during Childbirth: A Systematic Review', *Obstetrics and Gynecology* 95(3) (March 2000): 464–71; P. Flynn et al., 'How Can Second-Stage Management Prevent Perineal Trauma? Critical Review, (CME)' *Can Fam Physician* 43 (January 1997): 73–84.

CHAPTER 9:

1. R. Smith, 'The Timing of Birth', *Scientific American* 280(3) (1999): 68–75.

2. K. S. Olah et al., 'The Effect of Cervical Contractions on the Generation of Intrauterine Pressure during the Latent Phase of Labour', *British Journal of Obstetrics and Gynaecology* 101 (1994): 341–43.

3. V. C. Nikodem, 'Immersion in Water in Pregnancy, Labour and Birth', (Cochrane Review) in *The Cochrane Library* Issue 1, Update Software (2001); P. Simkin and M. A. O'Hara, 'Selected Non-pharmacologic Methods of Pain Relief in Labor', *American Journal of Obstetrics and Gynecology*, in press.

4. M. Eriksson et al., 'Early or Late Bath during the First Stage of Labour: A Randomised Study of 200 Women', *Midwifery* 13 (1997): 146–48.

5. J. M. Carlson et al., 'Maternal Position during Parturition in Normal Labor', *Obstetrics and Gynecology* 68(4) (October 1986): 443–47; P. Simkin and M. A. O'Hara, 'Selected Non-pharmacologic Methods of Pain Relief in Labor', *American Journal of Obstetrics and Gynecology*, in press.

6. M. Odent, 'Roundtable: The Fetus Ejection Reflex', *Birth* 14(2) (June 1987): 104–05; N. Newton, 'The Fetus Ejection Reflex Revisited', *Birth* 14(2) (June 1987): 106–08; L. Ginesi and R. Niescierowicz, 'Neuroendocrinology and Birth 1: Stress', *British Journal of Midwifery* 6(10) (October 1998): 659–63.

7. L. J. Mayberry et al., 'Maternal Fatigue: Implications of Second Stage Labor Nursing Care', *Journal of Obstetrical, Gynecological and Neonatal Nursing* 28(2) (March–April 1999): 175–81; L. Petersen and P. Besuner, 'Pushing Techniques during Labor: Issues and Controversies', *Journal of Obstetrical, Gynecological and Neonatal Nursing* 26(6) (November–December 1997): 719–26; J. Roberts and D. Wooley, 'A Second Look at the Second Stage of Labor', *Journal of Obstetrical, Gynecological and Neonatal Nursing* 25(5) (June 1996): 415–23.

8. C. Beynon, 'The Normal Second Stage of Labour: A Plea for Reform in Its Conduct', *Journal of Obstetrics and Gynaecology of the British Commonwealth* 64 (June 1957): 815, reprinted in *Episiotomy and the Second Stage of Labor*, 2nd ed., edited by S. Kitzinger and P. Simkin, Pennypress (1986): 23.

9. R. Caldeyro-Barcia, 'Influence of Maternal Bearing-Down Efforts during Second Stage on Fetal Well-Being', *Episiotomy and the Second Stage of Labor*, 2nd ed., edited by S. Kitzinger and P. Simkin, Pennypress (1986): 43; C. J. Aldrich et al., 'The Effect of Maternal Pushing on Fetal Cerebral Oxygenation and Blood Volume during the Second Stage of Labour', *British Journal of Obstetrics and Gynaecology* 102(6) (June 1995): 448–53.

10. P. Simkin, 'Active and Physiologic Management of Second Stage: A Review and Hypothesis', in *Episiotomy and the Second Stage of Labor*, 2nd ed., edited by S. Kitzinger and P. Simkin, Pennypress (1986): 7; H. Spiby, 'Early versus Late Pushing with Anesthesia in Second Stage of Labour', *Cochrane Updates on Disk,* Update Software (Disk Issue 1); D. Knauth and E. P. Haloburdo, 'Effect of Pushing Techniques in Birthing Chair on Length of Second Stage of Labor', *Nursing Research* 35 (February 1986): 49.

11. J. Roberts and D. Wooley, 'A Second Look at the Second Stage of Labor', *Journal of Obstetrical, Gynecological and Neonatal Nursing* 25 (June 1996): 415–23.

CHAPTER 10:

1. O. Irion and M. Boulvain, 'Induction of Labor for Suspected Fetal Macrosomia', (Cochrane Review) in *The Cochrane Library* Issue 1, Update Software (2000).

2. J. Yeast et al., 'Induction of Labor and the Relationship to Cesarean Delivery: A Review of 7001 Consecutive Inductions', *American Journal of Obstetrics and Gynecology* 180 (March 1999): 628–33.

3. Ibid.

4. D. Garry et al., 'Use of Castor Oil in Pregnancies at Term', *Alternative Therapies* 6 (January 2000): 77–79.

5. J. P. Elliott and J. F. Flaherty, 'The Use of Breast Stimulation to Prevent Postdate Pregnancy', *American Journal of Obstetrics and Gynecology* 149 (15 July 1984): 628.

6. Y. M. Salmon et al., 'Cervical Ripening by Breast Stimulation', *Obstetrics and Gynecology* 67 (January 1986): 21.

7. J. A. Duke, *The Green Pharmacy Handbook: Your Comprehensive Reference to the Best Herbs for Healing,* Rodale Press (2000).

8. M. Goldenberg et al., 'Stretching of the Cervix and Stripping of the Membranes at Term: A Randomised Controlled Study', *Eur J Obstet Gynecol Reprod Biol* 66(2) (June 1996): 129–32; V. Berghella et al., 'Stripping of Membranes As a Safe Method to Reduce Prolonged Pregnancies', *Obstetrics and Gynecology* 87(6) (June 1996): 927–31.

9. G. J. Hofmeyr and A. M. Gulmezoglu, 'Vaginal Misoprostol for Cervical Ripening and Induction of Labour', (Cochrane Review) in *The Cochrane Library* Issue 1, Update Software (2001).

10. L. Bricker and M. Lucas, 'Amniotomy Alone for Induction of Labour', (Cochrane Review) in *The Cochrane Library* Issue 1, Update Software (2001); W. D. Fraser et al., 'Amniotomy for Shortening Spontaneous Labour', (Cochrane Review) in *The Cochrane Library* Issue 1, Update Software (2001).

11. P. Simkin and M. A. O'Hara, 'Selected Non-pharmacologic Methods of Pain Relief in Labor: A Systematic Review', *American Journal of Obstetrics and Gynecolocogy*, in press.

12. J. L. Reynolds, 'Intracutaneous Sterile Water for Back Pain in Labour', *Can Fam Phys* 40 (October 1994): 1785–92.

13. J. G. B. Russell, 'The Rationale of Primitive Delivery Positions', *British Journal of Obstetrics and Gynaecology* 89 (September 1982): 712.

14. P. Simkin and R. Ancheta, *The Labor Progress Handbook: Early Interventions to Prevent and Treat Dystocia,* Blackwell Science (2000); P. Flynn et al., 'How Can Second-Stage Management Prevent Perineal Trauma? Critical Review', *Can Fam Phys* 43 (January 1997): 73–84.

15. G. Carroli and J. Belizan, 'Episiotomy for Vaginal Birth', (Cochrane Review) in *The Cochrane Library* Issue 1, Update Software (2001).

16. C. Smith et al., 'Knee-Chest Postural Management for Breech at Term: A Randomized Controlled Trial', *Birth* 26(2) (June 1999): 71–75.

17. G. J. Hofmeyr and R. Kulier, 'Cephalic Version by Postural Management for Breech Presentation', (Cochrane Review) in *The Cochrane Library* Issue 1, Update Software (2001).

18. M. E. Hannah et al., 'Planned Cesarean Section versus Planned Vaginal Birth for Breech Presentation at Term: A Randomised Multicentre Trial', Term Breech Trial Collaborative Group, *Lancet* 356(9239) (21 October 2000): 1375–83.

19. G. J. Hofmeyr and M. E. Hannah, 'Planned Cesarean Section for Term Breech Delivery', (Cochrane Review) in *The Cochrane Library* Issue 1, Update Software (2001).

20. G. W. Dahlenburg et al., 'The Relation between Cord Serum Sodium Levels in Newborn Infants and Maternal Intravenous Therapy during Labor', *British Journal of Obstetrics and Gynaecology* 87 (1980): 519; S. Singhi et al., 'Iatrogenic Neonatal and Maternal Hyponatraemia following Oxytocin and Aqueous Glucose Infusion during Labor', *British Journal of Obstetrics and Gynaecology* 92 (4) (April 1985): 356–63.

21. M. Eriksson et al., 'Warm Tub Baths during Labor: A Study of 1385 Women with Prelabor Rupture of Membranes after 34 Weeks of Gestation', *Acta Obstet Gynecol Scand* 75 (7) (August 1996): 642–44.

22. S. B. Thacker, D. F. Stroup and M. Chang, 'Continuous Electronic Heart Rate Monitoring for Fetal Assessment during Labor', (Cochrane Review) in *The Cochrane Library* Issue 2, Update Software (2001); N. F. Feinstein, 'Fetal Heart Rate Auscultation: Current and Future Practice', *Journal of Obstetrical, Gynecological and Neonatal Nursing* 29 (3) (May—June 2000): 306–15.

23. S. B. Thacker, D. F. Stroup and M. Chang, 'Continuous Electronic Heart Rate Monitoring for Fetal Assessment during Labor', (Cochrane Review) in *The Cochrane Library* Issue 2, Update Software (2001).

24. K. R. Simpson, 'Fetal Oxygen Saturation Monitoring during Labor', *Journal of Perinatal Neonatal Nursing* 12 (1998): 26–37.

25. K. R. Simpson, 'Fetal Oxygen Saturation Monitoring: An Adjunct to EFM', Presentation at 'Celebrate the Century!' The 2000 Convention of the Association of Women's Health, Obstetric and Neonatal Nurses (Seattle, WA, June 6, 2000).

26. G. Karroli and J. Belizan, 'Episiotomy for Vaginal Birth', (Cochrane Review) in *The Cochrane Library* Issue 2, Update Software (2001); M. C. Klein et al., 'Relationship of Episiotomy to Perineal Trauma and Morbidity, Sexual Dysfunction and Pelvic Floor Relaxation', *American Journal of Obstetrics and Gynecology* 171(3) (September 1994): 591–98.

27. G. Karroli and J. Belizan, 'Episiotomy for Vaginal Birth', (Cochrane Review) in *The Cochrane Library* Issue 2, Update Software (2001).

CHAPTER 11:

1. B. P. Sachs et al., 'The Risks of Lowering the Cesarean Delivery Rate', *New England Journal of Medicine* 340(1) (January 1999): 54–57.

2. V. Teridou and P. Bennett, 'Maternal Risk Factors for Fetal and Neonatal Brain Damage', *Biol Neonate* 79(3–4) (April 2001): 157–62; G. Jorch, 'Causes of Perinatal Brain Damage', *Zentralbl Gynakol* 117(4) (1995): 167–68; T. Sugimoto, 'When Do Brain Abnormalities in Cerebral Palsy Occur? An MRI Study', *Dev Med Child Neurol* 37(4) (April 1995): 285–92.

3. B. L. Flamm et al., 'Vaginal Birth after Cesarean Delivery: Results of a 5-Year Multicenter Collaborative Study', *Obstetrics and Gynecology* 76 (November 1990): 750; J. M. Mastrobattista, 'Vaginal Birth after Cesarean', *Obstet Gynecol Clin North Am* 26(2) (June 1999): 295–304; American College of Obstetricians and Gynecologists, 'Vaginal Birth after Previous Cesarean Delivery: Clinical Management Guidelines for Obstetricians-Gynecologists', *ACOG Practice Bulletin* Number 2 (October 1998).

CHAPTER 12:

1. C. M. Sepkoski et al., 'The Effects of Maternal Epidural Anesthesia on Neonatal Behavior during the First Month', *Dev Med Child Neurol* 34 (November 1992): 1072–80; D. B. Rosenblatt et al., 'The Influence of Maternal Analgesia on Neonatal Behaviour', *British Journal of Obstetrics and Gynaecology* 88 (April 1981): 407–13; E. Lieberman, 'The Unintended Effects of Epidurals during Labor: A Systematic Review', *American Journal of Obstetrics and Gynecology*, in press; B. L. Leighton, 'The Effects of Epidural Analgesia on Labor, Maternal, and Neonatal Outcomes', *American Journal of Obstetrics and Gynecology*, in press.

2. R. K. Boyle, 'Herpes Simplex Labialis after Epidural or Parenteral Morphine: A Randomised Prospective Trial in an Australian Obstetric Population', *Anaesth Intensive Care* 23 (1995): 433–37.

3. R. Russell and F. Reynolds, 'Epidural Infusion of Low-Dose Bupivacaine and Opiod in Labour: Does Reducing Motor Block Increase the Spontaneous Delivery Rate?' *Anaesthesia* 51(3) (March 1996): 266–73; J. D. Vertommen et al., 'The Effects of the Addition of Sufentanil to 0.125-percent Bupivacaine on the Quality of Analgesia during Labor and on the Incidence of Instrumental Deliveries', *Anesthesiology* 74 (1991): 809–14.

4. J. Loftus et al., 'Placental Transfer and Neonatal Effects of Epidural Sufentanil and Fentanyl Administered with Bupivacaine during Labor', *Anesthesiology* 83 (1995): 300–08.

5. H. Spiby, 'Early versus Late Pushing with Anaesthesia in Second Stage of Labour', *Cochrane Updates on Disk,* Update Software (Disk Issue 1); L. Petersen and P. Besuner, 'Pushing Techniques during Labor: Issues and Controversies', *Journal of Obstetrical, Gynecological and Neonatal Nursing* 26(6) (November–December 1997): 719–26.

CHAPTER 14:

1. T. L. Krebs, 'Cord Care: Is It Necessary?' *Mother Baby Journal* 3(2) (1998): 5–12; J. Rush, 'Care of the Umbilical Cord', *Midwifery Practice: Postnatal Care, A Research Based Approach*, edited by J. Alexander, V. Levy and S. Roch, University of Toronto Press (1994): 84–87.

2. S. Dore et al., 'Alcohol versus Natural Drying for Newborn Cord Care', *Journal of Obstetric, Gynecologic and Neonatal Nursing* 27 (1998): 621–27.

3. A. Henningsson et al., 'Bathing or Washing Babies after Birth?' *Lancet* (December 19/26 1981): 1401–03; T. Penny-MacGillivray, 'A Newborn's First Bath', *Journal of Obstetric, Gynecologic and Neonatal Nursing* 25 (1996): 481–87; S. G. Cole et al., 'Tub Baths or Sponge Baths for Newborn Infants?' *Mother Baby Journal* 4(3) (May 1999): 39–43.

4. M. Klaus and P. Klaus, *Your Amazing Newborn*, Perseus Books (1998).

5. J. G. Cole, 'What Can Babies See at Birth?' *Mother Baby Journal* 2(4) (1997): 45–47.

6. K. Barnard et al., 'Early Parent-Infant Relationships', *First Six Hours of Life*, No. 1., Module 3, National Foundation/March of Dimes (1978): 21; T. B. Brazelton, *Neonatal Behavior Assessment Scale,* J.P. Lippincott (1973).

7. A. Taddio et al., 'Efficacy and Safety of Lidocaine-Prilocaine Cream for Pain during Circumcision', *New England Journal of Medicine* 336 (1997): 1197–1201.

8. M. Frish et al., 'Falling Incidence of Penis Cancer in an Uncircumcised Population, Denmark 1943–90', *British Medical Journal* 311 (2 December 1995): 1471.

9. AAP Task Force on Circumcision, 'Circumcision Policy Statement', *Pediatrics,* 103(3) (March 1999): 686–93.

10. Ibid.

11. L. Pisacane et al., 'Breast-feeding and Urinary Tract Infection', *Journal of Pediatrics* 120 (1992): 87–89.

12. American Academy of Pediatrics, *2001 Family Shopping Guide to Car Seats,* American Academy of Pediatrics (2001).

13. G. Flo and M. Brown, 'Comparing Three Methods of Temperature Taking: Oral Mercury-in-Glass, Oral Diatek, and Tympanic First Temp', *Nursing Research* (March/April 1995): 120–22.

CHAPTER 15:

1. American Academy of Pediatrics, Work Group on Breastfeeding. American Academy of Pediatrics 1036.

2. American Academy of Pediatrics, Committee on Nutrition, *Pediatric Nutrition Handbook,* 4th ed., American Academy of Pediatrics (1998).

3. M. E. Fallot et al., 'Breastfeeding Reduces Incidence of Hospital Admissions for Infection in Infants', *Pediatrics* 65 (1980): 1121–24.

4. American Academy of Pediatrics, Work Group on Breastfeeding. American Academy of Pediatrics 1035.

5. Ibid.

6. U. M. Saarinen and M. Kajosaari, 'Breastfeeding as Prophylaxis against Atopic Disease: Prospective Follow-Up Study until 17 Years Old', *Lancet* 346 (1995): 1065–69.

7. G. Bauer et al., 'Breastfeeding and Cognitive Development of Three-Year-Old Children', *Psychological Reports* 68 (1991): 1281; R. A. Lawrence, 'Can We Expect Greater Intelligence from Human Milk Feedings?' *Birth* 19(2) (June 1992): 105–06; A. Lucas et al., 'Randomized Trial of Early Diet in Preterm Babies and Later Intelligence Quotient', *British Medical Journal* 28 (November 1998) 317: 1481–87; M. C. Temboury et al., 'Influence of Breastfeeding on the Infant's Intellectual Development', *J Pediatr Gastroenterol Nutr* 18 (1994): 32–36.

8. E. A. Mitchell et al., 'Results from the First Year of the New Zealand Cot Death Study', *New Zealand*

Medical Journal 104 (1991): 71–75.

9. P. A. Newcomb et al., 'Lactation and a Reduced Risk of Premenopausal Breast Cancer', *New England Journal of Medicine* 330 (1994): 81–87; NIH Consensus Conference, 'Ovarian Cancer: Screening, Treatment, and Follow-Up', *Journal of the American Medical Association* 273(6) (February 8, 1995): 491–97.

10. R. G. Cumming and R. J. Klineberg, 'Breastfeeding and Other Reproductive Factors and the Risk of Hip Fractures in Elderly Women', *International Journal of Epidemiology* 22 (1993): 684–91.

11. G. A. Weinberg, 'The Dilemma of Postnatal Mother-to-Child Transmission of HIV: To Breastfeed or Not?' *Birth* 27(3) (September 2000): 199–205; World Health Organisation Collaborative Study Team on the Role of Breastfeeding and the Prevention of Infant Mortality, 'Effect of Breastfeeding on Child Mortality Due to Infectious Diseases in Less Developed Countries: A Pooled Analysis', *Lancet* 355 (2000): 450–55; Committee on Infectious Diseases, American Academy of Pediatrics, *2000 Red Book: Report of the Committee on Infectious Disease*, 25th ed., American Academy of Pediatrics (2000).

12. L. Larson, 'Warnings Fail to Slow Low Iron Formula Sales', *AAP News* 11(3) (March 1995): 1, 14.

13. P. Fort et al., 'Breast and Soy-Formula Feedings in Early Infancy and the Prevalence of Autoimmune Thyroid Disease in Children', *Journal of the American College of Nutrition* 9(2) (1990): 164–67.

14. J. Riordan and K. G. Auerbach, *Breastfeeding and Human Lactation*, 2nd ed., Jones and Bartlett Publishers, Inc. (1998): 107.

15. J. Riordan and K. G. Auerbach, *Breastfeeding and Human Lactation*, 2nd ed., Jones and Bartlett Publishers, Inc. (1998): 127–28.

16. American Academy of Pediatrics, Work Group on Breastfeeding. American Academy of Pediatrics 1037.

17. Ibid.

18. J. Moon and S. Humenick, 'Breast Engorgement: Contributing Variables and Variables Amenable to Nursing Intervention', *Journal of Obstetric, Gynecologic and Neonatal Nursing* 18(4) (1989): 309–15.

19. Y. Yamauchi and H. Yamanouchi, 'Breast-feeding Frequency during the First 24 Hours after Birth in Full-Term Neonates', *Pediatrics* 86 (1990): 171–75.

20. S. Phillips, 'When Time Is of the Essence: Establishing Effective Breastfeeding before Early Discharge', *Mother Baby Journal* 1(1) (1996): 15–19.

21. J. Riordan and K. G. Auerbach, *Breastfeeding and Human Lactation*, 2nd ed., Jones and Bartlett Publishers, Inc. (1998): 284.

22. M. Neifert et al., 'Nipple Confusion: Toward a Formal Definition', *Journal of Pediatrics* 126(6) (1995): S125–S129.

23. J. Riordan and K. G. Auerbach, *Breastfeeding and Human Lactation*, 2nd ed., Jones and Bartlett Publishers, Inc. (1998): 294; P. Simkin, 'Intermittent Brachial Plexus Neuropathy Secondary to Breast Engorgement', *Birth* 15 (1988): 102–04.

24. V. Nicodem et al., 'Do Cabbage Leaves Prevent Breast Engorgement? A Randomized, Controlled Study', *Birth* 20 (1993): 61–64; K. Roberts, 'A Comparison of Chilled Cabbage Leaves and Chilled Gelpaks in Reducing Breast Engorgement', *Journal of Human Lactation* 11(1) (1995a): 17–20.

25. B. C. Bowles et al., 'Alternate Massage in Breastfeeding', *Genesis* 9 (1988): 5–9.

26. Institute of Medicine, *Nutrition during Lactation*, National Academy of Sciences (1992): 86; L. B. Duskieder et al., 'Is Milk Production Impaired by Dieting during Lactation?' *American Journal of Clinical Nutrition* 59 (1994): 833–40; A. Prentice et al., 'Energy Requirements of Pregnant and Lactating Women', *European Journal of Clinical Nutrition* 50(1) (1996): S82–S111.

27. G. Chan, *Lactation, the Breastfeeding Manual for Health Professionals*. Precept Press (1996); Institute of Medicine, *Nutrition during Lactation*, National Academy of Sciences (1992): 86.

28. E. Reifsnider and S. L. Gill, 'Nutrition for the Childbearing Years', *Journal of Obstetric, Gynecologic and Neonatal Nursing* 29(1) (2000): 50–51.

29. J. Mennella and G. Beauchamp, 'Maternal Diet Alters the Sensory Qualities of Human Milk and the Nursling's Behavior', *Pediatrics* 88(4) (1991): 737–44; J. Mennella and G. Beauchamp, 'Early Flavor Experience: Research Update', *Nutrition Reviews* 56(7) (1998): 205–11.

30. Institute of Medicine, *Nutrition during Lactation*, National Academy of Sciences (1992): 73.

31. J. Mennella and G. Beauchamp, 'Early Flavor Experience: Research Update', *Nutrition Reviews* 56(7) (1998): 205–11; J. Mennella and G. Beauchamp, 'Effects of Beer on Breast-fed Infants', *Journal of the American Medical Association* 269 (1993): 1635–36.

32. L. Righard and M. O. Alade, 'Breastfeeding and the Use of Pacifiers', *Birth* 24(2) (June 1997): 116–20.

33. V. Coiro et al., 'Inhibition by Ethanol of the Oxytocin Response to Breast Stimulation in Normal Women and the Role of Endogenous Opiods', *Acta Endocrinol,* 126 (1992): 213; C. Berlin, 'Disposition of Dietary Caffeine in Milk, Saliva, and Plasma of Lactating Women', *Pediatrics* 73 (1984): 59–63; A. Dahlstrom, 'Nicotine and Cotinine Concentrations in the Nursing Mother and Her Infant', *Acta Paediatr Scand* 79 (1990): 142–47.

34. M. Ziemer and J. Pigeon, 'Skin Changes and Pain in the Nipples during the First Week of Lactation', *Journal of Obstetric, Gynecologic and Neonatal Nursing* 22(23) (1993): 247–56.

35. J. Barger and P. Bull, 'A Comparison of the Bacterial Composition of Breast Milk Stored at Room Temperature and Stored in the Refrigerator', *International Journal of Childbirth Education* 2 (1987): 29–30; A. Pardou et al., 'Human Milk Banking: Influence of Storage Processes and of Bacterial Contamination on Some Milk Constituents', *Biol Neonate* 65 (1994): 302–09.

36. The Human Milk Banking Association of North America, *Recommendations for Collection, Storage, and Handling of a Mother's Milk for Her Own Infant in the Hospital Setting* (1993).

37. E. Buescher, 'Host Defense Mechanisms of Human Milk and Their Relations to Enteric Infections and Necrotizing Enterocolitis', *Clinical Perinatology* 21(2) (1994): 247–62.

38. A. Lucas et al., 'Breast Milk and Subsequent Intelligence Quotient in Children Born Preterm', *Lancet* 339 (1992): 261–64; A. Lucas et al., 'Randomized Trial of Early Diet in Preterm Babies and Later Intelligence Quotient', *British Medical Journal* 317(28) (November 1998): 1481–87.

39. S. Moscone and J. Moore, 'Breastfeeding during Pregnancy', *Journal of Human Lactation* 9(2) (1993): 83–88.

40. Centers for Disease Control, Practice Advisory Committee, 'General Recommendations on Immunizations', *Morbidity Mortality Weekly Report* 38 (1989): 205–27.

41. I. Matheson and G. Rivrud, 'The Effect of Smoking on Lactation and Infantile Colic', *Journal of the American Medical Association* 261 (1989): 42.

42. A. Woodward et al., 'Acute Respiratory Illness in Adelaide Children: Breastfeeding Modifies the Effect of Passive Smoking', *Journal of Epidemiology and Community Health* 44 (1990): 224–30.

43. A. Perez et al., 'Clinical Study of the Lactational Amenorrhoea Method for Family Planning', *Lancet* 339 (1992): 968–70.

44. P. Erwin, 'To Use or Not Use Combined Hormonal Oral Contraceptives during Lactation', *Family Planning Perspectives* 26(1) (1994): 26–33.

45. American Academy of Pediatrics, Committee on Nutrition, *Pediatric Nutrition Handbook,* 4th ed., American Academy of Pediatrics (1998): 236; L. Larson, 'Warnings Fail to Slow Low Iron Formula Sales', *AAP News* 11(3) (March 1995): 1, 14.

46. American Academy of Pediatrics, Committee on Nutrition, *Pediatric Nutrition Handbook,* 4th ed., American Academy of Pediatrics (1998): 36.

CHAPTER 16:

1. R. S. Isberg and W. E. Greenberg, 'Siblings in the Delivery Room: Consultations to the Obstetric Service', *Journal of the American Academy of Child and Adolescent Psychiatry* 26 (March 1987): 268; S. Van Dam Anderson and P. Simkin, eds., *Birth: Through Children's Eyes,* Pennypress (1981): 1.

2. M. Lewis and N. McCarthy, 'A Child's Strength', *Mothers Today* (November/December 1984): 6.

Recommended Resources

Following is a list of books, booklets and web sites that provide additional background on many of the topics discussed in this book.

Pregnancy and Birth

Campion, Mukti Jain. *The Baby Challenge: A Handbook on Pregnancy for Women with a Physical Disability,* 1990. Presents a positive and practical approach for women with a disability who are contemplating childbirth and for those who are involved in providing support.

England, Pam, and Rob Horowitz. *Birthing from Within: An Extra-Ordinary Guide to Childbirth Preparation,* 1998. Helps the reader prepare for childbirth by focusing on the art of birthing and the meaning of childbirth. Includes helpful suggestions for fathers and birth companions.

Enkin, Murray, et al. *A Guide to Effective Care in Pregnancy and Childbirth,* 2000. Conclusions of comprehensive studies of all aspects of care in pregnancy and childbirth.

Flanagan, Geraldine Lux. *Beginning Life,* 1996. Photographs illustrate the development of the baby from conception to birth.

Goer, Henci. *The Thinking Woman's Guide to a Better Birth,* 1999. Provides information about the full range of options for childbirth and the risks and benefits of each option.

Greene, Robin. *Real Birth: Women Share Their Stories,* 2000. Collection of thirty-six women's birth stories representing a range of childbirth experiences.

Haire, Doris et al. *The Pregnant Woman's Bill of Rights/The Pregnant Responsibilities,* 1975. Statement of the ICEA on informed consent and the equivalent responsibilities.

Keller, Trudy, and Ron Keller. *Pregnancy, Birth, and You,* 1994. Tightly written and nicely illustrated childbirth preparation booklet. Includes guides for early parenthood.

Kitzinger, Sheila. *Birth Over 35,* 1994. Focuses on the unique challenges of having a baby at age thirty-five or older.

Kitzinger, Sheila. *The Complete Book of Pregnancy and Childbirth,* 1996. A beautifully written guide for childbirth preparation. Well illustrated with drawings and photographs.

Kitzinger, Sheila. *New Pregnancy and Childbirth*, 1989. A classic guide to pregnancy, labour and early parenthood.

Korte, Diana, and Roberta Scaer. *A Good Birth, A Safe Birth,* 1992. What women need to know about options in pregnancy, birth and mothering to get what is best for them.

Lieberman, Adrienne B. *Easing Labor Pain: The Complete Guide to a More Comfortable and Rewarding Birth,* 1992. A practical guide on ways to reduce the pain of labour.

Lipson, Tony. *From Conception to Birth*, 1994. Reveals the world of the unborn baby.

Maternity Center Association. *Journey to Parenthood,* 1997. Provides information to help parents make thoughtful choices about their care, childbirth preparation and birth location.

Nathanielsz, Peter. *Life Before Birth and A Time to Be Born,* 1992. Describes the role of the foetus in determining the ideal time for birth.

Peterson, Barbara Edelston. *The Bed Rest Survival Guide,* 1998. Practical advice on how to survive bed rest during pregnancy. Includes resources for help.

Sears, Sears and Holt. *The Pregnancy Book,* 1997. Describes pregnancy month by month, informing the reader of what is happening to mother, baby and family.

Simkin, Penny. *The Birth Partner: Everything You Need to Know to Help a Woman through Childbirth,* 2001. Provides in-depth information and suggestions for the birth partner to support the woman in childbirth.

Simkin, Penny. *Simkin's Rating of Comfort Measures for Childbirth,* 1997. Describes eighteen different ways to relieve pain in labour.

Simkin, Penny, and Ruth Ancheta. *The Labor Progress Handbook,* 2000. Focuses on ways to prevent dystocia (difficult labour due to unfavourable position of baby and pelvis). Offers interventions to manage or treat dystocia.

Stewart, David. *Five Standards for Safe Childbearing,* 1997. Explores the safety of home birth and midwifery. Discussion based on a thorough scientific review of the literature.

Sundin, Julia. *Face to Face with Childbirth,* 1989. A comprehensive and active childbirth preparation program.

Wesson, Nickey. *Natural Mothering: A Guide to Holistic Therapies for Pregnancy, Birth, and Early Childhood,* 1997. Provides information about complementary therapies including aromatherapy, acupuncture and massage.

Caesarean Birth

Flamm, Bruce, and Edward Quilligan. *Cesarean Section: Guidelines for Appropriate Utilization,* 1995. Researched-based information and discussion.

Kaufmann, Elizabeth. *Vaginal Birth after Cesarean (VBAC),* 1996. Discusses issues to consider when electing a vaginal birth after a previous caesarean.

Korte, Diana. *The VBAC Companion: The Expectant Mother's Guide to Vaginal Birth after Cesarean,* 1997. Focuses on the mother's concerns about VBAC.

Teenage Pregnancy

Arthur, Shirley. *Surviving Teen Pregnancy,* 1996. Choices, decisions and survival tips for the teen mother.

Buckingham, Robert, and Mary Derby. *I'm Pregnant, Now What Do I Do?,* 1997. Presents options for pregnant teens and their families, including adoption and the realities of raising a child.

Simkin, Penny. *Cami Has a Baby,* 1990. A comic book written especially for pregnant teens.

Nutrition

Ash, S. and J. Allen. *Nutrition and Pregnancy, 1987.* A healthy start for your baby and an enjoyable diet for you.

Brown, Judith E. *Nutrition and Pregnancy: A Complete Guide from Preconception to Postdelivery,* 1998. Comprehensive, scientifically supported guidelines for the time spanning pre-pregnancy through post partum. Also contains guidelines for infant feeding.

Satter, Ellyn. *Child of Mine: Feeding with Love and Good Sense,* 2000. Encourages parents to use a common sense approach to feeding in order to foster good eating habits and reduce food arguments.

Swinney, Bridget. *Eating Expectantly,* 2000. Comprehensive, up-to-date, easy-to-read guide to pregnancy nutrition.

Exercise and Yoga

Balaskas, Janet. *Preparing for Birth with Yoga,* 1994. Designed for the beginner as well as the experienced.

Clapp, James. *Exercising through Your Pregnancy,* 1998. Comprehensive guide to exercise during pregnancy.

Noble, Elizabeth. *Essential Exercises for the Childbearing Year,* 1994. Describes exercises that focus on the muscles used for childbirth.

Family Planning and Infertility

Harkness, Carla. *The Infertility Book: A Comprehensive Medical and Emotional Guide,* 1992. Provides information about the emotional and social effects of infertility. Includes resources for help.

Hatcher, Robert, et al. *Contraceptive Technology,* 1998. Encyclopaedia of information about contraception and reproductive health.

Twins

Agnew, Connie. *Twins! Pregnancy, Birth, and The First Year of Life,* 1997. Provides comprehensive information and help for parents from the time they learn they will have twins through the first year of life.

Novotny, Pamela Patrick. *The Joy of Twins and Other Multiple Births,* 1994. A practical guide to parenting multiples.

Rothbart, Betty. *Multiple Blessings,* 1994. Information and advice for parents expecting multiples and for parents already facing the challenge of parenting twins or more.

Fathers

Goldman, Marcus Jacob. *The Joy of Fatherhood: The First Twelve Months,* 2000. Information and advice supported by shared experiences of fathers.

Shapiro, Jerrold Lee. *The Measure of a Man,* 1995. Help for today's father to become more involved.

Post-partum Adjustment

Dunnewold, Ann, and Diane Sanford. *Postpartum Survival Guide,* 1994. Addresses practical ways to survive the year following birth. Includes tips for fathers.

Gruen, Dawn, and Rex Gentry. *Beyond the Birth: What No One Ever Talks About,* 1997. Elegant, sensitive and information-filled booklet about post-partum mood disorder.

Kitzinger, Sheila. *The Year after Childbirth,* 1994. Focuses on the mother's experience during the first year following birth.

Kleiman, Karen, and Valerie Raskin. *This Isn't What I Expected: Overcoming Postpartum Depression,* 1994. Discusses how to recognise post-partum mood disorder, how to deal with the associated shame, ways to deal with panic attacks and more.

Misri, Shaila. *Shouldn't I Be Happy? Emotional Problems of Pregnant and Postpartum Women,* 1995. Written by a physician specialising in the emotional health of women during the perinatal period.

Parenting and Child Development

Brazelton, T. Berry. *Touchpoints: The Essential Reference,* 1993. Highlights the predictable challenges (touch-points) occurring in early baby and childhood development.

Fallows, Carol. *The Australian Baby and Childcare Handbook,* 1994. A book to help parents enjoy and manage the first five formative years.

Green, Christopher. *Babies,* 1994. A parents guide to surviving baby's first year.

Klaus, Marshall, and Phyllis Klaus. *Your Amazing Newborn,* 1998. Describes the amazing abilities of the newborn. Supported by beautiful photographs.

Leach, Penelope. *Your Baby and Child: From Birth to Age Five,* 1997. Complete guide to parenting from birth to age five.

Leboyer, Frederick. *Loving Hands: The Traditional Art of Baby Massage,* 1997. Describes how to use massage to communicate love and care to the baby.

Peterson, Gayle. *Making Healthy Families,* 2000. Describes the elements needed to make and sustain healthy families.

Sears, William. *Keys to Calming the Fussy Baby,* 1991. Common sense discussion of some of the causes of fussiness. Offers some effective solutions.

Sears, William. *Nighttime Parenting: How to Get Your Baby and Child to Sleep,* 1999. A classic, supportive guide for parents.

Sears, William, and Martha Sears. *The Baby Book,* 1993. Comprehensive guide to baby care.

Small, Meredith. *Our Babies, Ourselves: How Biology and Culture Shape the Way We Parent,* 1999. A fascinating look into the effect of culture and evolution on the choices we make as parents.

Stray-Gundersen, Karen. *Babies with Down Syndrome,* 1995. Discusses the special challenges for parents whose babies have Down Syndrome.

For Children

Carroll, Teresa. *Mommy Breastfeeds Our Baby,* 1990. A charming story that helps children ages three to ten understand breastfeeding as a natural and special way to feed their new sibling.

Taylor, Geraldine. *Baby* (Ladybird. series). For parents and children to read together.

Ziefert, Harriet. *Waiting for Baby,* 1998. A story about Max, a boy who has a hard time waiting for his sister to be born. For children ages three to seven years.

Breastfeeding

Cox, Sue. *Breastfeeding—I Can Do That,* 1997. This book, which is reader-friendly and beautifully illustrated, promotes confidence and enjoyment for new mothers. It also provides knowledge and understanding about breastfeeding.

Gromada, Karen Kerkhoff. *Mothering Multiples: Breastfeeding and Caring for Twins or More,* 1999. Provides excellent practical information about breastfeeding multiples.

Hale, Thomas. *Medications and Mothers' Milk,* 2000. Concise, easy-to-use and well-documented book about the presence of medications in breast milk.

Howard, Virginia. *Your Breastfeeding Handbook,* 1990. Practical answers for the Australian mother.

Huggins, Kathleen. *The Nursing Mother's Companion,* 1999. User-friendly, complete guide to helping parents understand the importance of breastfeeding, how to breastfeed and how to approach and treat some common and not-so-common challenges.

Huggins, Kathleen. *The Nursing Mother's Guide to Weaning,* 1994. Very supportive and practical guide to weaning.

Kitzinger, Sheila. *Breastfeeding Your Baby,* 1998. Practical advice about breastfeeding. Supported by many beautiful photographs.

La Leche League International. *The Womanly Art of Breastfeeding,* 1997. Written especially for mothers. Includes many women's stories about their breast-feeding experiences.

Mohrbacher, Nancy, and Julie Stock. *The Breastfeeding Answer Book,* 1997. Well-documented, practical and complete answers to questions about breastfeeding.

Nursing Mothers' Association. *Breastfeeding and Hospitalisation,* 1999. A booklet with hints on the management of breastfeeding when mother, baby or another child is hospitalised.

Nursing Mothers' Association. *Breastfeeding...Naturally,* 1997. A guide to expectant parents on breastfeeding and associated parenting. It explores the feelings and reactions of mothers and fathers to the responsibilities of parenthood coordinated through the central theme of breatsfeeding.

Nursing Mothers' Association. *Breastfeeding Twins,* 1999. Support, encouragement and the right information is provided in this comprehensive booklet.

Sears, William. *The Breastfeeding Book,* 2000. A realistic, up-to-date encyclopaedia on breastfeeding.

Wiggins, Pamela. *Why Should I Nurse My Baby? And Other Questions Mothers Ask About Breastfeeding,* 1998. Well-written book addressing the most common questions and concerns of breastfeeding mothers.

Loss and Grief

Ilse, Sherokee. *Empty Arms,* 2000. Support for parents and their families who have experienced a miscarriage, stillbirth or neonatal death.

Ilse, Sherokee, and Lori Leininger. *Grieving Grand-parents,* 1994. Practical discussion of the emotions grandparents experience at the death of a grandchild.

Schwiebert, Pat. *A Grandparent's Sorrow,* 1996. Guides to understanding the grief experienced by the family and ways to hold on to the memory of the baby.

Schwiebert, Pat. *Still to Be Born,* 1993. Suggestions for coping with stillbirth.

Schwiebert, Pat. *Strong and Tender,* 1996. Insights for fathers who have experienced the loss of a baby.

Schwiebert, Pat, and Paul Kirk. *When Hello Means Goodbye,* 1993. Resource for parents and others who have experienced the death of a baby.

Premature and Ill Infants

Gotsch, Gwen. *Breastfeeding Your Premature Baby,* 1999. Provides complete information about pumping, milk storage and tips for breastfeeding the premature baby.

Kitchen, Ryan et al. *Premature Babies—A Guide for Parents* (1998). Questions are answered, difficulties explored, positive suggestions for help are discussed and technical terms and procedures explained.

Manginello, Frank, and Theresa Foy DiGeronimo. *Your Premature Baby,* 1998. A book for those expecting a premature baby or for parents whose baby is premature.

Walker, Marsha, and Jeanne Driscoll. *Breastfeeding Your Premature or Special Care Baby: A Practical Guide for Nursing the Tiny Baby,* 1994. Provides excellent resources for parents and care providers.

Zaichkin, Jeanette. *Newborn Intensive Care,* 1996. Easy-to-read information guide for parents whose babies are in the neonatal intensive care unit.

Adoption

Lindsay, Jeanne Warren. *Pregnant? Adoption Is an Option,* 1996. Explores adoption from the birth parents' perspective.

Rogers, Fred. *Let's Talk about It: Adoption,* 1998. Addresses questions children might have about being adopted.

Web Sites

Australian College of Midwives: www.acmi.org.au

Australian Department of Health and Ageing: www.health.gov.au

Child Support Agency: www.csa.gov.au

Family Planning Australia: www.fpa.net.au

National Health and Medical Research Council: www.health.gov.au/nhmrc

Royal Australian and New Zealand College of Obstetricians and Gynaecologists: www.ranzcog.edu.au

Penny Simkin: www.pennysimkin.com

Support after Stillbirth and Neonatal Death: www.sands.org.au

The Australian Breastfeeding Association: www.breastfeeding.asn.au

The Children's Hospital at Westmead: www.chw.edu.au

More Contacts

Australian Society of Independent Midwives
41 Parklands Rd, Ryde, NSW. Ph: 02 9888 7829

Billings Family Life Centre
27 Alexandra Pararde, Fitzroy North, VIC 3068.
ph: 1800 335 860

Childbirth Education Association
PO Box 413, Hurstville Business Centre, Hurstville, NSW 1481. Ph: 02 9580 1481

Homebirth Australia
PO Box 1085, Bryon Bay, NSW 2481.
ph: 1800 222 180
Email: homebirthaust@one.net.au

Postnatal Depression Support
ACT: Postnatal Depression Support Network
ph: 02 6286 4082
NSW: Postnatal Depression Personal Support Network
ph: 02 9744 6646
NT: Casuarina Community Care Centre
ph: 08 8945 4804
OLD: Postnatal Depression Support
ph: 07 3358 4224
SA: Overcoming Postnatal Distress
ph: 08 8267 1191
VIC: Post- and Antenatal Depression Association
ph: 03 9882 5766
WA: Postnatal Depression Support Association
ph: 08 9340 1622

Index

Boldface numbers refer to pages on which definitions or descriptions of key terms are provided.